Neoplasms of the Colon, Rectum, and Anus

Mucosal and Epithelial

John S. Spratt, M.D.

Professor of Oncology
Department of Surgery
University of Louisville
Health Science Center
School of Medicine and
J. Graham Brown Cancer Center
Louisville, Kentucky

NORMA BRAVER
Editorial Assistant

W.B. SAUNDERS COMPANY

Philadelphia London Toronto
Mexico City Rio de Janeiro
Sydney Tokyo

1984

W. B. Saunders Company: West Washington Square
Philadelphia, PA 19105

1 St. Anne's Road
Eastbourne, East Sussex BN21 3UN, England

1 Goldthorne Avenue
Toronto, Ontario M8Z 5T9, Canada

Apartado 26370—Cedro 512
Mexico 4, D.F., Mexico

Rua Coronel Cabrita, 8
Sao Cristovao Caixa Postal 21176
Rio de Janeiro, Brazil

9 Waltham Street
Artarmon, N.S.W. 2064, Australia

Ichibancho, Central Bldg., 22-1 Ichibancho
Chiyoda-Ku, Tokyo 102, Japan

Library of Congress Cataloging in Publication Data

Main entry under title:

Neoplasms of the colon, rectum, and anus, mucosal and epithelial.

1. Colon (Anatomy)—Cancer. 2. Rectum—Cancer. 3. Anus—Cancer. I. Spratt, John Stricklin, 1929– [DNLM: 1. Anus neoplasms. 2. Colonic neoplasms. 3. Rectal neoplasms. WI 435 N438]

RC280.C6N47 1984 616.99′4347 83–14311

ISBN 0–7216–8534–X

Neoplasms of the Colon, Rectum, and Anus ISBN 0–7216–8534–X

Last digit is the print number: 9 8 7 6 5 4 3 2 1

To my father and greatest teacher,
John Stricklin Spratt, Sr.,
B.A. (American history), M.A. (American government),
Ph.D. (Economics),
Emeritus Professor of Economics
5 July 1902–16 July 1976
Deceased, from colon cancer

CONTRIBUTORS

ROBERT ADCOCK, B.S.

Senior Research Technologist, Price Institute of Surgical Research; Department of Surgery, University of Louisville School of Medicine, Louisville, Kentucky
Pseudomyxoma Peritonei

JOSEPH C. ALLEGRA, M.D., F.A.C.P.

Professor of Medicine, Chairman, Department of Medicine, University of Louisville School of Medicine; Chief of Medical Service, Humana Hospital University, Louisville, Kentucky
Chemotherapy of Colorectal Cancer

JONATHAN R. AUSOBSKY, M.D., F.R.C.S.

Price Fellow in Surgical Research, Department of Surgery, University of Louisville School of Medicine, Louisville, Kentucky; Senior Surgical Registrar, The General Infirmary at Leeds, Leeds, United Kingdom
Preoperative Preparation and Antibiotic Utilization in Operations for Carcinoma of the Colon and Rectum

JOHN J. BUCHINO, M.D.

Assistant Professor of Pathology and Pediatrics, University of Louisville School of Medicine; Chief of Pathology, Attending Pediatrician, Kosair-Children's Hospital, Louisville, Kentucky
Epithelial Tumors of the Large Intestine in Children

VICTOR W. FAZIO, M.B., B.S., F.R.A.C.S., F.A.C.S.

Chairman, Department of Colon and Rectal Surgery, The Cleveland Clinic Foundation, Cleveland, Ohio
Advances in the Surgery of Rectal Carcinoma Utilizing the Circular Stapler

RICHARD A. GREENBERG, Ph.D.

Professor of Epidemiology and Biostatistics, Acting Chairman, Department of Community Health, University of Louisville, Louisville, Kentucky
Epidemiology and Etiology

DILLER B. GROFF, M.D.

Professor of Surgery, University of Louisville School of Medicine; Surgeon-in-Chief, Kosair-Children's Hospital, Louisville, Kentucky
Epithelial Tumors of the Large Intestine in Children

DANIEL G. HALLER, M.D.

Assistant Professor of Medicine, University of Pennsylvania; Staff Physician, Hospital of the University of Pennsylvania, Philadelphia, Pennsylvania
Chemotherapy of Colorectal Cancer

CARL O. KNUTSON, M.D., F.A.C.S., F.A.C.G.

Chief of Surgery, Humana Hospital Audobon, Louisville, Kentucky
Flexible Endoscopic Examinations and Treatment

GERALD LARSON, M.D., F.A.C.S.

Assistant Professor of Surgery, Department of Surgery, University of Louisville School of Medicine; Teaching Staff, Department of Surgery, Humana Hospital University, Louisville, Kentucky
Chemosensitivity of Human Colon Cancer Cells in Culture

THERESA LEAKE, R.N., G.I.A.

Endoscopy Nurse, Norton Hospital, Louisville, Kentucky
Flexible Endoscopic Examinations and Treatment

PATRICIA MARTIN, B.S.N., E.T.

Surgical Nurse Clinician for Enterostomal Therapy, Norton Hospital, Louisville, Kentucky
Stomas and Their Care

MARIA C. MICHAELIDES, Ph.D.

Research Associate, Department of Surgery, Mount Sinai Medical Center, Miami Beach, Florida
Immunology and Immunotherapy of Colorectal Tumors

ROSCOE E. MILLER, M.D., F.A.C.R.

Distinguished Professor of Radiology, Indiana University School of Medicine; Chief of Gastrointestinal Radiology, Indiana University Hospital, Indianapolis, Indiana
Radiology of Neoplastic Colon Disease

JEAN PAPILLON, M.D.

Professor of Radiology, University of Lyon; Head of Radiotherapy Department, Centre Léon Bérard, Lyon, France
Place of Radiotherapy in the Management of Cancer of the Rectum and the Anal Canal

HIRAM C. POLK, JR., M.D., F.A.C.S.

Professor and Chairman, Department of Surgery, University of Louisville School of Medicine, Louisville, Kentucky
Preoperative Preparation and Antibiotic Utilization in Operations for Carcinoma of the Colon and Rectum; Recurrent Carcinoma of the Colon and Rectum; Screening and Follow-up

HARLAN J. SPJUT, M.D.

Clarence and Irene Fulbright Professor of Pathology, Baylor College of Medicine; Attending Physician in Pathology, Ben Taub General Hospital and The Methodist Hospital, Houston, Texas
Pathology of the Neoplasms

JOHN A. SPRATT, M.S., M.D.

Research Fellow, Department of Surgery, Duke University Medical Center, Durham, North Carolina
Growth Rates

JOHN S. SPRATT, B.S., M.S.P.H., M.D., F.A.C.S.

Professor of Surgery and Community Health, Head, Division of Health Systems, University of Louisville School of Medicine; Associate, James Graham Brown Cancer Center; Associate, Systems Science Institute; Surgical Staff, Humana Hospital University, Norton's Hospital, Kosair-Children's Hospital, Veterans Administration Hospital, Kentucky Baptist Hospitals, Louisville, Kentucky
A Rationale of Practice for Polypoid Lesions of the Colon; Adenocarcinoma of the Colon and Rectum (Primary Anatomic Extent, Histopathology, and Management Factors Correlating with Prognosis); Carcinoids; Carcinomas and Precancerous Dermatoses of the Anus and Perianal Area; Epidemiology and Etiology; Flexible Endoscopic Examinations and Treatment; Good Health and Avoidance of Cancer; Growth Rates; Hepatic and Pulmonary Metastases; Misadventures with Sigmoidoscopes, Flexible Endoscopes, Barium Enemas, and Colorectal Surgery; Pseudomyxoma Peritonei; Screening and Follow-up; Special Problems Associated with Colorectal and Anal Cancers; Stomas and Their Care

MICHAEL T. TSENG, Ph.D.

Associate Professor of Anatomy, Director of Tumor Evaluation Laboratory, University of Louisville School of Medicine, Louisville, Kentucky
Chemosensitivity of Human Colon Cancer Cells in Culture

DONALD J. VANDERTOLL, M.D., F.A.C.S.

Assistant Professor of Surgery, University of Louisville School of Medicine, Louisville, Kentucky
Recurrent Carcinoma of the Colon and Rectum

†HERBERT WALD, Ph.D., M.D., F.A.C.S.

Clinical Associate Professor of Surgery, Associate, Anatomy, University of Louisville School of Medicine, Louisville, Kentucky
†Deceased
Pseudomyxoma Peritonei

MARC K. WALLACK, M.D.

Assistant Professor of Oncology, Department of Oncology, University of Miami School of Medicine; Chairman, Department of General Surgery, Mount Sinai Medical Center, Miami Beach, Florida
Immunology and Immunotherapy of Colorectal Tumors

JAMES A. WOLF, M.D.

Research Fellow in Surgical Oncology, Department of Surgery, Washington University School of Medicine, St. Louis, Missouri
Immunology and Immunotherapy of Colorectal Tumors

NORMAN WOLMARK, M.D., F.A.C.S.

Assistant Professor of Surgery, University of Pittsburgh; Surgeon-in-Charge of Oncology, Assistant Chief of Surgery, Montefiore Hospital, Pittsburgh, Pennsylvania
Chemotherapy of Colorectal Cancer

Foreword

I have known John Spratt for over 30 years and have worked with him on problems of the gastrointestinal tract particularly in the field of polyps and cancer. The broad sweep of this book in the continuing problem of cancer of the large bowel is obviously needed in view of the high incidence and continuing high mortality of cancer. Prevention, epidemiology, pathology, and treatment are beautifully covered. The discussion of the uses of chemotherapy and radiation therapy brings balance to the book. The references are well chosen. At present there is no other book that covers this subject in such an adequate fashion. Granted, I am prejudiced. However, I have read practically all of this book with care, and I make my recommendations for its high value with full knowledge of its contents. The expert in gastroenterology, the surgeon, the radiologist, and the pathologist need this book in their practice of medicine.

LAUREN V. ACKERMAN, M.D.
PROFESSOR OF PATHOLOGY
STATE UNIVERSITY OF NEW YORK AT STONY BROOK

PREFACE

The first paper I ever published, while still a surgical resident in 1958, dealt with the relationship between colon polyps and cancer. That paper, the controversy that surrounded it, and the complexity and significance of neoplasms of the colon, rectum, and anus have challenged me to remain a careful student for thc subsequent twenty-five years. During this period I have either completed or participated in many additional studies. In parallel, I have witnessed steady progress in the basic understanding of the epidemiology, etiology, pathophysiology, natural history, and discovery of these neoplasms and in the treatment and rehabilitation of people with these disorders. However, even with all this progress, our impact on cancer deaths has probably reached a plateau. Disseminated colorectal and anal cancers are among the most resistant to effective chemotherapy. The endogenous microflora of the large bowel always places patients with these cancers at the brink of catastrophe owing to many types of spontaneous or iatrogenic misadventures.

The purpose of this book is to organize at least a part of the large body of knowledge of neoplasms of the large intestine and the achievements and pitfalls of cancer control and to present the clinician and his basic science colleagues with information on some of the opportunities that exist for future progress in the control of colorectal and anal cancers. This control also includes prevention. For this reason, I include an appendix on behavior, fitness, and diet, which is used for public health education.

This book was written without a rigid outline. It addresses areas of importance. Each author was requested to direct content and organization toward areas of real or potential clinical value. Since there are many excellent texts on surgical technique, I saw no reason to duplicate these. In a few chapters, technique is presented if it has not been broadly covered in the literature or if it is relatively new or if there is a need for special instrumentation.

In addressing the enormous body of knowledge now in existence about these neoplasms, there are undoubtedly some gaps in coverage. For these I take full responsibility.

I am particularly grateful to my colleagues who participated in the preparation of this book, each one being an expert in his area. By providing a timely review, I hope that, collectively, we have met the book's objectives.

I wish to express my gratitude to Ms. Susan Dudas, Associate Professor, College of Nursing, University of Illinois at Chicago, for providing a detailed and constructive critique of Chapter Twenty. Many of her suggestions have been incorporated into this chapter.

Special appreciation is extended to the people at the University of Louisville who have provided indispensable technical assistance—Marlene Humphrey at the

Word Processing Center; Norma Braver, research librarian; Betsy Hagan, my secretary; and Rhonda Hawley, my office manager. I wish to thank my eldest son, John Arthur Spratt, a surgical research fellow at Duke University, who helped me organize my extensive files in preparation for writing this book and who co-authored the chapter on growth rates. Pat Bensinger, manuscript editor of the Department of Surgery, provided invaluable assistance in proofreading.

The staff at W. B. Saunders Company has, as always, been impressive in their enthusiasm, support, and efficiency. Working with them makes the writing of a book a pleasure. Meriting specific designation for their great help with this book are Carroll Cann, the medical editor; Ann Binder, in Copy Editorial; Susan Hunter, in Marketing; Anthony Frizano, in Design; and Frank Polizzano, in Production.

Contents

ONE

Epidemiology and Etiology

J. S. Spratt, M.D.
R. A. Greenberg, Ph.D.

All residents of the United States must be considered at high risk for the development of adenocarcinomas of the colon and rectum (Correa and Haenszel, 1978). The anus, however, is a relatively infrequent site of cancer. Worldwide, these cancers are ubiquitous among all ethnic groups and geographic regions, although the incidence varies widely. Areas with the highest risk for colonic and rectal cancers are North America and Western Europe; those with the lowest risk are Latin America, Africa, and Asia. The epidemiologic studies on which these observations are based, plus excellent studies using animal models, provide many clues as to the etiology of these cancers. Determining the potential for premalignant, or presumed premalignant, neoplasms or states to become cancers is important since their timely eradication might prevent cancers. Any factors that can help differentiate high- and low-risk groups (e.g., family history, genetics, diet, and environment) become of practical consideration in planning control programs. The entire disease problem is, in fact, ecogenetic—a by-product of environmental and genetic interaction.

For both sexes, there is a striking North–South differential within the United States, with high incidence and mortality rates of cancer of the colon and rectum throughout the Northeast and low rates throughout the South. The higher mortality rates tend to be associated with urbanization, income, and ethnicity. When migrants move from low-risk to high-risk areas, they tend to become part of the high-risk population in about one decade (Blot et al., 1977).

HOSPITAL MORBIDITY AND MORTALITY

In 1977, a nationwide survey of the current state of hospital-based colon cancer management in the United States was made by the Commission on Cancer of the American College of Surgeons (Murphy, 1977). The survey contained a short-term evaluation and included patients with histologically confirmed adenocarcinoma of the colon and rectosigmoid who were admitted to a hospital during 1976 and who had had no prior treatment for their cancers. Patients with carcinoma in situ, carcinoma in a pedunculated polyp, or carcinoma within 15 cm from the anal orifice (i.e., rectal cancer) were excluded. The cancer program accreditation categories were subdivided, classifying hospitals according to levels of cancer program activities and number of beds. Statistics were remarkably similar in all categories as to duration of pretreatment symptoms, methods of work-up and treatment, length of stay, and stage of disease. From 35.5 to 42.1 percent of the patients had symptoms for less than 1 month, and 13.5 to 16.4 percent had pretreatment symptoms for more than 6 months. Postsurgical deaths ranged from 5.1 to 7.4 percent, and 1.9 to 2.3 percent of the patients died before surgery. Methods of treatment and categories of complications were also remarkably similar in all groups. From 27.9 to 35.5 percent of the patients were hospitalized for less than 14 days and 17 to 19.9 percent were hospitalized for longer than 30 days. From 28.2 to 30.5 percent of the cancers were localized; 20.6 to 22.3 percent had invaded the pericolic fat, 9.5 to 12 percent had spread to

Table 1–1. **SOCIAL AND ECONOMIC IMPLICATIONS OF CANCER IN THE UNITED STATES: ABSTRACTED DATA FOR LARGE INTESTINE AND RECTUM***

Days in short-stay hospitals (000)	2,629.1
Estimated hospital expenditures (000,000)	$425.3
Person-years lost owing to neoplasms (000)	682.7
Lost earnings (000,000)	$1,510.3

*Adapted from Rice DP, Hodgson TA: Social and economic implications of cancers in the United States. Vital Health Stat 3:1–43, 1981.

Table 1–2. **AGE-ADJUSTED CANCER INCIDENCE RATES FOR CANCERS OF THE COLON AND RECTUM BY SEX AND RACE PER 100,000 POPULATION, IN 1977***

	Black	White
Colon		
Male	42.9	38.5
Female	29.8	32.1
Rectum		
Male	14.1	19.1
Female	10.7	11.2

*Adapted from National Cancer Program, 1980: Director's Report and Annual Plan, FY 1982–1986. NIH Publ No. 81-2290. V: 25–28, 1981.

the regional lymph nodes, and 14.0 to 16.0 percent had invaded both pericolic tissues and nodes; and 20.3 to 25.5 percent exhibited distant metastases at the time of surgery. Absolute 5-year survival rate for all stages was 35.29 percent.

The conclusions of the audit were that the results of treatment were "essentially similar in hospitals throughout the country regardless of their size, location, and the presence or lack of residency training programs in major specialties" (Murphy, 1977). Older patients tolerated surgical management remarkably well, with an operative mortality of only 6 percent. Less than one third of all cancers were discovered while still restricted to the intestinal wall. The uniformity of results among reporting hospitals suggests that the biologic properties of colonic cancers may be the fundamental determinant of outcome.

INCIDENCE

The social and economic consequences attributable to cancers of the colon and rectum are very striking problems. Rice and Hodgson (1981) provide comprehensive documentation from which the data in Table 1–1 for cancers of the colon and rectum have been abstracted. Data from the National Cancer Program (1981) on the age-adjusted cancer incidence rates by race and sex further emphasize the magnitude of the problem (Table 1–2).

The American Cancer Society statistical staff edits data from various sources to provide estimates of new cancer cases and changes in rates of occurrence over time. The estimates of new cases and deaths for 1980 are given in Table 1–3 (American Cancer Society, 1979). Table 1–4 shows a downward trend in mortality from cancer of the colon and rectum when the periods from 1950 to 1952 and 1975 to 1977 are compared. Factors associated with the occurrence of anal cancers are discussed in the chapter on those cancers, since these factors often have implications for management.

The Statistics, Epidemiology and End Results (SEER) data for 1973 to 1976 show the relative rarity of anal cancer. For all races, the incidence of cancers of the anus and anal canal is about 0.6 new cases per 100,000 persons. The number of cases reported is too small to show significant race and sex differences (Table 1–5).

The available data on prevalence and age-specific incidence rates in similar cohorts are incomplete. The very high prevalence rate of colonic and rectal adenocarcinomas in elderly people, as measured at autopsy or at first screening, suggests a long duration of the growth of the cancers. The range of this duration can be crudely estimated from a compilation of data previously reported from autopsy series, screening examinations, and the vital statistics on annual incidence rates reproduced in Table 1–6 (Spratt and Ackerman, 1962).

Table 1–3. **ESTIMATED NEW CANCER CASES AND DEATHS BY SEX (1980)***

Site	Estimated New Cases *Total*	*Male*	*Female*	Estimated Deaths *Total*	*Male*	*Female*
Large Intestine	79,000	36,000	43,000	44,000	20,500	23,500
Rectum	35,000	19,000	16,000	8,800	4,800	4,000
Total	114,000	55,000	59,000	52,800	25,300	27,500

*Adapted from American-Cancer Society: Cancer Facts and Figures. New York, American Cancer Society, 1979.

Table 1–4. TWENTY-FIVE-YEAR TRENDS IN AGE-ADJUSTED CANCER DEATH RATES PER 100,000 POPULATION, 1950–1952 TO 1975–1977*

Sex	Site	1950–1952	1975–1977	Changes (%)
Male	Colon and rectum	19.4	19.0	− 2.1
Female	Colon and rectum	18.9	14.9	−19.5

*From American Cancer Society: Cancer Facts and Figures. New York, American Cancer Society, 1979.

By dividing the prevalence rate of adenocarcinomas found by Helwig (1947) in autopsied colons by the annual incidence rates for adenocarcinomas of the large intestine in the United States, as reported by Dorn and Cutler (1959), an estimate of duration before diagnosis was calculated:

$$\frac{\text{Prevalence of 1.7}}{\text{Age-adjusted incidence of 0.026}} = 65 \text{ years}$$

$$\frac{\text{Prevalence of 1.7}}{\text{Annual incidence at age 80 of 0.25}} = 6.8 \text{ years}$$

These estimates are quite compatible with the very slow rates of growth reported for colorectal cancers. Extreme variance from these estimated values can be anticipated, based on the observed variance in growth rates.

ETIOLOGY

Intense study of the causes of colon cancer has been underway through programs directed toward (1) defining the metabolism and mechanisms of action of colon carcinogens and colon cancer promoters, modifiers, and inhibitors; (2) studying the interactions of colon carcinogens with macromolecules and cytoplasmic proteins of colon mucosal cells; and (3) investigating biochemical variations in the colon cancer cell, which might be exploited as markers; and (4) studying the geographic epidemiology of the cancers. Many of the more recent studies have been funded through the National Large Bowel Project (National Cancer Program, 1981).

The numerous leads concerning potential causes of colon and rectal cancers have come so quickly from laboratory and epidemiologic studies that acquiring an even better understanding of cause and prevention merits a very high priority.

Current research emphasizes causation of large bowel cancer, identification of high-risk individuals, and pharmacologic control and prevention. Animal models have been used to (1) identify potential inhibitors of carcinogens, (2) examine methods of immunoprevention, (3) elucidate events associated with transformation of colon epithelium to precancerous lesions and ultimately overt carcinoma of the large bowel, and (4) examine the effects of dietary factors and influence of microflora in the development of large bowel cancer. Endogenous formation of mutagens and carcinogens is under investigation. The molecular genetics of these neoplasms are also under continuing study for knowledge exploitable for treatment or prevention.

Research efforts are directed toward seeking to elucidate the metabolic activities of the intestinal microflora in an effort to better understand their potential role in the genesis of colon cancer. Metabolic and epidemiologic studies and evaluation of fecal mutagenic activity in healthy controls and in low- and high-risk subjects are being conducted in an effort to identify compounds and biochemical processes that may be related to the etiology of human colon cancer.

Programs in progress seek to identify colon

Table 1–5. ANNUAL INCIDENCE RATES OF CANCERS OF THE ANUS AND ANAL CANAL PER 100,000 POPULATION*

All Races			White			Black		
Total	*Male*	*Female*	*Total*	*Male*	*Female*	*Total*	*Male*	*Female*
0.6	0.5†	0.7†	0.6	0.5†	0.7†	0.8‡	0.6‡	0.9‡

*From SEER Program: Cancer Incidence and Mortality in the United States, 1973–1976. Biometry Branch, Division of Cancer Cause and Prevention. National Cancer Institute. DHEW Publ No. (NIH) 78-1837, 1978.

†Standard error of the rate is between 5 and 10 percent.

‡Standard error of the rate is 10 percent or greater.

Table 1–6. THE FREQUENCY OF RECTAL AND COLONIC ADENOCARCINOMAS IN NECROPSY AND CANCER. DETECTION SERIES COMPARED WITH THE INCIDENCE OF RECTAL AND COLONIC ADENOCARCINOMAS REPORTED BY THE U.S. PUBLIC HEALTH SERVICE*

Source	Type of Series	No. Cases in Series	No. Adenocarcinomas Detected	Accumulative Frequency (%)	Mean No. Examinations per Person, Annual	Frequency of Adenocarcinomas per Single Examination, Annual (%)
Helwig	Necropsy	1,460	25	1.7	1	1.7
Lawrence	Necropsy	7,000	105	1.5	1	1.5
Susman	Necropsy	1,100	34	3.09	1	3.09
Bolt, Mallery, and Tupper	Proctosigmoidoscopy of asymptomatic GM executives	500	1	0.2	0.95	0.2
	Barium enema of asymptomatic GM executives	500	2	0.4	1.48	0.27
Jenson, Shahon, and Wagensteen	Minnesota Cancer Detection Center, examination of colon and rectum	9,123	33†	0.36	<3.6	>0.10
Rider, Kirsner, and Moeller	Asymptomatic persons having no associated polyps in the same colon, examined once	9,123	182	2.0	1	2.0
	Asymptomatic persons having adenomatous polyps discovered in the colon or rectum	537	32	5.8	3.5	1.3
Portes and Majarakis	Proctosigmoidoscopy of asymptomatic persons	50,000	19	0.038	1	0.038
Wilson, Dale, and Brines	Proctosigmoidoscopy of asymptomatic persons	20,847	29	0.14	1.07	0.13
Young	Proctosigmoidoscopy of asymptomatic persons	500	5	1.0	1	1.0

Site	Annual Incidence of Adenocarcinoma in the United States‡	
Large intestine, entire population, age-adjusted incidence	Male	0.025
	Female	0.027
Large intestine, at age 80§	Male	0.24
	Female	0.26
Rectum, entire population, age adjusted incidence	Male	0.021
	Female	0.015
Rectum, at age 80§	Male	0.17
	Female	0.10

*From Spratt JS Jr, Ackerman LV: Small primary adenocarcinomas of the colon and rectum. JAMA 179:337–346, 1962. Copyright 1962, American Medical Association.

†Twenty discovered in the Cancer Detection Center and 13 additional colonic cancers discovered by family doctor within 2 months after screening the Cancer Detection Center.

‡From Dorn and Cutter, 1959, pp. 30, 36, and 37.

§The incidence of rectal and colonic adenocarcinoma is highly age-dependent, and the maximum incidence for all ages is attained at age 80.

carcinogens and the factors that contribute to their formation and activation. The ability of an agent to induce cellular mutation can be assayed by an array of microbial mutagenicity tests, such as those popularized by Ames and co-workers (1973). Practical application of microbial mutagenic testing on a large scale is now available, as exemplified by the work of Shirasu and associates (1977).

A positive test finding with these bacterial systems establishes only that the tested substance has the *ability* to induce cellular mutation. The metabolism of the same substance in humans may negate its mutagenicity. Also, a substance providing a negative test result might still act as a procarcinogen whose metabolites might be carcinogenic.

Programs aimed at preventing large bowel cancer have primarily been directed toward (1) assessment of high-risk populations and dietary factors believed to exert an influence on large bowel carcinogenesis, (2) development of immunologic approaches, and (3) examination of drugs that may interfere with the carcinogenic process. Research goals are directed toward the ultimate control of large bowel cancer through the following objectives: (1) elucidation of etiologic and modifying factors associated with human large bowel cancer; (2) elucidation of processes that control the behavior of normal and malignant cells; (3) identification of factors that mediate the conversion of cells from normal to malignant and their mechanisms of action; (4) identification of the properties of malignant cells, with special emphasis on their vulnerabilities, and development of procedures that exploit those vulnerabilities while sparing the greatest possible amount of normal cells; (5) elucidation of the tumor-host interaction, with emphasis on understanding and augmenting the body's defense systems against cancer cells; (6) improvement of cell-culture techniques and establishment of normal colonic epithelium and colonic neoplasms in culture; and (7) application of new knowledge for disease prevention and control as rapidly and as effectively as possible.

Current research in colon carcinogenesis includes studies on the mechanism of action of procarcinogens and carcinogens and the promoting or inhibiting effects of various factors such as dietary fiber and fat, bile acids, and selenium, disulfiram, vitamin C, and other antioxidants. The role of diet in large bowel carcinogenesis is under investigation. The presence of mutagens arising from cooked meats has been confirmed, and work is now focusing on isolating and identifying these mutagens or carcinogens. The purification of fecal mutagens is also being pursued to determine their structures. Other work includes determining whether feeding antibiotics and *Lactobacillus acidophilus* in a dose approximating that in yogurt can change human fecal enzyme activity. The effects of specific types of bran on the chemical induction of colon tumors are being examined. The intestinal formation of nitrite in humans and its alteration by fat intake, fiber, and vitamins C and E are also being studied.

The relation of DNA repair to colon carcinogenesis is under study. DNA repair in colon cells has been compared with that in other cell types, and the local factors that effect specific inhibition of DNA repair have been investigated. Expanding knowledge of the cellular and molecular mechanisms that regulate cell division in normal and malignant cells opens new possibilities for improved prevention, diagnosis, prognosis, and treatment of large bowel cancer.

Methods have been developed for long-term tissue culture of human colonic carcinoma using density-gradient centrifugation. The conditions required for initial growth of most malignant epithelial cells have been determined. Isolation of subpopulations of cells from cultures of a single colonic carcinoma with different functional properties, as assessed by in vitro markers for malignancy, and transplantation of these cells into athymic nude mice have also been described.

Topographic studies have been initiated using lectins as specific molecular probes to define the labeling patterns of carbohydrate-containing components of colonic goblet cells. Alterations in the structure of membrane mucin glycoproteins in colonic cancer have also been determined and localized. Identification, isolation, and characterization of tumor-associated or tumor-specific cell surface membrane glycoproteins or glycolipids of homogeneous cultured human colon cancer cell lines could not only enable physicians to use glycoproteins or glycolipids as diagnostic tumor markers but also provide an explanation of the molecular processes involved in malignant transformation, growth control of cells, and metastasis.

The molecular basis of malignant transformation in cells of the colonic epithelium exposed to dimethylhydrazine (DMH) has been investigated. DMH induction of colonic tumors in rodents is accompanied by alterations in the composition of metabolism of DNA-binding proteins in the nucleus and by abnormal postsynthetic modifications of chromosomal proteins. Parallel investigations have focused on postsynthetic modifications of proteins at early stages in carcinogenesis, with attention to protein phosphorylation.

SPECIFIC STUDIES OF CARCINOGENS IN HUMANS AND ANIMALS

Early work by Spjut and Spratt (1965) established the remarkable similarity existing between the endemic of colon cancers seen naturally in humans and those producible in rats with 3:2′-dimethyl-4-aminobiphenyl (DMAB).

Experimental Studies with Amines and Anthracenes

Many investigators have reported on the carcinogenicity of different aromatic amines and anthracenes. Several of these compounds possess the well-documented capacity for inducing papillomas and cancers of the urinary bladder in both rat and humans (Melick et al., 1955; Melick and Naryka, 1960; Walpole and Williams, 1958). A number of these amines were shown to induce adenomatous polyps and adenocarcinomas of the colon in the rat and hamster (Table 1–7). No strong epidemiologic evidence has been presented that would incriminate any industrially produced amine in the etiology of colonic neoplasms of humans, as in the case of bladder tumors (Bridbord et al., 1978). The extremely slow rate of growth measured for colonic neoplasms in humans (Welin et al., 1963) and the advanced age of many persons ultimately developing the symptoms of colonic neoplasms would necessitate a very long period of follow-up of an exposed population to establish epidemiologic evidence of causality. In fact, among workers exposed to 4-aminobiphenyl, only 1.4 percent had developed urinary bladder tumors 5 to 10 years after exposure; however, 16 to 20 years after exposure, the accumulative incidence had reached 35.6 percent (Melick and Naryka, 1960). Various aromatic amines occur in nature and industry, and man's exposure to this family of chemical compounds begins in the

Table 1–7. **DRUGS THAT HAVE PRODUCED INTESTINAL NEOPLASMS IN SMALL ANIMALS***

		Tumors of Large Intestine or Rectum			
		Polyps Only	*Polyps and Cancer*	*Cancers Only*	*"Intestinal Tumors," No Detailed Reports on Morphology of Colonic or Rectal Tumors*
Animal Drugs	*Hamster*				
	9,10-Dimethyl-1,2-benzanthracene	X			
	2-Acetylaminofluorene			X	
	Urethan	X			
	20-Methylcholanthrene			X	
	O-Amine-azotoluene		X		
Animal Drugs	*Rats*				
	4:4′-Diaminobiphenyl (Benzidine)			X	
	3,2′-Diomethyl-4-aminobiphenyl		X		
	4′-Fluoro-4-aminobiphenyl				X
	3:3′-Dimethyl-4-aminobiphenyl				X
	3-Methyl-4-aminobiphenyl				X
	3:3′-Dihydroxybenzidine				X
	2-Acetaminofluorene				X
	4-Aminobiphenyl (xenylamine)				X
	4′-Methyl-4-aminobiphenyl				X
	3:2′,5′,-Trimethyl-4-aminobiphenyl				X
	3:2′,4′,6′-Tetramethyl-4-aminobiphenyl				X
	3-Chloro-4-aminobiphenyl				X

*From Spjut HJ, Spratt JS Jr: Endemic and morphologic similarities existing between spontaneous colonic neoplasms in man and 3:2′-dimethyl-4-aminobiphenyl induced colonic neoplasms in rats. Ann Surg 161:309–325, 1965.

newborn nursery (Fisch et al., 1963). The minimal dose that can produce human neoplasms has not been determined for most of the compounds listed in Table 1–7, although the carcinogenicity of a single application of a microgram dose has been shown for some (Klein, 1956; Lawrence, 1936). Increasing the dose of a carcinogen seemingly shortens the latency period between drug exposure and the appearance of a neoplasm and increases the total number of resulting tumors (Klein, 1956). Finally, the ubiquity of the colon cancer problem in man and the variegated dose-dependent forms and latency of presentation would compromise the identity of specific workplace causative factors.

The amine DMAB was implicated early as having great capacity for producing colonic neoplasms in the rat (Walpole et al., 1952). One study was undertaken to ascertain the similarities that might exist between colonic neoplasms produced in rats by DMAB and the colonic neoplasms occurring spontaneously in humans. No causal relations for human cancer could be inferred by the demonstration of a few elements of similarity. However, with sufficient similarity, animal tumors can serve as models for improving understanding of the natural history of colonic neoplasms. Also, as Rashevsky (1960) stated, "There should be a rational biophysical theory to interpret and explain the various statistical relationships which are found empirically."

This report confirmed the elements of similarity existing between the frequency, intracolonic distribution, and morphologic appearance of colonic adenocarcinomas and adenomatous polyps occurring spontaneously in humans and those induced in rats by the daily injection of DMAB.

It also compared the distributions of extracolonic cancers occurring in rats dosed with a known colon carcinogen and the distribution of extracolonic cancers occurring in humans with colon cancers and adenomas (Tables 1–8 and 1–9). The anatomic distributions are striking in their similarity, suggesting that the carcinogens that induce colonic neoplasms in man produce a pattern of multiorgan carcinogenicity remarkably similar to that which occurs in rats dosed with the known colon carcinogen DMAB.

Twenty-eight adult male and 50 female white Wistar rats (total of 78) of varying ages were given this drug in USP peanut oil, by subcutaneous injection, at a dosage of 2 mg/day/100 gm body weight for 5 days per week. Control animals received an equivalent amount of peanut oil.

The cecum, left in continuity with the ileum and ascending colon (Spjut and Eichwald, 1957), was transplanted to a subcutaneous location in another group of 15 female rats. The same daily dosage of DMAB was given to 14 of these animals by percutaneous injection into the cecal pouches. One control animal received daily intracecal injections.

The total dose per animal varied from 20 to 923 mg. The time elapsing between onset of treatment and the sacrifice or spontaneous death of the rats varied from 145 to 250 days. All animals were examined by autopsy. The greatest dimension of each bowel lesion was measured. The lesions were localized in relation to their distance from the stomach, ileocecal valve, and anus. Representative sections of all tumors and most organs were taken unless autolysis made sections useless. Tissue sections were stained with hematoxylin and eosin; step sections of the bowel lesions were made when needed. Twenty-six of 78 rats (33.3 percent) that received subcutaneous injections and four of 14 rats (28.5 percent) that received intracecal injections developed colonic adenomatous polyps or adenocarcinomas or both. Fifty-one of the 78 (65 percent) and ten of the 14 (71.4 percent) developed one or more neoplasms of some organ, but none of the animals receiving the carcinogen developed tumors at the sites of injection. Breast carcinomas, the most frequent extracolonic tumors, occurred in 64 percent of the females. None was observed in males. Other tumors that developed are shown in Table 1–9.

The animal data were compared with the morphology, distribution, and frequency of colonic neoplasms occurring in several populations of men. The similarities between animal and human tumor populations are considered in the following discussions.

Morphology of Tumors Produced by DMAB

The first polyps were found in a rat that died of pneumonia with abscess formation. The rat had received a total dose of 186 mg over a 145-day period. Three polyps were found, two in the cecal area and one in the rectosigmoid portion of the colon. Each was a pedunculated adenomatous polyp, with only slight atypical change.

Grossly, the large intestinal polyps and carcinomas were nearly all pedunculated or

Table 1–8. **TYPES OF EXTRACOLONIC NEOPLASMS OBSERVED AMONG PATIENTS WITH COLONIC AND RECTAL NEOPLASMS SEEN CONSECUTIVELY AT THE ELLIS FISCHEL STATE CANCER HOSPITAL, 1940–1961***

	Number of Patients Affected			
	Colonic or Rectal Cancers†		*Adenomas Only*†	
	Male (%)	*Female (%)*	*Male (%)*	*Female (%)*
Total with colonic neoplasms	615	526	69	51
Total with extracolonic neoplasms	63 (10.2)	58 (11.0)	30 (43.4)	18 (35.2)
Type of extracolonic neoplasms				
Lymphocytic leukemia	1 (0.16)	1 (0.19)		
Lymphosarcoma	1 (0.16)	1 (0.19)	1 (1.4)	
Plasma cell myeloma				1 (2)
Melanocarcinoma, skin		1 (0.19)		
Epidermoid carcinoma, skin	16 (2.6)	2 (0.38)	8 (11.6)	1 (1.92)
Basal cell cancer, skin	27 (4.4)	16 (3.0)	8 (11.6)	3 (5.9)
Mucoepidermoid, parotid	1 (0.16)			
Epidermoid cancer, larynx	1 (0.16)		1 (1.4)	
Epidermoid cancer, piriform sinus	1 (0.16)			
Carcinoid, ileum	2 (0.32)			
Adenocarcinoma, lung	2 (0.32)			
Adenocarcinoma, breast		12 (2.3)		4 (7.8)
Adenocarcinoma, prostate	15 (2.4)		6 (8.7)	
Adenocarcinoma, stomach		3 (0.57)	2 (2.9)	
Adenocarcinoma, ovary		3 (0.57)		
Adenocarcinoma, uterus		6 (1.14)		2 (4)
Epidermoid cancer, cervix uteri		7 (1.3)		
Epidermoid cancer, vagina or vulva		2 (0.38)		1 (2)
Basal-squamous cancer, anus			1 (1.4)	
Adenocarcinoma, kidney			1 (1.4)	
Transitional cancer, urinary bladder			2 (2.9)	
Dermatofibrosarcoma, lip			1 (1.4)	
Leiomyosarcoma, uterus				1 (2)
Lipoma, soft tissue	2 (0.32)	1 (0.19)		1 (2)
Adenomatous polyp, stomach	1 (0.16)		1 (1.4)	
Fibroadenomata, breast		1 (0.19)		2 (4)
Leiomyoma, uterus		7 (1.3)		4 (7.8)
Papilloma, epiglottis				1 (2)
Fibroma		1 (0.19)		1 (2)
Total number of tumors	70	64	32	22

*From Spjut HJ, Spratt JS Jr: Endemic and morphologic similarities existing between spontaneous colonic neoplasms in man and 3:2′-dimethyl-4-aminobiphenyl induced colonic neoplasms in rats. Ann Surg 161:309–325, 1965.

†Includes both simultaneously and nonsimultaneously occurring neoplasms.

broad-based. An occasional one was sessile. None of the lesions was ulcerated and none appeared to have penetrated the bowel wall. Several of the animals did have flat plaques in the rectosigmoidal mucosa. These turned out to be lymphoid masses. Adenomatous polyps could not be distinguished from carcinomas by gross examination. Only one of the carcinomas was a sessile lesion. In the small bowel, the carcinomas were flat, superficially ulcerated plaques. The serosa was often involved. The polyps were pedunculated. One adenomatous polyp in the terminal ileum had produced ileoileal intussusception.

Histologically, the polyps presented a variety of alterations. Most exhibited a moderate-to-marked glandular and cellular atypia. The polyps were similar to the adenomatous polyps in humans. However, in the rat, none of the polyps was entirely bland; all had definite and at least moderate cellular atypism. Most of the polyps were glandular; a few had a papillary component. The combination of papillary and glandular growth has been designated as a villoglandular polyp by Spjut (Welin et al., 1963). No entirely villous tumors were found in the rats.

Although many random sections of normal-appearing colon were made, no epithelial alterations other than those recognizable as polyps or carcinoma were seen. At the edge of both polyps and carcinomas, transition from normal to abnormal epithelium was sharply distinguishable. In one polyp, the mucosa near

Table 1–9. **TYPES OF NEOPLASMS OTHER THAN INTESTINAL OR MAMMARY OBSERVED IN RATS***

Type of Tumor	No. Times Observed†
Urinary bladder, papillary hyperplasia	3
Buccal mucosa, epidermoid cancer	1
Gingiva, sarcoma	1
Ear canal, epidermoid cancer	1
Skin, sebaceous gland carcinoma	1
Vagina, sarcoma 2	1
Breast or soft tissue, sarcoma with pulmonary metastases	1
Breast, fibromatosis	1
Stomach, squamous papilloma	1

*From Spjut HJ, Spratt JS Jr: Endemic and morphologic similarities existing between spontaneous colonic neoplasms in man and 3:2′-dimethyl-4-aminobiphenyl induced colonic neoplasms in rats. Ann Surg 161:309–325, 1965.

†These 11 growths occurred in eight different female rats.

it was thicker than normal but not otherwise altered. In 1959, King and Varasdi described diffuse hyperplasia of colonic mucosa in several of their rats, but this was not seen by Spjut. Often the smaller polyps contained deep-lying glands, which were the most atypical glands present. This suggested that the genesis of the altered glands was not necessarily a surface phenomenon. Similar observations were made in the human by Lane and Lev (1963). Two of the smallest polyps were studied by step sections. These demonstrated surface change, although the underlying mucosal glands were normal. This may indicate that some of the polyps began with surface epithelial alterations.

Diagnosis of Tumors Produced by DMAB

The diagnosis of carcinoma, except for a polyp with carcinoma in situ, was not made unless invasiveness was demonstrated. The route of invasion was into or through the muscularis mucosae, into the muscularis propria, or occasionally into the serosa. The carcinomas were similar to those found in the human and were like those described by Walpole, Williams, and Roberts (1952) and King and Varasdi (1959). None of the carcinomas in the Spjut and Spratt study (1965) had a mucinous component; all were adenocarcinomas. No metastases were demonstrable. King and Varasdi, in contrast, noted that some colonic cancers induced by DMAB tended to produce excessive mucin. They described lymph nodal metastases of the mucin-producing component of these cancers. Many human colonic adenocarcinomas produce mucin, and frequently it is the mucinous component of the cancer that metastasizes (Spratt and Spjut, 1967).

It could not be confirmed that residual adenomatous polyps existed in any of the carcinomas, large or small. No conclusive evidence could be found supporting a transition from polyp to carcinoma in the rats. Carcinoma in situ may represent a transition phase, but this remains to be proved. The frequency and rate of evolution of carcinoma in situ to cancer also need definition. This definition would be essential in the case of the elderly patient with small adenomatous polyps who would probably never be bothered by them even if the polyps contained carcinoma in situ. If the transition from carcinoma in situ to invasive cancer occurs, both the rate and frequency of transition remain unknown.

Of the 14 female rats that had percutaneous injection of DMAB into their cecal pouches, four (29 percent) developed colonic neoplasms, two had adenomatous polyps only, and two had adenomatous polyps and invasive carcinomas. Histologically these neoplasms were indistinguishable from those in rats receiving subcutaneous injections.

Ten of the rats given the drug (one male and nine female) had lymphoid masses in the large bowel, and all these masses except one were in the left side of the colon. The plaques measured up to 10 mm in their greatest dimension. One rat had three such lesions. Microscopically, the lesions appeared to be hyperplastic lymphoid tissue, with poorly defined secondary centers. Two of the lesions had irregular and atypical mucous glands in their depths. These glands were few and were not considered to be polyps or carcinomas.

Tumor Distribution

Similarities between the distributions of tumors within the colons of rats and humans are difficult to consider because of anatomic incongruities. The mean length of the rat colon is 18 cm, and it has only one identifiable flexure at its midpoint. The cecum and rectum are identifiable. However, segmental anatomy of the colon of the rat is not defined, and the determination of segments of the 18-cm rat colon corresponding to the anatomic segments of the 150-cm human colon can only be speculative. Because of this only the distributional data in the rat were analyzed, using a method previously employed for analysis of colonic tumors in man in which the tumors were plotted per centimeter of colorectal length. The colorectum of man averages 150 cm in length. In the rat, a proportionality was used to correct for the discrepancies in length. The resulting distributions of tumors were similar (Fig. 1–1). A predominance of cancers were found in the rectum and cecum, and a predominance of adenomatous polyps were found in the intervening colon. However, cancers and polyps in the terminal ileum of the rat far exceeded the occurrence of tumors in the terminal ileum of humans in relative frequency. In the rat, the upper rectum was particularly vulnerable to the carcinogenic effect. In 1950, Spitz, Maguigan, and Dobriner reported seven adenocarcinomas of the colon induced by benzidine among 385 rats, and they also noted the susceptibility of the upper rectum to the carcinogen. The cause of these distributions is not known. The upper rectum or rectosigmoid junction is the lowest and most consistently occupied point of fecal storage. Periodic defecation occurs when fecal storage capacity of the pelvic and descending colon is reached and material is forced into the rectal ampulla, stimulating the urge to defecate. The cecum is the area most active in liquid absorption.

Among the rats in this study, 42.8 percent of the males (12 of 28) and 28 percent of the females (18 of 64) had colonic neoplasms. In a series of this size this difference is not significant. However, the variance was great, i.e., $p\ (-6.1 < \Delta < 35.5 \text{ percent}) = 95$ percent. A significantly greater number of tumors occurred in all other sites in the females. Except for one small intestinal polyp, the male rats developed only colonic tumors. In female rats, tumors occurred in numerous and varied sites, the breast and small intestine predominating. The disposition of male rats to develop colonic neoplasms has been described also in associa-

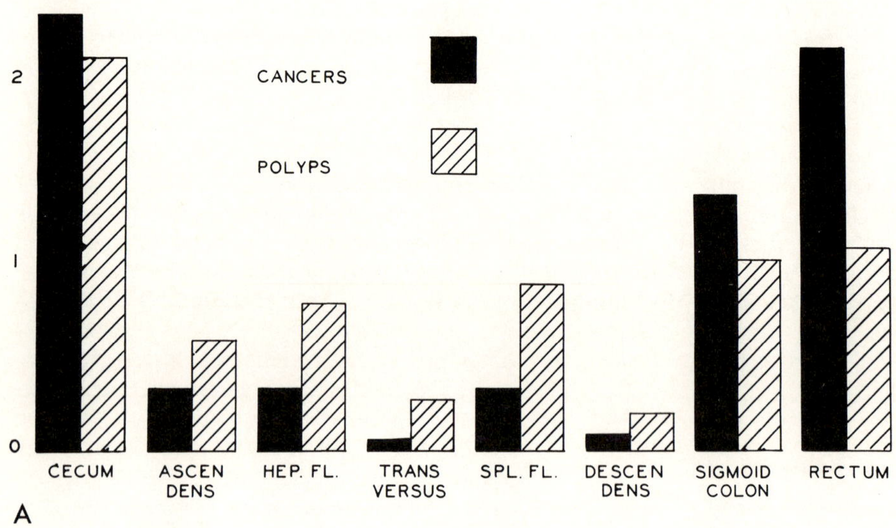

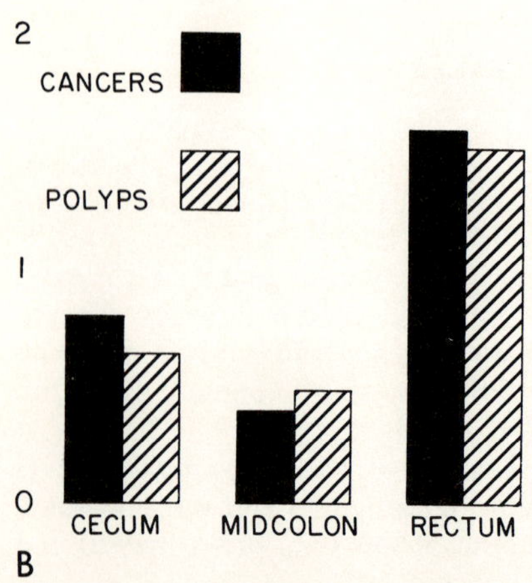

Figure 1–1. *A*, Distribution of 100 colonic cancers and 100 adenomatous polyps per centimeter of segmental length, based on a human colonic length of 150 cm, and the distribution of a proportionate number of colonic cancers and adenomatous polyps (18/150) per centimeter of segmental length, based on a murine colonic length of 18 cm. (From Spjut HJ, Spratt JS Jr: Endemic and morphologic similarities existing between spontaneous colonic neoplasms in man and 3:2′-dimethyl-4-aminobiphenyl induced colonic neoplasms in rats. Ann Surg 161:309–325, 1965.)

tion with the administration of benzidine (Spitz et al., 1950) and acetylaminofluorene (Bieleschowsky, 1944).

Of 1141 consective patients with carcinoma of the colon and rectum seen at the Ellis Fischel State Cancer Hospital between 1940 and 1961, 615 (53.9 percent) were men (see Table 1–8). If carcinomas of the skin were excluded, 27 of the 615 men (4.4 percent), but 46 of the 526 women (8.7 percent), had had extracolonic neoplasms during their lifetime. This greater frequency of extracolonic neoplasms among women was significant, i.e., p (1.4 percent $< \Delta <$ 7.2 percent) = 95 percent. However, the predominant extracolonic locus for spontaneous cancers in women, exclusive of skin, was the breast. In the female rat, the breast was also the predominant locus for extracolonic cancers induced by DMAB.

The human data from a cancer hospital were obviously selective and could represent a greater prevalence of multiple tumors than would be encountered in the general population. This was particularly true with reference to the extracolonic cancers found in the same patients having adenomatous polyps, since these patients generally presented with the extracolonic cancer, and the polyps were discovered only incidentally. However, with only 5 percent of the clinical group coming to autopsy, the prevalence of multiple tumors could also be greater than that ascertained by a clinical study. Furthermore, the accumulative percentage of multiple cancers observed in a population is dependent on the duration of observation. For example, Polk and associates (1965) obtained a 90 percent follow-up on the patients who survived surgical therapy for colonic cancers at Barnes Hospital between 1916 and 1939, and 27 percent of these survivors ultimately developed additional colonic or extracolonic cancers. In fact, the second cancer was the major cause of death among those patients who survived longer than 5 years after the successful surgical therapy of their first colonic cancer. Whether this frequency could be accounted for simply by accumulation attributable to the expected annual incidence of cancers was not determined. The important point is that both the rat and human populations, when observed during most of the life span, are prone to develop multiple extracolonic as well as multiple colonic neoplasms. The breast is the major extracolonic organ affected in the females of both groups. Both groups are susceptible to cancers about the head and neck.

The distribution of colonic tumors in an adult rat population exposed to DMAB was similar to that observed in an adult human population examined at necropsy. The frequency of observation of various types of colonic tumors and tumor combinations found in 92 adult rat colons and 899 colons of human adults over 20 years of age examined at autopsy by Helwig (1947) is shown in Table 1–10. No significant differences between the distributions in rats and humans were found for

Table 1–10. COMPARISON OF THE PREVALENCE OF COLONIC TUMORS IN MAN AND RAT*

Type of Tumors in Colon	*Host*	Number of Hosts with Contingency: *With the Tumor Type*	Number of Hosts with Contingency: *Without the Tumor Type*	*Chi-Square*	*Probability that Distribution of Contigencies Is the Same in Rat and Man*	*Conclusion*
Cancers with or without polyps	Rat	7 (7.6%)	85			Greater frequency in the rats
	Man§	27 (3.0%)	872	4.04	<0.05‡	
Cancers and polyps	Rat	6 (6.5%)	86			Greater frequency in the rats
	Man§	13 (1.4%)	886	8.8	<0.005‡	
Cancers, no polyps	Rat	1 (1.0%)	91		<0.5, >0.25†	No difference
	Man§	14 (1.5%)	885	0.64		
Polyps, no cancers	Rat	17 (18.4%)	75		<0.25, >0.1†	No difference
	Man§	118 (15.1%)	781	1.6		
Polyps with carcinoma in situ	Rat	2 (2.2%)	90		<0.75, >0.5†	No difference
	Man§	10 (1.1%)	889	0.14		
Polyps with or without cancer	Rat	23 (25%)	69			Greater frequency in the rats
	Man§	131 (15.6%)	837	3.8	<0.05‡	

From Spjut HJ, Spratt JS Jr: Endemic and morphologic similarities existing between spontaneous colonic neoplasms in man and 3:2′-dimethyl-4-aminobiphenyl induced colonic neoplasms in rats. Ann Surg 161:309–325, 1965.

†The prevalence of the contingent tumors is the same among a population of adult rats as among a population of humans over 20 years of age.

‡The prevalence of the contingent tumors is not the same among a population of adult rats as among a population of humans over 20 years of age. By comparing older populations of humans from Helwig's autopsy series, the prevalent frequency of these contingent tumors in humans become the same as the prevalent frequencies of those in rats.

§From Helwig, 1947, Table V, p. 46.

(1) cancers in the absence of adenomatous polyps occurring concurrently in the same colon, (2) adenomatous polyps in the absence of cancers occurring concurrently in the same colon, or (3) the relative infrequency with which colons are found containing polyps with carcinoma in situ. In rats there was a greater prevalence of cancers and polyps in combination than was observed in the human autopsy series of either Helwig (1947) or Blatt (1961) (see Fig. 1–2). The autopsied humans and the rats both represent adult populations of unselected ages. The adult rats were exposed for 5 to 7 months to the carcinogen; how comparable this period and dosage are to those of the unknown carcinogens producing colonic tumors in man is not known. Only 30 of the 92 rats exposed to the carcinogen developed tumors of the colon during the period of study.

Age as a Factor in Tumor Development

One factor common to both rats and humans is the increase in the frequency of tumors that occurs with aging (Figs. 1–2 and 1–3). In 1960,

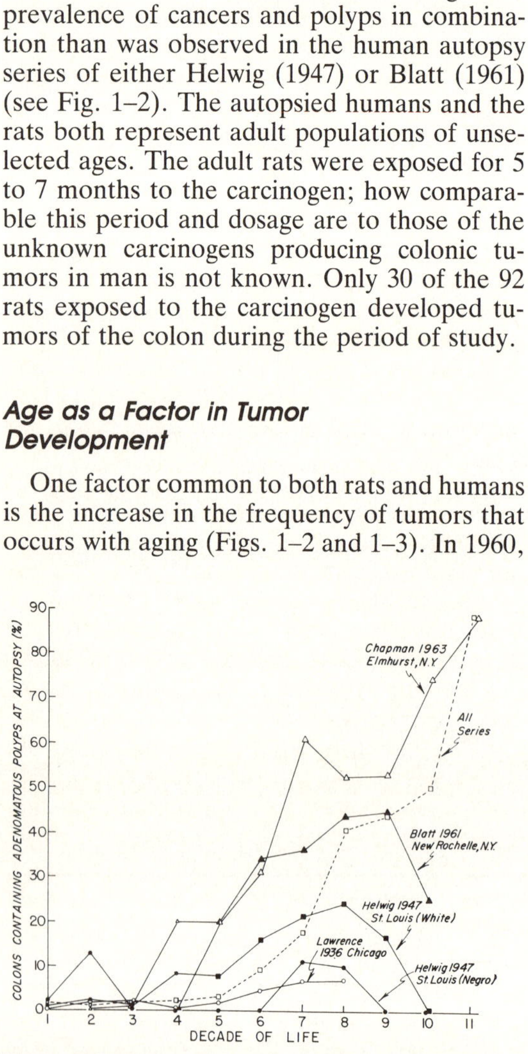

Figure 1–2. The number of persons reported by the prosector to have adenomatous polyps within the colon, divided by the total number of patients examined in each decade of life, multiplied by 100 percent, yields the age-specific percentage of human colons containing adenomatous polyps. The dotted line represents the summation of 9348 different autopsies by four different prosectors, who examined all cases consecutively in their own departments but worked at different times and places in the United States. The summation shows that the age-specific prevalence of adenomatous polyps increases progressively in older people until the affliction is nearly ubiquitous at the terminus of life. (W.U. 63–8002) (From Spjut HJ, Spratt JS Jr: Endemic and morphologic similarities existing between spontaneous colonic neoplasms in man and 3:2′-dimethyl-4-aminobiphenyl induced colonic neoplasms in rats. Ann Surg 161:309–325, 1965.)

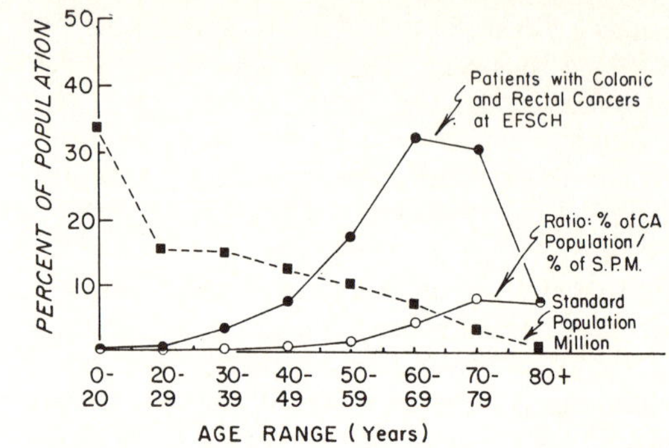

Figure 1–3. The proportion of patients of different ages is given for 1141 persons seen consecutively at the Ellis Fischel State Cancer Hospital between 1940 and 1961. The age-specific portion of a standard population million is divided into the former to show that the number of patients presenting with colonic cancer increases with age relative to the number of persons at risk. (W.U. 63–8003) (From Spjut HJ, Spratt JS Jr: Endemic and morphologic similarities existing between spontaneous colonic neoplasms in man and 3:2′-dimethyl-4-aminobiphenyl induced colonic neoplasms in rats. Ann Surg 161:309–325, 1965.)

Rashevsky, commenting on the incidence of cancer as a function of age, estimated, using some now-outdated human age-specific cancer incidence data, that there would be little chance of a human living past 88 years without developing a cancer somewhere. Spratt and Hoag (1966) estimated that the accumulative chance of developing one primary cancer by age 90 was 51.6 percent; two primary cancers, 17.5 percent; and three primary cancers, 5.97 percent. The chance of finding two separate primary cancers in the same person at the same time averaged 3.77 percent.

A recent autopsy study on a human population, updating the trends in cancer incidence, has been carried out in Oslo (Vatn and Stalsberg, 1982). The colons and rectums from 445 consecutive autopsies were examined under an illuminating magnifying lens. The lesions discovered included seven cancers undiagnosed before death, 329 adenomas, 174 hyperplastic polyps, 59 mucosal tags, 34 other polypoid lesions, and 54 polyps of which histologic diagnosis was not possible, usually as a result of autolysis. This provided a total of 7 cancers and 650 polypoid lesions, for a ratio of 1:93. In this series, adenomas were present in 34 percent of the men and 32 percent of the women. The prevalence of adenomas exhibited a steady increase with age in men but the prevalence was biphasic in women, with peaks at 50 to 59 years and at over 70 years.

The anatomic distribution of cancer in the colon changed with age, with a predominance on the left side before age 60 and a predominance on the right side after age 80.

Hyperplastic polyps were present in 27 percent of the men and 18 percent of the women. In men, the prevalence increased with increasing age, but in women, it did not. Multiple polyps were more frequent in women, and these tended to be larger, more atypical, and more villous than the polyps occurring in men. The study compared results with those of a similar study from northern Norway. There was no difference in the adenoma distribution, although the cancer incidence was 70 percent higher in the North.

No conclusions about cause and effect regarding a transition from polyp to cancer can be drawn from these studies. However, the study again shows the great prevalence of polypoid tumors existing at death and their vastly greater number in proportion to the number of cancers, i.e., a ratio of 93:1. The histologic diagnosis of a "polyp" visualized by endoscopic examination or barium enema study is not known to the examining clinician until removal. If all polyps had been removed to determine the histopathology and, presumably, to prevent cancer in these Norwegians, the mortality rate from polyp removal would have to be very low just to "break even." The logistic, financial, and compliance obstacles to such a preventive medicine program are staggering.

The frequency with which adenocarcinomas and adenomatous polyps are observed at autopsy may well be the basis of a simple method of assaying the exposure of human populations to carcinogens. The decade-specific frequencies of adenomatous polyps observed in four geographically and temporally different populations of autopsied Americans are plotted in Figure 1–2. In all four, the frequency of these polyps increased steadily with age. The decrease in frequency in the final decades observed by Blatt (1961) and Helwig (1947) can be attributed to the very small number of patients studied by them in these decades. The observation that the frequency of benign polyps increased, according to four successive American autopsy series, performed at different times and places on people of varied background and habits, may be pertinent. Helwig (1947) even observed a significant difference in the frequency of adenomatous polyps between Caucasian and Black populations in the same hospital and time period. In fact, the series of rats given DMAB in Houston rather than in St. Louis exhibited different distributions of the neoplasms (Spratt and Spjut, 1967). The strain of rats and dose of DMAB were the same in both groups, but numerous environmental factors were different.

Summary

The endemic of adenomatous polyps and adenocarcinomas induced in 92 rats by the injection of DMAB in peanut oil was remarkably comparable with the endemic of colonic neoplasms occurring in man. The following similarities were observed:

1. Morphologically, the adenomatous polyps and adenocarcinomas were similar in both rats and humans. The neoplasms of rats were homogeneous on step sections and were sharply demarcated from adjacent normal mucosa. No morphologic evidence of transition from benign to malignant could be found. Only one instance of carcinoma in situ in a benign adenomatous polyp was observed. All morphologic types were observed to the limits of visual distinction.
2. The tumors within the rat colon had a segmental distribution similar to that observed in human colons. The percentile distribution of cancers per unit length of colon was greater than that of adenomatous polyps in the rectum and cecum, and the ratio was reversed in the intervening colon.
3. Essentially, the male rats developed only colonic neoplasms, but extracolonic neoplasms were very frequent in the female rats. The sex distribution of concurrent or sequential extracolonic or colonic neoplasms occurring in 1141 consecutive patients with colonic cancer showed similar trends. In both the rat and the human, multiple neoplasms occurred with great frequency in aging populations.
4. In both rat and man, the prevalence of neoplasms increased sharply with the aging of the host populations.
5. Many polycyclic hydrocarbons reported to induce intestinal neoplasms in small animals have also been reported to induce urinary bladder tumors in both rats and humans. In humans, bladder tumors continued to appear with increasing prevalence 15 to 20 years later after exposure to 4-aminobiphenyl. The very slow rates of growth of many human colonic neoplasms are associated with equally long periods between exposure to a carcinogen and the appearance of a symptomatic neoplasm.

In 1964 Arminski and McLean presented further evidence that the prevalence of adenomatous polyps increased progressively with age in a human population and emphasized once again the almost ubiquitous affliction of older Americans with these tumors.

If adenomatous polyps are induced by the same carcinogen or carcinogens that induce adenocarcinomas of the colon and cancers of other organs, then it follows that the American population is being exposed almost universally to carcinogens having similar actions. There will be a continuing need to monitor the environment for causative agents.

Additional Animal and Human Studies

Numerous extensions of these early studies have been and are continuing to be conducted. In 1971, Spjut and Noall evaluated various dosage schedules from studies testing DMAB. All the neoplasms induced in rats were morphologically similar to those seen in man. The segmental distribution in the colon and rectum remained similar. Transition from benign neoplasms to malignant neoplasms was not seen; rather, the histologic growth pattern seemed set from the inception of the neoplasms. Fecal diversion by colostomy prevented the development of neoplasms in the bypassed segment.

Several areas of similarity between the experimentally produced neoplasms and the human colonic adenomatous polyps were observed. The rather uniform distribution of large intestinal neoplasms in the rat was similar to that in the adult human. In addition, the gross morphologic appearance, the histologic features, and the electron microscopic appearance (Spjut and Smith, 1967) of the experimental lesions were similar in many respects to those in humans. One major variation was the absence of metastases from the adenocarcinoma in rats. Others have reported metastases in rats from the carcinomas produced by DMAB (King and Varasdi, 1959).

Researchers failed to demonstrate the stepwise genesis of adenomatous polyps and their transition to carcinomas. By the time the lesions were discovered, they were already polyps or carcinomas. The random sections of nearby and distant colonic epithelium were always normal, with no evidence of neoplastic transformation of individual glands or parts of glands. Although no evidence was found of transition of a benign neoplasm to a malignant one, carcinoma in situ was observed. Whether this was a step in the transition from benign polyps to invasive carcinoma could not be ascertained.

In animal studies, various methods of compound administration have been used, resulting in some alteration in the frequency of occurrence of colonic neoplasms. In 1967, Druckrey and associates demonstrated that colonic neoplasms, although uncommon, could be induced by one injection of DMAB given to newborn rats. Varied methods of administration were used on the premise that in the human it is possible that exposure to a tumor-inducing agent is not continuous and may occur only once.

An important facet of this study was the use of DMAB-H, which demonstrated the distribution of the carcinogen, along with information about its excretion. It was concluded that the effective carcinogen from DMAB was a metabolite, probably produced in the liver.

In 1967, Navarrete and Spjut established that the performance of a colostomy before subcutaneous administration of DMAB protected the portion of colon and rectum distal to the colostomy from neoplasms. They concluded that in this experimental situation, the diversion of the fecal stream protected these regions of the Wistar rats.

Cleveland and Cole demonstrated, in 1969, that laxatives, which shorten transit time in the intestinal tract, reduced the potency of the carcinogenic effect of DMAB.

In 1971, Spjut and Noall established that metabolites of DMAB were present in bile of test animals injected with DMAB.

Rubio and Nylander, in 1981, showed that DMH, or its metabolites, could reach an isolated and frequently irritated colonic loop by way of the bloodstream and induce neoplasms there. Thus, a colon with no intraluminal passage of food or bile acids could be the target organ for some carcinogens. The mucosal lining of the bowel, which is a very metabolically active organ with a high cell replacement rate, was hypothesized to be a factor in carcinogenesis that needs more in-depth study.

Detailed histologic analyses were performed on tumors of the large intestine obtained from 152 DMH-treated rats. Of a total 539 glandular neoplasms, 45 were benign and 494 (92 percent) were locally invasive; 222 of these (41 percent) had invaded the muscularis propria. Of the 141 tumors less than 3 mm in diameter, 127 (90 percent) were invasive. In addition to macroscopic nodules, several microscopic carcinomas were observed on serial sections of flat mucosa. The benign polyps usually appeared after longer latency periods than did carcinomas. A review of the literature indicated that in the majority of rat experiments, most or all DMH-induced tumors were invasive carcinomas, often in the absence of adenomas. Microscopic invasive carcinomas were frequently reported. All these data constitute strong evidence that most experimental adenocarcinomas do arise de novo in flat mucosa, i.e., without a prior adenomatous stage. However, in mice, most DMH-induced tumors were reported to be adenomas. It was suggested that "de novo arising carcinomas" and adenomatous polyps, both of which are inducible by the same carcinogens and can coexist in some experimental systems, nonetheless constitute independent and distinct pathologic entities; they can be separated by genetic susceptibility (Maskens and Dujardin-Loits, 1981).

There is a growing list of chemicals capable of inducing colorectal neoplasms in animal models. A complete review of this subject is beyond the scope of this chapter. However, a few studies should be cited because of their implications.

In 1977, Lijinsky confirmed that *N*-nitroso compounds can be formed by the interaction of nitrites and secondary amino compounds. This reaction can occur in vivo in the stomach. *N*-nitroso compounds, especially nitrosamides, can reach the colon and contribute to the induction of colonic tumors. The implications of this observation are significant because of the ubiquity of precursors of these reactions in our environment (National Research Council, 1978).

Venitt (1982) concluded that the roles of nitrates, nitrites, and nitrosamines in carcinogenesis are not resolved. Studies with conflicting results exist. Among other things, conditions in the lower gastrointestinal tract may even favor denitrification rather than nitrification, and the reported identification of nitrosamines in feces is subject to question.

Sugimura and co-workers established, in 1977, that carcinogens were produced by the incomplete pyrolysis of such common precursors as tryptophan and phenylalanine.

Toth (1977), Fiala (1977), and Moon and Fricks (1977) have reviewed the capacity of common hydrazines to induce colonic neoplasms. Two of these hydrazines occur in nature, one in tobacco and one in wild mushrooms. Synthetic hydrazines are used as rocket fuels. Both genetic and sexual differences in susceptibility were shown in the study of Moon and Fricks.

In many animal tumor models, the two-step nature of chemical carcinogenesis has been demonstrated. The first step is caused by the carcinogen, and the effect is additive with repetitive doses. The changes are transmissible within renewable mucosa for prolonged periods. The affected cells have no proliferative advantage. The second step does not require the presence of the carcinogen, although continued exposure to the carcinogen may yield more cancers after a shorter latency period. This second step affects only cells that have undergone the first change at a constant rate within the considered tissue.

Maskens (1981) confirmed the two-step nature of chemical carcinogenesis in one animal model. The cancers produced had no prior benign polyp stage. Tumor growth tended to be Gompertzian and, in the case of large primary tumors, was slow enough to allow the accumulation of up to 20 multiple carcinomas in the same colon. The carcinogen used in the study, DMH, was potent enough to cause cancers with a single injection.

The concise quantitative nature of Maskens' experiment and the mathematical models he used give data consistent with the hypothesis that the DMH induces a recessive mutation followed by the conversion of the recessive mutant to a homozygous state. The rate of conversion to neoplasm is an intrinsic property of the colon tissue. This second step can be promoted by a variety of noncarcinogenic agents. Any factor increasing the number of cells that have undergone the first-step change or that will enhance mitotic activity can serve as a promoter, even though it may not be a carcinogen.

Weisburger and associates (1977) grouped the following chemicals that have been shown to produce colonic neoplasms in animals: 3-methyl-4-aminobiphenyl and 3-methyl-2-naphthylamine; derivatives and analogs of cycasin and methylazoxymethanol (MAM); intrarectal direct-acting carcinogens, such as MAM acetate; alkyl nitrosoureas, such as *N*-methyl-*N*-nitrosurea (MNU) and methly-*N'*-nitro-N-nitrosoguanidine (MNNG); and 3-methylcholanthrene administered orally in large doses. Potential mechanisms of action include (1) ingestion of complex carcinogens with diet, with the liberation of the active agent by bacterial or intestinal enzymes; (2) ingestion of procarcinogens that are absorbed, metabolized largely in the liver, secreted in the bile, and freed in the gut; and (3) production of active agents by the bacterial flora. Another possible mechanism is the primary production of carcinogenic mycotoxins by the intestinal bacterial flora.

In fact, direct studies of the mutagenicity of

fecal contents have established that fecal mutagens are widely prevalent and subject to manipulation by a very wide range of factors (Bruce and Dion, 1980; Weisburger et al., 1981).

DIETARY FACTORS

Epidemiologic studies in humans suggest that colon cancer may be related to a high standard of living. There is evidence to suggest an association between colon cancer and diets containing a high proportion of fat or meat (Doll and Peto, 1981). Correlations between the national consumption of fat and meat per head of household and incidence of colon cancer are impressive (Armstrong and Doll, 1975). The relationship is not consistent, however. Mormons, who are not vegetarians, have as low an incidence of colon cancer as Seventh Day Adventists, who are vegetarians (West et al., 1980; Lyon et al., 1980a and 1980b).

One suggestion is that certain fats contribute to the production of carcinogens in the body by increasing the amounts of bile acid and cholesterol metabolites in the feces (Reddy et al., 1980). Larger amounts of deoxycholic and lithocholic acids are found in the stools of populations on western-type diets, in whom colon cancer is relatively common. Larger amounts are also found in the stools of patients with colorectal cancer than in the stools of patients with other intestinal diseases or in the stools of healthy controls. The amounts of these acids in the stools can also be increased experimentally in humans by a high fat–high meat diet.

Despite these observations, the relation of high cholesterol levels to human colorectal cancer remains uncertain. There is no evidence that increased levels of any form of cholesterol in the blood is correlated with an increased risk of developing cancer. On the contrary, there is evidence to suggest that people with a low blood level of cholesterol suffer a high mortality from colon cancer. This has been reviewed by Laskarzewski (1982) and also by Feinlieb (1982). If, indeed, cholesterol or bile acids or both are risk factors for colon cancer, it is most likely because they are acted upon by bacteria in the colon to produce intermediate carcinogenic metabolites.

Hirai and associates (1982) reported a potent mutagen isolated from human feces, (S)-3-(1, 3, 5, 7-dodecapentaenyloxy)-1, 2-propanediol, produced by at least five species of intestinal bacteria from an unknown precursor. About 3 percent of the population thus far tested contained high levels of the carcinogen in their feces. Incubation of the bacteria in the presence of bile acids increased production of the mutagen, whereas fiber in the diet decreased production. Higher levels of the mutagen in the feces were present in high-risk populations. The authors considered that the low levels of the mutagen in the feces from colons with polyps was evidence contradictory to the theory that polyps are precancerous. Actually, their finding is simply more evidence that benign colonic polyps are *not* premalignant.

Burkitt (1969) observed that colon cancer and several other intestinal diseases were rare in rural Africa, where unprocessed food is consumed and stools tend to be soft, bulky, and frequent. In 1971, Burkitt popularized the idea that many common diseases of the bowel, such as neoplasms, diverticular disease, and appendicitis, might have a common cause. He concluded that these conditions might be associated with a diet low in fiber content. Dietary fiber was conceived of as regulating or influencing fecal transit time, bulk, consistency, and bacterial flora. Variations in incidence rates associated with variations in dietary fiber content were used to support his hypothesis. The hypothesis still remains controversial. Studies relating to specific types of fiber and colon cancer are now being pursued.

All dietary fibers are not the same, and many other variables may exist simultaneously that effect carcinogenesis. Rigidly designed studies establishing the role of dietary fiber content in cancer prevention are inconsistent in their conclusions. Burkitt's observations were followed by a series of conflicting studies. Talbot (1981) reviewed the status of dietary fiber in diverticular disease and colon cancer in a report for the Federation of American Societies for Experimental Biology.

He first observed that an accepted definition and classification system for "fiber" are lacking, as are clear end points for measuring the impact of fiber as an isolated variable in colonic carcinogenesis and diverticular disease. Dietary fiber is part of a very complex interaction pattern involving nutrients, gut flora, metabolites, enteric secretions, and transit time. None of the reported epidemiologic studies allowed for numerous genetic, environmental, or other uncontrolled variables. Thus, conclusive evidence on the role of fiber in colon carcinogenesis does not yet exist. Clinical trials have been conducted on the relationship between the symptoms of diverticular disease and supplementary dietary fiber, and the results have generally been favorable.

The complexity of determining the role of fiber is shown in two studies on rats. Freeman and co-workers (1978) compared the protective role of a chemically defined fiber-free diet with a nutritionally and calorically equivalent diet containing purified microcrystalline cellulose. In this study, cellulose ingestion was associated with a reduction both in the number of animals afflicted and the total number of colonic neoplasms. The protective effect seemed time-dependent and was associated with a shift in the distribution of tumors from the proximal to the distal colon. The fiber content had no apparent effect on the histopathology or size of those neoplasms that did develop. Although the mechanism of benefit was not elucidated, this study was strongly supportive of the protective role of fiber.

Bauer and co-workers (1979) identified other problems. The type of fiber made a difference in the protective effect. For example, citrus pectin was associated with an increase in neoplasms, not only in the colon but also elsewhere, and wheat bran may have provided a weak protective effect.

Harvey (1981) presented evidence supporting the interesting hypothesis that any benefit accruing from a high-fiber diet may be indirect, such as by restriction of caloric intake. The mechanical effects of the fiber might be of no consequence.

The role of dietary fat content in carcinogenesis has also been the subject of numerous studies that reaffirm the multifactorial origin of most cancers. Dietary fats, for example, affect the immunocompetence of rats (Newberne, 1981). Epidemiologic evidence indicating that fats play a role in the etiology of human cancer is not clear-cut. Despite an increasing number of studies, the exact nature of the fats and other dietary components purported to influence neoplastic induction remains unknown. Contradictory or inconclusive results have yet to be reconciled so as to be useful in preventing human cancer (Enig et al., 1978; Leveille and Rogers, 1981).

In 1980, Sherlock and associates reviewed the potential for colon cancer prevention by dietary modification. They concluded that a diet low in cholesterol and fat might be protective. When control of environmental carcinogen uptake is not possible, blocking agents might be helpful. Factors that have been shown to serve as blocking agents for some carcinogens include vitamins A, C, and E (Newberne and Suphakarn, 1977; DeCosse et al., 1975; Cook and McNamara, 1980). The exact role of these vitamins is not known. Vitamin A is important in maintaining epithelial integrity. Vitamins C and E are antioxidants, and accelerate the decay of many carcinogens.

As the 1982 review by Sugimura confirms, our daily food intake contains numerous mutagens, carcinogens, procarcinogens (e.g., substances convertible to carcinogens by bacterial action), and tumor promoters. Reduction in their prevalence or inactivation is possible, although this would require lifelong modification of certain life styles and dietary habits, as summarized by the author (J. S. S.) in 1974, and earlier in 1967 (see Appendix). These studies recommend the following: temperance; a balanced diet; avoidance of overweight; minimum intake of processed or over-cooked foods; avoidance of all known carcinogens, including direct sunlight and tobacco; adequate daily vitamin and mineral intake (particularly vitamins A, C, and E); avoidance of excessive salt, sugar, and other condiments; and adequate daily rest. There is no "controlled experiment" in humans that proves that the incidence of cancer would be reduced by these practices, but there is abundant animal evidence and epidemiologic studies of humans that verify the importance of life style and diet in cancer prevention.

In a succinct review concerning the effect of social and cultural dietary habits on cancer prevention, Randeria (1981) concluded that well-documented results of worldwide research on hazardous life-style factors pertaining to harmful food habits can be put to beneficial use. During pregnancy, lactation, childhood, and adolescence, the oral intake of various substrates, patterns of diversion of the fecal stream, possibly prior cholecystectomy, and other unidentified factors may cause cancer. It is encouraging that some sources of these cancers are avoidable, and the effect of others may be ameliorated by chemoprevention.

There have been an increasing number of studies, using animal models, that have specifically sought to determine the roles of various modifications in diet and of specific inhibitors in reducing the development of neoplasms. These studies, which augment epidemiologic studies that show geographic and cultural variations in cancer incidence, attempt to establish associations between various practices subject to modification. Whenever a high degree of similarity can be identified between these epidemiologic and animal studies, a strong case can often be developed for recommending changes in human behavior as a method of cancer prevention. However, to take the next step in scientific inquiry and actually set up a human controlled trial is very difficult. The factors that would have to be controlled and the duration and cost of the experiment would be very great. The ethics of such a trial would also be subject to question. In this situation, the available course of action is to cite pertinent and representative studies in various areas. If recommended behavioral modifications associated with a reduction of cancer are followed (all other factors staying static over time), evidence will accumulate supporting the value of such changes. Since none of the recommended changes is of known harm, this approach may be the only ethical one available for putting much new knowledge to use.

INTESTINAL FLORA

The effect of the intestinal flora and dietary fat consumption on the induction of colon neoplasms by DMAB was investigated by Reddy and Ohmori (1981). They used weanling germ-free and conventional rats fed semipurified diets with low- and high-fat content. The incidence of colon, small intestinal, ear duct, and skin tumors was lower in the germ-free group. Both the incidence and multiplicity of neoplasms were higher in the conventional rats fed high-fat diets than in those fed low-fat diets. However, the level of dietary fat had no effect on tumor incidence in the germ-free rats. A positive association between the consumption of high-fat diets, and its secondary effect of increasing fecal bile acid excretion, and the development of colon cancers in man has also been shown (Hill et al., 1971; Nigro et al., 1976; Reddy et al., 1980).

Sonoda and associates (1983) reviewed the accumulating evidence that the bacterial degradation of bile acids may lead to endogenous formation of carcinogens and that cholecystectomy may enhance this formation. They speculated that the apparent shift of colonic cancers toward the right hemicolon may be an expression of this enhancement in patients with surgically absent gallbladders. Kingston and associates (1982) have reported the isolation of a potent mutagen from some human feces, (s)-3-(1,3,5, 7-dodecapentaenyloxy)-1,1-propanediol. They have produced this mutagen by the incubation of bile acids with fecal bacteria.

OTHER CARCINOGEN INHIBITORS

Inhibitors of colon carcinogens include selenium and disulfiram (Jacobs, 1977; Wattenberg et al., 1977). The carcinogenic potential of DMH for colonic neoplasms was significantly reduced in mice by the addition of aminocaproic acid to their drinking water. The investigators suggested that this action could have been induced by the interference with the binding of some substance to the strong lysine-binding site of plasminogen. Aminocaproic acid is normally antifibrinolytic (Corasanti et al., 1982). Indomethacin had a similar inhibitory effect on DMH-induced rat colon tumors (Pollard and Luckert, 1980).

ETIOLOGIC CONSIDERATIONS IN CHILDREN

Colorectal cancer occurs only infrequently in children and adolescents. As of 1977, only about 300 cases had been reported in the world's literature (Pratt et al., 1977).

Since in adults colorectal cancers do not become a major problem until after age 40, Pratt and associates (1977) questioned whether some causation unique to children might exist, such as unique carcinogen exposure. Pratt's study was updated by the St. Jude's group (Caldwell et al., 1981). The authors of both studies looked at place of residence, family clusters, exposure to carcinogenic pesticides, water source, and other factors. The possibilities raised as to the causes of childhood colorectal cancer merit attention, and continued surveillance of all childhood cases should be maintained. The implications of these studies are interesting, although no cause-and-effect relationships between the various factors and cancer have been established.

ECOGENETICS

The phenotypic characteristics reported to exist in populations with increased susceptibility to colonic cancers are important considerations in the assessment of causation. Many carcinogens or procarcinogens probably express themselves through patterns of metabolism influenced by genetic factors, giving rise to the observation that most cancers are ecogenetic in origin. Awareness of these patterns is essential when designing any clinical or epidemiologic study. Studies of the complex subject of metabolic interaction with nutrients, carcinogens, and other factors are really in their infancy.

Genetic expression is by protein synthesis. The identification of abnormal proteins or proteins in abnormal amounts may permit the diagnosis of hereditary or mutant disorders more accurately than can the usual family history or the analysis of chromosome morphology. Also, these defects may be identified early in life. As knowledge grows, specific prevention programs for susceptible individuals may become possible.

In 1981, Lyko and Hartman reported a 100-fold increase in plasma protease activity ($p < 0.001$) in 9 of 12 persons with heritable adenomatosis of the colon and rectum (ACR). The three people without increased protease were found to have a 400 percent increase in plasmin inhibitor activity when compared with controls. The protease-positive samples, when added to a culture of normal colonic epithelial cells, caused a transformation in cell morphology. From further evaluation of their data, the authors concluded that protease and protease inhibitors in people with ACR permitted identification of individuals with the disorder and that both protease and protease inhibitors were implicated in the development of cancer. In patients with ACR, diversion of the fecal stream by ileostomy or proximal colostomy does not prevent the development of either polyps or cancers in colon, and cancers were not prevented in these cases when all polyps were removed as often as every 6 months (Bussey, 1975; Schuchardt and Pousky, 1979; McKusick, 1974).

RADIATION

The role of radiation in the induction of colorectal neoplasms has been the topic of many anecdotal papers reporting the development of cancers of the colon and rectum in patients who have had previous radiotherapy (Castro et al., 1973). These studies show a time lag of 5 to 30 years between irradiation and the appearance of the cancers in the field of radiation. The cancers were more frequently mucinous, with concomitant evidence of radiation proctocolitis.

Adenocarcinomas can be induced in the colons of rats by irradiation. Denman and associates (1978) set up an experiment to determine if x-irradiation could induce tumors of the colon in outbred Holtzman rats. Only the descending colon was irradiated with a collimated x-ray beam that delivered tumorogenic exposures in the kilo-roentgen range. The male Holtzman rats were divided into six exposure groups of 15 animals each. In the first group, the colon was exposed to 2500 rad; in the second group, the colon was exposed to 3500 rad; the exposures were increased by 1000-rad increments up through 6500 rad in the third, fourth, and fifth groups. The sixth group was sham irradiated. Animals in each of the irradiated groups developed mucoid adenocarcinomas, with the highest incidence (47 percent) occurring in the 4500-rad group.

Histopathologically, the induced tumors bore a close resemblance to human colon adenocarcinoma. The development of pulmonary metastases in one of the animals with multiple primary tumors demonstrated their malignancy.

The issue, however, with all multiple cancers is always the same. By chance alone, common cancers in different organ sites are going to occur in the same individual. The question is whether the additional cancers occur with more, or less, or the same incidence per person-year of risk. This question was addressed in a follow-up study of 1853 women with a first cancer of the cervix uteri treated by radiation (Spratt and Hoag, 1966). These women, who were a median age of 54 years, were followed for a total of 6264 person-years. Only 36 developed new cancers, for an incidence of 0.0057 per person-year. The expected range was 0.00481 to 0.01256 per person-year, based on Connecticut tumor registry data. The 6264 person-years of follow-up were spread over a 20-year span. Only two cases of colorectal cancer occurred among the 36 patients with second primary cancers. Clearly, rectal cancer may occur after irradiation, but a cause-and-effect relationship between radiotherapy and the subsequent appearance of adenocarcinoma of the colon in the field of radiation was not established.

PREVENTION

The prevention of cancer may be divided into primary prevention and secondary prevention. Primary prevention includes that set of interventions that keeps cancerous processes from ever developing and includes environmental controls, such as the elimination of exposure to known carcinogens, and behavioral changes through health counseling and education. Secondary prevention is that set of interventions leading to the discovery and control of cancerous and precancerous processes while they are still localized. Secondary prevention includes screening, early detection, and effective treatment (Spratt 1977; 1981).

This chapter has attempted to review current knowledge that is potentially useful in primary prevention. Secondary prevention is discussed in the chapter on screening and follow-up (see Chapter Four).

The day may well be approaching when the assay of feces for the presence of mutagens will become a clinically useful test. The methodology for the quantitative titration of the levels of chemopreventive agents necessary to inactivate carcinogens can then be perfected for clinical application. Finally, methods of dietary modification, specific for the reduction of the fecal mutagens in each individual with demonstrable mutagens, would have to be designed and tested for efficacy. This process would have to start in infancy and possibly even in utero. At least this type of thinking is necessary to make the primary prevention of cancer a reality.

A review of the current state of knowledge concerning the cause of cancers of the colon and rectum presents a very complex picture. Clearly, there is no single cause; rather, many factors are implicated in an increased incidence. These factors include genetics; diet; an increasing list of chemical procarcinogens, carcinogens, and cocarcinogens; fecal mutagens; and colonic bacteria and their reactions with unessential hazardous food items. Sensitivity to carcinogenic initiators is known to be great during the active growth periods found in utero and in early childhood. Safe levels of exposure to these initiators during these periods are largely undefined in humans. Examples of products that should be excluded from maternal and early childhood intake include many nonessential items: alcohol; tobacco, betel, and related chewing products; fungal contaminants; nitrosatable ingredients; products of pyrolysis; and an array of food additives. The evidence supporting the protective effects of antioxidants during this critical period is inadequate. Overdependence upon chemopreventive agents during these critical periods could provide a false sense of security. Continuation of bad dietary habits in later life can serve to promote neoplasms. Obesity and excessive caloric intake may also serve promotional roles (Carroll, 1981). There exist many exciting leads for future research into primary prevention. The multifactorial origin of cancers might simultaneously require a profiling of genetic risk, a lifelong reduction in exposure to known carcinogens and promotors, fundamental and sustained modifications of diet, and use of chemoprevention for some carcinogens and carcinogenic metabolites. The cataloging of potential carcinogens is improving annually (Public Health Service, 1981). The transformation on this knowledge into effective public policy and health education curricula is a major challenge for the future.

Whether or not dietary fiber is important in preventing cancer is uncertain, and further study into the benefits of different types of fibers is required. Prolonged fecal transit time is undesirable. A number of complex chemopreventive agents, such as vitamins A, C, E, and indomethacin, reduce the cancer risk in animal models. Stools can now be assayed for mutagen content, and future studies must explore what can be done to reduce the mutagen content in stools. Even then, timing is important. How soon and how rigorously must we start to establish a lifelong strategy that might indeed prevent colorectal cancers?

At present, the part played by fecal mutagens in the induction of colorectal cancers remains to be determined (Venitt, 1982). Venitt has provided an excellent review of the enormous complexity of this possibility as a research problem. Feces, bacterial flora, metabolism, enterohepatic circulation, and diet of the host; genetic variations; and an array of still to be defined factors all complicate experimental design, implementation, and interpretation. Many years of patient investigation will be required to sort out the issues confronting investigators. However, all this work may result in a level of understanding that could lead to prevention of a major part of the neoplastic disease problem.

In the interim, over a period of several years, the author (JSS) has updated a handout used for his own patients to inform them of steps they might take to reduce their risk of cancer. This handout, entitled "Good Health and the Avoidance of Cancer," appears as an appendix on page 429.*

*The author solicits critical feedback on this appendix and waives all rights to its content, permitting unlimited duplication and use by any interested parties.

References

American Cancer Society: Cancer Facts and Figures, 1980. New York, N.Y., American Cancer Society, 1979.

Ames BN, Lee FD, Durston WE: An improved bacterial test system for the detection and classification of mutagens and carcinogens. Proc Natl Acad Sci USA 70:782–786, 1973.

Arminski TC, McLean DW: Incidence and distribution of adenomatous polyps of the colon and rectum based on 1,000 autopsy examinations. Dis Colon Rectum 7:249–261, 1964.

Armstrong BK, Doll R: Environmental factors and cancer incidence and mortality in different countries, with special reference to dietary practices. Int J Cancer 15:617–631, 1975.

Bauer HG, Asp NG, Oste R, et al: Effect of dietary fiber on the induction of colorectal tumors and fecal β-glucuronidase activity in the rat. Cancer Res 39:3752–3756, 1979.

Beilschowsky F: Distant tumours produced by 2-amino- and 2-acetyl-amino-fluorene. Br J Exp Path 25:1–4, 1944.

Berlinger NT, Lopez C, Lipkin M, et al: Defective recognitive immunity in family aggregates of colon carcinoma. J Clin Invest 59:761–769, 1977.

Blatt LJ: Polyps of the colon and rectum: incidence and distribution. Dis Colon Rectum 4:277–282, 1961.

Blot WJ, Mason TJ, Hoover R, Fraumeni JF Jr: Cancer by county: etiologic implications. *In* Hiatt HH, Watson JD, Winsten JA (eds): Origin of Human Cancer. Book A. Incidence of Cancer in Humans. Cold Spring Harbor Conference on Cell Proliferation. Cold Spring Harbor, NY, Cold Spring Harbor Laboratory, 1977, pp 21–32.

Bridbord K, Decoufle P, Fraumeni JF Jr, et al: Estimates of the fraction of cancer in the United States related to occupational factors. Presented at the Occupational Safety and Health Hearings, 1978.

Bruce WR, Dion PW: Studies relating to fecal mutagen. Am J Clin Nutr 33(11 Suppl):2511–2512, 1980.

Burkitt DP: Related disease—related cause? Lancet 2:1229–1231, 1969.

Burkitt DP: Epidemiology of cancer of the colon and rectum. Cancer 28:3–13, 1971.

Bussey HJ: Familial Polyposis Coli. Family studies, Histopathology, Differential Diagnosis, and Results of Treatment. Baltimore, Johns Hopkins University Press, 1975.

Caldwell GG, Cannon SB, Pratt CB, Arther RD: Serum pesticide levels in patients with childhood colorectal cancer. Cancer 48:774–778, 1981.

Carroll KK: Dietary promotion of carcinogenesis. Cancer Detect Prev 4:117–120, 1981.

Castro EB, Rosen PP, Quan SH: Carcinoma of large intestine in patients irradiated for carcinoma of cervix and uterus. Cancer 31:45–52, 1973.

Chapman I: Adenomatous polypi of large intestine: incidence and distribution. Ann Surg 157:223–226, 1963.

Cleveland JC, Cole JW: Relation of experimentally induced intestinal tumors to laxative ingestion. Cancer 23:1200–1203, 1969.

Cook MG, McNamara P: Effect of dietary vitamin E on dimethylhydrazine-induced colonic tumors in mice. Cancer Res 40:1329–1331, 1980.

Corasanti JG, Hobika GH, Markus G: Interference with dimethylhydrazine induction of colon tumors in mice by aminocaproic acid. Science 216:1020–1021, 1982.

Correa P, Haenszel W: The epidemiology of large bowel cancer. Adv Cancer Res 26:1–141, 1978.

Danes BS, Krush AJ: The gardner syndrome: a family study in cell culture. J Natl Cancer Inst 58:771–775, 1977.

Darchun V, Hadler HI: Metabolic and carcinogenic studies with 9, 10-dimethyl-1, 2-benzanthracene. Cancer Res 16:316–323, 1956.

DeCosse JJ, Adams MB, Kuzma JF, et al: Effect of ascorbic acid on rectal polyps of patients with familial polyposis. Surgery 78:608–612, 1975.

Denman DL, Kirchner FR, Osborne JW: Induction of colonic adenocarcinoma in the rat by X-irradiation. Cancer Res 38:1899–1905, 1978.

Deschner E, Lewis CM, Lipkin M: In vitro study of human rectal epithelial cells. I. Atypical zone of H3 thymidine incorporation in mucosa of multiple polyposis. J Clin Invest 42:1922–1928, 1963.

Deschner EE, Lipkin M: Study of human rectal epithelial cells in vitro. III. RNA, protein, and DNA synthesis in polyps and adjacent mucosa. J Natl Cancer Inst 44:175–185, 1970.

Doll R, Peto R: The causes of cancer: quantitative estimates of avoidable risks of cancer in the U.S. today. New York, Oxford University Press, 1981.

Dorn HF, Cutler SJ: Morbidity from Cancer in the United States. Pub Health Monograph No. 56, Washington, GPO, 1959.

Druckrey H, Preussman R, Matzkies P, Ivankovic S: Selektive Erzengung von Darmkrebs bei Ratten durch 1,2-Dimethyl-hydrazin. Naturwissenschaften 54:285–286, 1967.

Enig MG, Munn RJ, Keeney M: Dietary fat and cancer trends: a critique. Fed Proc 37:2215–2220, 1978.

Feinlieb M: Summary of a workshop on cholesterol and noncardiovascular disease mortality. Prev Med 11:360–367, 1982.

Fiala ES: Investigations into the metabolism and mode of action of colon carcinogens 1,2-dimethylhydrazine and azoxymethane. Cancer 40(5 Suppl):2436–2445, 1977.

Fisch RO, Berglund EB, Bridge AG, et al: Methemoglobinemia in a hospital nursery: a search for causative factors. JAMA 185:760–763, 1963.

Freeman HJ, Spiller GA, Kim YS: A double-blind study on the effect of purified cellulose dietary fiber on 1,2-dimethylhydrazine-induced rat colonic neoplasia. Cancer Res 38:2912–2917, 1978.

Harvey JS: Mechanism of fibre prophylaxis of chemically induced colonic carcinoma in rat. *In* European Society for Surgical Research 16th Congress Garmisch-Partenkirchen, 1981. Eur Surg Res 13:96, 1981.

Helwig EB: The evolution of adenomas of the large intestine and their relation to carcinoma. Surg Gynecol Obstet 84:36–49, 1947.

Hiatt HH, Watson JD, Winsten JA: Origins of Human Cancer. Cold Spring Harbor, NY, Cold Spring Harbor Laboratory, 1977.

Hill MJ, Drasar BS, Hawksworth G, et al: Bacteria and the etiology of cancer of the large bowel. Lancet 1:95–100, 1971.

Hirai M, Kingston DGI, Van Tassle RL, Wilkins TD: A structure elucidation of a potent mutagen from human feces. J Am Chem Soc 104:6149–6150, 1982.

Jacobs MM: Inhibitory effects of selenium on 1,2-dimethylhydrazine and methylazoxymethanol colon carcinogenesis. Cancer 40(5 Suppl):2557–2564, 1977.

King ESJ, Varasdi G: Experimentally induced tumors of the intestine. Aust NZ J Surg 29:38–53, 1959.

Kingston DGI, Wilkins, TD, Van Tassel, RL: Potent mutagen from human feces. Reported at the 184th National Meeting of The American Chemical Society, 12–17 Sept 1982, Kansas City, Mo.

Klein M: Induction of skin tumors in the mouse with minute doses of 9,10-dimethyl-1,2-benzanthcacene alone or with croton oil. Cancer Res 16:123–127, 1956.

Kopelovich L, Conlon S, Pollack R: Defective organization of actin in cultured skin fibroblasts from patients with inherited adenocarcinoma. Proc Natl Acad Sci USA 74:3019–3022, 1977.

Lane N, Lev R: Observations on the origin of adenomatous epithelium of the colon: serial section of minute polyps in familial polyposis. Cancer 16:751–764, 1963.

Laskarzewski P, Khoury P, Kelly K: Prevalence of familial

hyper- and hypolipoproteinemias in blacks: the Princeton School District Family Study. Prev Med 11:142–161, 1982.

Lawrence JC: Gastrointestinal polyps; statistical study of malignancy incidence. Am J Surg 31:499–505, 1936.

Leveille GA, Rogers AE: Working group II: fatty acids, steroids, and cancer. Introduction. Cancer Res 2:3752–3754, 1981.

Lijinsky W: Nitrosamines and nitrosamides in the etiology of gastrointestinal cancer. Cancer 40(5 Suppl):2446–2449, 1977.

Lijinsky W, Shubik P: Benzo(a)pyrene and other polynuclear hydrocarbons in charcoal-broiled meat. Science 145:53–55, 1964.

Lipkin M: Growth kinetics of normal and premalignant gastrointestinal epithelium. *In* Drewinko B, Humphrey RM (eds): Growth Kinetics and Biochemical Regulation of Normal and Malignant Cells. Baltimore, Williams and Wilkins Company, 1977, 569–589.

Lyko HC, Hartmann JX: Familial polyposis coli plasma causes a transformation-associated morphology of cells in vitro: hyperproteinaemia and colorectal polyps. Cancer Detect Prev 4:401–405, 1961.

Lyon JL, Gardner JW, West DW: Cancer in Utah: risk by religion and place of residence. J Natl Cancer Inst 65:1063–1071, 1980a.

Lyon JL, Gardner JW, West DW: Cancer incidence in Mormons and non-Mormons in Utah during 1967–75. J Natl Cancer Inst 65:1055–1061, 1980b.

McKusick VA: Genetics and large bowel cancer. Am J Dig Dis 19:954–957, 1974.

Maskens AP: Confirmation of the two-step nature of chemical carcinogenesis in the rat colon adenocarcinoma model. Cancer Res 41:1240–1245, 1981.

Maskens AP, Dujardin-Loits R: Experimental adenomas and carcinomas of the large intestine behave as distinct entities: most carcinomas arise de novo in flat mucosa. Cancer 47:81–89, 1981.

Mathews JJ, Walpole AL: Tumors of the liver and kidney induced in Wistar rats with 4′-fluoro-4-amino-diphenyl. Brit J Cancer 12:234–241, 1958.

Melick WF, Escue HM, Naryka JJ, et al: First reported cases of human bladder tumors due to new carcinogen—xenylamine. J Urol 74:760–766, 1955.

Melick WF, Naryka JJ: Xenylamine (para-aminobiphenyl) bladder tumors in man. Acta Un Int Contre Cancer 16:277–283, 1960.

Moon RC, Fricks CM: Influence of gonadal hormones and age on 1,2-dimethylhydrazine-induced colon carcinogenesis. Cancer 40(5 Suppl):2502–2508, 1977.

Morson BC, Bussey HJ: Predisposing causes of intestinal cancer. Curr Probl Surg 1–46, 1970.

Murphy GP: Short-Term Patient Care Evaluation of Cancer of the Colon. Commission on Cancer, Chicago, American College of Surgeons, 1977.

National Cancer Program, 1980. Director's Report and Annual Plan, FY 1982–1986. NIH Publ No. 81–2290. V:25–28, 1981.

National Research Council: Nitrates: An Environmental Assessment. Scientific and Technical Assessments of Environmental Pollutants. Washington DC, National Academy of Sciences, 1978.

Navarrete A, Spjut HJ: Effect of colostomy on experimentally produced neoplasms of the colon of the rat. Cancer 20:1466–1472, 1967.

Newberne PM: Dietary fat, immunological response and cancer in rats. Cancer Res 2:3783–3785, 1981.

Newberne PM, Suphakarn V: Preventive role of vitamin A in colon carcinogenesis in rats. Cancer 40(5 Suppl):2553–2556, 1977.

Nigro ND, Campbell RL, Singh DV, Lin YN: Effect of diet high in beef fat on the composition of fecal bile acids during intestinal carcinogenesis in the rat. J Natl Cancer Inst 57:883–888, 1976.

Polk HC Jr, Spratt JS Jr, Butcher HR Jr: Frequency of multiple primary malignant neoplasms associated with colorectal carcinoma. Am J Surg 109:71–75, 1965.

Pollard M, Luckert PH: Indomethacin treatment of rats with dimethylhydrazine-induced intestinal tumors. Cancer Treat Rep 64:1323–1327, 1980.

Pratt CB, Rivera G, Shanks E, et al: Colorectal carcinomas in adolescents; implications regarding etiology. Cancer 1977 40(5 Suppl):2464–2472, 1977.

Public Health Service: Second Annual Report on Carcinogens. Washington, DC, U.S. Department of Health and Human Services, Public Health Service, December 1981.

Randeria JD: Dietary modulation in cancer prevention with reference to social and cultural food habits. Cancer Detect Prev 4:141–148, 1981.

Rashevsky N: Outline of a physio-mathematical approach to the cancer problem. *In* Mathematical Biophysics; Physico-Mathematical Foundations of Biology. 3rd revised ed. New York, Dover Publications. 1:299–306, 1960.

Reddy BS, Cohen L, McCoy GD, et al: Nutrition and its relationship to cancer. Adv Cancer Res 32:237–345, 1980.

Reddy BS, Mastromarino A, Gustafson C, et al: Fecal bile acids and neutral sterols in patients with familial polyposis. Cancer 38:1694–1698, 1976.

Reddy BS, Ohmori T: Effect of intestinal microflora and dietary fat on 3,2′-dimethyl-4-aminobiphenyl-induced colon carcinogenesis in F344 rats. Cancer Res 41:1363–1367, 1981.

Rice DP, Hodgson TA: Social and economic implications of cancer in the United States. Vital Health Stat 3:1–43, 1981.

Roffo AH: Tumeurs malignes développeés dans l'appareil digestif par l'ingestion de graisses oxydeés par chauffage. Bull Assoc Fr Etude Cancer 28:556–588, 1939.

Rubio CA, Nylander G: Further studies on the carcinogenesis of the colon of the rat with special reference to the absence of intestinal contents. Cancer 48:951–953, 1981.

Schoentel R: Carcinogenesis by polycyclic aromatic hydrocarbons and by certain other carcinogens. *In* Polycyclic Hydrocarbons, New York, Academic Press, 1964.

Schuchardt WA Jr, Pousky JL: Familial polyposis coli. Surg Gynecol Obstet 148:97–103, 1979.

SEER Program: Cancer Incidence and Mortality in the United States 1973–1976. Biometry Branch, Division of Cancer Cause and Prevention, National Cancer Institute. DHEW Publ No. (NIH) 78–1837, 1978.

Sherlock P, Lipkin M, Winawar SJ: The prevention of colon cancer. Am J Med 68:917–931, 1980.

Shirasu Y, Moriya M, Kato K, et al: Mutagenicity screening on pesticides and modification products: a basis of carcinogenicity evaluation. *In* Hiatt HH, Watson, JD, Winsten JA, (eds): Origin of Human Cancer. Book A. Incidence of Cancer in Humans. Cold Spring Harbor Conferences on Cell Proliferation. Cold Spring Harbor, NY, Cold Spring Harbor Laboratory, 4:267–285, 1977.

Shubik P, DellaPorta G, Pietra G, et al: Factors Determining the Neoplastic Response Induced By Carcinogens. Biological Interactions in Normal and Neoplastic Growth. Boston, Little, Brown and Co, 1961.

Sonada T, Youngman DJ, Reynolds RD: Cholecystectomy and carcinoma of the colon. Milit Med 148:721–722, 1983.

Spitz S, Maguigan WH, Dobriner K: Carcinogenic action of benzidine. Cancer 3:789–804, 1950.

Spjut HJ: Malignant potential of large bowel polyps (adenomatous and villous). *In* Program and Abstracts of Papers of the 1977 Workshop on Large Bowel Cancer. Modern Methods of Biomedical and Clinical Research Toward Control and Cure of Large Bowel Cancer. Houston. 61:21–23, 1977.

Spjut HJ, Eichwald EJ: Induction of mammary tumors by injection of N-2 fluorenylacetamide into artificial cecal pouches in rats. J Nat Cancer Inst 18:473–480, 1957.

Spjut HJ, Noall MW: Experimental induction of tumors of the large bowel of rats: A review of the experience with 3-2′-dimethyl-4-aminobiphenyl. Cancer 28:29–37, 1971.

Spjut HJ, Smith MN: A comparative electron microscopic study of human and rat colonic polyps and carcinomas. Exp Molec Path 6:11–24, 1967.

Spjut HJ, Spratt JS Jr: Endemic and morphologic similarities existing between spontaneous colonic neoplasms in man and 3:2′-dimethyl-4-aminobiphenyl induced colonic neoplasms in rats. Ann Surg 161:309–324, 1965.

Spratt JS Jr: Avoidable cancers. Mo Fam Doctor 7:10, 11, 13, 1967.

Spratt JS Jr: Your behavior and cancer. Mo Med 71:22A–24A, 1974.

Spratt JS: Cybernetics of cancer control by prevention. Mo Med 74:213–217, 1977.

Spratt JS: The primary and secondary prevention of cancer. J Surg Oncol 18:219–230, 1981.

Spratt JS Jr, Ackerman LV: Relationship of the size of colonic tumors to their cellular composition and biological behavior. Surg Forum 10:56–61, 1960.

Spratt JS Jr, Ackerman LV: Small primary adenocarcinomas of the colon and rectum. JAMA 179:337–346, 1962.

Spratt JS Jr, Ackerman LV, Moyer CA: Relationship of polyps of the colon to colonic cancer. Ann Surg 148:682–698, 1958.

Spratt JS Jr, Hoag MG: Incidence of multiple primary cancers per man-year of follow-up; 20-year review from the Ellis Fischel State Cancer Hospital. Ann Surg 164:775–784, 1966.

Spratt JS Jr, Spjut HJ Jr: Prevalence and prognosis of individual clinical and pathologic variables associated with colorectal carcinoma. Cancer 20:1976–1985, 1967.

Sugimura T: Mutagens, carcinogens and tumor promoters in our daily food. Cancer 49:1970–1984, 1982.

Sugimura T, Kawachi T, Nagao M, et al: Mutagenic principles in tryptophane and phenylalanine pyrolysis products. Proc Jpn Acad 53:58–61, 1977.

Sula JP: The carcinogen 3,4-benzpyrene in the living environment and human organism. Neoplasma (Bratislava) 10:571–579, 1963.

Talbot JM: Role of dietary fiber in diverticular disease and colon cancer. Fed Proc 40:2337–2342, 1981.

Toth B: The large bowel carcinogenic effects of hydrazines and related compounds occurring in nature and in the environment. Cancer 40(5 Suppl):2427–2431, 1977.

Varghese AJ, Land P, Furrer R, Bruce WR: Evidence for the formation of mutagenic n-nitroso compounds in the human body. Proc Am Assoc Cancer Res 18:80, 1977.

Vatn MH, Stalsberg H: The prevalence of polyps of the large intestine in Oslo: An autopsy study. Cancer 49:819–825, 1982.

Venitt S: Mutagens in human feces: Are they relevant to cancer of the large bowel. Mut Res 98:265–286, 1982.

Walpole AL, Williams MHC: Aromatic amines as carcinogens in industry. Br Med Bull 14:141–145, 1958.

Walpole AL, Williams MHC, Roberts DC: Carcinogenic action of 4-aminodiphenyl and 3:2′-dimethyl-4-aminodiphenyl. Br J Indust Med 9:255–263, 1952.

Watne AL, Lai HY, Mance T, Core S: Fecal steroids and bacterial flora in patients with polyposis coli. Am J Surg 131:42–46, 1976.

Wattenberg LW, Lam LKT, Fladmoe AV, Borchert P: Inhibitors of colon carcinogenesis. Cancer 40(5 Suppl):2432–2435, 1977.

Weisburger JH, Reddy BS, Wynder EL: Colon cancer: its epidemiology and experimental production. Cancer 40(5 Suppl):2414–2420, 1977.

Weisburger JH, Spingarn NE, Wang YY, Vuolo LL: Assessment of the role of mutagens and endogenous factors in large bowel cancer. The Cancer Bulletin 33:124–128, 1981.

Welin S, Youker J, Spratt JS Jr, et al: The rates and patterns of growth of 375 tumors of the large intestine and rectum observed serially by double contrast enema (Malmö technique). AJR 90:673–687, 1963.

West DW, Lyon JL, Gardner JW: Cancer risk factors: an analysis of Utah Mormons and non-Mormons. J Natl Cancer Inst 65:1083–1095, 1980.

Wilkins TD, Hackman AS: Two patterns of neutral steroid conversion in the feces of normal North Americans. Cancer Res 34:2250–2254, 1974.

TWO

Growth Rates

J. S. Spratt, M.D.
J. A. Spratt, M.D.

Growth is a fundamental property of lethal neoplasms. All growth proceeds at a *rate,* and knowledge of the rates and mathematical patterns of growth of cancers is fundamental to the understanding of the behavior and lethality of neoplasms of the large intestine, rectum, and anus. The purpose of this chapter will be to review the growth kinetics of cancers and benign neoplasms of these organs.

In most cases, the growth of a new daughter cell proceeds until it reaches the size and age at which binary division occurs. This process is cyclic, except that some cells die, desquamate, or become nonproliferating. With successive generations, cells also become heterogeneous in all their properties.

The cell cycle can be divided into four phases: the presynthetic (G1), the DNA synthesis (S), the postsynthetic (G2), and the mitotic (M). The mitotic time is the shortest segment of the entire cell cycle and may be regarded either as the fourth phase of the cell reproductive cycle or simply as the point in the cycle when two daughter cells appear. The duration of each phase is subject to biologic variation, leading to frequency distributions of cell cycle times, which Steel (1967, 1972) classified as normal, lognormal, gamma, or other.

The three principal parameters determining the net rates of growth of cancer are the cell cycle time of proliferating cells, the proportion of cells proliferating, and the extent of cell loss. Cell loss may be by exfoliation, metastasis, or cell death (Pearlman, 1976; Spratt and Ackerman, 1961). Only a very small percentage of all cancer cells that metastasize actually survive. Mathematical models of tumor kinetics, as they become better tested with data from human cancer, may become essential in the planning of optimum strategies for screening, treatment, follow-up, and management of cancers.

The range of cell cycle time has been measured for various colonies of cancer cells. The median value (or geometric mean) of this spread is the usually quoted value. Cell cycle time is measured using tritiated thymidine to label DNA during synthesis. This method of measurement provides a wealth of information on the cytokinetics of both normal and neoplastic tissues (Steel, 1972). Cytokinetic terms and their relationships are as follows:

t_c = cell cycle time.

t_s = duration of DNA synthesis of proliferating cells.

LI = the labeling index defining the ratio of the number of cells incorporating tritiated thymidine into DNA during mitosis over the total number of cells. This ratio is expressed as the percentage of cells in mitosis during the time period of thymidine incorporation.

LI = $\mu t_s/t_c$ for proliferating cells; when doubling time (DT) > 19 days, μ, the constant, is in the range of 0.7 to 0.8.

$DT_{(Pot)}$ = potential doubling time or time required for the cancer to double its volume once, in the absence of cell loss, i.e., when all dividing cells survive.

$DT_{(Act)}$ = actual doubling time or actual time required for a cancer to double its volume once.

The actual doubling time represents the net

effect of all cytokinetic parameters. Cell loss is a major and variable factor, and $DT_{(Act)}$ is of longer duration than $DT_{(Pot)}$. $DT_{(Act)}$ frequently can be calculated from gross serial measurements of a growing human cancer taken either from roentgenograms or from the direct measurement of the tumor mass. In measuring gross rates of tumor growth, there is always a variable margin of error.

If cell loss is a major and variable factor, and $DT_{(Act)}$ is therefore of longer duration than $DT_{(Pot)}$, the relationship between them can be defined by a parameter ρ for the rate of cell loss defined as a fraction of the rate at which cells are entering mitosis. For a 100 percent loss of new cells, $DT_{(Act)}$ would be static. The relationship is given by the following:

$$\rho = 1 - \frac{DT_{(Pot)}}{DT_{(Act)}}$$

The lognormal frequency distribution that best describes the frequency distribution of many cytokinetic parameters, as well as other characteristics of cancers and their hosts, is simply a normal frequency distribution of the logarithm of the variate. Such a distribution occurs whenever the random errors of the variate are geometric or logarithmic rather than arithmetic or linear.

All standard statistical tests applicable to the commonly displayed arithmetic normal distribution can be applied (Spratt, 1969). The probability that a frequency distribution is in fact lognormal can be calculated by testing against a distribution of normal ordinates (Spratt et al., 1977).

Various growth equations express the pattern of growth within a cancer. The pattern is determined by the complex and changing interaction of variables affecting the division and accumulation of cancer cells. The equations that define the more commonly observed growth patterns of colonic and rectal neoplasms follow.

LINEAR GROWTH EQUATION

A cancer whose growth is defined by the linear growth equation has its linear dimensions increased by a specific increment each day, regardless of the size of the cancer. Jensen's rat sarcoma (Mayneord, 1932) and some human lung cancers are examples of this growth form (Spratt and Spratt, 1976). This pattern is thought to occur when all cellular proliferation is restricted to the periphery of the cancer. The equation has the following form:

$$R = \frac{d_1 - d_0}{t}$$

R = linear rate of change in the diameter, and $\frac{\Delta d}{t}$, usually expressed as mm per day, is defined as follows:

d_0 = greatest chordal dimension or, in the case of spherical tumors, the diameter at first observation.

d_1 = preceding dimension at second observation.

t = time elapsing between measurement of d_0 and d_1. If the rate of a single growth vector or radius is desired, R must be divided by 2.

This pattern may also apply to colon cancers that grow as flat discs (cylinders). In these cancers, increasing volume is primarily attributable to radial growth of a cylinder of cancer in which the altitude of the cylinder (thickness of the cancer) remains relatively constant.

EXPONENTIAL GROWTH EQUATION

Cancer growing exponentially or geometrically would have a randomly steady increase in volume per unit volume per unit time. Any cell population increasing in number by the randomly steady binary division of cells, with negligible or at least steady-state cell loss, would follow this equation. For the expression of an exponential increase in volume, the equation has the following forms:

$$V_1 = V_0e^{bt} \text{ or } d_1^3 = d_0^3e^{bt}$$

$$b = \frac{\ln V_1 - \ln V_0}{t} \text{ or } b = \frac{3(\ln d_1 - \ln d_0)}{t}$$

$$DT_{(Act)} = \frac{\ln 2}{b} = \frac{0.69315}{b}$$

V_0 = volume at first measurement expressed in mm^3.

V_1 = volume at second measurement expressed in mm^3.

d_0 = diameter at first measurement expressed in mm.

d_1 = diameter at second measurement expressed in mm.

t = time in days elapsing between the measurement of V_0 and V_1 or between the measurement of d_0 and d_1.

b = exponential growth constant with the dimension of mm^3 per mm^3 per day.

ln = natural logarithm of the variate.

e = base of the natural logarithm i.e., 2.71828.

By moving the decimal point of b three places to the right, the constant becomes a measure of the number of new cells per 1000 existing cells per day. Also, as noted previously when b is divided into the natural logarithm of 2 (0.69315), $DT_{(Act)}$ is obtained in days. When more than two measurements exist, the growth equation that best fits the measurements can be more accurately determined by the use of regression analysis (Spratt and Ackerman, 1961).

The actual method of calculating will vary with the geometric shape of the cancer (spherical, spheroid, and cylindrical being the most frequent shapes). By using $V_1 \propto d_1^3$, for example, the value for the volume is proportionally correct (i.e., it differs only by a constant) for spherical tumors. For cylindrical tumors, the volume increase is proportional to the square of the diameter of the base. It is directly proportional to the altitude of the cylinder. The altitude is equivalent to the thickness of the cancer.

GOMPERTZIAN AND LOGISTIC GROWTH EQUATIONS

A cancer following a Gompertzian (Gompertz, 1825) or logistic growth curve grows rapidly while small but grows more slowly as its size increases. The curve approaches a horizontal asymptote determined by a size that the cancer never exceeds. The growth curve is upwardly concave until it reaches a point of inflection, after which it is downwardly concave as it approaches the asymptote.

Both Gompertzian and logistic curves have a sigmoidal shape that characterizes many growth processes and have three adjustable parameters for matching growth. A close approximation of the Gompertzian or logistic curve may be obtained by matching the segments of the curve at either side of the point of inflection to exponential functions. The Gompertzian growth curve follows the general equation

$$S = S_0 e^{(1-e^{-\alpha t})\beta/\alpha}$$

where S is the tumor size at time t, S_0 is the initial tumor size, and α and β are constants. The size may be expressed in any unit of measurement, including number of cells. The Gompertzian curve has upper and lower asymptotes. The lower asymptote is assumed to be a single cell or its volume, and the upper asymptote of the Gompertz function is obtained by letting t become arbitrarily large

$$S_\infty = \lim_{t\to\infty} (S_0 e^{(1-e^{-\alpha t})\beta/\alpha}) = S_0 e^{\beta/\alpha}$$

This theoretic limit is probably never actually attained. The constant β is the specific growth rate at t = 0. At any time t, the growth rate is

$$\lambda = \beta e^{-\alpha t}$$

where λ is a proportionality factor that is dependent on t. By differentiating the preceding general Gompertzian equation, the following is obtained.

$$\frac{dS}{dt} = kS - \theta$$

where $k = \alpha \ln S_\infty$ and $\theta = \alpha S \ln S$. In this form, k can be interpreted as an intrinsic growth rate, and θ measures the incremental decrease in actual growth rate that occurs with increasing size. This intrinsic rate would reasonably be determined by a randomly steady rate of binary fission inherent in an asynchronously dividing clone of neoplastic cells. The actual doubling time of the neoplasm may then be determined by the following:

$$DT_{(s)} = \frac{1}{\alpha} \ln \left(1 - \frac{\ln 2}{\ln(S_\infty/S)}\right), \text{ where } S < 1/2\, S_\infty$$

The resulting curve has a point of inflection that is rarely a concern at the gross levels of clinical measurement. This point of inflection is attained before the cancer is generally detected. Verhagen (Verhagen, 1960) estimates the point of inflection to be at about 37 percent of the upper asymptote. The segment of the total growth curve measured clinically can "fit," within the random errors of measurement, almost any of the known possibilities. In the laboratory where the kinetics of very small numbers of dividing cancer cells can be measured, Gompertzian growth is commonly found (Lloyd, 1975).

A fundamental question regarding in vivo human cancers is, at what size is the point of inflection reached? If the point of inflection is reached at or before most cancers are grossly visible, then the exponential function applied to measurements made past the point of inflection might be sufficiently accurate for the gross analysis, but these rates could not be used to extrapolate back and estimate the time of origin of the cancer with any accuracy. However, knowing that more rapid growth may have occurred while the cancer was smaller is of great significance. A method of determining the frequency of this situation in the clinical setting is to measure the number of cancers that surface in the intervals between screening examinations, as has been done for breast cancer (Spratt et al., 1982).

RATES OF GROWTH OF PULMONARY METASTASES

As early as 1956, Collins and associates reported the time required for pulmonary metastases from four rectal adenocarcinomas to double in volume. The time ranged from 49 to 123 days. In 1962, Collins updated his investigation and by that time was studying 25 cases of rectal cancer. The doubling times of these cancers ranged from 34 to 210 days with a median of 96 days.

Spratt and Spratt (1964) reported the growth rates of ten pulmonary metastases from adenocarcinomas of the colon and rectum. Doubling times ranged from 9 to 1300 days, with 95 percent confidence with mean of the log-normal frequency distribution of doubling times of 109 days. The exponential growth constant was 0.0064, with a 95 percent confidence ranging from 0.0005 through 0.077. By moving the decimal point three places to the right, an estimate of the *net* number of new cancer cells per 1000 existing cancer cells per day is obtained, i.e., 6.4 new cells per 1000 cells per day, ranging from 0.5 new cells to 77 new cells per 1000 cells per day, with 95 percent confidence.

The characteristics of the studied population of metastases were described by the parameters of the frequency distributions of their sizes. The frequency distributions of the tumor diameters of 656 nonsimultaneous radiographic measurements of 1 to 4 pulmonary metastases from cancers and sarcomas in 138 consecutive patients were reported. The distributions of the diameters formed lognormal distributions, giving them a large positive skew. The lower limits of resolution were about 3 mm, but tumor nucleus shadows were not generally diagnosed by the radiologist until their diameter exceeded 6 mm, a size equivalent to 26.7 net doublings of a cell 1000 μ^3 in size. A malignant intrathoracic neoplasm that had attained a diameter of 200 mm, a size equivalent to 40.8 doublings of a cell 1000 μ^3, in size, put the host at death's door since death occurred before a cancer attained a size that would be produced by 40.8 net doublings. The maximum life expectancy of the untreated host from the time that an intrathoracic tumor is radiographically visible until it reaches antemortem size is equal to about 40.8 doublings (200-mm tumor) minus 26.7 doublings (6-mm tumor) or about 14 doublings multiplied by the doubling time of the cancer.

Collins and associates (1956) speculated on time of origin of pulmonary metastases by extrapolating backward using the doubling time data. They took the doubling times of pulmonary metastases and made the assumption that if the doubling time remained constant from the moment of metastasis and if the original size of a metastasis was a single cell, the time of occurrence of the metastasis could be estimated. By their estimates, pulmonary metastases could have occurred from 3 to 18 years before discovery of the primary cancer. He considered this a fundamental reason why mortality rates were not changing despite other advances in the period. He observed that the prescriptions for earlier and more radical surgery and earlier detection as means of lowering mortality rates should "offer some assurance that the techniques and tools at hand are equal to the demand placed upon them" (Collins, 1962). Although this conclusion may be correct, his extrapolations of duration were probably too long because he did not consider the Gompertzian growth function just discussed. A more definitive method of estimating duration before diagnosis is to divide the prevalence rate by the annual incidence rate, assuming that the incidence rate remains constant (see Chapter One) (Spratt, 1982).

Mensuration similar to that used by Collins was applied to 18 spherical pulmonary metastases observed in the serial thoracic roentgenograms of 11 patients having primary adenocarcinomas of the colon and rectum who were being treated at the Ellis Fischel State Cancer Hospital. The doubling times of these and 25 additional metastases are given in Table 2–1 (Welin et al. 1963).

As mentioned earlier, the basic assumption that exponential growth is constant from the inception of the neoplasm is probably false. The extremely early phases of cancer growth may proceed at a much faster rate. The rate then slows with increasing size and as the tumor becomes grossly measurable.

Table 2–1. **THE ACTUAL DOUBLING TIME OF PULMONARY METASTASES FROM COLONIC AND RECTAL ADENOCARCINOMAS***

Actual Doubling Time (days)	Total
0–100	22
101–200	16
201–300	2
301–400	0
401–500	1
No growth	1
Total	43

*From Welin S, Youker J, Spratt JS: The rates and patterns of growth of 375 tumors of the large intestine and rectum observed serially by double contrast enema study (Malmö Technique). AJR 90:673–687, 1963. ©1963, American Roentgen Ray Society.

RATES OF GROWTH OF PRIMARY CANCERS

The first reported case in which the rate of growth of a primary cancer of the colon and rectum was measured, was provided by Spratt and Ackerman (1961).

The case involved a man who was 67 years old when first seen in 1952. On the first double contrast enema, a polypoid filling defect (2.9 cm in diameter) was found in the descending colon. A left colectomy was performed, and the intestinal continuity was restored by colocolostomy between the midtransverse and the midsigmoid colon. The tumor was a well-differentiated adenocarcinoma, with no metastases in 15 mesocolic lymph nodes. A small, round filling defect located in the right transverse colon was not removed. Eight subsequent barium enemas performed during the subsequent 7.5 years demonstrated growth of this lesion (Fig. 2–1). By the ninth examination, the tumor had encompassed the bowel and had extended 17 mm longitudinally. The patient had consistently guaiac-negative stools. A resection of this still asymptomatic tumor was performed. It was an adenocarcinoma arising in the transverse colon, 6 cm proximal to the old anastomosis. No gross intra-abdominal or hepatic metastases were found.

This cancer is shown in Figure 2–2. It had grown as a rodent plaque of cancer, 50 mm around the circumference of the bowel and 27 mm longitudinally. Its thickness was uniformly 5 mm. The tumor was well differentiated. Its deep margin extended through all layers of the colonic wall and just into the mesenteric fat. No metastases were found in 16 lymph nodes removed from the adjacent mesocolon.

It was thought that the 7.5 years of observation were justified. The man's physical condition was poor. He had had a myocardial infarction during the fifth postoperative day after his first colon resection. He was obese and hypertensive. He had cholelithiasis and prostatism, which had required a transurethral resection. He was an old man. Actually, he tolerated his second operation without difficulty and lived 6 more years after this resection. He died at age 80 with, but not from, hepatic metastases.

Many small, well-differentiated adenocarcinomas of the colon grow predominantly as plaques. While quite small, the plaques may wrinkle over submucosal stroma and some even develop pedicles, making them grossly indistinguishable from pedunculated benign adenomatous polyps (Spratt and Ackerman, 1960a). Later, the central part of the plaque desquamates while the cancer grows beneath and around the erosion, with a tendency toward circumferential spread. This patient's first cancer, removed in 1952, was also an erosive convoluted exophytic plaque. The volume of such a cancer can be calculated from the roentgen films, correcting for magnification simply by treating the lesion as a cylinder having a diameter (d) ascertained from the roentgeno-

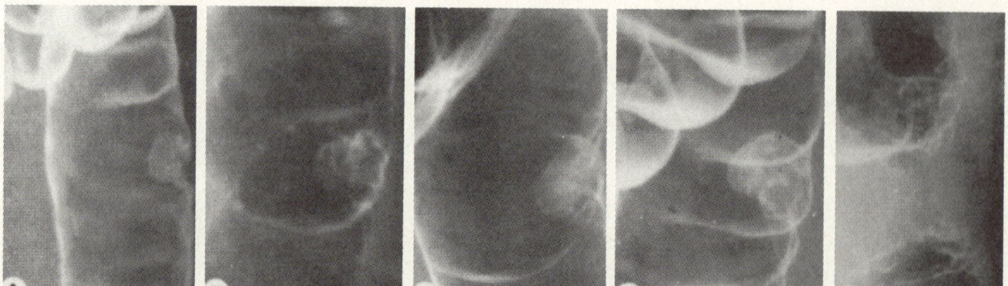

Figure 2–1. Five of nine barium enemas performed over a 7.5-year period, showing growth of an adenocarcinoma of the colon. (From Spratt JS Jr, Ackerman LV: The growth of a colonic adenocarcinoma. Am Surg 27:23–28, 1961.)

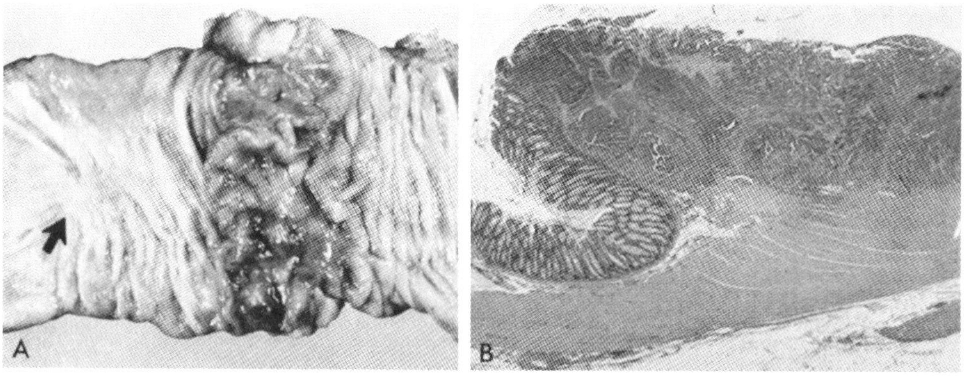

Figure 2–2. *A*, Gross photograph of the transverse colon cancer shown in Figure 2–1 at the time of resection (1960). The arrow points to scarring from a colon resection in 1952. *B*, Photomicrograph of the cancer. (From Spratt JS Jr, Ackerman LV: The growth of a colonic adenocarcinoma. Am Surg 27:23–28, 1961.)

gram and a depth (h) equal to the thickness of the tumor measured after its removal (Spratt and Ackerman, 1961).

Correction for the roentgen magnification of the diameter of the tumor could be effected because all roentgenograms had been taken with essentially the same radiographic technique. Fortunately, in three of the barium enema examinations made at Mallinckrodt Institute of Radiology, using the same technique in 1952 and in 1953, the ratio of actual size to roentgen size (0.86) could be estimated from the size of the first tumor shown by the barium enema study of August 14, 1952 (2.9 cm) and the actual size of the tumor removed on August 19, 1952 (2.5 cm). The remaining six barium enema studies were performed using similar techniques (1953 to 1960). The extension of the tumor along the long axis of the bowel measured 27 mm both on the last barium enema study and in the freshly resected colon. Consequently, no correction for roentgen magnification of the six barium enemas was needed. Correction for roentgen magnification is unnecessary in calculating growth, as long as the magnification is roughly the same in all views. With a constant thickness, the volume of the tumor increases as its surface area increases.

The plot of these volumes on a logarithmic ordinate and the corresponding time on a linear abscissa is practically linear (Fig. 2–3), suggesting an exponential relationship between time and volume. However, additional computations were done to determine the line of best fit and to establish that there was a significant correlation between time and volume. By converting the exponential growth equation to its logarithmic form, the method of least squares of linear regression analysis was used to find the line of best fit. A highly significant correlation between the volume (logarithmic function) and the duration of the cancer was found.

The regression coefficient of a growth curve represented the relative rate of growth. The rate of growth of this cancer was 0.001089 mm^3 per mm^3 of existing cancer per day. Expressed in terms of cells, this rate was equivalent to an increase of one cell per 1000 existing cancer cells per day. The cellular content of the cancer had randomly doubled every 636 days.

This first case raised many questions. For instance, did not necrosis of the tumor invalidate the calculation of the true growth rate? Microscopically, there was no necrosis in this cancer. Did not the desquamation that continually took place from the tumor render calculation of growth rate superfluous? Unless desquamation is cyclic, it does not seriously affect the calculation. In a cancer having a uniform thickness of 5 mm, a constant proportion of the cells of the cancer are exposed for possible desquamation. In this cancer growing as a plaque, the rate of desquamation had to be constantly related to the total number of cells on the surface of the cancer. Consequently, desquamation had to proceed according to the exponential growth equation but with a negative regression coefficient. The regression coefficient, determined from the observed growth of the reported cancer, therefore represented the algebraic sum of the regression coefficient of actual growth (total growth less desquamation) but was still exponential. This method enables the calculation of the regression coefficient and the coefficient of correlation for the measurable data.

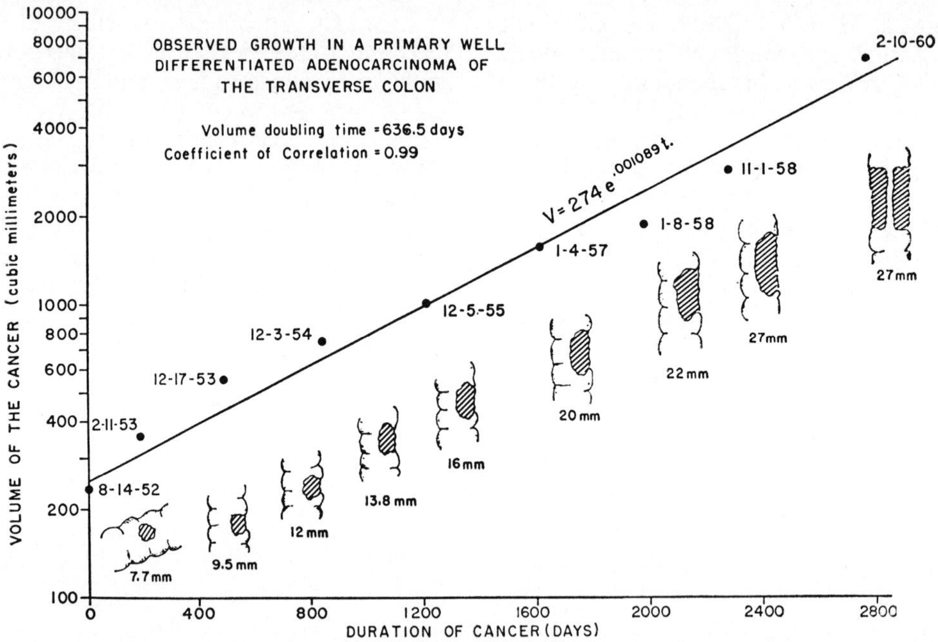

Figure 2–3. Observed increases in the volume of a transverse colonic adenocarcinoma in a man 67-years old at the time of the first barium enema and 75-years old at the time of the ninth, which was performed just before resection. The tumor volumes, calculated from measurements of the cancer on the roentgenograms, are plotted against time in days on a semilogarithmic scale. The line of best fit was characterized by a $DT_{(Act)}$ of 636 days (coefficient of correlation = 99). (From Spratt JS Jr, Ackerman LV: The growth of a colonic adenocarcinoma. Am Surg 27:23–28, 1961.)

Following this isolated case, in 1962, the opportunity arose to calculate the rates and patterns of growth of 375 primary tumors of the colon and rectum and to study the association between these rates and the histopathology of the tumors. A series of high-quality double contrast enema studies in which similar measurements had been made were found in the possession of Solve Welin, Director of the Roentgendiagnostik Institute, Malmö Allmanna Sjukhuset, University of Lund, Sweden (Table 2–2). He offered his material for study. Youker measured all the tumors that were observed on more than one date. From these measurements, the rates of growth were calculated (Welin et al., 1963). Folke Linnell, a

Table 2–2. TOTAL EXPERIENCE IN THE OBSERVATION OF TUMORS OF THE LARGE INTESTINE AND RECTUM BY DOUBLE CONTRAST ENEMA STUDY (MALMÖ MODIFICATION) (DECEMBER 1, 1953 TO JUNE 30, 1962)*

No. of patients examined	16,177
Total no. of double contrast enema studies performed	21,043
No. of patients having tumors demonstrated	2,118
No. of patients having resections for tumors after first observation	479
No. of patients having presence of tumors verified at autopsy	53†
No. of tumors observed two or more times in 109 patients before resection of tumor	136‡
No. of tumors observed two or more times in 194 patients (tumors still under observation)	239§
No. of patients having polypoid tumors observed roentgenographically without confirmation by resection, autopsy, or second roentgen examination	1,282‖

*Welin, S, Youker J, Spratt JS: The rates and patterns observed serially by double contrast enema study (Malmö Technique). AJR 90:673–687, 1963. © 1963, American Roentgen Ray Society.

†Obligatory autopsy examinations are performed on all persons dying in the city of Malmö at the Pathological Institute of the Malmö Allmanna Sjukhuset.

‡Total number patient-days of observation = 113,430.
Minimal period of observation = 26 days.
Mean period of observation = 834 days.
Maximum period of observation = 3,859 days.

§Total number patient-days of observation = 225,450.
Minimal period of observation = 65 days.
Mean period of observation = 939 days.
Maximum period of observation = 3,745 days.

‖Most not re-examined because tumors were smaller than 6 mm in diameter.

pathologist at Malmö, provided his pathologic readings and also permitted all histopathologic slides to be reviewed independently by three American surgical pathologists, H. J. Spjut, R. E. Johnson, and L. V. Ackerman. This collaboration resulted in the first large-scale effort to ascertain whether an association existed between the rates of growth and the histopathology of primary neoplasms of the large intestine (Welin et al., 1963).

The Malmö Roentgendiagnostik Department performed all the roentgen diagnostic studies required on a stable population of 235,000 inhabitants of the city of Malmö. All persons included were referred by physicians within the city or from other departments of the hospital. No systematic effort was made to perform cancer detection examinations on asymptomatic persons.

Between December 1, 1953 and June 30, 1962, all examinations of the large intestine and rectum were made using a double contrast enema technique (see Table 2–2). The preparation and examination involved the following steps: (1) On the day before the examination, the patient was fed a light diet and 30 ml of castor oil; (2) on the evening before the examination, the patient was given one plain water enema; (3) on the morning of the examination, the patient was given atropine, 1 mg orally, followed 30 minutes later by a cleansing enema of plain water with Clysodrast* added; (4) the colon was filled initially to the splenic flexure with thick barium-containing Clysodrast; (5) after each use of Clysodrast, a complete colonic evacuation occurred within one minute; (6) after the last evacuation, the colon was filled only to the sigmoid flexure; (7) the colon was insufflated with air through a straight balloonless rectal tube until good distention was obtained; (8) the patient was rotated to ensure filling to the cecum; (9) residual barium in the rectum was evacuated with a tube; and (10) multiple roentgenograms including lateral decubitus, oblique, upright, and anteroposterior projections, were obtained.

Fluoroscopy was employed only briefly to monitor the presence of barium throughout the colon. A standard tube film distance of 150 cm was used for all projections, permitting comparison of changes in size on serial views and minimizing magnification (Welin, 1958, 1962; Welin and Lorinc, 1962). The quality of the studies was dependent on the thoroughness with which the colon was cleansed by the Clysodrast, the degree of colonic relaxation induced by the atropine, and the number of projections giving clear contrast views of the entire colon including the cecum. Of the 21,043 examinations performed, only two (0.009 percent) were complicated by perforation of the colon. Both perforations were below the peritoneal reflection and both healed spontaneously (Lorinc and Brahme, 1959).

When the roentgenographic projection was made tangential to the intestinal wall from which the tumor was rising, intramural infiltration could be diagnosed. This infiltration resulted in indistinct or "infiltrative" margins of the roentgen shadow of the tumor and, in time, produced "indentation" of the intestinal wall (Figs. 2–4 and 2–5, *A–F*). When these roentgen diagnostic signs of infiltrating cancer were detected at the first examination, tumors were resected in all but a few instances. Typical marginal infiltration was seen and the correct diagnosis of cancer was made for tumors as small as 3 mm (Fig. 2–4). Of the 20 cancers shown in Figure 2–6, marginal infiltration by four was diagnosed at first examination, marginal infiltration by ten was diagnosed during the period of observation, the bases of five were never viewed by tangential roentgeno-

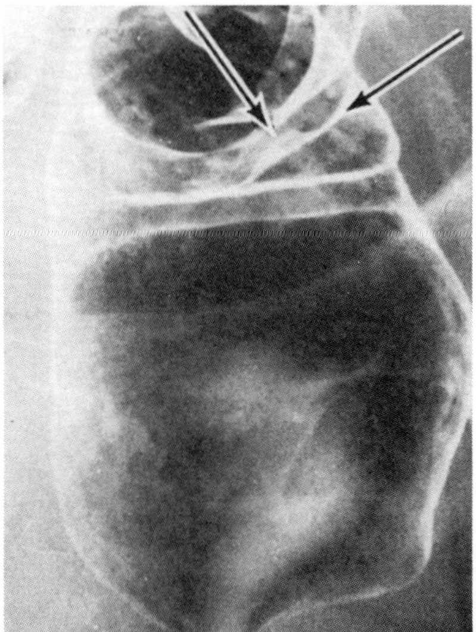

Figure 2–4. An infiltrating primary cancer of the rectosigmoid, 3 mm on its long axis, was diagnosed correctly as a cancer using the "indentation sign." (From Welin S, Youker J, Spratt JS Jr: The rates and patterns of growth of 375 tumors of the large intestine and rectum observed serially by double contrast enema study (Malmö technique). AJR 90:673–687, 1963. © 1963, American Roentgen Ray Society.)

*Clysodrast: Ferrosan Malmö, Malmö, Sweden.

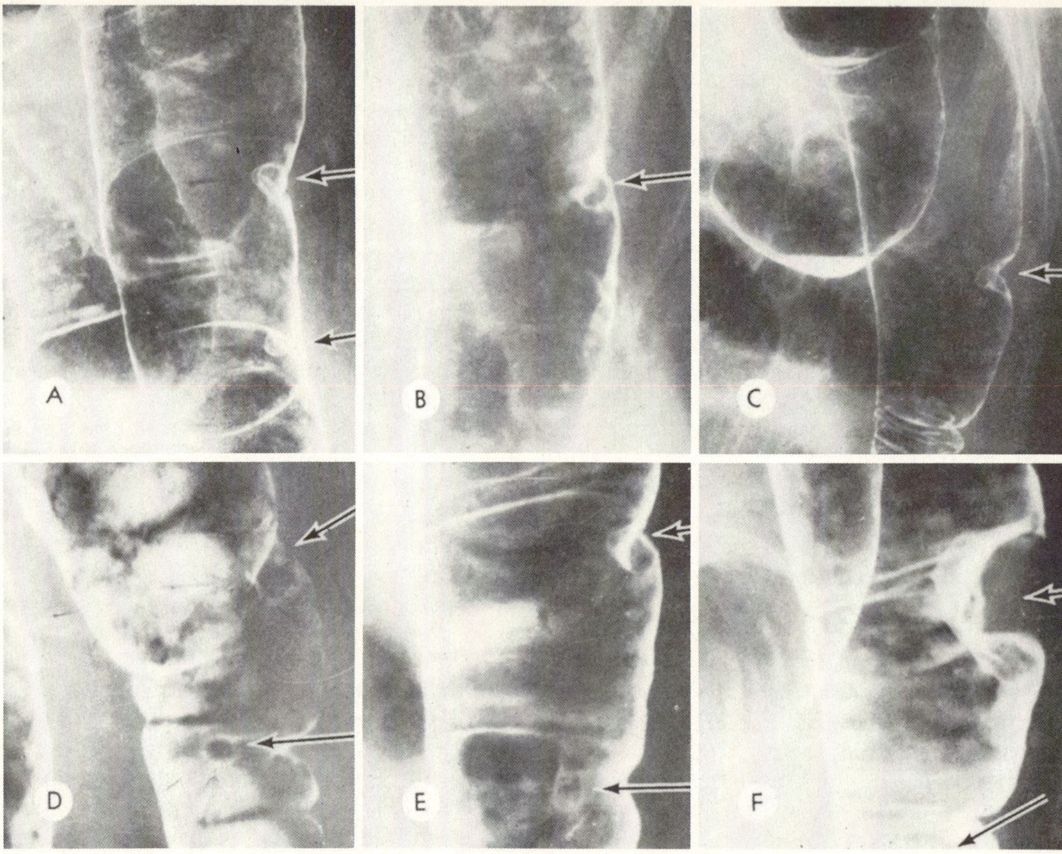

Figure 2–5. These double contrast enema studies span a 3.5-year period, during which an 8-mm tumor grew into a 32-mm tumor in an asymptomatic man. From the very first observation, the marginal infiltration with indentation at the base was diagnostic of cancer. (From Welin S, Youker J, Spratt JS Jr: The rates and patterns of growth of 375 tumors of the large intestine and rectum observed serially by double contrast enema study (Malmö technique). AJR 90:673–687, 1963. © 1963, American Roentgen Ray Society.)

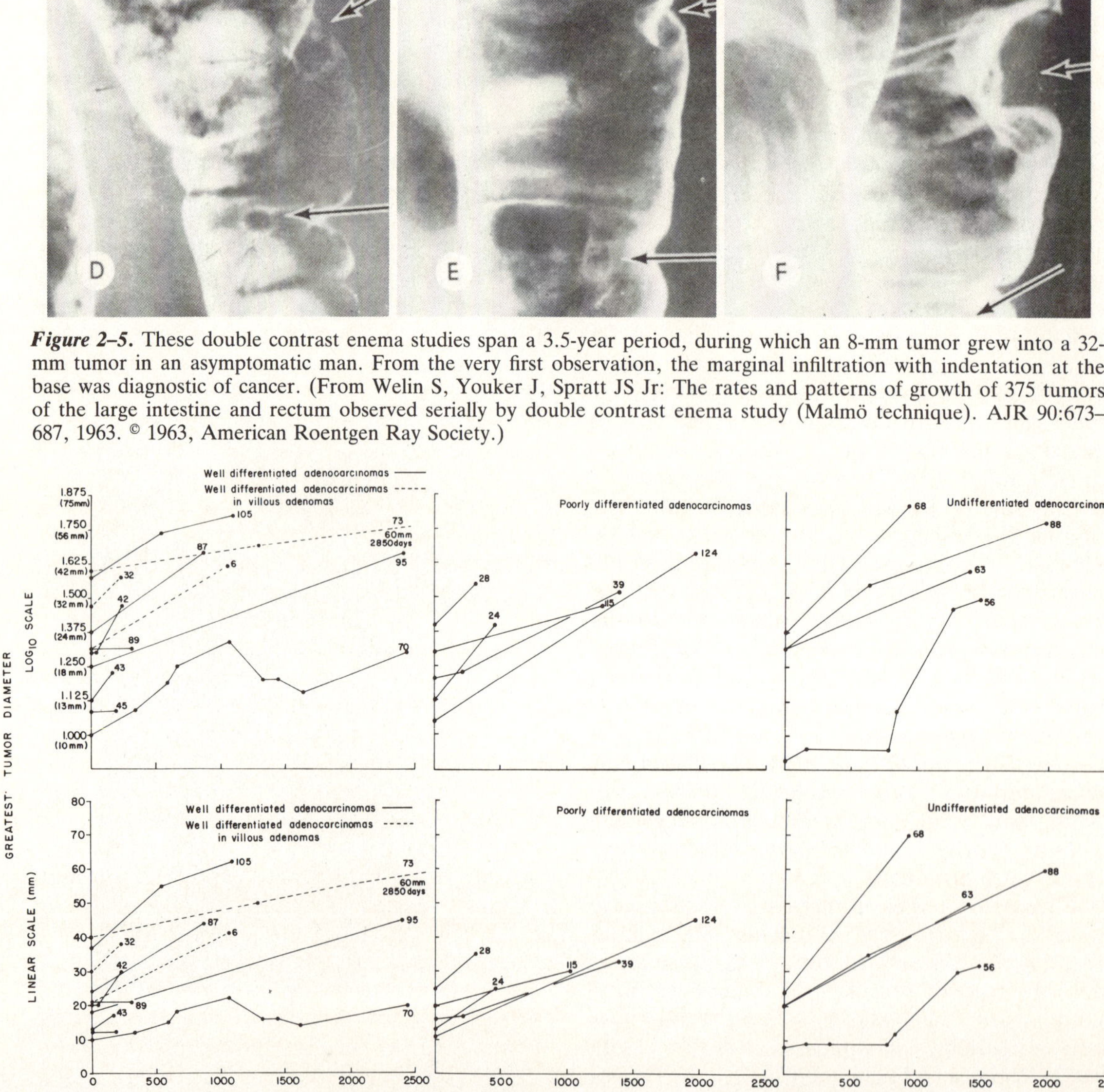

Figure 2–6. Diameters of tumor shadows measured on tangential views of double contrast barium enemas and plotted against time of observation. The upper plots are semilogarithmic, and the lower ones arithmetic. (From Welin S, Youker J, Spratt JS Jr: The rates and patterns of growth of 375 tumors of the large intestine and rectum observed serially by double contrast enema study (Malmö technique). AJR 90:673–687, 1963. © 1963, American Roentgen Ray Society.)

graphic projections, and one, a polypoid carcinoma on a stalk, did not develop signs of infiltration. Thus, there existed a bias in the selection of tumors observed serially. Only the more polypoid-shaped or protuberant tumors with distinct roentgenographic margins were available for serial observations.

The largest tumor diameter and the dates of measurements on two or more double contrast enema studies were recorded for 136 tumors excised from 109 patients. For 239 tumors in 194 patients, defects appearing on roentenograms still remained untreated at the time measurements were made. The tumor outline was measured to the nearest millimeter on each margin. The margin of error in determining diameter approximated ±2 mm. The error could vary from as much as 50 percent for a 4-mm tumor to as little as 3 percent for a 60-mm tumor. Only the same roentgenographic projections from each examination were measured to enhance the chance that serial measurements were comparable.

The time intervals between examinations were recorded in days. At Malmö semiannual re-examination of patients with tumors was encouraged, but this policy was not followed strictly. The number of double contrast enema studies for each patient varied from two (215 patients) to ten (one patient). Only ten tumors were observed for a total period of less than 6 months.

INTERPRETATION

The collected data defined changes in diameter of tumors over measured periods of time. The authors recognized that they were measuring the net results of new cell formation (the fundamental requisite for growth), cell death, cell dissemination away from the primary cancer, and surface desquamation. Generally, when cellular proliferation is unrestrained, growth proceeds by geometric progression or by the exponential increase in the numbers of cells, and the rate of increase is constantly proportional to the size the tumor already attained. When growth-limiting factors slow the growth of increasingly large neoplasms, Gompertzian or logistic growth occurs. Other variables acting simultaneously could alter the exponential growth to produce any of the variety of types of growth mentioned previously including arithmetic or linear growth in the diameter, random variation in growth, continued deceleration in growth, continued acceleration in growth, Gompertzian growth, or no growth (Davis, 1960; Defares and Sneddon, 1960; Gompertz, 1825; Hoffman, 1953; Mayneord, 1932; Spratt and Spratt, 1964; Verhagen, 1960). The ability to determine the growth curves best fitting the collected data was hampered by the limited number of measurements.

First, the geometric configuration of growing colonic neoplasms had to be known to relate the chordal dimensions to changes in tumor volume. Most cancers of the colon and rectum grew over the mucosal surface of bowel as circumferentially spreading plaques. The plaques became ulcerated, sessile, or pedunculated (Spratt and Ackerman, 1962). The plaques approached the geometric shape of cylinders ("medallion cancers") until they achieved a diameter of several centimeters. At this size, some of them tended to involve the entire circumference of the bowel ("napkin ring" cancers). These surface-spreading growths remained fairly constant in thickness, and the changing volumes of the growing cancers were mainly proportional to the surface areas. In analyzing these Malmö data, the authors regarded the diameters measured as being the diameters of the bases of cylinders of uniform thickness. More simply, for the purpose of calculating exponential growth constants and doubling times, they regarded change in surface area as being directly proportional to change in volume of cancers of constant thickness.

Figure 2–7 shows graphically the inability of these measurements to permit the differentiation between linear growth and exponential diametric growth. An error of diametric measurement of only ±2 mm produces an overlap of exponential and linear growth curves during five-eighths of the time necessary for a tumor to grow from a diameter of 3 mm to a diameter of 60 mm. With a sigmoid-shaped curve (a Gompertz or logistic curve), an overlap of the linear and exponential growth curves, owing to random errors in measurement, might be present throughout the entire period that the neoplasms are roentgenographically visible. Actually, no single tumor was observed long enough to exclude this overlap of growth curves in the presence of random errors in measurement estimated as ±2 mm. The differentiation between linear growth and exponential growth was indeterminable for all tumors observed only twice in 215 patients. Also, some tumors exhibited variations in growth rates, further complicating efforts to confirm a particular growth curve. The growth curves for the 20 cancers, plotted successively on linear

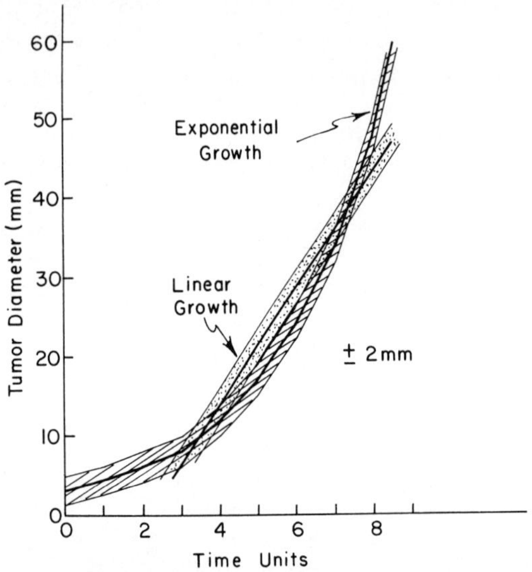

Figure 2–7. Overlap of the straight line or linear growth curve and exponential growth curve during the segment of tumor growth grossly visible on double contrast enemas (3 mm to 60 mm), with a margin of error in the measurement of the diameters of ± 2 mm. (From Welin S, Youker J, Spratt JS Jr: The rates and patterns of growth of 375 tumors of the large intestine and rectum observed serially by double contrast enema study (Malmö technique). AJR 90:673–687, 1963. © 1963, American Roentgen Ray Society.)

and semilogarithmic graphs (see Fig. 2–6), illustrate these points quite well. Consequently, the authors considered that these neoplasms might have grown by either an exponential progression or a linear progression in tumor diameter, and calculated the mean rates of growth for both possibilities in their simplest mathematical forms.

An additional concern with these data was that nothing was known about the rate of growth of tumors seen only once on a barium enema study before removal. If these were faster growing neoplasms, then frequency distributions of growth rates would be truncated. Also not known is the number of cancers that surfaced in the intervals between barium enema examinations and produced symptoms leading to discovery and resection. These interval-surfacing cancers could grow even faster than the previously mentioned tumors. They might well come to emergency operations with no roentgen measurements at all.

CORRELATION BETWEEN HISTOPATHOLOGY AND GROWTH RATES

There was little difference in the interpretations of the histopathologic sections made by each of the pathologists. Neither the presence nor the absence of atypical changes in benign adenomatous polyps had any effect on the distribution of growth rates; in fact, morphological alteration was probably of no consequence as far as rate of tumor growth was concerned. Spjut (Welin et al., 1963) diagnosed a variant of a polyp that he called "villoglandular polyp." Histologically the villoglandular polyp was a mixture of adenomatous polyp and villous adenoma. These polyps were generally larger than adenomatous polyps and villous adenomas, and the distribution of their growth rates resembled that of villous adenomas. Consequently, they were grouped with the pure villous adenomas. Not enough cancers were present in each category of differentiation to permit statistically significant conclusions regarding the association of cancerous "differentiation" with growth rate.

The percentile frequencies of invasive cancers, villous adenomas and villoglandular polyps, adenomatous polyps, and unresected tumors among the observed exponential and linear rates of growth are given in Figures 2–8 and 2–9. Figure 2–10 gives the percentage of invasive cancers among all tumors observed in each growth rate range. Obviously, a distinctive range existed that encompassed the mean rates of growth of 80 percent of the invasive cancers and smaller percentages of the noninvasive tumors. On the linear scale, this range extended from .003 to .025 mm per day and, on the exponential scale, from .0003 to .0025 mm per mm per day for the exponential diametric growth ranges. The latter are equivalent to a doubling time ranging from 1155 to 138 days. These rates of growth were exceedingly slow. The fastest growing cancer required 100 days to increase only 2.5 mm in diameter. Consequently, in seeking a change in size of the neoplastic roentgen shadow, it would not be useful to perform double contrast enema studies more often than every 100 days unless truncation existed in these data. A faster growing subset of cancer could exist with truncation. The value of more frequent examinations would be justified only if there are faster growing cancers than could be documented by this study. As already noted, nothing is known about the rate of growth of cancers observed only once. Little is known about the net growth rate of cancers that exhibited predominantly infiltrative or ulcerative growth (Spratt and Ackerman, 1962). These cancers have no protuberant mass that could be measured on double contrast enemas. Growth was measurable in all cancers observed for at least 500 to 1,000

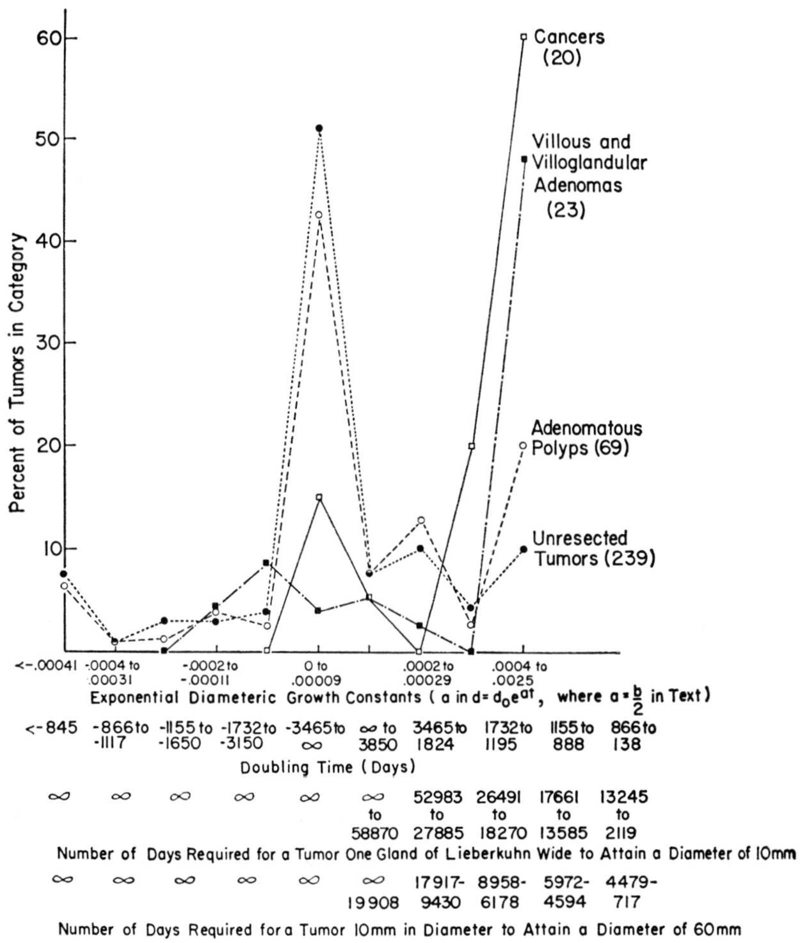

Figure 2–8. Patterns of exponential diametric tumor growth. (From Welin S, Youker J, Spratt JS Jr: The rates and patterns of growth of 375 tumors of the large intestine and rectum observed serially by double contrast enema study (Malmö technique). AJR 90:673–687, 1963. © 1963, American Roentgen Ray Society.)

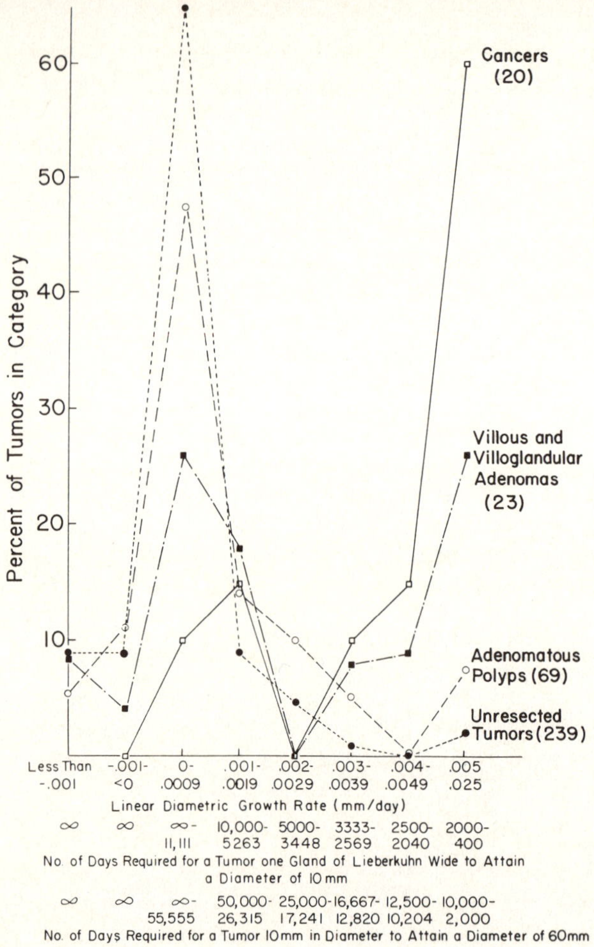

Figure 2–9. Patterns of linear diametric tumor growth. (From Welin S, Youker J, Spratt JS Jr: The rates and patterns of growth of 375 tumors of the large intestine and rectum observed serially by double contrast enema study (Malmö technique). AJR 90:673–687, 1963. © 1963, American Roentgen Ray Society.)

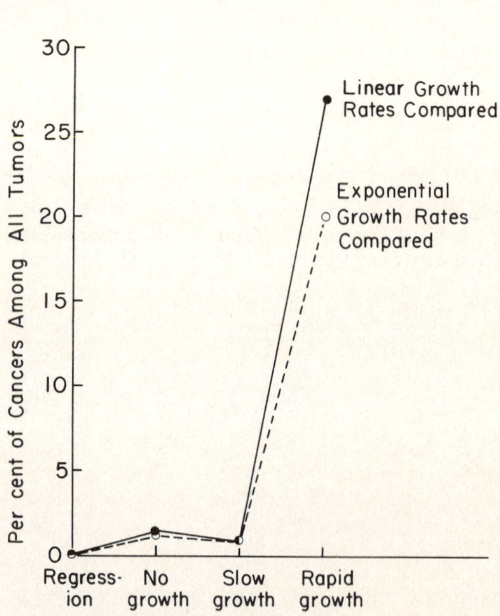

Figure 2–10. Graphic representation of the percentage of cancers counted among all tumors in each growth rate range. Rapid growth of the tumor diameter is defined in three ways: .003 to .025 mm/day (linear scale), .0003 to .0025 exponential growth constant or 138 to 1155 days volumetric doubling time (exponential scale). (From Welin S, Youker J, Spratt JS Jr: The rates and patterns of growth of 375 tumors of the large intestine and rectum observed serially by double contrast enema study (Malmö technique). AJR 90:673–687, 1963. © 1963, American Roentgen Ray Society.)

days, although many noncancerous tumors observed for much longer either demonstrated no growth or regressed.

The duration and changes in size of all neoplasms in an entire population must be known if the full spectrum of growth behavior is to be defined. The time required for a tumor growing steadily at a known rate to increase a given amount in size is easily calculated. For tumors growing by an exponential increase in the diameter, this interval is calculated

$$t_b - t_a = \frac{\ln d_b - \ln d_a}{a}$$

where a is the exponential growth constant for a cylinder of cancer of constant thickness.

For a tumor growing by a linear increase in diameter, this interval is calculated

$$t_b - t_a = \frac{d_b - d_a}{R}$$

The exponential diametric growth constant, a, and the linear rate of diametric growth, R, were calculated using the Malmö data and are provided in Figures 2–8 and 2–9, respectively. Whether these rates of growth were constant from the inception of the tumor is not known. Consequently, any estimation of the time required for a tumor to grow from the size of a single neoplastic gland of Lieberkühn to 10 mm in diameter would be speculative. On the other hand, any estimation of the time required for a tumor 10 mm in diameter to grow to a size 60 mm in diameter would be based on more reliable data. The times required for colonic or rectal neoplasm to grow from the size of a gland of Lieberkühn to a diameter of 10 mm and from 10 mm to 60 mm was calculated using the corresponding rates of growth scales shown in Figures 2–8 and 2–9.

Obviously, tumors could have very long periods of silent evolution before they become large enough to produce symptoms regularly. The fastest growing cancer observed in the Malmö data would have required 6 to 8 years to grow from glandular size to a diameter of 60 mm.

A life span of about 70 years is equivalent to about 25,550 days. Obviously, many elderly people would be expected to die with, although not from, these indolent slow-growing neoplasms in their colon and rectum. The fact that this occurs is confirmed by the prevalence of asymptomatic colonic neoplasms prevalent in colons of elderly patients examined at autopsy. These cancers were generally not known to exist before death (see Chapters One and Ten for further discussion of this observation).

The vast majority of the benign adenomatous polyps and the unresected tumors in the Malmö study grew so slowly that they could not have achieved a significant size during the longest human life span (see Figs. 2–8 and 2–9). These tumors were producing and desquamating new glandular cells without increasing in mass. To this extent they were behaving as normal intestinal epithelium. However, sometime in the life history of these tumors, they had enlarged enough to become visible.

A total of 17 adenomatous polyps had mean exponential rates of growth calculated to be in the same range as those of cancers. Twelve of these tumors were completely benign adenomatous polyps and five showed slight atypical change. Sixteen of the 17 benign polyps were of small size and were observed for relatively short periods of time. The seventeenth polyp was a large atypical adenomatous polyp that grew from a diameter of 34 mm to a diameter of 42 mm in 181 days, the doubling time being 304 days. Neither invasion nor metastasis had occurred from this tumor, but if such growth was permitted to continue, a bulky tumor would have developed. Only eight of the adenomatous polyps, including the one just described, had linear diametric rates of growth of the same magnitude as those of cancers. Only five of these polyps were observed three or more times and none of them showed accelerating growth.

Forty-five percent of the villous and villoglandular adenomas grew as fast as cancers, and these tumors regularly became large. Associated with their great size, extensive surface area involvement, and cancerous rates of growth, villous adenomas have a greater statistical chance of becoming invasive, and indeed, the large villous tumors observed frequently contained areas of invasive cancers. Two of the 20 cancers in this study arose in villous adenomas. Neither of the villous adenomas containing invasive cancers underwent an acceleration in growth rate during the period of observation. In fact, only one cancer among all 20 observed underwent a seemingly abrupt acceleration of growth rate during the period of observation (see Fig. 2–6). However, the roentgen shadow showed typical marginal infiltration (Welin's roentgen diagnostic sign of cancer) by the second of the seven double contrast enema studies when the cancer was only 9 mm in diameter. In the specimen removed, this was a highly invasive undifferentiated carcinoma with lymph node metastases. No morphologic evidence of an antecedent benign tumor was found. The observation of the abrupt increase in growth rate depended on the accuracy of only two measurements of a tumor with an infiltrating indistinct margin and is therefore subject to question.

A gradation of growth rates corresponding to gradations of malignancy existed, but there was an overlap of the spectrum of observed rates in each morphologic category. Furthermore, a few tumors of no cancerous significance were found in each growth rate range (Table 2–3). Consequently, rate of growth is not the only factor that determines whether a neoplasm of the large bowel or rectum becomes or is an invasive cancer. True primary cancers invade while they are still small (Spratt and Ackerman, 1962). As mentioned previously, large-sized, rapidly growing villous adenomas have a greater statistical chance of becoming invasive. From the standpoint of growth rate and frequency of invasive cancer with increasing size, the villous adenoma might more accurately be named "villous adenocarcinoma," with subclassifications of "invasive" and "noninvasive." This type of tumor is definitely implantable in open wounds, as reported by Wheat and Ackerman (1958).

The same possibility might apply to the occasional, although relatively rare, rapidly growing adenomatous polyp. Other purely physical factors that might affect the propensity to invade or metastasize or both are the mechanical resistance of the host tissue, the rupturing pressure within the expanding neoplasm, the mutual adhesiveness of the neoplastic cells, and the fragmentation of the basement membrane (Coman, 1944; Kellner, 1961). The gross morphologic configuration of the tumor could affect and be affected by these physical factors. Greater cellular adhesiveness is associated with a more protuberant growth pattern (Coman, 1944). Also, a polypoid tumor on a well-formed pedicle, such as the polypoid cancer in Figures 2–3 and 2–11, has a greater ratio of surface area to volume than have the more penetrating tumors. For 7 years, the cancer in Figures 2–6 and 2–11 was in an equilibrium state, varying between 10 and 20 mm in diameter, and it invaded only through the muscularis mucosae and never metastasized. A pedunculated morphologic configuration could increase the likelihood of an equilibrium between the rate of cellular loss by desquamation and the rate of cellular gain from neoplastic cellular proliferation. The lateral growth of a polypoid cancer could expand into the lumen of the bowel rather than into the host. Conversely, a neoplasm with a more rapid rate of growth composed of less adhesive cells might begin in the depths of a crypt of Lieberkühn, rupture into the submucosa, and begin reticular or infiltrative submucosal growth. Such a cancer might first present on the surface as an ulceration or might infiltrate extensively as linitis plastica.

Failure of slowly growing or non-growing noninvasive tumors to attain significant size during the human life span has practical significance in the diagnosis of colonic tumors demonstrated by double contrast enema studies. Very slow growing tumors do not get very big. The measurement of fresh tissue specimens of consecutively resected benign and malignant tumors showed that benign tumors rarely exceeded a diameter of 12 mm (Spratt and Ackerman, 1960b). With an error in roentgenographic measurement of ± 2 mm, the critical dimension should lie in the vicinity of 10 to 14 mm. An analysis of the diameters of the 375 tumors in the Malmö study that were

Table 2–3. RATES OF GROWTH OF MISCELLANEOUS TUMORS MEASURED ON SERIAL DOUBLE CONTRAST ENEMAS*

Tumor	Rapid Growth†	Slow Growth	No Growth	Regression	Total
Amyloid tumor	1				1
Hyperplastic polyp	2		2		4
Leiomyoma			1		1
Lipoma			1		1
Normal mucosa	3	1		1	5
Retention polyp	2	1			3
Histologic section not available‡		2	5	2	9
Total	8	4	9	3	24

*From Welin S, Youker J, Spratt JS: The rates and patterns observed serially by double contrast enema study (Malmö Technique). AJR 90:673–687, 1963. ©1963 American Roentgen Ray Society.

†Rapid growth = 0.003–0.025 mm/day or a DT_{Act} <1,155 days.

‡Classified as adenomatous polyps on original review.

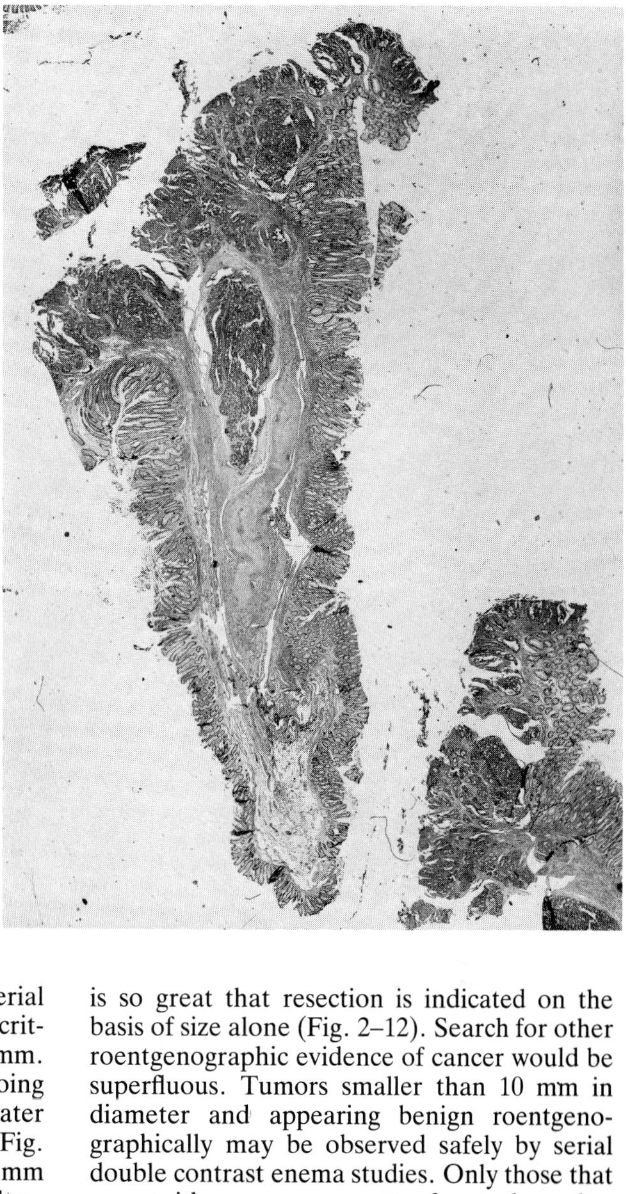

Figure 2–11. This cancer on a well-formed pedicle fluctuated between 10 and 20 mm in diameter, as measured on double contrast enema studies made at intervals over 7 years of observation. (From Welin S, Youker J, Spratt JS Jr: The rates and patterns of growth of 375 tumors of the large intestine and rectum observed serially by double contrast enema study (Malmö technique). AJR 90:673–687, 1963. © 1963, American Roentgen Ray Society.)

measured on the first and the last of the serial double contrast enema studies showed the critical roentgenographic diameter to be 10 mm. Tumors larger than 10 mm were undergoing sustained growth, and there was a greater chance of their being invasive cancers (see Fig. 2–12). One of the two cancers that was 10 mm or less in diameter developed marginal infiltration before it attained a diameter of 10 mm, permitting the diagnosis of cancer, based on its roentgenographic appearance.

As previously observed, the diagnosis of cancer has been made correctly on the basis of infiltrating margins observed on roentgenograms in tumors as small as 3 mm in diameter. However, pedunculated cancers, cancers with well-circumscribed or pushing margins, and cancers arising in villous adenomas may not develop this sign until they are quite large. In these cases, when biopsy is not possible, we must rely on size and growth to make the diagnosis of cancer. The statistical chance that any polypoid tumor attaining a roentgenographic diameter greater than 10 mm is cancer is so great that resection is indicated on the basis of size alone (Fig. 2–12). Search for other roentgenographic evidence of cancer would be superfluous. Tumors smaller than 10 mm in diameter and appearing benign roentgenographically may be observed safely by serial double contrast enema studies. Only those that grow with a cancerous rate of growth or that exceed a diameter of 10 mm on subsequent examinations will require resection. Among the numerous very small tumors (less than 8 mm in diameter) with no premalignant significance (Koppel et al., 1962; Spratt et al., 1958), new cancers have been found with the same age-specific incidence rates observed for the general population (Spratt and Ackerman, 1962). However, in children, single and multiple retention polyps regularly exceed a diameter of 10 mm. Roentgenographically, these tumors appear benign. They have been observed until disappearance (Welin, 1958). Transendoscopic removal of all tumors, no matter how small, for histopathologic evaluation is possible, as long as they are visible by

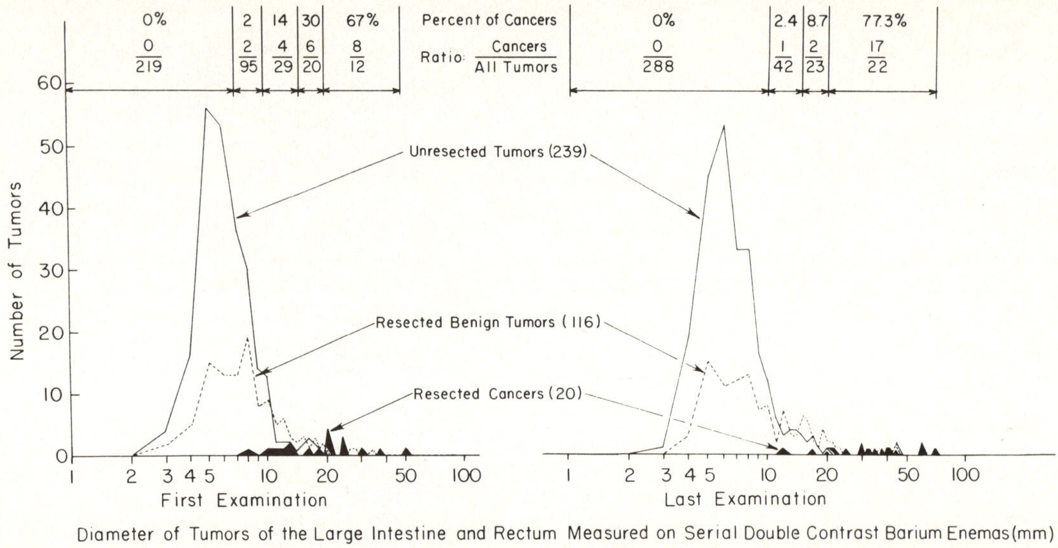

Figure 2-12. The frequency distributions of 375 colonic tumors measured on the first (left figure) and the last (right figure) of a series of double contrast enemas. The upper scale provides the percentage of tumors in each size range that were cancers. The period of observation averaged 834 days for the benign tumors and cancers to 939 days for tumors still unresected after the last observation. These data support the conclusion that tumor size is a critical characteristic in the presumptive diagnosis of cancer. Benign tumors generally grew very slowly, exceeding 8 mm in diameter with a steadily decreasing frequency. By the last observation, no cancer was less than 12 mm in diameter. (From Welin S, Youker J, Spratt JS Jr: The rates and patterns of growth of 375 tumors of the large intestine and rectum observed serially by double contrast enema study (Malmö technique). AJR 90:673–687, 1963. © 1963, American Roentgen Ray Society.)

sigmoidoscope. This is also possible if a tumor can be reached by a flexible endoscope, but no controlled clinical trial exists proving the optimum strategy. The benignity and frequency of small, non-growing colonic tumors is so great that no morbidity or mortality as a result of their removal as a means of cancer prevention is justified.

Among the Malmö data was information that permitted the calculation of $DT_{(Act)}$ for an assortment of infrequently seen colonic tumors (see Table 2–3) (Welin et al., 1963).

RELATION BETWEEN $DT_{(Act)}$ OF PRIMARY CANCERS AND PULMONARY METASTASES

It was speculated that primary cancers might grow at the same rate as pulmonary metastases (Collins, 1962; Spratt and Ackerman, 1960b). The doubling times of 43 spherical pulmonary metastases from carcinomas of the colon and rectum in 36 patients are shown in Table 2–1. The median doubling time for the pulmonary metastases (see Table 2–1) was 109 days and for the 20 primary carcinomas, 620 days, a sixfold difference. The median linear radial growth was .02 mm per day for the pulmonary metastases and .004 mm per day for the primary cancers, the former rate being five times faster than the latter (Spratt, 1965). However, the pulmonary metastases shown in Table 2–1 and the primary cancers shown in Figures 2–8 and 2–9 did not occur in the same patients. Only two of the 20 primary cancers having doubling times of 323 and 550 days, respectively, produced pulmonary metastases and in neither patient was the doubling time of the metastases measured. Furthermore, interval-surfacing cancers and cancers of possibly greater malignancy with roentgen signs of infiltration could be faster growing primaries and might produce faster growing metastases.

In summary, the rates of growth of 375 tumors of the colon and rectum were calculated from the diameters of tumors observed more than once on double contrast enema studies (Malmö technique). There was a spectral overlap of growth rates for different histopathologic types of tumors, with cancers being distinctly predominant in the group that had the more rapid rate of growth. The cancerous rates of growth were in the range of .003 to .025 mm per day, for linear diametric growth. If the growth was predominantly exponential, a point that could not be resolved with certainty, the exponential diametric growth constant would vary from .0003 to .0025 mm per mm per day, which is equivalent to a doubling time of 1115 to 138 days. These very slow rates of growth characterize tumors that had many years of silent growth before attaining symptomatic size. Slower growing benign neoplasms of the colon and rectum might never attain significant size within the human life span. The mean rates of growth of metastases in the lung from colonic and rectal cancers were five- to sixfold faster than the mean rates of growth of the primary cancers growing in the colon or rectum.

These Malmö data, and perhaps data on pulmonary metastases, are all subject to a length bias in their selection. Only tumors that persisted long enough to permit serial observation could be included. The author (J.S.S.) specifically asked Solve Welin about the incidence of cancers in his study population that might surface in the intervals between examinations. These might come to surgery with one or no roentgen measurements, i.e., as interval-surfacing cancers. He said that accurate numbers were not available. Also, there was no knowledge on the growth rate of neoplasms diagnosed and resected at the first observation. Thus, the possibility does persist that neoplasms exist that could grow faster or slower than those reported in this study. This problem has been studied in relation to breast cancer, and these interval-surfacing cancers are frequent, different, and more aggressive than the tumors that grow at a slower rate (Spratt et al., 1982). Possibly, the ulcerating cancer of the large intestine falls in this more acute subset. Observations in the final part of this chapter give support to the possibility that very acute variants of colorectal cancers may exist.

Additional Observations

Additional observers (Figiel et al., 1965) have confirmed the feasibility of performing measurements of growth using barium enemas. As a result of Figiel's assessment of the growth behavior of small polypoid colonic tumors on serial barium enema examinations, a highly accurate differentiation of the benign from the malignant tumor was possible. A polypoid tumor that did not grow or increase in size during progress studies could be safely presumed to be benign. In one polypoid tumor, sudden acceleration of growth occurred. Volumetric doubling of a polypoid tumor in 6 to 12 months or less indicated a high cancer potential. Case material and growth data relating to the growth of colonic carcinoma were presented, and a review of about 300 cases in which follow-up study of colonic polypoid tumors was undertaken was summarized.

Burnett and Greenbaum (1981) recently reported colonic primary cancers exhibiting more rapid growth than had been previously reported. In these cases, the doubling times were 53, 67, and 150 days. The linear growth rates were 0.137, 0.133, and 0.057 mm per day.

Mueller (1982) observed a major variation in the rates of dying among persons with cancers of the colon that could be attributable to variations in the rates of growth. When rates of dying were plotted on semilogarithmic scales, he observed a biphasic distribution composed of people who died very rapidly and of people who died very slowly. For several cancers studied, this biphasic pattern was found among all histologic grades. However, the more undifferentiated the cancer, the greater the percentage of rapidly dying. Long-term survivors were still present among all histologic grades. One plausible explanation of this phenomenon could be a spectrum of growth rates ranging from the very fast to the very slow. Other factors, however, such as a propensity to metastasize, could also account for this observation.

Stragand and associates (1982) provided an interesting observation on the $DT_{(Act)}$ of two human colonic adenocarcinoma cell lines propagated in Rowett athymic rats. The $DT_{(Act)}$ were 5.5 days for one cancer and 8.5 days for the other. The implants grew as adenocarcinomas without metastases but with necrosis, and they invaded underlying muscle.

When the measurement of very rapid growth is possible by radiologic methods, the "window" of time in the life history of a cancer becomes ever shorter as the rate of growth increases or the doubling time shortens. A way of quantifying the existence and prevalence of acute cancers is to discover all the colorectal cancers that occur in a population followed at specified intervals. The cancers that are diagnosed in the intervals between screening examinations are, by definition, interval-surfacing cancers and are presumably more acute or rapidly growing.

As an example for such a study, complete identification of all the breast cancers occurring in a population of 10,120 women screened in the Breast Cancer Detection and Demonstration Project at the University of Louisville supported the position that there was a significant subset of acute cancers and that they were biologically more aggressive (Heuser et al., 1979). Spratt (1982) has compiled evidence indicating that this may be a serious and general problem in cancer screening and detection.

GROWTH RATES ASSAYED BY RADIOISOTOPIC LABELING

Radioisotopic labeling studies have added even more insight into the growth of colorectal neoplasms. Meyer and Prioleau (1981) measured the S-phase fraction (SPF) of epithelial cells in 100 resected colorectal carcinomas by in vitro exposure to tritiated thymidine and autoradiography. The frequency distribution of the SPFs was gaussian for 90 unirradiated cancers, with a median count of 17.8 per hundred. For ten cancers given radiation therapy preoperatively, the distribution was positively skewed, with a median SPF of 6.9 per hundred. No significant association could be identified between SPF and age, race, sex, site, size, Dukes' stage, histologic grade, number of metastasis-bearing lymph nodes, presence of adenomas in the colon, survival or relapse-free interval of the patient, or the SPF of adjacent normal colorectal crypts. The authors were unable to divide colorectal cancers into kinetic subsets. Many tumors contained a very significant fraction of nonproliferative cells. Hoffman (1949) provided theoretical considerations necessary to relate the traditional mitotic figure counts done by light microscopy to the total number of cells in mitotic cycle. The ratio is estimated to be 1:10.

Malaise (1982) has informed the author (J.S.S.) that he has measured the tritiated thymidine labeling indices on colorectal adenocarcinomas. The values range from 2.3 to 27.97, with a geometric mean of 7.63. These values may be used to estimate the $DT_{(Pot)}$. In Malaise's total experience in comparing potential with actual doubling times of solid tumors of many types, he observed the log mean $DT_{(Act)}$ to be 83 days but the $DT_{(Pot)}$ from thymidine labeling data to be 23.8 days. Many primary cancers in his study were, however, growing in nonsurface sites, where desquamation is not a factor, as it is with primary colorectal adenocarcinomas.

Using the median tritiated thymidine labeling index (4.5 percent), Steel calculated the potential doubling time for 31 human colon cancers to be 13.5 days (Steel, 1967, 1972). In 1967, Steel estimated that cell loss could exceed 50 percent. On an epithelial surface as the colon, where epithelial desquamation is a normal and rapid phenomenon, the magnitude of cell loss from a cancer would be expected to drop dramatically when the same cancer metastasized to lymph node, liver, or lung, where desquamation no longer occurs. This $DT_{(Pot)}$ for colonic cancers is certainly vastly faster than the gross or net doubling times that have been measured on roentgenograms. Even on roentgenograms, the average $DT_{(Act)}$ for pulmonary metastases is about sixfold faster than the $DT_{(Act)}$ measured by double contrast enema. Surface desquamation could account for a major part of this difference.

The proliferative compartment of normal colonic mucosa is limited to the lower two thirds of the crypts, but it increases in various states. The rate of mitosis in neoplasms is not increased when compared with that in normal mucosa. Actual growth of neoplasms can be accounted for by a decrease in cell loss (Camplejohn, 1982).

An obvious conclusion from all studies to date is that this heterogeneity of colonic and rectal neoplasms is a major factor affecting growth rates and possibly limiting treatment response to drugs. The kinetic data from a tumor in one patient cannot be used for another. The kinetics of metastases are dissimilar from the kinetics of the primary. The degree of heterogeneity recorded for colonic and rectal neoplasms is consistent with the 10 to 20 percent responses recorded for 5-fluorouracil and methotrexate (Lesher et al., 1977).

Fialkow (1979) reported an indirect approach to cancer origin, taking advantage of naturally occurring cell labels to determine whether a neoplasm had single or multiple cell origin. The assumption was made that a cancer arising from a rare "spontaneous" somatic mutation would originate from a single cell. On the other hand, a multicellular origin would be anticipated in neoplasms arising primarily as a result of a highly infectious oncogenic virus (or a similar-acting carcinogen). By this method, most studied neoplasms seemed to be of clonal origin. One case of carcinoma of the colon seemed to be of multicellular origin.

Heterogeneity of cellular characteristics in human colonic carcinomas has also been demonstrated in other ways. Brattain and associates (1981) isolated three subpopulations of a single human colonic carcinoma from a primary cell culture. Although all cell lines had a near diploid number of chromosomes, each cell line showed a distinct histologic pattern when grown in xenografts of athymic nude mice.

GROWTH RATES OF ANAL CANCERS

No data have been located that specifically measure the net or gross growth rates of anal cancers. To date, the doubling time of all epidermoid cancers metastatic to the lung and primary epidermoid carcinomas of the lung have all exhibited similar rates. Primary epidermoid cancers of the lung exhibited a mean $DT_{(Act)}$ (of a lognormal frequency distribution) of 70 days with a range of 21 to 233 days (95 percent confidence). Metastatic epidermoid cancers from numerous sites exhibited a mean $DT_{(Act)}$ (of a lognormal frequency distribution) of 46 days with a range of 7 to 298 days (95 percent confidence). This is equivalent to about 15 new cancer cells per 1000 existing cells per day, ranging from 2.3 to 99 (95 percent confidence). Linear radial growth would average 0.034 mm per day, ranging from 0.0027 to 0.43 mm per day (Spratt and Spratt, 1964).

Malaise (1973) did observe that squamous cell cancers grew more slowly than mesenchymal sarcomas, although they had higher labeling indices. He hypothesized that the rapidity of cell loss from the squamous cell carcinomas could account for this difference.

SUMMARY

In summary, there is a wide, natural variance in doubling times and tritiated thymidine labeling indices of neoplasms of the lower bowel. There is a crude correlation between growth rate and histopathology. The difference between $DT_{(Act)}$ and $DT_{(Pot)}$ is manifold. Primary surface desquamating cancers probably grow much slower than their metastases. These factors are of importance in understanding neoplastic behavior and in designing detection and treatment protocols. The rates of growth are very relevant to screening and diagnostic strategies.

References

Brattain MG, Fine WD, Khaled FM, et al: Heterogeneity of malignant cells from a human colonic carcinoma. Cancer Res 41:1751–1756, 1981.

Burnett KR, Greenbaum EI: Rapidly growing carcinoma of the colon. Dis Colon Rectum 24:282–286, 1981.

Camplejohn RS: Colorectal cancer: cell kinetics. Recent Results in Cancer Res 83:21–30, 1982.

Collins VP: Time of occurrence of pulmonary metastases from carcinoma of colon and rectum. Cancer 15:387–395, 1962.

Collins VP, Loeffler RK, Tivey H: Observations on growth rates of human tumors. AJR 76:988–1000, 1956.

Coman DR: Decreased mutual adhesiveness, a property of cells from squamous cell carcinomas. Cancer Res 4:625–629, 1944.

Davis HT: Problem of growth in two populations conflicting with one another. *In* Introduction of Nonlinear Differential and Integral Equations. Washington, D.C., U.S. Government Printing Office, 1960, 99–102.

Defares JG, Sneddon IN: Common growth and biology. *In* An Introduction to the Mathematics of Medicine and Biology. Chicago, Year Book Medical Publishers, 1960, 227–234.

Fialkow PJ: Clonal origin of human tumors. Annu Rev Med 50:135–143, 1979.

Figiel LS, Figiel SJ, Wietersen FK: Roentgenologic observations of growth rates of colonic polyps and carcinoma. Acta Radiol (Diagn) 3:417–429, 1965.

Gompertz B: On the nature of the function expressive of the law of human mortality, and on a new method of determining the value of life contingencies. Philos Trans R Soc Lond 513–585, 1825.

Heuser L, Spratt JS, Polk HC Jr: Growth rates of primary breast cancer. Cancer 43:1888–1894, 1979.

Hoffman JG: Theory of the mitotic index and its application to tissue growth measurement. Bull Math Biol, 11:139–144, 1949.

Kellner B: Progression of tumor growth and formation of metastases. Acta Morphol Acad Sci Hung 10:337–356, 1961.

Koppel M, Bailar JC III, Weakley FL, Shimkin MB: Incidence of cancer in colon and rectum among polyp-free patients. Dis Colon Rectum 5:349–355, 1962.

Lesher S, Schiffer LM, Phanse M: Human colonic tumor cell kinetics: potential for therapy. Cancer 40(5 Suppl):2706–2709, 1977.

Lloyd HH: Estimation of tumor cell kill from Gompertz growth curves. Cancer Chemother Rep 59(2 Pt 1)267–277, 1975.

Lorinc P, Brahme F: Perforation of colon during examination by double contrast method. Gastroenterology 37:770–773, 1959.

Malaise EP: Personal communication 4 March 1982.

Malaise EP, Chavaudra N, Tubiana M: The relationship between growth rate, labelling index and histological type of human solid tumours. Eur J Cancer 9:305–312, 1973.

Mayneord WV: On a law of growth of Jensen's rat sarcoma. Am J Cancer 16:841–846, 1932.

Meyer JS, Prioleau PG: S-phase fractions of colorectal carcinomas related to pathologic and clinical features. Cancer 48:1221–1228, 1981.

Mueller CB: Personal communication 6 Dec 1982 (based on unpublished studies of the Upstate Medical Center Cancer Registry, 12th Annual Report, Syracuse, New York, 1967).

Pearlman AW: Breast cancer—influence of growth rate on prognosis and treatment evaluation. A study based on mastectomy scar recurrences. Cancer 38:1826–1833, 1976.

Spratt JS Jr: The rates and patterns of growth of neoplasms of the large intestine and rectum. Surg Clin North Am 40:1103–1115, 1965.

Spratt JS Jr: The lognormal frequency distribution and human cancer. J Surg Res 9:151–157, 1969.

Spratt JS: Epidemiology of screening for cancer. Curr Probl Cancer 6:1–58, 1982.

Spratt JS Jr, Ackerman LV: Pathological significance of polyps of the rectum and colon. Dis Colon Rectum 3:330–335, 1960a.

Spratt JS Jr, Ackerman LV: Relationship of size of colonic tumors to their cellular composition and biological behavior. Surg Forum 10:56–61, 1960b.

Spratt JS Jr, Ackerman LV: The growth of a colonic adenocarcinoma. Am Surg 27:23–28, 1961.

Spratt JS Jr, Ackerman LV: Small primary adenocarcinomas of colon and rectum. JAMA 179:337–346, 1962.

Spratt JS Jr, Ackerman LV, Moyer CA: Relationship of polyps of colon to colonic cancers. Ann Surg 148:682–698, 1958.

Spratt JS, Heuser L, Kuhns JG, et al: Variations and associations in histopathology, clinical factors, mammographic patterns and growth rates among breast cancers confirmed in a screened population. *In* Issues in Cancer Screening Communications. New York, Alan R Liss, 1982, 295–299.

Spratt JS Jr, Kaltenback ML, Spratt JA: Cytokinetic definition of acute and chronic breast cancer. Cancer Res 37:226–230, 1977.

Spratt JS Jr, Spratt JA: The prognostic value of measuring the gross linear radial growth of pulmonary metastases and primary pulmonary cancers. J Thorac Cardiovasc Surg 71:274–278, 1976.

Spratt JS Jr, Spratt TL: Rates of growth of pulmonary metastases and host survival. Ann Surg 159:161–171, 1964.

Steel GG: Cell loss as a factor in the growth rate of human tumours. Eur J Cancer 3:381–387, 1967.

Steel GG: The cell cycle in tumours: an examination of data gained by the technique of labeled mitoses. Cell Tissue Kinet 5:87–100, 1972.

Stragand JJ, Drewinko B, Henderson SD, et al: Growth characteristics of human colonic adenocarcinomas propagated in the Rowett athymic rat. Cancer Res 42:3111–3115, 1982.

Verhagen AMV: Growth curves and their functional forms. Aust J Stat 2:122–127, 1960.

Welin S: Modern trends in diagnostic roentgenology of colon. The Mackenzie Davidson Memorial Lecture. Br J Radiol 31:453–464, 1958.

Welin S: Uber die rongenologische Untersuchung des Dickdarmes mit der Doppelkontrastmethode (Die Malmomodifikation). Radiologe (Berlin) 2:87–100, 1962.

Welin S, Lorinc P: Das Rontgenbild des villosen (zottenformigen) tumors in Bereich des colons. Radiologe (Berlin) 2:107–112, 1962.

Welin S, Youker J, Spratt JS Jr, et al: The rates and patterns of growth of 375 tumors of the large intestine and rectum observed serially by double contrast enema study (Malmö Technique). AJR 90:673–687, 1963.

Wheat MW Jr, Ackerman LV: Villous adenomas of the large intestine. Ann Surg 147:476–487, 1958.

THREE

A Rationale of Practice for Polypoid Lesions of the Colon

J. S. Spratt, M.D.

Polyps of the colon and rectum have been of great interest to me since my days as a house officer at Barnes Hospital. An early tradition of the Barnes program was an "at the dissecting bench and microscope" rotation in surgical pathology for surgical residents. When I was a resident, this tradition was continued under Dr. Lauren Ackerman. Most residents completed a project in surgical pathology. I was assigned the project to "go look up colon polyps," which culminated in my first publication (Spratt et al., 1958). Many years later I am still "looking them up" because the knowledge I gained proved to be the tip of the iceberg of a very complex health problem. Since that time, much has been learned about polyps—their etiology, pathology, growth rates, incidence, prevalence, and epidemiology; the technology of discovery and removal; and misadventures in their pursuit—but many gaps in knowledge still remain. There has not been a controlled clinical trial testing hypotheses concerning the superiority of one strategy of management over another, particularly in regard to frequency and method of examination. Confronted with this reality, efforts have been made to define a rationale of management based on the best available data. Such a rationale has been published previously (Spratt and Watson, 1971), and this present chapter constitutes a review and update of this subject.

The 1965 edition of Webster's Dictionary defines rationale as "an explanation of controlling principles of opinion, belief, practice or phenomenon." The controlling opinion or belief is that medical knowledge and technology should be used in a systematic way to minimize the morbidity and mortality attributable either *directly* or *indirectly* to polypoid lesions of the colon at a cost in time and money tolerable to the individual patient and the public. A polyp is defined as any "projecting mass of swollen and hypertrophied or tumorous membrane."

In the absence of a well-tested method of prevention, a control system must follow a systematic strategy in the application of the available technology to alter the natural history of the polypoid lesions so that they have a less adverse pattern, without substituting morbidity from the technology itself. The resulting system becomes the rationale of practice regarding polypoid lesions of the colon. Data on gross and microscopic taxonomies, etiology, epidemiology, and natural history are used to support this rationale. The details of histopathologic classification, radiologic detection, endoscopic management, and the nature and management of perforation are discussed in other chapters.

The growing body of knowledge about the etiology and epidemiology of polypoid lesions of the colon is summarized in Chapter One. A comprehensive review of growth rates is presented in Chapter Two. Growth rates determine the time required for a tumor to attain a visible and a symptomatic size. In so doing, growth rates also influence and affect optimum intervals for periodic re-examination.

FACTORS AFFECTING THE RATIONALE OF PRACTICE

Because of the variation in biologic behavior and growth rates of polypoid lesions and colorectal cancers, the ubiquity of these growths, the problem of patient compliance in even the best system, and the epidemiology of colonic polyps, it is doubtful that early diagnosis alone will eliminate the problem of polypoid lesions and colorectal neoplasms in humans (Spratt, 1969). Consequently, the complexities of polyp and cancer induction in the human colon must be further unraveled so that steps in the induction process can be changed to reduce the magnitude of the problem (see Chapter One).

Exciting possibilities for the chemoprevention of polyposis coli are beginning to reach the published literature. For example, Bussey and associates (1982) carried out a two-year human clinical trial to determine the efficacy of ascorbic acid (3 gm per day) in reducing colonic polyps. The ascorbic acid was compared with a placebo. Ascorbic acid is a potent antioxidant that inactivates many known carcinogens, and it has been shown to inhibit murine large bowel carcinogens (Reddy and Hirota, 1979; Logue and Frommer, 1980).

By the ninth month of the trial, there was a significant reduction of polyps in the treated group. By 18 months, the tritiated thymidine labeling index of the colonic mucosa in the treated group was lower than in the controls. Further studies in chemoprevention and reduction of exposure to inducing conditions hold exciting promise for the future. Further possibilities in this area are discussed in Chapter One.

DIAGNOSIS OF COLONIC POLYPS AND RATIONALE OF PRACTICE

Asymptomatic colonic polyposis is rarely diagnosed unless it is visualized by endoscopy, barium or barium–air contrast roentgenographic studies, or pathologic examination after the colon has been removed by surgical resection or at autopsy. The appearance of blood or excess mucus in the stools or a strong family history of colonic polyps may initiate the clinical process of discovery. By each method of diagnosis, characteristics of both the gross polypoid lesions and the patient are revealed that permit a presumptive diagnosis of the microscopic taxonomy and the probable behavior of the polyps if left untreated. However, the nature of the grossly diagnosed polyps is never known with certainty until histopathologic sections are examined. The gross characteristics of polypoid lesions that can be measured or described are the number, size, area, shape, and location. These observed characteristics are combined with other characteristics of the patient in the descriptions of certain syndromes (Watne et al., 1982).

When several gross measurements are recorded at different points in time, the mean rate of change in size that occurs between the two measurement points can be estimated, providing still another parameter for taxonomy, i.e., the gross rate of growth (see Chapter Two).

Microscopic taxonomy correlated with the gross rates of growth and the observed prevalence has shown that the most frequent polyps are the scattered slow-growing adenomatous polyps that increase in incidence with age. Although frequent, most never reach a symptom-producing size during the human life span (Spratt and Ackerman, 1960b; Spratt et al., 1958; Welin et al., 1963), and many are suspected to disappear spontaneously.

By relating the time required for the fastest growing colon cancer measured in the Malmö study (Welin et al., 1963) to attain clinically significant size to the remaining life span (Spratt, 1965; 1971), the conclusion can be drawn that people past age 85 years probably do not benefit from diagnostic evaluation for either benign neoplasms or colorectal cancer if they are *asymptomatic*. Most benign colonic polyps grow even more slowly than do cancers, and many have been observed to regress on serial roentgenographic observation (Welin et al., 1963). Furthermore, elderly people are less tolerant of the occasional complications of proctosigmoidoscopy and barium enema (Kiser et al., 1968). Infrequent colonic polyps that have been observed on sequential barium enema studies show variable rates and patterns of growth (Welin et al, 1963) (see Chapter Two).

Because of the correlation between the presence of cancerous morphologic findings in colonic filling defects (either polypoid or sessile initially) and a faster rate of growth, the cancers are more likely than the polyps to attain significant size during the human life span. Consequently, size at any observation is highly significant in making a presumptive diagnosis of cancer in polypoid lesions of the colon (see Fig. 2–12 in Chapter Two) (Welin et al., 1963). Radiographically diagnosed "polyps" larger than 1 to 2 cm in greatest chordal dimension usually merit laparotomy or flexible endoscopic biopsy or removal because the chance that the larger polyps are indeed cancers exceeds the risk of removal (Welin et al., 1963). Many lesions formerly accessible only by laparotomy are now accessible to visualization and biopsy or removal with the flexible endoscope.

MULTIPLE ADENOMATOUS POLYPOSIS

Multiple polyposis of the large intestine and rectum is a gross diagnosis. On the basis of age, family history, and other syndrome-specific variables, a presumptive diagnosis may be made regarding the histologic composition of a polyp. However, the final diagnosis cannot be made until the polyp is biopsied. Types of multiple colon polyp syndromes encountered include familial adenomatous polyposis (Watne et al, 1982; Smith, 1959; Smith and Jackman, 1956), Peutz-Jeghers syndrome involving the colon (Staley and Schwarz, 1957; Waugh et al., 1964), lymphoid polyposis (Welin et al., 1963), and other less frequent types (Kaplan, 1961; Welin et al., 1963; Watne, 1982). The prognosis and method of management vary with each type of multiple polyposis (Localio, 1962; Spratt and Ackerman, 1960a, 1960b, 1964; Waugh et al., 1964; Williams and Fish, 1966; Watne et al., 1982). Both overtreatment and undertreatment can result from failure to make judgment decisions that would minimize adverse host effects under various circumstances.

Familial Adenomatous Polyposis

In the rationale for treatment of familial adenomatous polyposis, a condition known to be precancerous, a frequent question is, "After diagnosis, what is the 'safe' period of time before colectomy is recommended?" This question can be answered accurately only if the age-specific incidence rate of cancer diagnosis in a followed population is known. The reported rates are inadequate and vary with the person-years of follow-up and the age of the patient. However, when the diagnosis of familial adenomatous polyposis is established, the neoplastic transition is also predictable. In numerous studies of animal and human systems, it is evident that cancer develops at a measurable rate (Localio, 1962; Polk and Spratt, 1971; Watne et al., 1982); that is, a percentage of those at risk will develop cancer during each time interval of observation. Thus, some will always be developing cancer, and there is no absolutely "safe" period after diagnosis. Frequently, students of the subject have mistakenly assumed that the average period between diagnosis of familial polyposis and the diagnosis of cancer is a "safe" period for all patients.

Eventually all patients with bona fide cases of familial adenomatous polyposis develop invasive carcinomas in the rectum and colon. Preservation of the rectum and fulguration of polyps in cases of familial adenomatous polyps have not proved to be satisfactory or effective therapeutic approaches. Too many procedures, unusually close follow-up, and too much morbidity, expense, and uncertainty plague this approach, which is often incorrectly called the "conservative" approach. The unequivocal diagnosis of precancerous familial adenomatous polyposis requires a proctocolectomy, hopefully, before invasive metastasizing cancer develops.

The only feasible method of identifying asymptomatic people at risk for familial polyposis is to obtain a careful family history of a patient known to have this condition. The history should extend through as many generations as possible, since the trait is transmitted as a mendelian dominant. All people identified as being at risk in the family study should be advised of the genetic predisposition and should undergo periodic rectocolonic examination. Those who are known transmitters should be advised of the risk to their offspring. They may elect sterilization as a preventive measure. Familial adenomatous polyposis should be suspected in any individual, particularly those under 40 years, having multiple polyposis diagnosed by either proctosigmoidoscopy or barium enema. A representative polyp must be biopsied using the simplest method possible. The polyps of familial polyposis are adenomatous.

Gardner's Syndrome

Gardner's syndrome is a well-studied condition involving hereditary colonic polyposis. It has many features in common with the neurocristopathies, although I know of no studies confirming the association. A number of developmental anomalies seen with Gardner's syndrome are of neural crest origin, such as fibromatosis, pigmentation, and developmental anomalies (Riccardi et al., 1981). An alternate explanation for the phenomena of Gardner's syndrome may lie with the fibroblasts rather than with cells of the neural crest (Kopelovich, 1977). Growth abnormalities in fibroblasts from cutaneous biopsies of patients with this syndrome can be regularly demonstrated in tissue culture. The fibroblasts, unlike those from unaffected individuals, show a lack of contact inhibition, decreased requirements of serum for growth, elevated levels of plasminogen activator, and alterations in the intracellular distribution of actin cables. The cells grow without anchorage, do not form palpable tumors in athymic mice (BALB/c nu/nu) and are much more susceptible to conversion to sarcoma. Observations such as these may potentially lead to the earlier identification of individuals susceptible to colon neoplasia.

Other Benign Polyps

Other types of single and multiple polyps, occurring mainly in the young, are juvenile and lymphoid polyps. The latter requires no surgical intervention. The absolute indications for surgical intervention to alleviate or prevent adverse host effects caused by juvenile polyposis include the following:

1. Intestinal obstruction usually associated with intussusception.
2. Persistent symptoms of intermittent intestinal obstruction.
3. The coincidental diagnosis of intestinal cancer (an infrequent possibility).

In each surgical operation for juvenile polyposis, conservatism is in order. The simplest operation that will totally remove the troublesome polyps is the preferred treatment. These polyps are not neoplastic and could be of allergenic or hamartomatous origin. A careful allergenic work-up should be performed on children with juvenile polyposis.

Polyps in Peutz-Jeghers syndrome involve both the small and large intestines (Dozois, 1969; Horn et al., 1963). Patients may have other manifestations of the Peutz-Jeghers syndrome, such as circumoral pigmentation, and they are at risk of being over-irradiated as a result of diagnostic studies and overtreated as a result of the resection of excessive lengths of intestine, resulting in malabsorption syndrome. Consequently, diagnostic tests and treatment should be restricted to symptomatic patients. Once patients are educated about their disease, they will make the logical demands for the required services. Intermittent colic can be effectively treated, and if treated promptly, crisis episodes of intussusception may be avoided.

Burdick and Prior (1982) provide an informative longitudinal study of the scope of afflictions associated with Peutz-Jeghers syndrome. They followed a family for 27 years. One died of surgical complications from a bypass of an unresectable jejunal cancer. Two family members developed breast cancer, one arising in a fibroadenoma. Both patients died, one of breast cancer and one of a jejunal cancer. Three family members had benign ovarian tumors, one a benign breast tumor, and one a benign colloid thyroid nodule. The authors concluded that the jejunal cancer could have arisen from a polyp in Peutz-Jeghers syndrome. In reviewing the literature, the authors observed some similarity between these neoplasms and sex cord tumors with annular tubules (SCTAT), described earlier by Scully (1970).

Despite these rare reports, the relationship between Peutz-Jeghers syndrome and cancer is doubtful. A review by Dozois (1969) presented the following conclusions:

1. Carcinoma has been reported in the intestines of people with proven Peutz-Jeghers syndrome.
2. The sites most frequently affected by the Peutz-Jeghers syndrome (i.e., the jejunum and ileum) are least affected by cancers. Cancers in those people with this syndrome occur in those sites most frequently involved by cancer in the general population.
3. There are only three cases that showed a reported contiguous relationship between a polyp from Peutz-Jeghers syndrome and a cancer. Other cancers have arisen in polyp-free segments of the colon.

Consequently, extensive resections as a method of cancer prevention are not acceptable practice. Additional comments on the pediatric polyp problem are provided in Chapter Sixteen.

THE SINGLE OR SCATTERED POLYP IN THE ADULT

The rationale of practice for the single or scattered adenomatous polyps and villous adenomas of the colon that are not part of a recognized syndrome is a more frequent or general problem. These polyps are so frequent in older people that a considerable percentage of the elderly die *with* them, but few die *from* them (Spratt and Ackerman, 1960a, 1960b, 1964; Spratt et al., 1958). The significant clinical questions concern not their presence but the symptoms and adverse effects that they may cause during the normal life span. Symptoms and effects known to be attributable either directly or indirectly to colonic polyps are shown in Tables 3–1 and 3–2.

Variables influencing the selection of diagnostic and therapeutic methods to avoid these adverse effects are listed in Table 3–3. No absolute values can be given for the variables in this table for the reason that they vary among different populations and in the hands of different practitioners.

The rationale of practice for these single or scattered polyps is based on various data (Fielding and Lumsden, 1973; Kiser et al., 1968; Polk and Spratt, 1971; Polk et al., 1964, 1965; Sperling et al., 1963; Spratt, 1965, 1969; Spratt and Ackerman, 1960b, 1960d, 1961, 1962, 1964; Spratt et al., 1958, 1970; Spratt and Spjut, 1967; Turnbull et al., 1967; Welin et al., 1963). The sequential action and observation processes are partially shown in Figures 3–1 and 3–2. The rationale of practice is a single action sequence based on the possibility of finding and of removing harmful or potentially harmful pathological conditions, using as guidelines records of morbidity and mortality previously experienced as a result of similar clinical actions. The action sequence is predicated on the assumption that each action will be conducted with a high order of skill to keep morbidity and mortality of the action sequence itself to an absolute minimum. In patients in whom results of the action sequence are negative, it is doubtful that the sequence should be repeated more often than every 3 to 5 years. Thorough examinations performed less frequently may well prove more cost-effective than annual examinations. Further, if the results of the examination part of the action sequence are really negative for gross pathological conditions, the slowness of the neoplastic growth rate reduces but does not eliminate chances of abnormal findings for at least 3 to 5 years (see Chapters Two and Four). The really acute or rapid growing cancers may arise too quickly to be detected effectively by the periodic screening of asymptomatic persons.

A strong family history of colonic neoplasms might merit more frequent evaluation (Watne et al., 1982). The development of interval symptoms merits prompt re-evaluation. Relevant screening strategies in the asymptomatic patient are discussed in Chapter Four. The most significant new developments in the diagnosis and management of polyps are discussed in Chapter Five, which covers diagnostic radiology, and in Chapter Six, which covers the flexible endoscope, now permitting direct visualization and biopsy of lesions beyond the 25-cm reach of the proctosigmoidoscope. The place of this new technology in the "rationale of practice" is being sorted out.

The following provides an example of the uncontrolled "sorting out" process occurring with respect to the role of the flexible endoscope.

SUMMARY OF DESCRIPTIVE STATISTICS WITH THE FLEXIBLE ENDOSCOPE FROM A TYPICAL CLINICAL SERIES

There have been many clinical series on the status of flexible endoscopy. I will discuss one that is typical of the studies being done. In 1981, Colacchio and Forde reviewed 733 patients who had undergone endoscopic removal of pedunculated adenomatous polyps. Forty-three (5.9 percent) had polyps containing carcinoma-in-situ and 47 (6.4 percent) had polyps with carcinoma invasive through muscularis mucosae. In this latter group, 31 had a colon resection and 16 had endoscopic polypectomy only. Eight of the 31 (26 percent) had lymph nodes that contained metastatic cancer in the resected mesentery. All 31 pedunculated tumors had been resected with a segment of uninvolved stalk. The authors concluded that colonic resection must follow endoscopic polypectomy whenever invasive cancer is found. Out of the entire series, the patients in whom the cancer metastasized to the lymph nodes constituted only 1.1 percent of those studied (8 of 733). All conclusions of this study are based on descriptive statistics of clinical data from a nonrandomly selected series with no controls. Thus, conclusions are not based on the testing of an hypothesis to ascertain whether the recommended course of action resulted in enhanced survivorship of the studied population. As is documented in Chapter Ten, survivorship is independent of cancer size. Some small colorectal neoplasms with positive lymph nodes will not be cured. In a large series, some patients would experience operative mortality. End-result evaluation would have to consider both lead time and length bias. As the preceding discussion indicates, there are many questions in the man-

Table 3–1. PATIENT SYMPTOMS ATTRIBUTABLE TO POLYPOID LESIONS OF THE COLON DURING DIFFERENT PHASES OF THEIR EXISTENCE*

Symptom	Type of Polyp
None	All
Bleeding	All
Occult	All
Gross	All
Colic†	Polyps large enough to produce partial obstruction and serve as obturator for an intussusception.

*From Spratt JS Jr, Watson FR: The rationale of practice for polypoid lesions of the colon. Cancer 28:153–159, 1971.
†Primarily as symptom of partial obstruction. Large villous adenomas add to diarrhea by surface exudation and mucous production malabsorption.

Table 3–2. ADVERSE HOST EFFECTS PRODUCED BY POLYPOID LESIONS OF THE COLON*

1. Continued growth of polypoid lesion to symptom-producing size before normal life span terminates.
2. Blood loss anemia—acute and chronic.
3. Fluid and electrolyte imbalance.
4. Intussusception.
5. Partial intestinal obstruction.
6. Complete intestinal obstruction.
7. Perforation of intestine with obstruction or intussusception.
8. Polypoid lesion may be a cancer when first observed and may invade, metastasize, and shorten patient's life span.
9. Polypoid lesion may progress from a benign to a malignant state, as in:
   a. Polypoid lesions associated with familial adenomatous polyposis.
   b. Villous adenomas.
10. A benign polypoid lesion that would cause no trouble during the human life span may be incorrectly diagnosed as a cancer or precancerous condition, and the patient may suffer harm from prophylactic, diagnostic, or therapeutic effort.
11. Polypoid lesions may be part of a colonic or systemic syndrome, and host effect may be polyp dependent or syndrome dependent.
12. Surgical implantation in wound or as pseudomyxoma peritonei.
13. Time consumed in diagnosis and treatment.
14. Cost of diagnosis and treatment.

*From Spratt JS Jr, Watson FR: The rationale of practice for polypoid lesions of the colon. Cancer 28:153–159, 1971.

Table 3–3. VARIABLES INFLUENCING THE SELECTION OF DIAGNOSTIC AND THERAPEUTIC METHODS TO AVOID ADVERSE EFFECTS OF POLYPOID LESIONS*

I. Clinical management information for the following:
   A. Age-specific annual mortality for colon cancers:
      1. Arising de novo.
      2. Arising in a previous benign polypoid lesion.
   B. Age-specific incidence rates of polypoid lesions that can produce adverse host effect.
   C. False-negative diagnostic rates.
   D. False-positive diagnostic rates.
   E. Morbidity and mortality rates of diagnostic procedures.
   F. Morbidity and mortality rates of therapeutic procedures.
   G. Rate of growth by type.
   H. Critical size:
      1. Permitting diagnosis.
      2. Producing symptoms.
      3. Producing adverse effects.
   I. Age-specific person-years of life remaining.
II. Clinical skills and equipment available for a control program:
   A. Availability of safe and adequate equipment.
   B. Availability of trained personnel.
   C. Availability of a population group at risk to develop adverse effects from polypoid lesions of the colon with a frequency great enough to make economic and efficient use of equipment and trained personnel.

*From Spratt JS Jr, Watson FR: The rationale of practice for polypoid lesions of the colon. Cancer 28:153–159, 1971.

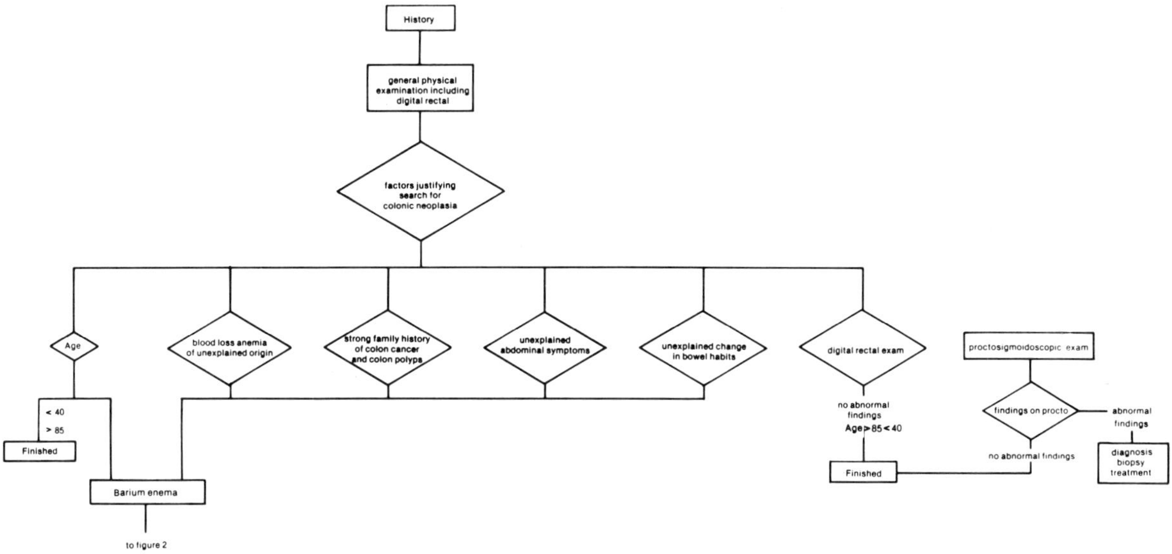

Figure 3–1. The decision-making process associated with a rationale of clinical practice that is intended to maximize patient benefit is complex and requires a logic diagram. Diagrams of this type are for the most frequent problems of colonic polyps and do not contain all the possible diagnostic, pathologic, and therapeutic variables. They should be regarded as a framework for further improvement in the logic behind the rationale of practice. Other special techniques could be integrated into these diagrams to become an established part of the rationale of practice. (From Spratt JS, Watson FR: The rationale of practice for polypoid lesions of the colon. Cancer 28:153–159, 1971.)

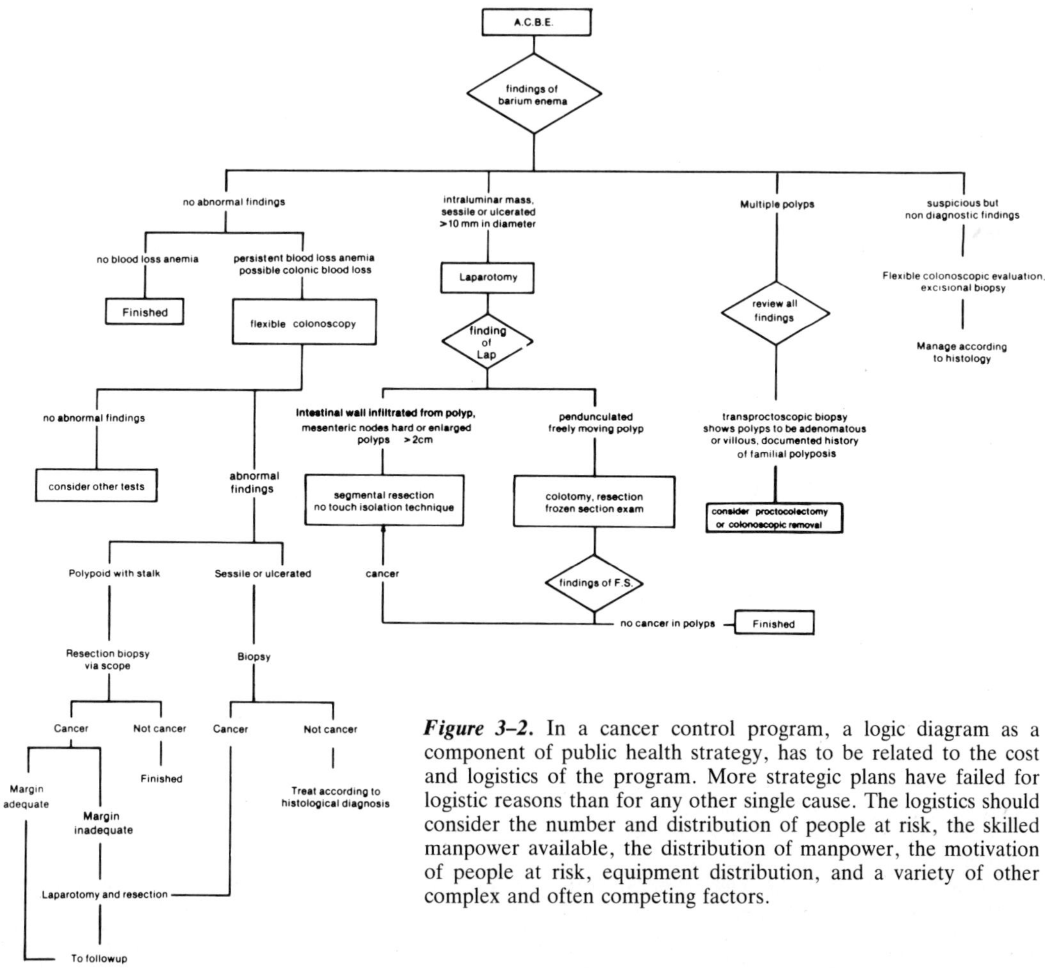

Figure 3–2. In a cancer control program, a logic diagram as a component of public health strategy, has to be related to the cost and logistics of the program. More strategic plans have failed for logistic reasons than for any other single cause. The logistics should consider the number and distribution of people at risk, the skilled manpower available, the distribution of manpower, the motivation of people at risk, equipment distribution, and a variety of other complex and often competing factors.

agement of colorectal neoplasms that can only be answered by a controlled clinical trial with prolonged follow-up.

Occasional polyps remain beyond the access of the endoscope for removal or biopsy and are of a size or shape large enough to carry a significant risk of cancer. The size and shape of these polyps often can be determined by barium enema study. If the polyp is larger than 12 mm or exhibits Welin's sign (see Chapter Two) or if an increase in size is demonstrated on a second barium enema study done 3 months later, periodic transabdominal exploration will be necessary. Welch (1964) provided an excellent review of the basic surgical techniques essential for investigation and removal of polyps transabdominally. Gentle transmural palpation of the base of the polyp and the adjacent mesentery provides much information. Invasion of the bowel wall and the presence of small *firm* lymph nodes suggest cancer. In the absence of these findings, the polyp head can be milked along the bowel, placing traction on the stalk. The serosa will be pulled in at the base of the stalk, as shown in Figure 3–3. A longitudinal colotomy opposite this point opens the bowel over the base of the pedicle. The polyp head is delivered through the colotomy, and the base of the pedicle is transected between clamps and is then suture ligated. The colotomy is then closed transversely to avoid narrowing of the bowel. While closure is in progress, the polyp is sent for frozen section examination by the pathologist. The pathologist must make at least two sections. One is through the head of the polyp to ascertain its histopathologic diagnosis. The other is made across the transected proximal end of the pedicle. If the polyp contains cancer and if the base of the pedicle is free from cancer, no further resection is required. If cancer is in the base of the pedicle, particularly if it is in the lymphatic vessels, a colonic resection should be done that is adequate for removal of the contiguous lymph node–bearing mesentery. A significant percentage of colonic cancers are nonmetastasizing (Spratt et al., 1970), and these are locally curable while small.

With the development of the flexible colonoscope, it is no longer necessary to use a rigid scope through several colotomies to examine the lumen of the entire colon to remove polyps. If a portion of the colonic lumen cannot be seen using the endoscope before laparotomy, the patient can be positioned in a modified lithotomy position so that the endoscopist can pass the flexible instrument per anus during the course of the laparotomy. The surgeon can then direct the scope and orient the en-

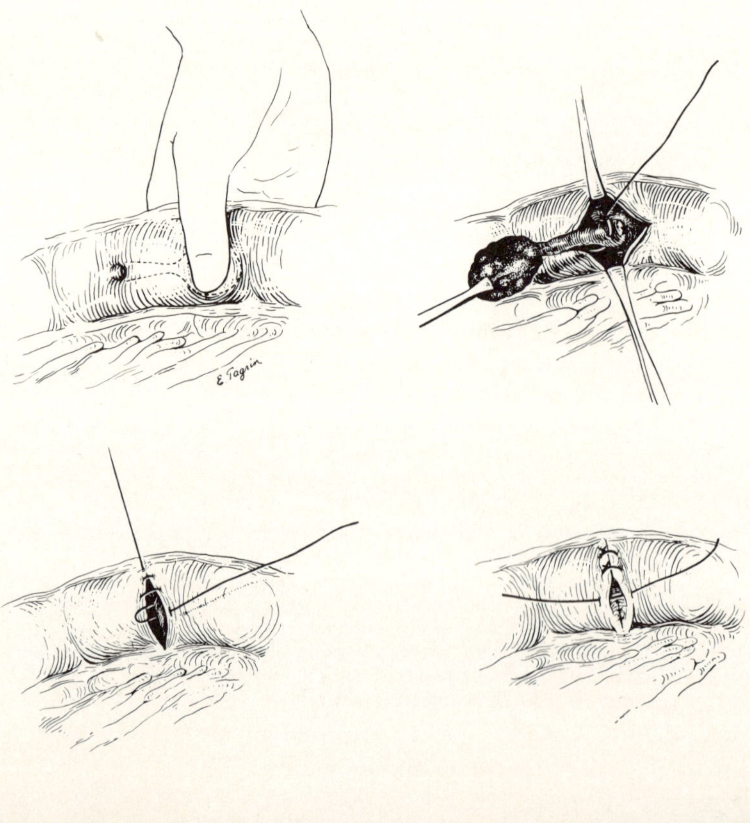

Figure 3–3. Colotomy and polypectomy. The base of the pedicle is determined by traction upward and downward. The colon is opened longitudinally, and the pedicle is doubly transfixed before excision. Coloscopy is carried out before closure, which is done in a transverse direction with two layers of sutures. (From Welch CE, Hedberg SE: Polypoid lesions of the Gastrointestinal Tract. 2nd ed. Philadelphia, W. B. Saunders Company, 1975.)

doscopist, making possible complete and rapid examination. In some cases, tumors may be biopsied or removed in this way, without opening the bowel. The great frequency of multiple primary cancers of the colon and rectum may ultimately increase the use of this technique (Polk et al., 1965).

References

Burdick D, Prior JT: Peutz-Jeghers syndrome—a clinicopathologic study of a large family with a 27-year follow-up. Cancer 50:2139–2146, 1982.

Bussey HJ, De Cosse JJ, Deschner EE, et al: A randomized trial of ascorbic acid in polyposis coli. Cancer 50:1434–1439, 1982.

Colacchio TA, Forde KA: Endoscopic polypectomy: inadequate treatment for invasive colorectal cancer. Gastrointest Endosc 27:133, 1981.

Dozois PR, Judd ES, Dahlin DC, Bartholomew LG: The Peutz-Jeghers syndrome. Arch Surg 98:509–517, 1969.

Fielding JF, Lumsden K: Large-bowel perforations in patients undergoing sigmoidoscopy and barium enema. Br Med J 1:471–473, 1973.

Horn RC Jr, Payne WA, Fine G: The Peutz-Jeghers syndrome. Arch Pathol (Chicago) 76:29–37, 1963.

Kaplan BJ: Gardner's syndrome: heredofamilial adenomatosis associated with "soft and hard" fibrous tumors and epidermoid cysts. Dis Colon Rectum 4:252–262, 1961.

Kiser JL, Spratt JS Jr, Johnson CA: Colon perforations occurring during sigmoidoscopic examinations and barium enemas. Mo Med 68:969–974, 1968.

Kopelovich L: Phenotypic markers in human skin fibroblasts as possible diagnostic indices of hereditary adenomatosis of the colon and rectum. Cancer 40:2534–2541, 1977.

Localio SA: Spontaneous disappearance of rectal polyps following subtotal colectomy and ilioproctostomy for polyposis of the colon. Am J Surg 103:81–82, 1962.

Logue T, Frommer D: The influence of oral vitamin C supplements on experimental colorectal tumour induction. Aust NZ J Med 10:588, 1980.

Polk HC Jr, Spratt JS Jr: Recurrent colorectal carcinoma: detection, treatment and other considerations. Surgery 69:9–23, 1971.

Polk HC Jr, Spratt JS Jr, Bennett D, et al: Surgical mortality and survival from colonic carcinoma. Arch Surg 89:16–23, 1964.

Polk HC Jr, Spratt JS Jr, Butcher HR Jr: Frequency of multiple primary malignant neoplasms associated with colorectal carcinoma. Am J Surg 109:71–75, 1965.

Reddy BS, Hirota N: Effect of dietary ascorbic acid on 1,2-dimethylhydrazine-induced colon cancer in rats. Fed Proc 38:174, 1979.

Riccardi VM, Mulvihill JJ (eds): Neurofibromatosis (von Recklinghausen Disease) Genetics, Cell Biology and Biochemistry, Vol 29, Advances in Neurology. New York, Raven Press, 1981.

Scully RE: Sex cord tumors with annular tubules: A distinctive ovarian tumor with Peutz-Jeghers syndrome. Cancer 25:1107–1121, 1970.

Smith WG: Desmoid tumors in familial multiple polyposis. Proc Staff Meetings Mayo Clin 34:31–38, 1959.

Smith WG, Jackman RJ: Results of treatment in familial multiple polyposis. Proc Staff Meetings Mayo Clin 31:304–308, 1956.

Sperling D, Spratt JS Jr, Carnes VM: Adenocarcinoma of the large intestine with perforation. Mo Med 60:1104–1107, 1963.

Spratt JS Jr: The rates and patterns of growth of neoplasms of the large intestine and rectum. Surg Clin N Am 45:1103–1115, 1965.

Spratt JS Jr: Cancer detection: curability of symptomatic and advanced cancers. Cancer Bull 21:7–14, 1969.

Spratt JS Jr: The measurement of the value of the clinical process to individuals by age and income. J Trauma 11:966–973, 1971.

Spratt JS Jr, Ackerman LV: Relationship of the size of colonic tumors to their cellular composition and biological behavior. Surg Forum 10:56–61, 1960a.

Spratt JS Jr, Ackerman LV: Treatment of polyps of the colon as benign lesions. Curr Surg Management 37:37–41, 1960b.

Spratt JS Jr, Ackerman LV: The growth of a colonic adenocarcinoma. Am Surg 27:23–28, 1961.

Spratt JS Jr, Ackerman LV: Small primary adenocarcinomas of the colon and rectum. JAMA 179:337–346, 1962.

Spratt JS Jr, Ackerman LV: Colonic cancer and colonic polyps. Hosp Med 1:4–8, 1964.

Spratt JS Jr, Ackerman LV, Moyer CA: Relationship of polyps of the colon to colonic cancer. Ann Surg 148:682–698, 1958.

Spratt JS Jr, Spjut HJ: Prevalence and prognosis of individual clinical and pathologic variables associated with colorectal carcinoma. Cancer 20:1976–1985, 1967.

Spratt JS Jr, Watson FR: The rationale of practice for polypoid lesions of the colon. Cancer 28:153–159, 1971.

Spratt JS Jr, Watson FR, Pratt JL: Characteristics of variants of colorectal carcinoma that does not metastasize to lymph nodes. Dis Colon Rectum 13:243–246, 1970.

Staley CJ, Schwarz H II: Gastrointestinal polyposis and pigmentation of the oral mucosa (Peutz-Jeghers syndrome). Surg Gynecol Obstet 105:1–15, 1957.

Watne AL: Syndromes of polyposis coli and cancer. Curr Probl Cancer 7:1–31, 1982.

Waugh JM, Harp RA, Spencer RJ: The surgical management of multiple polyposis. Ann Surg 159:149–154, 1964.

Welch CE: Polypoid Lesions of the Gastrointestinal Tract. Philadelphia, WB Saunders Company, 1964.

Welin S, Youker J, Spratt JS Jr, et al: The rates and patterns of growth of 375 tumors of the large intestine and rectum observed serially by double contrast enema study (Malmö technique). AJR 90:673–687, 1963.

Williams RD, Fish JC: Multiple polyposis, polyp regression, and carcinoma of the colon. Am J Surg 112:846–849, 1966.

FOUR

Screening and Follow-up

J. S. Spratt, M.D.
H. C. Polk, M.D.

SCREENING

Screening is the use of intervention techniques to discover asymptomatic cancers or precancerous conditions. Ideally, the yield of discoveries by these techniques can be increased by screening higher risk groups. Screening involves a very complex decision-making process, with rapid branching of actions. A typical screening model is shown in Figure 4–1. This branching model is an "unbounded horizon" in the mathematics of operations research. Partially as a result of the complexity of the screening problem and the very long time periods of population monitoring required to exclude sources of lead time and length bias, no really satisfactory studies have yet been done in the form of a controlled clinical trial establishing what screening strategy ensures the optimum survivorship free of colorectal cancer obtainable at a tolerable cost and risk.

The desire with any screening effort is to detect a cancer immediately after it is large enough to be found by the detection method employed, but before it disseminates beyond the region of origin. When dissemination beyond the resectable region occurs, the cancer is no longer curable by resection of bowel and the contiguous lymph node–bearing mesentery. This segment of time in the life history of a cancer is referred to as the cancer control window (Fig. 4–2) (Spratt, 1982). The duration of this window is primarily determined by the net rate of growth of the cancer and the size at which it disseminates. The threshold size of detection is dependent upon the limits of the diagnostic method used and the anatomic location, shape, and size of the cancer. The extreme natural variance in the growth rates of colorectal cancers and of the size at dissemination (terminal size) results in extreme variance in the duration of the cancer control window. The longer the interval between screenings, the higher the probability that screening will detect indolent neoplasms, resulting in length bias in the measurement of end results. The more acute, and presumably more lethal, cancers surface in the intervals between screenings. Thus, the longer the interval between screenings, the greater the number of interval-surfacing cancers. With this bias, the more favorable slow growing cancers are picked up at the screenings (Spratt, 1982). Thus, any controlled clinical trial intended to determine the optimum screening strategy would have to monitor *all* the cancers in a defined population occurring during a period of time long enough so that these groups can be differentiated. Follow-up would be required for the period necessary to rule out lead-time bias in comparing end results.

In identifying optimum screening strategies, it is not inhumane to look more realistically at an individual's potential longevity and the dollar resources society can allot. The census data have been translated into person-days of residual life by age and sex (Fig. 4–3). The issues associated with gain in survivorship are very complex in the fields of theoretic public health planning and health economics. The issues involve many considerations at a "macro" level; screening in clinical practice involves more considerations at a "micro" level. At this level the controlled clinical trial remains the major tool for evaluating impact. In either

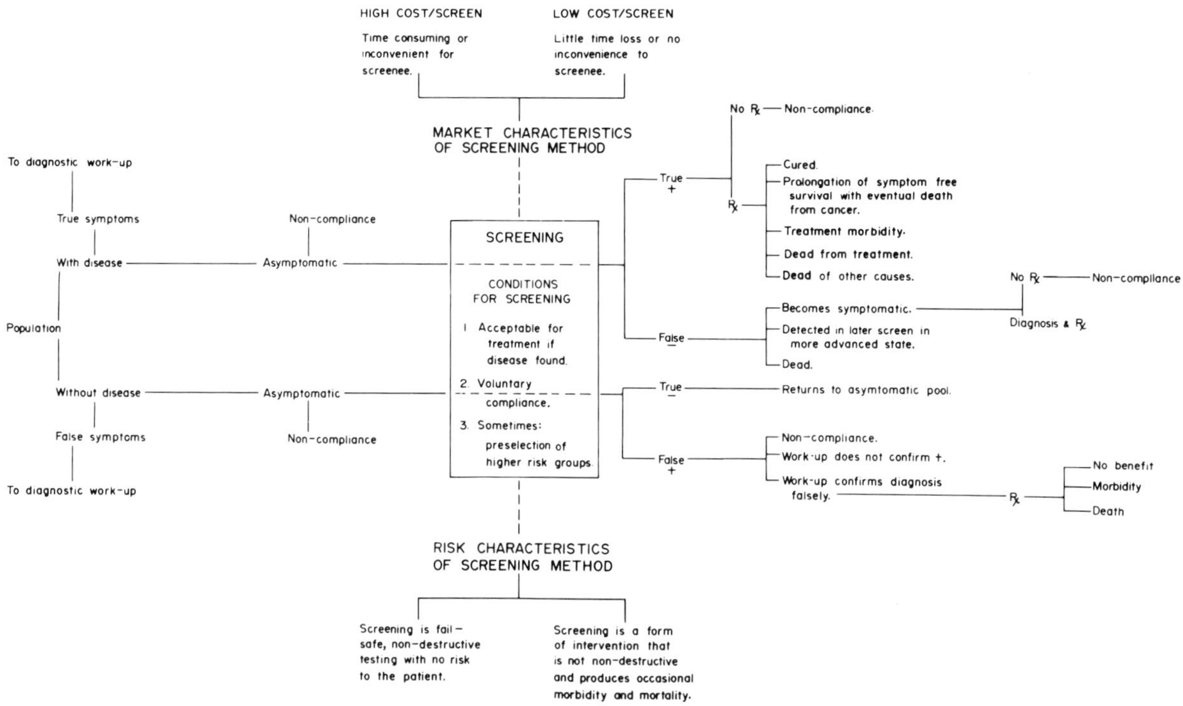

Figure 4–1. Flow diagram of representative decisions and outcomes existing in any screening program. Quality control at many points is essential to the reduction of errors. The existence of effective treatment determines the ultimate benefit of screening. A controlled clinical trial is generally essential to test hypotheses on the benefit of screening. (From Spratt JS Jr: Epidemiology of screening for cancer. *In* Hickey RC, et al (eds): Current Problems in Cancer. Copyright © 1982 by Year Book Medical Publishers, Inc., Chicago. Reprinted with permission.)

case, the limits of potential gain, i.e., the average number of days of useful life remaining according to age, sex, and ethnicity must be appreciated (see Fig. 4–3). Similar financial limits exist on the dollars that can be effectively spent in screening. At a macro level the issues concern the allocation of all health dollars and the ranking of the competitive priorities in terms of the potential gain from screening. Just "finding a cancer" or a precancerous condition does not confirm that screening, per se, enhances survivorship. For cancers with negative "cancer control windows," enhanced survivorship from screening is not possible. For other cancers, the presence of lead-time bias must be excluded by a controlled study before the conclusion can be drawn that screening and earlier discovery are responsible for enhanced survivorship (Spratt, 1981). When this cannot be shown, high-cost screening programs may have no public health value. When it can be shown, high costs for screening may be totally justifiable because of reduced treatment morbidity or costs, or enhanced survivorship.

The data generally support arguments that the strategies must be directed at optimizing the number of functional person-days an individual has remaining according to age and sex (Spratt, 1975a and b). This optimization has to come about within a cost framework that is surprisingly restrictive on the average. Not only is the determination of the cost effectiveness of public health screening complicated but also screening is only part of the process.

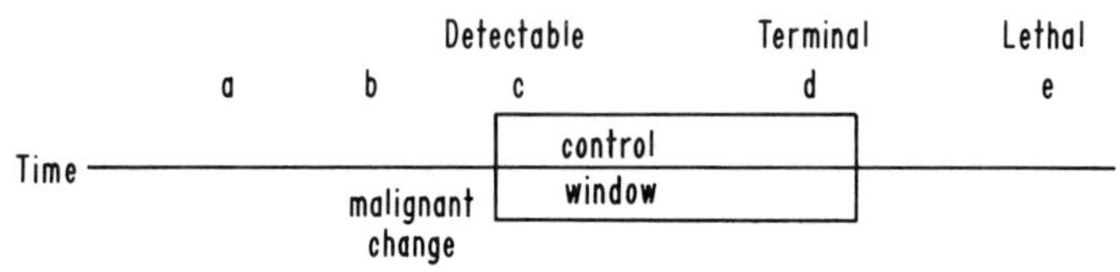

Figure 4–2. The "cancer control window" is the variable time segment in the life history of a cancer between the time cancer is large enough to detect (c) and the time it becomes terminal (d). At (a), the host is exposed to a cancer "starter" or carcinogen, and at (b), the malignant change is well established. The duration of intervals is highly variable, probably because of variations in growth rates and the sensitivity of screening methods. When dissemination (d) occurs before the cancer is large enough to detect (c), the cancer control window is negative and effective screening is not possible. (From Spratt JS Jr: Epidemiology of screening for cancer. *In* Hickey RC, et al (eds): Current Problems in Cancer. Copyright © 1982 by Year Book Medical Publishers, Inc, Chicago. Reprinted with permission.)

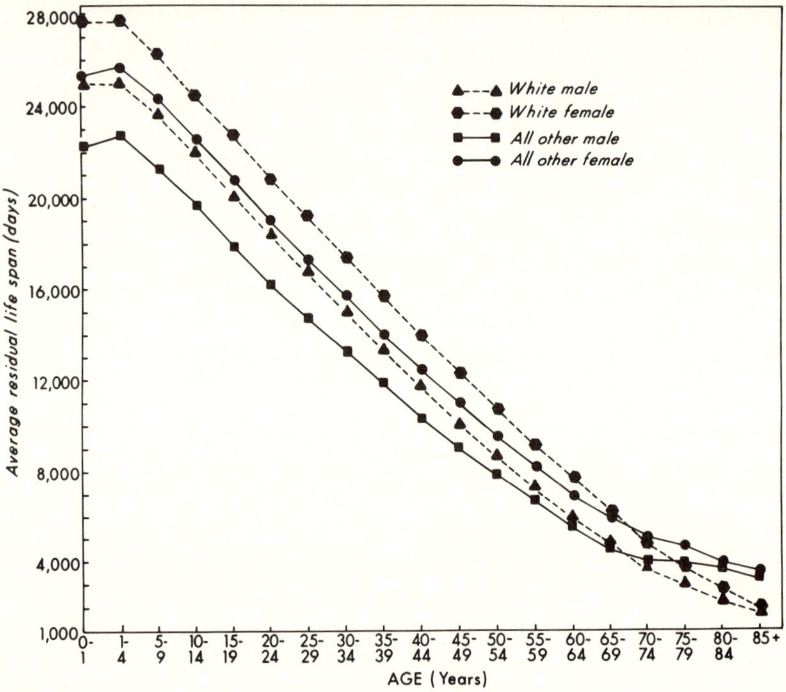

Figure 4–3. The average age-specific residual life-span (in days). (From Spratt JS: The relation of "human capital" preservation to health costs. Am J Econ Soc 34:295–307, 1975.)

Good screening has to be coupled with effective therapy and rehabilitation to be of any value.

The screening model for colorectal cancers by Thompson and Jacob (1977) led to the following conclusions: The age for screening and the number of screenings in a lifetime depend on the measure of screening effectiveness. The planners of screening programs would have to determine the objectives that they want the screenings to achieve and then consult the nomograms in Thompson and Jacob's work. For example, the optimum number of spaced lifetime proctosigmoidoscopic examinations beginning at age 40 is somewhere between five and ten. The value of occult blood measurements still has not been assessed adequately because of the lack of good data on false-negative and false-positive results and the duration of preclinical disease. The costs of screening and diagnosing should be outweighed by the reduction in treatment cost for earlier diagnosis and in wages lost through premature death. These cost measures are obviously sensitive to lead-time and length bias. Finally, Thompson and Jacob's model confirms that an improved base of data was needed, with accepted objectives of screening, in order to give further refinement to policies. The authors noted that even the best policies may fall short of what may be achieved with available equipment, skilled manpower, and public compliance.

The barium contrast enema study, although not a screening test, remains the primary diagnostic modality for confirming colonic lesions. Yet, frequently the clinical significance of a study is minimal because of inadequate colon preparation prior to the examination. The frequency of false-positive results of routine barium contrast enema examinations has been reported as 17 per cent in 230 consecutive patients who underwent endoscopy for removal of specific roentgenographically identified polypoid colon lesions (Knutson et al., 1979; Knutson and Max, 1980). The inaccuracy of these pre-endoscopic barium contrast enema studies was shown by postendoscopic air contrast roentgenography in colons that were physically clean, as demonstrated by endoscopic examination, following a 2-day colon preparation, as discussed in Chapters Five and Six. These results suggest that more emphasis on a 2-day colon preparation before the initial barium contrast enema would significantly reduce the frequency of false-positive results and minimize the need for repeat contrast studies and needless colonoscopic examinations (Knutson et al., 1979). In the case of colorectal neoplasms, there have already been several studies that relate morphologic findings to both prognosis and growth rates (Spratt and Spjut, 1967; Wagner, 1974) and that are relevant to the modeling of the natural history of colorectal cancers. The methods for and results of high-quality barium enema studies are discussed in Chapter Five.

A major argument for the further development of an optimum lifetime colorectal screening strategy is that small nonmetastasizing colorectal cancers are often locally curable, have a slow growth rate associated with a long cancer control window, and if allowed to progress, are known to produce costly, morbid, and catastrophic events such as obstruction, hemorrhage, perforation, transserosal implantation, and invasion, all of which may be preventable by earlier treatment (Spratt et al., 1970). The prevention of these complicating factors could be a justification for screening, even in the absence of enhanced survivorship.

In 1978, Barrows and associates developed a method for reducing the risk of false-positive and false-negative results, when testing for occult blood in the stool in hopes of increasing the specificity of more complicated screening methods. Previous tests have been sensitive to hemoglobin, regardless of the animal source. Thus, mass screening for occult blood has been both cumbersome and expensive because abstention from meat for the time necessary to clear the gastrointestinal tract of exogenously ingested hemoglobin was essential to reduce false-positive results. The earlier tests generally used peroxidase oxidation of chemical indicators such as guaiac and benzidine.

Barrows and co-workers (1978) developed an immunochemical test for human blood in feces using goat antibodies to hemoglobin. When used in radial immunodiffusion, the test is not complicated by cross reaction with common foods or other nonhemorrhagic fecal constituents. This method provides a lower limit of sensitivity for hemoglobin in stool samples of 10 mg per 100 ml. The threshold for the peroxidase methods is 100 mg per 100 ml in stool.

In clinical trials in humans, no cross reactivity between species has been demonstrated (Songster et al., 1980). The minimum of hemoglobin detected was 0.5 mg per gm of stool. Neither dietary constituents, drugs, nor chemicals interfered with the results. In the first clinical trial, 29 percent of the patients with known cancer exhibited no bleeding by either Hemoccult test or Barrow's method. In patients with known cancer, trace bleeding was detected by the Hemoccult test (40 percent) and by the immunochemical method (64 percent). The immunochemical method was ten times more sensitive than the Hemoccult test and gave complete specificity.

This unique and very promising approach needs to be developed further to become accessible at a reasonable cost. Even after perfection of the methodology, the applied research for determining its optimum use pattern remains to be defined by clinical trials establishing that host survivorship will be enhanced through earlier diagnosis. The major advantage of the test is its greatly reduced false-positive rate.

Knutson and Max (1980) determined that rectal blood loss can serve as an indication for a second phase in screening. They identified a consecutive series of patients who had rectal blood loss but who had examinations with negative findings, using a 25-cm proctoscope and a standard barium enema. This group of 168 patients was encouraged to undergo colonoscopic examination. Of these, 139 patients (83 percent) were so examined and 110 had the total colon examined to the cecum. A total of 41 unsuspected lesions were detected in 35 patients (21 percent), including nine cancers (22 percent), two of the cancers being in one patient. Lesions ranged in size from less than 1 cm to as large as 2.9 cm. Proof of the significance of this approach in terms of improved survivorship requires a controlled trial. The high number of cancer cases found approaches the prevalence rate noted at autopsy and is reviewed in Chapter One. The first question to be answered in a trial would be, What is the age-specific prevalence of lesions in people with no rectal blood loss? Proof of enhanced survivorship by such a program would again necessitate a randomized clinical trial. The extremely slow growth rates of many benign and malignant colonic neoplasms (Welin et al., 1963) makes these lead-time and length-bias considerations of major importance in evaluating enhanced survivorship. This is particularly true in the very elderly (see Chapter One).

In 1978, Eddy conducted a thorough study that required programming a simulation model of the complex problem of screening and searching the literature thoroughly for quality clinical data that could be used in the model. The conclusions of his study led to the modification of guidelines for screening endorsed by the American Cancer Society (Eddy, 1980). He concluded that men and women over 50 years should have the stools tested for occult blood annually. This same group should have a sigmoidoscopic examination every 3 to 5 years after two initial examinations with negative findings 1 year apart. Eddy (1979a) provides considerable background research and analysis to justify these seemingly simple guidelines.

As Neuhauser (1979) noted, the major advantage of a good model is that it forces people to test assumptions. If the model is correct, many different assumptions can be tested against it. All models ultimately should raise the following questions:

1. How confident are we that the intervention benefits patients?

2. Is the intervention cost effective when compared with other interventions?

The Achilles' heel of many screening strategies is the false-positive rate and the lead-time bias. Neuhauser credits Dales (1974) with observing that of all the diseases for which screening has been provided, only two have shown a significant reduction in mortality—hypertension and colon cancer. Neuhauser considered these results encouraging but was not totally convinced that there was a cause-and-effect relationship.

The results of and methods for radiologic screening and diagnosis of primary colorectal cancers are provided in Chapter Five of this text.

FOLLOW-UP

Follow-up is a special screening problem for a high-risk group. For many years, follow-up after treatment of cancer was considered by the Commission on Cancer of the American College of Surgeons as being highly desirable in patient care and necessary for College approval of a hospital cancer program. For years, follow-up was primarily associated with cancer registries. It generated the information for many end-result studies and accessioned data useful for longitudinal audits of cancer patient management. Problems were managed as they were encountered. In time, a number of new factors became molded into policy for complete follow-up (frequency, types of exam, etc.) and became solidified in *The Patient with Cancer: Guidelines for Follow-up,* published by the Commission on Cancer of the American College of Surgeons in 1976. Although the recommendations represented the consensus of experienced clinicians from multiple disciplines, many of the recommendations were not supported by controlled clinical trials or models that could define optimum follow-up strategies nor did they emphasize the essential importance of effective patient and family education.

The patient, the health care institutions, and the physician all can benefit from patient education. Instruction may reduce readmission days, provide more informed and cooperative patients, accelerate rehabilitation, allow a more effective use of staff time, and remove some of the burden of patient teaching from already overworked physicians (Monaco et al., 1972). It also may facilitate postdischarge management of treatments and conditions to which the patient and his or her family must adapt and, when well planned and executed, can reduce errors of omission in communication.

Levoy (1966) provided a different but relevant perspective of benefits accruing to the physician as a result of a planned program of patient education. He viewed the services provided by physicians (e.g., knowledge, skill, and experience) as intangible and believed that most physicians take for granted that patients appreciate these skills. Levoy proposed that the patient without education sees "fees" rather than "value," "time or lack of it" rather than "results," and "disinterest" rather than "more benefits for me." A planned patient education program both preoperatively and as an integral part of postoperative rehabilitation and follow-up helps correct this perception and benefits both patient and physician.

Patient education in follow-up is particularly relevant in regard to an important biologic characteristic of cancer. The extreme variance in the growth rates of human cancers ensures that any follow-up system based solely on examinations at arbitrary intervals will potentially result in a significant number of cases lost to cancer due to the failure to detect recurrent disease while it is possibly retreatable but before it is terminal. For slower growing recurrent cancers, earlier diagnosis in follow-up may introduce a lead-time bias. For acute cancers, arbitrary intervals may be associated with high-interval recurrence rates. Thus, determining optimum intervals for post-treatment follow-up examinations is a very important area for applied research.

At any clinic, the demands of follow-up can exceed institutional resources. Follow-up that is not cost-effective can add greatly to the economic morbidity of cancer without improving outcome. This first became a subject of study for me (J.S.S.) when the Ellis Fischel State Cancer Hospital (EFSCH) faced a serious problem. The staff was effectively striving to maintain a 100 percent follow-up to death on all diagnosed cancer patients. The thousands of patients who came to the EFSCH each year from all parts of Missouri for follow-up simply exceeded the capacity of the staff and the facilities to accommodate them. The directors of ambulance services and other agents providing transportation from across the state complained about the cost, travel, and waiting time. Several questions needed answers: Could some of the follow-up be done in the community? How did the hospital staff determine the value of the follow-up *to the patient?* What categories of cancer cases benefit from follow-up and how often must they be evaluated? How should patients in these categories be examined so that they derive this benefit? Does the timely discovery of recurrences, metastases, and new primary tumors result in benefit to the patient? If discovery is beneficial, how can the greatest benefit be achieved at tolerable cost? How frequently should follow-up examinations be performed, and what elements of the examination provide information of ultimate benefit to the patient? What elements of follow-up are traditional and encyclopedic only? When is follow-up no longer necessary? (Spratt, 1971).

The logistics of the problem were not those of individual private office practice nor those of a voluntary general hospital. The logistics were related to the provision of a beneficial follow-up system at a tolerable cost for over 10 percent of the cancer population of a state with over 69,686 square miles and over 4 million people. The health planning challenge was to show that the follow-up effort was measurably beneficial to the citizens of the state at a realistic cost. The political decision makers were aware that economic observers were studying the utility value of different types of medical efforts (Harris, 1963; Fortune, 1970; Spratt, 1969). Tradition and professional opinion were not acceptable bases for cost justification.

The economic problem was immediate at the EFSCH, since the follow-up system had to be designed for a hospital with a legislatively fixed appropriation, whose budget could not be increased by charging for more frequent patient-physician contact or special laboratory and roentgenographic studies. In fact, without a plan for systematic follow-up, all fiscal resources could have been expended with little measurable benefit. The problem was to determine the utility value by answering, "How many person-years of productive life and how much comfort and function are added to a population as a result of follow-up?" Follow-up screening after treatment can be justified only on the basis of patient benefit, such as is the case with primary screening and treatment.

The data available for study included 39,526 records of cancer patients seen consecutively at the EFSCH from 1940 to 1960, with complete end-results data. Some of these patients had multiple neoplasms. All were legal residents of the state of Missouri. They composed about 10 percent of the expected cancer cases of the state and came from lower economic strata. Seventy-five percent were still residents of the county in which they were born. All case records were maintained in a unit file. They were all typed except for in-patient progress notes and contained complete medical and social histories; records of physical examinations; all laboratory, surgical, pathologic, and roentgenographic examination results; records of all follow-up examinations and autopsy reports, and documentations of death. The completeness of the records made accurate retrospective clinical management reviews more reliable than is often possible. The data had the shortcomings of selection bias, no controls, and variable clinic practices. The total number of cancers occurring among these 39,526 persons was 92,693, an arithmetic mean of 2.3+ cancers per patient. Many of these were skin cancers.

In studying the follow-up system that existed before 1961, the interval-recurrence rate was determined for different categories of cancer not cured by primary therapy. This was done by dividing the number of persons alive and free of gross neoplasms at the beginning of successive monthly intervals into the number of persons who developed symptomatic recurrences during the succeeding month. These interval rates were then matched to the existing follow-up system. Some gross disparities were found. In general, patients had been seen too infrequently during the first several post-treatment years when the interval recurrence rate is highest and too frequently after the third year. In the case of cancer of the cervix uteri treated by radiation therapy, an international survey of all institutions reporting results to the League of Nations was conducted, and this disparity was found to be rather general (Gary et al., 1964).

Sensitive prognostic indicators that were measurable at the time of initial therapy increased the likelihood of predicting recurrences (Polk and Spratt, 1979; Spratt, 1969; Welin et al., 1963). Studies have been made of the prodromal symptoms and signs of recrudescent cancer, which can be used for educating patients in self-surveillance and for follow-up histories. The development of pain is one of the most reliable indicators of recrudescence. The seven danger signals of cancer are also useful. Few laboratory studies in the period studied outweighed, in availability and effectiveness, the value of a careful interval history and physical examination coupled with self evaluation by an educated patient.

The studies on follow-up were also addressed to the efficacy of retreatment as a basis for establishing the value of follow-up in detecting treatable recrudescent neoplasms (Gilbertson, 1974; Lee et al., 1978; Polk and Spratt, 1971, 1979; Spratt et al., 1965, 1970; Spratt, 1967; Waggoner and Spratt, 1969). The question was to determine in whom the timely discovery of recrudescent cancer was succeeded by efficacious therapy that kept the follow-up effort from being an exercise in futility. When retreatment is effective and the benefits of retreatment are dependent on earlier diagnosis of recurrence, a follow-up schedule that is designed for most frequent and systematic patient examination is essential during those intervals when the recurrence rate is highest.

At the time these studies were done, the sole forms of effective treatment, both for primary and recidivated cancer, were surgery and radiotherapy. When chemotherapy is an adjuvant of proved value for colorectal cancers, a need exists for an accurate assessment of prognosis at the time of primary treatment. The subsets of patients at high risk for recidivation should be the major candidates for adjuvant treatment. For these patients, the follow-up program requires modification to monitor the value of adjuvant treatment.

Without reviewing all the studies done on the EFSCH population, the works confirmed the efficacy of retreatment of locally recrudescent cancer by additional surgery or radiotherapy, or both, and treatment of metastases in the liver, lung, lymph nodes, brain, and skin. The studies suggested that, in many cases, the opportunity for effective additional treatment could be lost by a delay in diagnosis. The ability to diagnose metastatic cancer while the total mass of residual neoplasm is at the threshold of diagnostic sensitivity may also prove of great importance in assuring the efficacy of various forms of chemotherapy. The objective of clinical management is to produce protracted periods of symptom-free survival by the methods most tolerable to the host from the standpoint of morbidity, time, and cost. Ideally, the total mass of neoplastic tissue must be kept below a symptom-producing size during these periods of symptom-free survival (Spratt, 1975a).

Frequency of Multiple Primary Cancers

Another traditional argument in favor of follow-up that was investigated was based on the belief that a person who has had a cancer is more likely to develop additional primary neoplasms than a person without a prior history of cancer. The frequency of simultaneous and nonsimultaneous multiple primary tumors was studied as a function of age, anatomic site of the cancers, and other demographic characteristics of the patient (Cook, 1966; Spratt, 1977). Basically, all people are subject to cancer with an incidence that increases exponentially with aging. The observed age-specific incidence rates can account for the development of one cancer in 51.6 percent, 2 cancers in 17.5 percent, and 3 cancers in 5.9 percent of the population living to age 90, without there being any host-specific predisposition to multiple cancers (Spratt and Hoag, 1966). In the case of specific sites, there are a few exceptions (Cook, 1966). Aside from these site-specific associations, one may ask whether the usefulness of following cancer patients to detect new primary tumors warrants preferential examinations of former cancer patients compared with the general population (Spratt and Hoag, 1966; Spratt, 1977).

In 1977, Schoenberg and Myers refined the patient-years-at-risk approach to search for significant fluctuations in the incidence of multiple primary cancers in Connecticut Cancer Registry data (Schoenberg, 1977). Collectively, the risk of an additional cancer in a person previously treated for cancer was about 1.29 times greater than in a population with no cancers. This predisposition was highly selective and not greatly different from the Missouri conclusions (see Table 4–1).

Detection of Recurrent Cancer

Later, Polk and Spratt (1971, 1983) provided a study (1) to determine the value of follow-

Table 4–1. **SIGNIFICANT ASSOCIATIONS OF ANATOMIC SITES DEVELOPING CANCERS IN THE SAME INDIVIDUAL—MULTIPLE PRIMARIES***

Site of One Primary Cancer	Site of Additional Primary Cancer
Endometrium	Breast
Hodgkin's	Soft Tissue
Larynx	Lung
Lip	Skin
Mouth	Esophagus
Ovary	Endometrium
Pharynx	Esophagus
Prostate	Urinary Bladder
Soft Tissue	Lymphoid Tissue
Tongue	Esophagus
Vagina	Endometrium
Vulva	Cervix

*Adapted from Spratt JS: Epidemiology of screening for cancer. Curr Probl Cancer 6:1–58, 1982.

up examinations in the detection and timely treatment of carcinomas of the colon and rectum that recur after resection intended for cure and (2) to evaluate the efficacy of the various methods of treatment of recurrent cancer. The contention was that follow-up examinations are expensive and time consuming; they should be scheduled to permit the timely discovery of those neoplasms not controlled by primary therapy. Any additional treatment should offer a chance for control of the recurrent cancer in some instances, and added duration of comfortable life in others. Discovery of complications arising from initial therapy and palliation of symptomatic but incurable carcinoma were considered additional justifications for follow-up examinations.

Problems were to determine (1) the time elapsing between resection intended for cure and the detection of recurrent carcinomas, (2) the signs and symptoms of recurrent cancer, and (3) the efficacy of additional treatment.

The group of cases reported by Spratt and Spjut in 1967, reviewed in detail in Chapter Ten, was the base population first studied (Polk and Spratt, 1971). Of the 1141 patients observed, 386 (34 percent) underwent resection thought to be curative. The clinic follow-up schedule employed was empirical according to the personal experience of the clinical staff, dictated in part by transportation problems and the availability of professional staff for follow-up examinations. The patients were asked to return to the hospital for examination at three- to six-month intervals, somewhat more frequently in the first 3 years after operation than subsequently. Variably, thoracic roentgenograms, fecal examinations for occult blood, barium enema studies, and/or intravenous pyelograms were obtained in addition to an interval history and a generally thorough physical examination. The interval between barium enema studies, for example, varied from 3 months to 2 years if ordered at all. As far as can be determined, this was the first systematic study of recurrent colorectal carcinomas for the purposes of designing a more efficacious follow-up program.

All carcinomas recidive after resection intended for cure were defined as recurrent. Gross persistence was precluded by limiting material to those patients having resections thought curative by the operating surgeon. In this report, recurrence was established by the presence of neoplasm, confirmed by biopsy, celiotomy, or autopsy examination. Probable recurrence was determined by way of roentgenographic or clinical (e.g., palpable abdominal mass) signs only. These were not confirmed to be cancer by histopathologic examination. The subsequent courses of patients with recurrent cancer determined by clinical assessment only were compatible with those of the group whose recurrences were confirmed histologically. The clinical courses and median survival time after detection of recurrent carcinoma did not differ significantly whether the disease was classified as certainly or probably recurrent.

By December 31, 1962, recurrent colorectal carcinoma had developed in 121 of the 386 patients who had been subjected to resection intended for cure (Table 4–2). Twelve patients were found to harbor "recurrent" carcinoma on their first postoperative visit, which took place 1 to 11 months after resection. Sixty-five percent of all recurrences had been detected by the end of the second postresection year, and 88 percent were noted by the completion of the fourth year after operation (Polk and

Table 4–2. **FOLLOW-UP STATUS: RESECTION INTENDED FOR CURE***

Patient Status After Resection	Total	Recurrent
Alive and free of cancer	138	4
Died after first operation	25	—
Lost to follow-up	1	—
Alive, status unknown	26	4
Alive with colorectal cancer	2	2
Dead from colorectal cancer	108	108
Dead from other cancer	12	2
Dead of cause other than cancer	19	1
Dead, status unknown	55	—
Total	386	121

*Adapted from Polk HC Jr, Spratt JS Jr: Recurrent colorectal carcinoma: Detection, treatment and other considerations. Surgery 69:9–23, 1971.

Spratt, 1971). The interval recurrence rate was calculated by dividing the number of patients at risk for each time interval into the number of patients developing recurrent carcinoma in that interval. When calculated on a monthly basis, peak interval recurrence rates corresponded precisely with the 3- to 6-month intervals commonly scheduled for re-examinations. However, when the interval recurrence rates were computed, 13 percent of those at risk were found to have recurrent cancer in the first year and 9 percent in the following year (see Fig 22–1, page 410.) On the other hand, if the 12 individuals in whom cancer was discovered on their first postoperative visit were excluded as having de facto persistent cancer, then the interval recurrence rates for the first 2 years approximated 10 percent. The interval recurrence rates for the third and fourth years after operation were similar to each other, but only about half that of the first 2 years (i.e., 5 percent). After the 48th month, the annual recurrence rate remained about 2 percent per annum.

If one accepts an interval recurrence rate of 2 percent as sufficient to justify examination, follow-up examinations should be performed about every 2 months in the first postoperative year, every 3 months in the second year, every 6 months in the third and fourth years, and annually thereafter. Obviously, beyond the end of the 48th month, patient education as to signs and symptoms of recrudescent neoplasm becomes the major method of detection of the infrequent late recurrence. Every patient must be educated and motivated to obtain an earlier examination should any suggestive signs or symptoms appear. Patients in this category with new complaints merit immediate evaluation by a physician.

Neoplasms remaining quiescent longer are thought to be associated with longer patient survival after detection of recurrence by virtue of more favorable biologic behavior, possibly leading to prolonged untreated host survival or improved responsiveness to retreatment. However, plotting the time that elapsed between primary resection and detection of recurrence against subsequent length of survival resulted in a random scatter of points, indicating no correlation between these two variables in the studied population.

Pathologic Examination

The effects of many pathologic characteristics upon host survival in this cancer population are reviewed in Chapters Nine and Ten. Those patients who developed recurrent cancer were analyzed with respect to these pathologic characteristics and were compared with those who remained free of cancer. Table 4–3 illustrates the significant differences that existed between those patients free of cancer and those developing recurrent neoplasms whose operations were initially performed at EFSCH. The previously described adverse effects of infiltrating elements in the tumor margins, regional lymph node metastases, absence of inflammatory response about the primary carcinoma, and limited excisions of regional lymph node–bearing tissue were confirmed (Spratt and Spjut, 1967).

Separate analyses as to the elapsed time between resection and detection of recurrence in the groups of patients found to have these unfavorable characteristics were not done. However, those individuals with infiltrating elements in the tumor margins or with no inflammatory response about the primary carcinoma, or with both, who did develop recurrent cancer did so locally and within 18 months of resection (89 percent cumulative recurrence as opposed to 52 percent for all recurrences). Because of the propensity for rapid, and often local, recurrence of cancer among that population whose resected neoplasms bear these unfavorable pathologic characteristics, this group warrants more frequent early follow-up examinations than the curative resection group as a whole. This group would also form the most logical subset for participation in controlled clinical trials intended to evaluate the effectiveness of surgical adjuvant treatments.

The initial symptoms of recurrent colorectal carcinoma were so nonspecific that they contributed to delayed diagnosis in many patients. However, some patterns were sufficiently repetitive to warrant description. Dull, aching perineal discomfort, aggravated by sitting, preceded detectable recurrence by 1 to 9 months in 16 of 20 individuals developing recurrent carcinoma in the perineal scar after abdominoperineal resection. Every patient with these perineal symptoms developed recurrent adenocarcinoma in or about the perineal scar or in the presacral space. Although the charts of these patients known to be free of cancer were not re-examined in detail for "false-positive" perineal pain, those remaining free of perineal recurrence after abdominoperineal resection did not complain of perineal discomfort after the healing of the wound.

Of those individuals initially treated by resection and anastomosis, gross bleeding from

Table 4–3. **PATHOLOGIC DETERMINANTS OF PATIENT SURVIVAL***

Characteristics	Patients		P
	Recurrence (A)	*Well (B)*†	*A = B*
Tumor margin—mixed‡	63/103	69/138	0.050§
Nodal metastases—absent	86/100	129/137	0.035
Inflammatory response—absent	16/96	9/133	0.020
Tumor margin—infiltrating	62/90	40/83	0.007
Nodes resected—six	37/100	10/84	0.005

*Adapted from Polk HC Jr, Spratt JS Jr: Recurrent colorectal carcinoma: Detection, treatment and other considerations. Surgery 69:9–23, 1971.

†In Group B (well patients), tests for significance were applied to the 5-year survivors initially and then to all patients free of cancer at the close of this study if the differences were of borderline significance upon the first determination.

‡Margin contains both pushing and infiltrating elements.

§Null hypothesis rejected at 0.05 level or less: The frequency of the characteristic is the same among those who developed recurrent colorectal carcinoma (A) as among those who remained well (B).

the rectum or melena was noted by 12 of the 15 who developed recurrent cancer in or about the anastomosis. Only five others among the 386 resection patients noted bleeding in the follow-up period, two having new colonic cancers and the other three having large adenomatous polyps.

Significant weight loss, once pre-illness weight level was regained, was found to be the first sign of recrudescent cancer in 23 of the 121 patients. Interpretation of anorexia and weight loss was especially difficult in an aging population, for it often occurred even in those without cancer. However, only four patients noted significant "dry" weight gains within the 3 months immediately preceding detection of their recurrent neoplasm, the individuals with clinically evident ascites being excluded from this group.

Crampy abdominal pain and constipation were recorded by 11 patients as early or primary signs of recurrent carcinoma. However, a similar number of those who remained free of cancer developed these symptoms secondary to adhesive obstruction. When examined, the majority of the former group had some other physical signs of cancer, often a dominant mass.

These patterns warranted incorporation into a follow-up system if earlier detection of recurrence was to result. The patient with perineal pain after excision of the rectum should be considered to harbor recurrent cancer until proved otherwise. Residual sinus tracks should be probed and material submitted for histologic study. Even in the absence of a palpable mass, needle biopsy of the area can be performed. Before biopsy, computed axial tomography (CAT) scans may demonstrate soft tissue recurrences in the perineum and guide the biopsy needle. Cancer was confirmed in two patients with no palpable mass whatsoever with this type of biopsy examination. Both were free of subsequent recurrence (after irradiation and wide re-excision of the perineal tissues) for 2 years, and one remained well after 4 years.

The patient who is found to have rectal bleeding or occult fecal blood should have the anastomotic site directly inspected, as it is usually within endoscopic view. Barium enema study is indicated if the suture line is beyond endoscopic range. The techniques and results of barium enema study in follow-up are discussed in Chapter Five. New primary lesions are second only to recurrence as a cause for such signs and symptoms.

The frequency of anorexia and weight loss in those patients free of cancer was similar to that noted as initial signs of recurrent neoplasm. However, weight gain in the absence of ascites or edema was strongly presumptive evidence that recurrence would not be detected in the next three months ($p=0.07$).

A palpable mass, often nodular, was the only sign uniformly indicative of recurrent carcinoma. The masses were found in the perineal scar after combined abdominoperineal resection in and about intestinal suture lines, in the abdominal incision, in the liver, in the rectal stump after Hartmann-type resections, in the original bed of the primary neoplasm, and in the superficial lymph nodes.

Four to six patients developing neoplastic inguinal lymphadenopathy also had recurrent perineal disease. Many extensive, grossly cancerous masses were detected in areas described as only firm or indurated on the previous examination. Suspicious firm or indurated areas warrant immediate biopsy examination, rather than continued observation. This procedure is also recommended for painful perineal scars in the absence of a discrete mass.

As the charts were reviewed, the types and

dates of examination revealing recurrent cancers were recorded, as well as the types and dates of the immediately preceding examinations not indicating recurrence. This allowed an assessment of several examination methods, in respect to both their usefulness in detecting cancer and their likelihood of having missed earlier manifestations of recurrent disease. A variety of methods were employed at irregular intervals. Those procedures resulting in initial detection of recrudescent neoplasm (Table 4–4) were interpretable only in view of common practices in the hospital within the period studied. Although data are not available regarding the frequency with which such examinations were carried out in the follow-up group as a whole, the negative findings of the immediately preceding examination provided some insight. For example, although proctosigmoidoscopy revealed only two recurrences not otherwise detected, it is possible that it was the fallible, negative prior examination on only three occasions. Similarly, barium enemas did not reveal a single recurrent cancer not apparent otherwise, although it was the immediately preceding study with negative results in six patients. However, the observations in Chapter Five are more valuable in defining the role of barium enema in follow-up. Early baseline postoperative studies were rarely obtained at the EFSCH, and the schedule of re-examination was erratic.

The thoracic roentgenogram proved most helpful in examination. It indicated that the frequency of isolated pulmonary metastases from large bowel cancer was inadequately appreciated. Reports of long-term survival and apparent cure after resection of pulmonary metastases from colorectal cancer are not rare (Halbein et al., 1959). One patient in this series was well and possibly cured 34 months after a left upper lobectomy performed 47 months after primary resection. Perineal needle biopsy examination failed only once to discover a neoplasm that became apparent at the subsequent clinic visit (see Chapter Twenty-Two).

On the basis of these observations, the following suggestions were made concerning a satisfactory physical examination of a patient surviving resection intended for cure. Careful palpation or digital examinations, or both, should be directed at the primary tumor bed, the liver, the superficial lymph nodes, the perineal scar if the rectum is absent, any surgically constructed stomas, and the vagina and rectum. The data neither support nor refute the usefulness ascribed to the results of early baseline and regular subsequent barium enema studies in the follow-up of a patient with anastomotic reconstruction. This procedure should be supplemented by proctosigmoidoscopic examination of every patient whose suture line is within conventional endoscopic view. The value of periodically observing higher lying anastomoses with a flexible colonoscope has yet to be defined. Semiannual thoracic roentgenograms seem indicated in addition to those studies suggested by the patient's interval history and physical examination. If hospital admission and celiotomy are required in search of recurrence, recognition of the patterns of recurrence previously outlined may preclude "false-negative" investigation.

Table 4–4. PROCEDURES TO DETECT RECURRENT CANCER*

Procedure	No. of Patients
Perineal examination	18
Rectal digital examination	17
Thoracic roentgenogram	12
Palpation of site of primary lesion	12
Palpation of superficial lymph nodes	10
Vaginal examination	9
Palpation of liver	9
Celiotomy	8
Cystoscopy	5
Intravenous pyelogram	3
Colostomy, digital examination	2
Proctosigmoidoscopy	2

*Adapted from Polk HC Jr, Spratt JS Jr: Recurrent colorectal carcinoma: Detection, treatment and other considerations. Surgery 69:9–23, 1971.

Survival With Untreated Recurrent Carcinoma

Description of the natural history of carcinoma recurrent after resection intended for cure was calculated from the review of 62 individuals whose initial operation and all subsequent care, including documentation of certain recurrence, were received at EFSCH. The median survival after initial detection of recurrence for the 48 individuals who received no treatment directed toward the ablation of residual neoplasms was about 5 months and is not changed significantly by the inclusion of the remaining 28 untreated patients who did not receive all care and documentation of recurrence at EFSCH. Although the philosophies of the several surgeons and radiotherapists caring for these patients largely determined the aggressiveness with which recurrence was sought and treated, perusal of hospital records indicated that the untreated group consisted of far less favorable subjects as to extent of neoplasm and general debility than those who underwent reoperation intended for cure. Those treated by irradiation fell between these two extremes, the primary indication for treatment being persistent pain.

Results of Treatment

The selected individual in whom limited recurrence was detected and in whom resection intended for cure was accomplished had a much better prognosis, quantitatively and qualitatively, than other patients. Among the dozen patients thus treated, there was one operative death and one patient who lived only 5 months after reoperation. Four others ultimately died of primary large bowel adenocarcinoma at 21, 21, 34, and 67 months after resection, respectively. Of the others, three remained well and were likely cured. Two survived about 4 years before succumbing to new primary extracolonic cancers, and one died of causes other than cancer almost 10 years after reoperation.

A substantial proportion of the patients who received initial treatment at other hospitals were still amenable to reresection intended for cure upon the detection of recurrence (Table 4–5). Review of the case material indicated that the greater prevalence of retreatment intended for cure and for improved survival among those initially treated at other hospitals was primarily associated with the discovery that there was localized recurrence in individuals whose initial resection had been less extensive than was usually considered adequate. This was supported by the observation that carcinoma, ultimately to recur, did so later if initially treated at EFSCH (median recurrence time after primary resection, 17 months) as compared with the other hospitals as a group (median recurrence time after primary resection, 12 months). Patients initially treated elsewhere were often amenable to complete excision of the recurrence by standard resections (e.g., abdominoperineal resection after transanal, Kraske-type excisions of rectal cancers). It is, of course, impossible to explain this observation fully, for many factors affected patient selection at EFSCH as well as at the other institutions frequently referring patients to EFSCH for follow-up. The observations are anecdotal and not the product of a controlled clinical trial.

The difficulties besetting attempts to define recurrence of neoplasm have been explored in detail. In 1966, Kuzma and Dixon found that the "diagnosis" of recurrent cancer depended upon a variable relationship among the time since cure was attempted, coexisting illnesses, and physician prejudices. In the 1971 study by Polk and Spratt, the patients experiencing recurrent carcinoma corresponded closely to Kuzma and Dixon's Categories I and II. Although every effort was made to ensure accuracy, the diagnosis of recurrent cancers described in this report was less certain than that verified by autopsy, but it was more certain than data derived from death certificates.

The attitudes of the several surgeons-in-chief and their associates at EFSCH greatly influenced the material studied. Pessimism as to the prognostic significance of recurrent colorectal cancer was responsible, in part, for the low rate of reoperation undertaken for cure. Similarly low rates have been reported elsewhere (Long et al., 1950). Most physicians participating in the follow-up program appeared to have done so in order to collect survival data, evaluate original treatment regimens, and gather data concerning palliation of symptomatic recurrent carcinoma when detected.

Meaningful survival data with and without treatment are known for many characteristics. The various standard treatment modalities have been thoroughly assessed. New treatment programs, including combinations of methods

Table 4–5. **SURVIVAL ACCORDING TO SITE OF PRIMARY RESECTION AND SUBSEQUENT RETREATMENT***

	Initial Operation			
	At EFSCH†		*At Another Hospital*	
Treatment of Residual Neoplasm	*Patients (%)*	*Median Survival Period (mo.)*	*Patients (%)*	*Median Survival Period (mo.)*
No treatment	48	7	29	8
Any treatment	52	7	71	21
Curative resection	11	21	30	34

*Adapted from Polk HC Jr, Spratt JS Jr: Recurrent cancer of the colon. Surg Clin North Am 63:151–160, 1983.
†Ellis Fischel State Cancer Hospital.

previously evaluated separately, would, of course, require further follow-up evaluation. Complications of treatment methods, as well as cases of symptomatic untreatable recurrent disease, will ultimately come to light without regular follow-up when symptoms sufficient to warrant treatment develop. Thus, aside from evaluation of new therapeutic schemes, there is no indication for continued follow-up of patients whose colorectal carcinomas were resected for cure *unless* one is seeking recurrent disease that is sufficiently limited to allow retreatment. The data presented allowed reasonably efficient planning for detection of treatable recurrent neoplasm in terms of both schedule of re-examinations and specific procedures indicated according to the site and the initial therapy for the original cancer. Such an approach toward the follow-up could yield more patients whose recurrent disease is treatable with intent to cure than the 10 percent (12 of 21 patients) discovered in this retrospective study.

Whereas the use of recurrent neoplasm as an index of effectiveness of a treatment modality has been exhaustively described, relatively few investigations of the problems described in this report have been undertaken. The existing studies do allow the following comparisons.

The time elapsing between resection intended for cure and the discovery of recurrent neoplasm has been mentioned in some precise reviews concerning efficacy of various treatment regimens, especially the merit of anterior resection (Cole, 1952; Dunphy et al., 1969; Judd and Bellegie, 1952; Williams et al., 1966). The tendency (Table 4–6) toward earlier recurrence in the collected cases than that in those reported from EFSCH may largely be due to the selection of material. In either case, the collected series emphasized the first 2 years as the most productive period for detection of recurrent disease.

The validity of the very early recurrence rate (see above) is in part supported by the observation made by Mayo and Schlicke (1942) that 7 percent of patients dying within 30 days of resection for cure, presumably of operative and postoperative complications, had grossly residual carcinoma discovered by autopsy. This represents the most accurate available estimate of the frequency with which seemingly curative operations are absolutely not curative. If a similar proportion obtained in the EFSCH material, then 27 individuals may not have undergone "curative resection." Recidivated cancer was detected in 13 individuals *less* than 6 months postoperatively. Whether these early failures are recurrent or persistent carcinoma seems pedantic because both groups were equally in need of additional treatment.

The propensity of tumors with unfavorable pathologic characteristics for prompt, often local recurrence has also been noted previously. In 1963, Morson and associates found that the frequency of recurrence varied directly with the presence of high-grade malignancy (Broders' index), lymph node metastases, and extensive local spread, but was not altered by an increasing rate of resectability over the years studied. In 1966, Talley and associates also correlated higher incidence of recurrences with penetration of cancer through the intestinal wall and with lymph node metastases.

Although little attention has been directed toward clinical signs or symptoms of recurrent cancer, the sites of recurrence have been thoroughly studied in an attempt to improve operative therapy. The bulk of the latter data concerns the controversy of sphincter-saving and -sacrificing operations for cancers of the lower sigmoid and upper rectum. Most reviews conclude that the low anterior anastomosis is commonly involved by recurrent neoplasm but disagree whether these "surgical failures" are primarily attributable to compromised excisions, implantation of tumor, biology of the neoplasm, or local extent of disease. There is a striking similarity between the frequency of anastomotic recurrence after anterior resection and pelvic recurrence following abdominoperineal resection (Gilbertsen, 1960). Furthermore, although not often specified, many alleged suture line recurrences after fully adequate anterior resections appear to arise in the pelvis about the suture line, invading the suture line only secondarily. Even at more proximal levels where length of distal large bowel excised is of no concern, anastomotic recurrence approaches 10 percent. Many neoplasms recurrent after nonrestorative resections of the rectum and lower sigmoid colon present as a mass within the confines of the pelvis and perineum. This appears to be no less true for those patients treated by continence-preserving procedures, since in 1955, Black and Kelly found that only four of 109 luminal recurrences extended above the pelvic brim.

The tendency of many adenocarcinomas of the large bowel to recur locally early is further supported by the findings of an autopsy study by Floyd and associates (1965) of patients who

Table 4–6. COLLECTED CUMULATIVE RECURRENCE RATES AFTER CURATIVE RESECTION*

No. of Months Since Resection	Nonrestrictive Resection of Rectum and Rectosigmoid (155 Patients Recurrent) (%)†	Anterior Resections Only (98 Patients Recurrent) (%)‡	Pelvic or Wound Recurrence in Rectum and Rectosigmoid (92 Patients Recurrent) (%)§	Anterior Hartmann's Resection (23 Patients Recurrent) (%)‖	Local Recurrence Only (15 Patients Recurrent) (%)
	Characteristics				
6			16	30	33
12			58	52	73
24	80	73	81	74	80
36		87		87	87
48				91	
60	97				100

*Adapted from Polk HC Jr, Spratt JS Jr: Recurrent colorectal carcinoma: Detection, treatment and other considerations. Surgery 69:9–23, 1971.
†Floyd et al (1965).
‡Gary et al (1964).
§Gilbertsen (1960).
‖Goligher et al (1951).

had had recurrent large bowel cancer at Charity Hospital. These data, as well as others, suggest that retreatment for cure in localized recurrent colorectal carcinomas is feasible.

For reasons previously noted, the authors were unable to determine the best strategy for barium enema and proctosigmoidoscopic examinations in detecting recurrent carcinoma of the colon and rectum. The examinations were likely to detect recurrent neoplasm only if applied to those groups most susceptible to intraluminal recurrence. Primarily, the performance of these studies in a patient who had undergone abdominoperineal resection was likely to disclose only new primary neoplasms. Since carcinoma in and about the anastomotic site was the most frequent site of recurrence after restorative operations on the lower colon, every examination of these patients should include a digital rectal examination along with digital palpation of all pararectal areas. The exact role of follow-up proctosigmoidoscopic examination for the timely discovery of recurrent cancers remains ill-defined. If, for example, one half of the patients develop recurrent cancer sometime after low anterior resection, and 15 percent of these cancers involve the suture line, proctosigmoidoscopy could disclose 75 recurrent cancers among an initially treated and followed population of 1000 individuals. Some recurrences thus located might be amenable to abdominoperineal resection or, occasionally, pelvic exenteration. However, the risk must be balanced against this yield. In 1968, Kiser and associates discovered five patients with perforations among 7000 who had proctosigmoidoscopic examinations at EFSCH. Although all survived with repair of the perforation without colostomy, the expense, morbidity, and potential mortality deserve constant consideration in developing such a scheme and must be evaluated in each practice setting.

The value of follow-up barium enema studies in detecting recurrent cancer is proportional to the regularity with which the studies are done; the initial examination should be performed 3 months after anastomosis (Cronqvist, 1957; Fleischner and Berenberg, 1956). A well-studied strategy for barium enema use and its results are described in Chapter Five. No data are available regarding the frequency with which the examination should be repeated. One group (Agnew and Cooley, 1962) discovered 12 recurrences of cancer among 111 anastomoses examined by barium enema. This yield is encouraging, but requires substantiation. Anastomoses within proctosigmoidoscopic view should seldom require confirmatory roentgenographic contrast study if recurrence was not suspected endoscopically. This question of radiologic follow-up is addressed in greater detail in Chapter Five. Indeed, this area is primarily the responsibility of the surgeon-endoscopist on whom the patient should depend rather than on barium enema study alone.

Rarely, primarily extraluminal cancer may be more apparent upon fluoroscopic examination (stiffening and rigidity of the bowel is seen) than upon sigmoidoscopic study. There can be little argument that barium enema is the only special study likely to disclose recurrence in and about the more proximally situated anastomoses. In 1968, Kiser and co-workers found only one perforation among 2150 patients having barium enema studies at EFSCH. The early and late morbidity of barium peritonitis is appreciable, and expense must be weighed against the benefits.

Data on retreatment is, of course, scant and reflects the attitude of the surgical staff attending the patient as well as the extent of disease and perhaps the adequacy of the initial excision. Dunphy (1947) was among the first to point out that reoperation in selected cases might prolong useful life and effect cure in some. The data tabulated in Table 4–7 indicate that reresection for cure can be accomplished in at least 10 percent of recurrences, and perhaps with prompt detection and a definitive surgical approach in up to 40 percent of selected cases. Despite isolated comments about the futility of reresection once recurrence is apparent, the majority of reports indicate that most patients can be helped, many can have their lives prolonged, and some can apparently be cured. Although we did not study irradiation per se in detail, other reports confirm that radiotherapy, often with adjunctive surgical diversion, may greatly improve and occasionally significantly prolong the remaining life of patients with recurrence.

Comparable data on results of retreatment are difficult to discover among English language publications. Black and Kelly (1955) studied 116 cases of recurrent cancer after continence-preserving resections of the rectum and rectosigmoid. Seventy were treated by irradiation, 20 with complementary colostomy; seven patients lived more than 3 years, and five lived more than 5 years. The former figure is very similar to survival time for patients with recurrent cancer treated at EFSCH, but the latter is much better. Thirty of the 116 patients with recurrence underwent re-exploratory operation. Seventeen of them had reresections. Lofgren and associates (1957) subsequently described reoperation upon 56 of 108 recurrences, 37 of which were reresected. Although neither of these reports from the Mayo Clinic seemed enthusiastic about reresection, in 1955, Black and Kelly found that four of 12 patients undergoing reresection for cure lived for more than 3 years after the procedure. The bulk of the group described by Lofgren and associates had been operated on too recently to assess results fairly. They did mention some long-term survivals and apparent cures obtained by fulguration and irradiation.

Although, in 1967, Kiselow and co-workers did not specify patient distribution as to advanced primary neoplasm or recurrence, they successfully retreated patients with recurrent cancer after sigmoid or abdominoperineal resection by total pelvic exenteration. Among the entire group of patients with large bowel cancers thus treated, a 30 percent 5-year survival rate had been obtained. This experience has recently been updated and confirmed in a more comprehensive review (Spratt et al., 1973).

On the basis of the material reviewed herein, Table 4–8 outlines a suggested schedule of examinations after curative resection of colorectal carcinoma. This table provides the timing and types of examinations that are most likely to result in the discovery of treatable recurrent cancer, based on observed interval discovery rates. Those patients with unfavorable pathologic characteristics (see Table 4–3) probably should be examined at 2-month intervals through the second postoperative year and at 3-month intervals in the third year after operation. The expense of such a schedule can be justified: (1) If localized recurrent cancer is detected, retreatment can be undertaken (specifically reresection if not contraindicated by other illness). (2) At least 20 percent of recurrent cancers can be subjected to additional

Table 4–7. **RERESECTIONS FOR CURE OF RECURRENT CANCER**

Reference	Initial Resections (No.)	Total Recurrences	No. Reresected	Percent Reresected
Green and Black (1963)	242	25	2	8
Scudamore et al (1960)	213	66	9	14
Goligher et al (1951)	162	16	9	—
Beal and Cornell (1956)	140	21†	5	24
Black and Kelly (1955)	—	116	12	11
Lofgren et al (1957)	—	108	37	34
Bacon and Berkley (1959)	—	93‡	38	41

*Adapted from Polk HC Jr, Spratt JS Jr: Recurrent colorectal carcinoma: Detection, treatment and other considerations. Surgery 69:9–23, 1971.

†Anastomotic recurrence only.

‡Local recurrence only.

Table 4–8. **PROPOSED SCHEDULE OF EXAMINATION***

Initial Treatment and Special Examinations	Months After Resection Intended for Cure 2	4	6	8	10	12	15	18	21	24	30	36	42	48
Abdominoperineal														
Pelvic, women	X	X	X	X	X	X	X	X	X	X	X	X	X	X
Perineum, (?) biopsy	X	X	X	X	X	X	X	X	X	X	X	X	X	X
Groin adenopathy	X	X	X	X	X	X	X	X	X	X	X	X	X	X
Intravenous pyelogram, men						X				X				X
Chest x-ray			X			X		X		X		X		X
Resection and Anastomosis Below 25 Cm														
Proctosigmoidoscopy	X	X	X	X	X	X	X	X	X	X	X	X	X	X
Feces for occult blood	X	X	X	X	X	X	X	X	X	X	X	X	X	X
Urinalysis			X			X		X		X		X		X
Pelvic, women	X	X	X	X	X	X	X	X	X	X	X	X	X	X
Chest x-ray			X			X		X		X		X		X
Resection and Anastomosis Above 25 Cm														
Barium enema	X	X	X	X	X	X	X	X	X	X	X	X	X	X
Feces for occult blood	X	X	X	X	X	X	X	X	X	X	X	X	X	X
Primary tumor site	X	X	X	X	X	X	X	X	X	X	X	X	X	X
Chest x-ray			X			X		X		X		X		X

*Adapted from Polk HC Jr, Spratt JS Jr: Recurrent colorectal carcinoma: Detection, treatment and other considerations. Surgery 69:9–23, 1971.

treatment intended for cure. (3) One third of those subjected to such retreatment are cured.

Polk and Spratt (1971) provided monetary calculations by which the value of follow-up was determined to justify the system. It was based on a 2 percent discovery per interval encounter. Data were insufficient to project the results in terms of added person-years, which is the ultimate yardstick. Further discussion on both prevention of postresective recurrences and the treatment is found in Chapter Twenty-Two.

The concept of patient responsibility, which is always so necessary after the fourth postoperative year, has been subjected to a very limited trial among highly selected patients, as an extension of the follow-up scheme. The signs and symptoms most indicative of early recurrent carcinoma of the large bowel were thoroughly explained when the final necessary postoperative examination occurred (usually about 3 months after operation). No regular pattern of visits was prescribed, and the patients were encouraged to call the physician when signs or symptoms of any other problems arose. This program did not consider the emotional reassurance and support derived from repeated "negative" re-examinations. When this limited investigation was 3 years old, only 23 patients had been admitted to the study group. There had been seven recurrences, only one of which seemed to be advanced. Three patients had been treated by reresection intended for cure and two were free of neoplasm. Of greatest interest was the sparsity of physician visits, averaging only two per patient year for the first year and less than that for the second.

Biologic Markers in the Follow-Up

The use of biologic markers from cancer in follow-up is now being studied. Pregnancy-associated alpha$_2$glycoprotein (alpha$_2$PAG) is a high molecular weight glycoprotein, approximately 206,000 MW (Gold and Freedman, 1965), that is found in high serum concentrations throughout pregnancy (Horne et al., 1973), yet during the puerperium it decreases drastically to insignificant levels (Stimson, 1975a and b). Alpha$_2$PAG is also referred to as pregnancy zone protein and as alpha$_2$ macroglobulin. It is synthesized by circulating leucocytes (Stimson and Blackstock, 1975), and its production is stimulated by estrogens (Horne et al., 1973). It may function as an immunosuppressive factor (Stimson, 1972). Alpha$_2$PAG is also present in high serum concentrations in the following conditions: rheumatoid arthritis, psoriasis, primary biliary cirrhosis, malignant lymphoid neoplasms and cancer involving the gastrointestinal tract, bronchus, breasts, and female genital tract.

Carcinoembryonic antigen (CEA) is a family of heterogenous but related glycoproteins. The molecular weight of these glycoproteins approximates 200,000, and they have both shared and distinct antigenic properties. CEA was first identified by Gold and Freedman (1965) in extracts of cancerous large bowel and in the digestive organs of human fetuses. Researchers detected this antigen in embryonic and fetal gut, pancreas, and liver during the first two trimesters of gestation, which resulted in the name carcinoembryonic antigen of the human digestive system. CEA was not detectable in fetal tissue during the third trimester of gestation.

CEA is also detectable in primary and metastatic tissue arising from entodermally derived digestive system epithelium. CEA concentrations appear greater in lower bowel cancers than in those of the upper gastrointestinal tract (Gold et al., 1978). It is thought that 90 to 95 percent of all malignant lesions of the colon and rectum are able to produce CEA. The presence of CEA is dependent upon tissue of origin rather than tissue of growth of the cancer. Therefore, tumor metastasis to the colon does not produce a clinically elevated CEA level (Gold and Freedman, 1965).

Testing of large populations has shown CEA elevations in diverticulitis, cirrhosis, pancreatitis, ulcerative and granulomatus bowel disease, chronic bronchitis, emphysema, and cancers arising from all parts of the gastrointestinal tract, the pancreas, lungs, breasts, prostate, ovary, and urinary bladder. CEA elevations in healthy heavy smokers have also been found (Mach et al., 1974).

Since laboratory tests are available to determine the presence and concentrations of both $alpha_2PAG$ and CEA levels, an important concern is to compare and differentiate the clinical usefulness of these two glycoproteins in screening, diagnosis, and recurrence of large bowel carcinoma. The upper limit of normal of $alpha_2PAG$ for men is 5 ng/l; for women the upper limit of normal is significantly higher, about 30 ng/l at age 30, rising to 60 ng/l by age 75 (Wood et al., 1978a and b). The most commonly used procedure in measuring CEA levels is radioimmunoassay. The cutoff limit of quantitative significance was determined to be 5 ng/ml (Mach et al., 1974). Most nonsmokers have a CEA level less than 2.5 ng/ml, whereas smokers have a slightly higher level.

The initial hope was that altered plasma levels of $alpha_2PAG$ and CEA would be useful screening tools for the early detection of colorectal cancer. However, elevated levels of each have been found in numerous other malignant diseases, benign diseases, and in populations of "normal" people. Likewise, normal levels of each have been measured in patients in the early stages of colorectal cancer. Therefore, the two tests have been rendered nearly useless for screening purposes. Wood and coworkers (1978a and b) found elevated $alpha_2PAG$ levels in 32 of 54 patients (59 percent). Thirty-one of the 54 patients had cancer subjectable to curative resection. Sixteen of the 31 (52 percent) had elevated $alpha_2PAG$ levels and 17 of the 31 (55 percent) had elevated CEA levels. Wood and associates found elevated $alpha_2PAG$ levels in 32 of 54 patients with colorectal cancer (59 percent) and elevated CEA levels in 35 of the 54 patients (65 percent). Reversing these figures will reveal considerable percentages of false-negative results from measurement of both the $alpha_2PAG$ and CEA levels.

By these assays, 31 of the 54 patients were candidates for curative resections. A similar percentage of patients had preoperative elevations of $alpha_2PAG$ and CEA; that is, 52 percent and 55 percent, respectively (Wood et al., 1978a and b). A spot chart review at a hospital in Louisville, Kentucky, indicated that 50 percent, seven of 14 patients with colonic cancers, had elevated CEA levels preoperatively. No patients were found to have $alpha_2PAG$ assays run preoperatively.

Interest in screening colonic secretions for CEA levels as a means of early colon cancer detection has also been considered. In 1976, Molnar and associates found elevated CEA levels in the plasma of 16 of 23 patients and elevated CEA levels in the colonic mucus of all 23 patients. When colonic mucus samples were obtained by sigmoidoscopy for CEA levels, cancer was found in 22 per cent of the patients in whom the diagnosis would have been otherwise missed by noninvasive procedures.

Using CEA levels to screen high-risk patients has also been suggested. High-risk candidates for colorectal cancer include those with familial polyposis, sporadic adenomatous or villous polyps, and inflammatory bowel disease. Elevated CEA levels are seen in these high-risk patients, often without a further increase in the levels with the development of cancer. Therefore, CEA levels are not a definitive screening tool for high-risk patients.

Preoperative assessment of plasma CEA has been reported to assist in establishing the prognosis of patients. In 1978, Wanebo and associates studied 358 patients with colorectal cancer and found the recurrence rate was higher in patients with Dukes' B and Dukes' C lesions who had preoperative CEA levels greater than 5 ng/ml. It was also seen that recurrence was earlier in patients with elevated CEA levels. Patients without preoperative elevations of

CEA have a greater proportion of Dukes' A lesions, less risk of recurrence, and a longer disease-free interval.

A chart review, conducted on patients with colorectal cancer at Norton's Hospital in Louisville, Kentucky, between the years 1976 and 1979, revealed the following: 11 patients with Dukes' B and one with Dukes' C lesions were found to have documented CEA levels obtained prior to curative resection. Six of the 11 and the patient with Dukes' C lesion had CEA levels less than 5 ng/ml. Of these six patients, three developed metastasis within 2 years and the patient with Dukes' C lesions remained free of evidence of cancer recurrence. Of the five patients with Dukes' B lesions and CEA levels greater than 5 ng/ml, one developed metastasis. The findings in this small series do not concur with those of Wanebo and associates (1978).

Preoperative assessment of plasma alpha$_2$-PAG by Stimson (1975a and b) showed that patients with metastasis tended to have higher levels than those with localized tumors. Patients with metastasis had a median value of 100 ng/ml compared with a median value of 45 ng/ml in those with localized tumors. Wood and associates (1978) found that patients undergoing curative resection had postoperative mean alpha$_2$PAG levels that were virtually unchanged from the preoperative mean values. Of patients with extensive local tumor spread for whom curative surgery was unlikely, 16 of 23 tested patients (70 percent) had elevated levels of alpha$_2$PAG and 18 of 23 tested patients (78 percent) had elevated levels of CEA (Wood et al., 1978).

Koch and McPherson (1979), as well as Arnaud and associates (1980), reported that failure of CEA levels to drop within normal range postoperatively was a bad prognostic sign in relation to recurrence rates. Koch and McPherson (1979) found that 187 patients (23 percent) presenting as disease-free after curative surgery had CEA levels greater than the cutoff of 5 ng/ml. Of these, 116 (62 percent) eventually showed disease progression. The Louisville chart review showed six of 47 patients (13 percent) had CEA levels that did not fall within normal range 6 months postoperatively. All six of these patients showed disease progression.

In 1975, Stimson believed that the failure of alpha$_2$PAG levels to decrease following treatment signals a need to re-evaluate the patient or the need to introduce a different mode of therapy. Wood and associates (1978a and b), however, found a large percentage of false-positive elevated postoperative alpha$_2$PAG levels.

Currently, the greatest use of serum CEA levels involves serial monitoring of postoperative plasma levels for early detection of recurrent colorectal cancer. The goal of such early detection is the discovery of recurrent cancer when additional therapy might still result in cure. Staab and associates (1978) found that obtaining plasma CEA samples a few days before surgery, 8 to 10 days following surgery, then at 2-month intervals for 2 years, and at 4-month intervals thereafter provided a reliable basis for earlier detection of recurrence. The value of early detection by this method is controversial. In cases of tumor recurrence, the rise of CEA levels preceded a positive clinical diagnosis by a mean of 4 months. A 30 to 50 percent increase in the CEA level during postoperative follow-up as compared with preceding CEA determination should be confirmed by a second CEA determination within a month and should promote a search for recurring disease. This search should always begin with a review of the pathologic characteristics of the original cancer.

When consecutive CEA values showed a persistent increase, tumor recurrence became highly probable. A slow rise in CEA levels not exceeding 30 to 50 percent in consecutive readings was generally correlated with local tumor recurrence or limited metastasis, or both. A second curative resection was sometimes possible provided that the delay time was short (Staab et al., 1978). A 1978 study by Minton and associates found that by decreasing the delay time for a "second-look" operation from 7 months to 1.4 months, the proportion of patients with recurrent resectable carcinoma increased from 27 percent to 78 percent.

A rapid increase in CEA, with consecutive increases of greater than 50 percent so that it exceeds 10 ng/ml of serum, was correlated with generalized tumor spread, predominantly liver metastasis. In such cases, there is only a minimal chance for a second radical resection (Staab et al., 1978).

Stimson and co-workers (1975a and b) do agree that serial determinations of alpha$_2$PAG levels may be useful in detecting patients with tumor recurrence. In adequately treated patients, the alpha$_2$PAG levels fell below the pretreatment values. In patients who later developed recurrence, the alpha$_2$PAG levels usually increased before the recurrence was diagnosed clinically. Wood and associates (1978a and b) found that the measurement of alpha$_2$PAG concentrations is a less reliable means of detecting tumor recurrence than the measurement of serial CEA samples. Postoperatively, it was found that alpha$_2$PAG assays gave a false-positive value in 56 percent of the patients showing elevated values, and only 16 percent of these patients showed elevated CEA levels. Also, all patients with tumor recurrence after curative resections showed elevated CEA levels, yet the alpha$_2$-PAG levels yielded false-negative results in 38 percent of the patients (Wood et al., 1978a and b; Stimson, 1975a and b).

Another suggested use of serum alpha$_2$PAG and CEA levels is in assessing the response of recurrent or metastatic colorectal cancer to radiation therapy or chemotherapy. Wood and associates (1978a and b) pointed out that there may be a quantitative relationship between serum alpha$_2$PAG and tumor load because it was noticed that patients with distant metastasis receiving adjuvant therapy did not show the characteristic rise in alpha$_2$PAG levels. Studies monitoring CEA levels during adjuvant therapy may not provide a totally reliable parameter, but generally there is a correlation between levels and the amount of tumor mass present. The determination of CEA levels may be useful in assessing the response to treatment of metastatic colorectal cancer not clinically measurable, such as during irradiation therapy, to assure that the bulk of the tumor mass is regressing under treatment.

Based on this review, several conclusions were drawn regarding the use of serum CEA and alpha$_2$PAG concentrations. Assays at this time are too insensitive and nonspecific to recommend the use of alpha$_2$PAG and CEA levels as screening tests for colorectal cancer. In the absence of obvious metastatic disease, preoperative measurement of alpha$_2$PAG and CEA should be performed, since markedly elevated values suggest metastasis and indicate a possible need for evaluation of liver for the presence and extent of metastases before laparotomy. Conflicting data exist regarding the value of postoperative CEA levels for the detection of tumor recurrence prior to clinical evidence, allowing for earlier and more successful "second-look" operations. Alpha$_2$PAG levels are less reliable in detecting tumor recurrence, but may be of value when measured alongside CEA levels in reducing false-positive and false-negative results. If serial measurements are to be used, the same laboratory should perform all assays, eliminating interlaboratory variations (Taylor et al., 1977). Serial measurements of alpha$_2$PAG and CEA can be helpful in monitoring responsiveness to chemotherapy and radiotherapy of otherwise unmeasurable disease. And finally, if a single serum value of either glycoprotein is to be used, CEA is apparently more reliable than alpha$_2$PAG.

Approaches to Follow-Up

In conclusion, the patient whose colorectal carcinoma has been treated with the expectation of cure can reasonably derive benefit from a follow-up program designed according to the primary site of the cancer, the pathologic properties of the cancer, and the surgical technique employed. Tailoring of the schedule and the method of examination to the particular patient may allow improvement in (1) timely detection, (2) retreatment for cure, and (3) prolongation of comfortable and productive life.

The timely detection of recurrent cancer has as its optimum goal detection of the recurrence at a stage in which there is a large possibility of successful retreatment. There was a time when follow-up activity was concerned with defining the course of the disease, the impact of pathologic factors, and the adequacy of primary treatment. In fact, the need for this has long since passed, and the outcome of standard surgical resections for the various pathologic types of colorectal cancer has long since been defined. New approaches that seek to improve end results are the subject for future controlled clinical trials.

Based on reviewed experience and careful analysis of the options, the follow-up period must be designed considering the following factors: (1) half of all treatment failures after resection for cure occurred within 18 months of the primary resection; therefore, follow-up should be concentrated in that period, with increasing dependency on self-surveillance later; (2) certain patterns of recurrence and the relative value of retreatment were associated with definable characteristics of the primary cancer, and these characteristics were helpful in designing follow-up systems based on the interval risk for recurrence, and (3) certain symptoms, signs, and examinations were more helpful at some intervals than at others.

The role of CEA in the care of the patient with colon cancer remains debatable (Goslin et al., 1980; Wanebo, 1981). It certainly is not a useful primary screening technique, and its many false-positive results make it suspect even as a secondary or tertiary screening procedure. Its expense is also a major concern.

However, some researchers believe that the CEA is of value in the follow-up of a patient whose CEA is initially elevated but then returns to very low or nonmeasurable levels following resection (Balz et al., 1977; Martin et al., 1979; Minton and Martin, 1978). They believe that a subsequent elevation of CEA in a patient with this pattern indicates very early recurrent disease. They have reoperated on a number of patients and found early evidence that such promptly detected disease was more amenable to reresection for cure and, by inference, ultimate control of disease.

An alternative approach to follow-up is based on one author's (H.C.P.) personal experience with a selected *non*–follow-up system in a group of well-motivated, intelligent patients cared for at the University of Miami in the latter half of the 1960s. This approach was practiced on a limited basis and was not formally reported. The patients were selected for evidence of cooperativeness, emotional stability, intelligence, and a willingness to understand the risks and rewards of a predominantly self-surveillance scheme. For their given tumor locus, they were given a list of signs and symptoms that were known harbingers of recurrent disease (Table 4–9). They were asked to check with the investigating physician (H.C.P.) by phone or in person when any question arose. Although the program was terminated before a valid outcome could be assured for all these patients, several points became clear. First, the frequency of extensive recurrent disease clearly was not increased in these patients. The proportion of early or localized recurrent disease was identical to that of a separate group of patients undergoing the "ideal" follow-up scheme previously outlined. Patient anxiety was the commonest cause of visits, but these patients as a group in their first 3 years of care averaged only two phone calls and 1.8 visits per year, compared with an average of one phone call and 4.3 visits per year for patients undergoing the "ideal" follow-up (Polk, 1982; Polk and Spratt, 1983).

The expense involved in the "ideal" follow-up is obvious, as well as the risk in conducting endoscopy, barium enema, and so forth. Patient benefit must include a high probability of assurance far in excess of any risk from diagnostic interventions.

Table 4–9. SIGNS OF RECURRENT CANCER THAT THE PATIENT MAY BE TAUGHT TO DISCOVER*

Perineal pain and discomfort developing after abdominoperineal resection
Renewed rectal bleeding
Mass in incision or in vicinity of the site of the primary cancer
Change in bowel habits
Weight loss

*Adapted from Polk HC Jr, Spratt JS Jr: Recurrent cancer of the colon. Surg Clin North Am 63:151–160, 1983.

The second-look concept, popularized in 1959 by Wangensteen and his school of surgery, requires comment in this review. Wangensteen hypothesized that certain variants of colon cancer predisposed to local recurrence and such recurrent disease could best be detected and retreated for cure by empirically planned repeat laparotomy. The basic hypothesis involved in this was interesting, since our data and others (Griffin et al., 1969) suggest that, even in the hands of those extremely interested and knowledgeable in the field, the discovery of early or favorable recurrent disease while asymptomatic is the exception rather than the rule. However, there were a number of problems in the implementation of this approach. These are reviewed in Chapter Twenty-Two.

In a curative sense, management is dictated by the site of recurrence. Recidivated cancer is more likely to be successfully treated when the interval from primary treatment to detection of recurrence is lengthy. This implies some favorable biologic characteristics of the tumor, which enhances its responsiveness to retreatment.

Types of Cancer Seen at Follow-Up

Hepatic and Pulmonary Metastases

The most frequent focus of metastatic colorectal cancer is the liver. Hepatic as well as pulmonary metastases are covered in a separate chapter (see Chapter Fourteen). Curability of some pulmonary metastases from colorectal cancer is not often discussed or appreciated; however, an abnormal chest film was the second most common sign of metastatic cancer in the group of patients reported by Polk and Spratt (1971). Many of the principles discussed for the identification of patients with hepatic metastases apply to the occasional patient that will benefit from pulmonary resection of isolated metastases. The risk of pulmonary resection is less than that of hepatic resection in most surgeons' hands; therefore, in the authors' opinion, it can be pursued somewhat more optimistically.

Local Disease

Another frequent site of recurrent colorectal cancer is in and about the primary site of resection or about the anastomosis. The concerns regarding the basic pathologic type of tumor, the interval since original resection, and the absence of other disease are significant in such cases. The classic signs are the presence of a mass determined by an examiner, the presence of occult blood in fecal matter, increased anastomotic deformity evident on barium contrast study, and the patient's increasing difficulty with defecation.

Experience is growing in the delineation of recurrent cancer using the CAT scan. Not only can the CAT scan help delineate the extent and location of recidivated pelvic cancer, but the information gained from the scan is useful in directing percutaneous needle biopsies to continue the diagnosis (Zelas et al., 1980). The same principles of reasonable search for additional metastatic disease apply and include, in a specific search for hepatic disease, the presence of the latter, effectively ruling out an attempt at curative reoperation, and its absence, indeed, encouraging the surgeon to proceed.

When recurrences involve the pelvis, a complete urologic evaluation, including cystoscopy and study of the ureters, is valuable in planning attempts at reresection. The extent of the disease is better defined and the patient can be better prepared for significant eventualities that the findings might indicate (Eickenberg et al., 1976). Reoperation can be a highly effective form of palliation or, remotely, can offer some chance of cure.

The recurrent colorectal cancer that involved adjacent organs in the *primary* situation is the favorable recurrent situation and has no more ominous prognosis than the cancer with a limited number of regional lymph node metastases (Polk, 1972). Therefore, by analogy, if a fairly long period of time has elapsed before recurrence and if there is firm evidence of absence of other disease, recurrent disease that invades the trigone of the bladder should be treated by pelvic exenteration and urinary diversion.

Incisional Implants or Metastases

A particularly favorable variant of recurrent colon cancer is the one that presents with only an isolated implant, often in the incision. Patients with these cancers have been discussed on several occasions (Polk and Warren, 1969), and they should undergo the usual tests in search of additional metastases. If no metastases are found, the tumors can be approached through an incision remote from the original incision and/or the site of primary cancer, and extensive abdominal wall resection can be carried out following the principles of tumor surgery and reconstruction and using either simple abdominal flaps, myocutaneous flaps, or failing that, prosthetic material such as polypropylene mesh (Marlex) (Voyles et al., 1981). These tumors often have very favorable prognoses, and in the absence of other disseminated cancer, are among the most rewarding lesions to treat.

Multiple Primary Cancers

Multiple primary malignant neoplasms are also important considerations in the follow-up of the patient who has had colorectal cancer (Polk et al., 1965; Spratt, 1977). Neoplasms occurring simultaneously must be sought and appropriately treated primarily, particularly when colonic carcinoma exists (Bargen and Rankin, 1930; Brindley and Rice, 1952). However, the nonsimultaneous, subsequent carcinoma in patients cured of their initial neoplasm must also be considered in follow-up. In 1965, Polk, Spratt and Butcher reported on the follow-up of persons with histologically verified carcinoma of the colon and rectum. Their 2157 patients were distributed in the following three groups: (1) 170 Missouri residents consecutively treated surgically in the Barnes Hospital between 1914 and 1935 inclusive, (2) 1141 individuals observed at EFSCH between 1939 and 1961 inclusive, and (3) 856 patients attended in the Barnes Hospital between 1940 and 1951 inclusive.

These groups were congruous in terms of the maximum chordal dimension of the resected carcinomas, the frequency of nodal and distant metastases, and the cellular types of the primary tumor (Polk et al., 1964) (Table 4–10).

New primary cancers were distinguished from possible metastases by comparison of cellular types and by careful microscopic examination of all available tissues to rule out

Table 4–10. PATHOLOGIC CHARACTERISTICS OF CARCINOMA OF THE COLON AND RECTUM*

	Group 1†	Group 2	Group 3‡
Median maximum chordal dimension (cm.)	4.9	6.0	5.2
Frequency of nodal and distant metastases (operated cases)	54/170 (31.8%)	336/849 (39.6%)	136/325 (38.7%)
Cellular type			
Adenocarcinoma	140 (82.3%)	926 (81.1%)	280 (79.5%)
Mucinous carcinoma	16 (9.4%)	68 (5.9%)	28 (7.9%)
Undifferentiated carcinoma	14 (8.2%)	147 (12.9%)	44 (12.5%)

*Adapted from Polk HC Jr, Spratt JS Jr, Butcher HR Jr: Frequency of multiple primary malignant neoplasms associated with colorectal carcinoma. Am J Surg 109:71–74, 1965.

†Patients in Group 1 were probably understaged due to failure to regularly perform biopsy on hepatic and peritoneal metastases.

‡The pathologic data in Group 3 are based on examination of 352 cases operated on from 1948 to 1951. Pathology protocols in 1940 to 1947 were not satisfactory for evaluation.

submucosal spread in the case of multiple colonic carcinomas.

Excluded from this study were carcinomas complicating ulcerative colitis and multiple polyposis, villous adenomas with atypia, and adenomatous polyps with focal carcinoma in the tip. Each neoplasm included was frankly invasive, with the exception of epidermoid carcinoma in situ of the cervix uteri.

Three synchronous but separate primary carcinomas occurred in Group 1 (170 patients); two were colonic cancers and one an epidermoid carcinoma of the esophagus. Of the group, 153 (90 percent) were followed to death. Five others were followed 10 years or longer before being lost.

Sixty patients (35 percent) died within 30 days of operation and were considered operative deaths (see Table 4–2). Seventy-six others (45 percent) died of their initial colorectal carcinoma 1 week to 20 years after discharge from the hospital. Eight patients (5 percent) died of causes other than cancer. Nine (six women and three men) developed new primary carcinomas 2.5 to 22 years after resection of their initial colonic cancers. The second primary carcinomas occurred in the large bowel in four persons; the cancers in the remaining five arose from the esophagus, breast, endometrium, ovary, and urinary bladder. Three neoplasms were resectable when discovered. Only one patient survived without recurrence of the second primary lesion and that individual lived but a year before dying of heart disease. Of those surviving the initial carcinoma, a new primary cancer was the most frequent cause of death. The nine persons developing a second primary cancer represented 36 percent of the 25 who did not die of their first colonic carcinoma, and they were followed 2 or more years. Only five of the 1141 patients observed with colorectal carcinoma in Group 2 were lost to follow-up. Two hundred twenty-one were alive 5 years or longer after treatment.

No patient was known to have had a colorectal carcinoma before their initial treatment at EFSCH. Thirty-four had multiple simultaneously occurring malignant neoplasms of the large intestine. Six of these persons had three separate primary adenocarcinomas; two patients had four or more simultaneous adenocarcinomas. Table 4–11 indicates the frequency and types of extracolonic malignant neoplasms. In addition, 28 (3.3 percent) gave a history of cancer of an extracolonic site before the diagnosis of their colon cancer. Cook (1966) provides a compilation from the literature in Table 4–12.

Table 4–11. SEPARATE PRIMARY EXTRACOLONIC MALIGNANT NEOPLASMS (Simultaneous and Nonsimultaneous) IN 1,141 CASES*

Neoplasm	Number
Basal cell carcinoma, skin	43
Epidermoid carcinoma, skin	18
Adenocarcinoma, prostate	15
Adenocarcinoma, breast	12
Epidermoid carcinoma, cervix uteri	7
Adenocarcinoma, endometrium	6
Adenocarcinoma, stomach	3
Adenocarcinoma, ovary	3
Epidermoid carcinoma, vagina-vulva	2
Adenocarcinoma, lung	2
Lymphocytic leukemia	2
Lymphosarcoma	2
Carcinoid, ileum	2
Epidermoid carcinoma, larynx	1
Epidermoid carcinoma, piriform sinus	1
Mucoepidermoid carcinoma, parotid	1
Malignant melanoma, lower extremity	1
Total	121 (10.6%)

*Adapted from Polk HC Jr, Spratt JS Jr, Butcher HR Jr: Frequency of multiple primary malignant neoplasms associated with colorectal carcinoma. Am J Surg 109:71–74, 1965.

Table 4–12. **TEMPORAL RELATIONSHIP OF SEPARATE PRIMARY MALIGNANT NEOPLASMS TO COLORECTAL CARCINOMA***

Primary site	Diagnosis Relative to Colorectal Cancer Diagnosis *Before*	*After*
Skin	64	92
Breast	48	39
Endometrium	41	35
Stomach	41	27
Cervix uteri	29	9
Blood and bone marrow (leukemias)	18	8
Bladder	17	6
Lymphoid tissue	16	11
Ovary	6	43
Pancreatobiliary	6	16
Prostate	4	58
Lung	4	12
Kidney	3	9
Esophagus	2	24
Appendix	2	0
Brain	2	2
Larynx-pharynx	2	7
Soft somatic tissues	1	8
Vulva	1	6
Oral cavity	1	6
Small intestine	0	14
Urethra	0	3
Penis	0	3

*Collected from American medical literature by Galen B. Cook, M.D., Ellis Fischel State Cancer Hospital. Adapted from Polk HC Jr, Spratt JS Jr, Butcher HR Jr: Frequency of multiple primary malignant neoplasms associated with colorectal carcinoma. Am J Surg 109:71–74, 1965.

Among this group, 16 were discovered to have one or more simultaneous separate primary adenocarcinomas of the large bowel. Despite incomplete follow-up, ten patients had died of carcinoma originating in sites other than the colon and rectum at the time of publication.

The frequencies of multiple simultaneously occurring primary malignant neoplasms depend upon the thoroughness of examination and investigation. The number of new lesions detected after initial therapy for colonic carcinoma was dependent upon the duration of follow-up and accuracy of follow-up studies. The frequency of extracolonic neoplasms that were detected before or after the initial colorectal carcinoma was dependent upon (1) the prevalence of the particular neoplasm, (2) the age-adjusted attack rate compared with that of colonic cancer, and (3) the long-term survival rate for the particular cancer. For example, patients with pancreatobiliary cancer rarely survived long enough to develop a clinically evident colonic cancer.

Other studies of the association of multiple primary malignant tumors with colorectal carcinoma have been reported. Including 24 cases each of multiple polyposis and ulcerative colitis, 157 (2.6 percent) multiple simultaneous primary colonic neoplasms were encountered in the treatment of 6012 carcinomas of the colon and rectum in a 10-year period at the Mayo Clinic (Moertel et al., 1958, 1961). A new primary colonic carcinoma was known to have developed subsequently in 95 (1.6 percent), whereas in nine patients with simultaneously detected carcinomas, additional new primary colonic carcinomas also developed. An additional 21 patients had extracolonic carcinomas. It was not stated whether lesions such as villous adenoma with atypia and focal adenocarcinomas in the tip of the adenomatous polyp were included.

The frequency of subsequent new colonic carcinomas among those surviving initial therapy for colorectal cancer was studied by Rosenthal and Baronofsky (1960). Of 1628 patients who had resections in a 10-year period, 1100 were considered to have a good prognosis. Fifty-three (4.8 percent) of the 1100 patients had multiple simultaneous colonic carcinomas, excluding those with ulcerative colitis and multiple polyposis. Four hundred fifty-three of the 1100 resected patients were followed for variable periods of time, and 77 ultimately required further resection for new primary colorectal carcinoma. The authors noted an advanced stage of disease at the time of reoperation, as in the Group 1 presented previously.

The study reported the prevalence of separate primary malignant neoplasms among those patients with colorectal carcinoma and defined the likelihood of another cancer developing during the patient's remaining life. The conclusions were as follows: (1) 2 to 3 percent of colonic carcinomas will be multiple at the time of detection of the initial colonic cancer, (2) 3 percent of patients with these carcinomas had a previously detected malignant neoplasm of extracolonic origin, and (3) a new malignant neoplasm, of colonic or extracolonic origin, developed at some subsequent time in fully one third of patients surviving their initial colorectal carcinoma.

Two of the enigmas of the follow-up considerations are that a strong family history of colonic cancer is associated with improved end results, and neither physician nor patient delay in primary treatment, as measured from onset of symptoms, affected prognosis (see Chapter Ten).

SUMMARY

The status of a lesion shown in the original pathology report will substantially determine the patterns of recurrent disease and success in its retreatment. In 1967, Spratt and Spjut characterized those factors that truly influence outcome (see Chapter Ten). Although virtually no patient with recurrent disease will have all of the favorable characteristics indicated, the higher the proportion present, the more suitable the cancer is for another resection.

The importance of the time interval between original therapy and recurrence of cancer has been discussed. Although there have been occasional reports of very late recurrent disease, 50 percent of all patients initially treated for cure will develop recurrent cancer within 18 months of the first resection. The remaining half do so over the course of the next 5 to 6 years.

The major purpose of follow-up of the colorectal cancer patient is to retreat recurrent cancer in an effective and timely manner. An inadequate primary operation followed by radiotherapy is worse than no treatment at all, and the same applies to supplemental chemotherapy.

Follow-up always has to be viewed as a screening program for the discovery of cancer (new or old) in a high-risk group. Difficulties in experimental design, high cost, and the large number of cases needed over long periods have contributed to the lack of controlled clinical trials to prove or disprove the benefit and optimum strategy for follow-up. The complexity of this problem as well as the cumulative problem of multiple primary cancers at multiple sites in a steadily aging population at ever higher risk, largely from age alone, has been studied (Spratt, 1977, 1982).

With colorectal cancer, recurrence is a major medical problem. We are only moderately successful in treatment of the primary disease. Understanding the prognostic significance of the pathologic characteristics of the primary neoplasm, the importance of the original operation, and the periods of risk for recurrence are essential in planning both follow-up and further treatment. Reresection for cure after a standard operation only infrequently accomplishes cure. In the absence of cure, palliation is possible, and the lives of patients can be substantially extended. Whether early detection with CEA can convert these same patients to long-term cures remains to be determined. Further study is necessary to establish if changes in the levels of biologic markers can be monitored in a way that will enhance survivorship. The Achilles' heel in all follow-up is the large segment of cases whose outcome is already predetermined by the inherent pathologic properties of the original primary cancer.

It must be recognized when the limits of available technology have been reached with respect to a further reduction in the morbidity and mortality of these cancers, in order to avoid compounding the economic and physical morbidity of the disease and its management by ineffective overmanagement. The law of diminishing marginal returns is ever present. In system after system, more stringent efforts and expenditures beyond a certain optimum point are not associated with a better outcome. A great challenge in all systems is to define the strategy that provides the *optimum* benefit to the patient, as discussed in Chapter Four. Determining the most cost-effective, valuable, and humane strategy for the screening and follow-up merits continuing study.

References

Adson JA, Van Heerden JA: Major hepatic resections for metastatic colorectal cancer. Ann Surg 191:576–583, 1980.

Agnew CH, Cooley RN: Barium enema study of postoperative recurrences of carcinoma of the colon. JAMA 179:331–336, 1982.

Arnaud JP, Koehl C, Adloff M: Carcinoembryonic antigen (CEA) in diagnosis and prognosis of colorectal carcinoma. Dis Colon Rectum 23:141–144, 1980.

Bacon HE, Berkley JL: The rationale of reresection for recurrent cancer of the colon and rectum. Dis Colon Rectum 2:549–554, 1959.

Balz JB, Martin EW, Minton JP: CEA as an early indicator for second-look procedure in colorectal carcinoma. Rev Surg 34:1–4, 1977.

Bargen JA, Rankin FW: Multiple carcinomata of the large intestine. Ann Surg 91:583–593, 1930.

Barrows GH, Burton RM, Jarrett DD, et al.: Immunochemical detection of human blood in feces. Am J Clin Pathol 69:342–346, 1978.

Beal JM, Cornell GN: A study of the problem of recurrence of carcinoma at the anastomotic site following resection of the colon for carcinoma. Ann Surg 143:1–7, 1956.

Black BM, Kelly AH: Recurrent carcinoma of the rectum and rectosigmoid; results of treatment after continence-preserving procedures. Arch Surg 71:538–542, 1955.

Brindley G, Rice JS Jr: Multiple primary malignancies of the large intestine. Surg Clin North Am 32:1499–1510, 1952.

Cole WH: Recurrence in carcinoma of the colon and proximal rectum following resection for carcinoma. Arch Surg 65:264–270, 1952.

Cook GB: A comparison of single and multiple primary cancers. Cancer 19:959–966, 1966.

Cronqvist S: Changes in the colon following resection and end-to-end anastomosis. Acta Radiol 48:425–433, 1957.

Dales LG, Friedman GD, Collen MF: Evaluation of a

periodic multiphasic health checkup. Methods Inf Med 13:140–146, 1974.

Dunphy JE: Recurrent cancer of the colon and rectum: Report of cases with favorable results following radical surgery. N Engl J Med 237:111–113, 1947.

Dunphy JE, Pikula JV: Anterior resection. *In* Turrell R (ed): Diseases of the Colon and Anorectum. 2nd ed. Vol. 1. Philadelphia, WB Saunders Company, 1969, p. 533.

Eddy DM: Screening for Cancer: Theory, Analysis and Design. Stanford, Stanford University Press, 1978.

Eddy DM: Computer-Assisted Evaluation of Screening Tests and Early Detection of Colorectal Cancer. NIH Publication No. 80-2075 1979, 35–46.

Eddy D: ACS report on the cancer-related health checkup. CA 30:193–240, 1980.

Eickenberg HU, Amin M, Klompus W, Lich R Jr: Urologic complications following abdominoperineal resection. J Urol 115:180–182, 1976.

Fazio VW: The current status of the pullthrough procedure for rectal cancer. *In* Welvarrt K, et al (eds): Colorectal Cancer (Boerhaave Series for Postgraduate Education, No. 18) The Hague, Leiden University Press, 1980, pp. 205–216.

Fleischner FG, Berenberg AL: Recurrent carcinoma of the colon at the site of the anastomosis. Radiology 66:540–547, 1956.

Floyd CE, Corley RG, Cohn I Jr: Local recurrence of carcinoma of the colon and rectum. Am J Surg 109:153–159, 1965.

Foster JH: Survival after liver resection for secondary tumors. Am J Surg 135:389–394, 1978.

Gary RK, Sala JM, Spratt JS Jr.: The detection and treatment of post-irradiationally recidivated cancers of the cervix uteri. Radiology 83:208–218, 1964.

Gilbertsen VA: Adenocarcinoma of the rectum: Incidence and locations of recurrent tumor following present-day operations performed for cure. Ann Surg 151:340–348, 1960.

Gilbertsen VA: Proctosigmoidoscopy and polypectomy in reducing the incidence of rectal cancer. Cancer 34:936–939, 1974.

Gold P, Freedman SO: Specific carcinoembryonic antigens of the human digestive system. J Exp Med 122:467–481, 1965.

Gold P, Shuster J, Freedman S: Carcinoembryonic antigen (CEA) in clinical medicine: historical perspectives, pitfalls and projections. Cancer 42(3 Suppl):1399–1405, 1978.

Goligher JC, Dukes CE, Bussey HJR: Local recurrences after sphincter-saving excisions for carcinoma of the rectum and rectosigmoid. Br J Surg 39:199–211, 1951.

Goslin R, Steele G Jr, Macintyre J, et al: The use of preoperative plasma CEA levels for the stratification of patients after curative resection of colorectal cancers. Ann Surg 192:747–751, 1980.

Green WW, Blank WA: Perineal recurrence after abdominoperineal resection of carcinoma of the rectum. Dis Colon Rectum 6:125–129, 1963.

Griffin WO Jr, Humphrey L, Sosin H: The prognosis and management of recurrent abdominal malignancies. Curr Probl Surg April, 1969, pp. 3–41.

Habein HC Jr, Clagett OT, McDonald JR: Pulmonary resection for metastatic tumors. Arch Surg 78:716–723, 1959.

Harris SE: The Economics of American Medicine. New York, Macmillan Publishing Co., 1963, pp. 335–390.

Horne CHW, McLay ALC, Tavadia HB, et al: Studies on pregnancy-associated globulin. Clin Exp Immunol 13:603–611, 1973.

Johnson J Jr, Fantone J, Flye MW: Histological evaluation of the nodules resected in the treatment of pulmonary metastatic disease. J Surg Oncol 21:1–4, 1982.

Judd ES Jr, Bellegie NJ: Carcinoma of the rectosigmoid and upper part of rectum. Recurrence following low anterior resection. Arch Surg 64:697–706, 1952.

Kiselow M, Butcher HR, Bricker EM: Results of the radical surgical treatment of advanced pelvic cancer. Ann Surg 166:428–436, 1967.

Kiser JL, Spratt JS Jr, Johnson CA: Colon perforations occurring during sigmoidoscopic examinations and barium enemas. Mo Med 65:969–974, 1968.

Knutson CO, Fry DE, Barbie RD, Polk HC: Reassessment of intraoperative decisions; why operations for cancer of the large bowel fail. Ann Surg 187:549–554, 1978.

Knutson CO, Max MH: Value of colonoscopy in patients with rectal blood loss unexplained by rigid proctosigmoidoscopy and barium contrast enema examinations. Am J Surg 139:84–87, 1980.

Knutson CO, Williams HC, Max MH: Detection of intercolonic lesions by barium contrast enema. The importance of adequate colon preparation to diagnostic accuracy. JAMA 242:2206–2208, 1979.

Koch M, McPherson A: Predictive value of plasma CEA in patients with colorectal carcinoma. J Surg Oncol 12:319–325, 1979.

Kuzma JW, Dixon WH: Evaluation of recurrence in gastric adenocarcinoma patients. Cancer 19:677–688, 1966.

Lee YTN, Hori JM, Spratt JS Jr: Malignant lymphoma: Histologic types of multiple biopsies. Am Chin Scholar 1:16–23, 1978.

Levoy RP: The $100,000 Practice and How to Build It. Englewood NJ, Prentice-Hall, 1966, p. 1.

Lim BS, Dennis CR, Gardner B, Newman J: Analysis of survival vs. patient and doctor delay of treatment in gastrointestinal cancer. Am J Surg 127:210–214, 1974.

Lofgren EP, Waugh JM, Dockerty MB: Local recurrence of carcinoma after anterior resection of the rectum and sigmoid: relationship with the length of normal mucosa excised distal to the lesion. Arch Surg 74:825–838, 1957.

Long JW, Mayo CW, Dockerty MB, Judd ES Jr: Recurrent versus new and independent carcinomas of the colon and rectum. Proc Staff Meeting Mayo Clinic 25:169–178, 1950.

Mach JP, Jaeger P, Bertholet MM, et al: Detection of recurrence of large-bowel carcinoma by radioimmunoassay of circulatory carcinoembryonic antigen (CEA). Lancet 2:535–540, 1974.

Martin EW Jr, Cooperman M, King G, et al: A retrospective and prospective study of serial CEA determinations in the early detection of recurrent colon cancer. Am J Surg 137:167–169, 1979.

Mayo CW, Schlicke CP: Carcinoma of colon and rectum; study of metastasis and recurrences. Surg Gynecol Obstet 74:83–91, 1942.

Minton JP, James KK, Hurtubise PE, et al: The use of serial carcinoembryonic antigen determinations to predict recurrence of carcinoma of the colon and the time for a second-look operation. Surg Gynecol Obstet 147:208–210, 1978.

Minton JP, Martin EW Jr: The use of serial CEA determinations to predict recurrence of colon cancer and when to do a second-look operation. Cancer 42(3 Suppl):1422–1427, 1978.

Moertel CG, Bargen JA, Dockerty MB: Multiple carcinomas of the large intestine: a review of the literature and a study of 261 cases. Gastroenterology 34:85–98, 1958.

Moertel CG, Dockerty MB, Baggenstoss AH: Multiple primary malignant neoplasms. I. Introduction and presentation of data. III. Tumors of multicentric origin. Cancer 14:238–248, 1961.

Molnar IG, Vandevoorde JP, Gitnick GL: CEA levels in fluids bathing gastrointestinal tumors. Gastroenterology 70:513–515, 1976.

Monaco R, Salfen L, Spratt JS Jr: The patient as an education participant in health care. Mo Med 69:932–933, 937, 1972.

Morson BC, Gaughan EG, Bussey HJR: Pelvic recurrence after excision of rectum for carcinoma. Br Med J 2(5348):13–18, 1963.

Mountain CF, Khalil KG, Mermes KE, Frazier OH: The contribution of surgery to the management of carcinomatous pulmonary metastases. Cancer 41:833–840, 1978.

Neuhauser D: Economic Considerations, Screening and Early Detection of Colorectal Cancer. NIH Publication No. 80-2075, 1979, pp. 47–49.

Our ailing medical system. Fortune 81:79, 1970.

Polk HC Jr: Extended resection for selected adenocarcinomas of the large bowel. Ann Surg 175:892–899, 1972.

Polk HC Jr: Personal communication, 1982.

Polk HC Jr, Spratt JS Jr: Recurrent colorectal carcinoma: Detection, treatment and other considerations. Surgery 69:9–23, 1971.

Polk HC Jr, Spratt JS Jr: The results of treatment of perineal recurrence of cancer of the rectum. Cancer 43:952–955, 1979.

Polk HC Jr, Spratt JS Jr: Recurrent cancer of the colon. Surg Clin North Am 63:151–160, 1983.

Polk HC Jr, Spratt JS Jr, Bennett D, et al: Surgical mortality and survival from colonic carcinoma. Arch Surg 89:16–23, 1964.

Polk HC Jr, Spratt JS Jr, Butcher HR Jr: Frequency of multiple primary malignant neoplasms associated with colorectal carcinoma. Am J Surg 109:71–74, 1965.

Polk HC Jr, Warren WD: Incision and related considerations. *In* Turell R (ed): Diseases of the Colon and Anorectum. 2nd ed. Philadelphia, WB Saunders Company, 1969.

Racaberen JA, Lynch HT, Campbell AS, et al: Natural history of hereditary cancer of the breast and colon. Cancer 50:360–363, 1982.

Rosenthal I, Baronofsky ID: Prognostic and therapeutic implications of polyps in metachronous colic carcinoma. JAMA 172:37–41, 1960.

Schoenberg BS: Multiple Primary Malignant Neoplasm. The Connecticut Experience, 1935–1964. Berlin, Springer-Verlag, 1977.

Schoenberg BS, Myers MH: Statistical methods for studying multiple primary malignant neoplasm. Cancer 40(4 Suppl):1892–1898, 1977.

Scudamore HH, Corr WP Jr, Judd ES: Value of periodic medical examinations following operation for carcinoma of the colon or rectum. Proc Mayo Clin 35:258–268, 1960.

Songster CL, Barrows GH, Jarrett DD: Immunochemical detection of fecal occult blood—the fecal smear punch-disc test: a new non-invasive screening test for colorectal cancer. Cancer 45(5 Suppl):1099–1102, 1980.

Spjut HJ, Spratt JS Jr: Endemic and morphologic similarities existing between spontaneous colonic neoplasms in man and 3:2′-dimethyl-4-aminobiphenyl induced colonic neoplasms in rats. Ann Surg 161:309–324, 1965.

Spratt JS Jr: Locally recurrent cancer after radical mastectomy. Cancer 20:1051–1053, 1967.

Spratt JS Jr: The physician's obligation to the development of managerial skills in health care facilities. Mo Med 66:916–918, 965–969, 1969.

Spratt JS Jr: Cost effectiveness in the post-treatment of follow-up of cancer patients. J Surg Oncol 3:393–400, 1971.

Spratt JS Jr: The physician's role in minimizing the economic morbidity of cancer. Semin Oncol 2:411–417, 1975a.

Spratt JS Jr: The relation of "human capital" preservation to health costs. Am J Econ Soc 34:295–307, 1975b.

Spratt JS Jr: Multiple primary cancers: Review of clinical studies from two Missouri hospitals. Cancer 40:1806–1811, 1977.

Spratt JS Jr: The relationship between the rates of growth of cancers and the intervals between screening examinations necessary for effective discovery. Cancer Detect Prev 4:301–305, 1981.

Spratt JS: Epidemiology of screening for cancer. Curr Probl Cancer 6:1–58, 1982.

Spratt JS Jr, Ackerman LV: Colonic cancer and colonic polyps. Hosp Med 1:4–8, 1964.

Spratt JS Jr, Ackerman LV, Moyer CA: Relationship of polyps of the colon to colonic cancer. Ann Surg 148:682–698, 1958.

Spratt JS Jr, Butcher HR Jr, Bricker EM: Exenterative Surgery of the Pelvis. Philadelphia, WB Saunders Company, 1973.

Spratt JS Jr, Hoag MG: Incidence of multiple primary cancers per man-year of follow-up: 20-year review from the Ellis Fischel State Cancer Hospital. Ann Surg 164:775–784, 1966.

Spratt JS Jr, Shieber W, Dillard BM: Anatomy and Surgical Technique of Groin Dissection. St Louis, CV Mosby Company, 1965.

Spratt JS, Jr, Spjut HJ: Prevalence and prognosis of individual clinical and pathological variables associated with colorectal carcinoma. Cancer 20:1976–1985, 1967.

Spratt JS Jr, Spratt TL: Rates of growth of pulmonary metastases and host survival. Ann Surg 159:161–171, 1964.

Spratt JS Jr, Watson FR, Pratt JL: Characteristics of variants of colorectal carcinoma that do not metastasize to lymph nodes. Dis Colon Rectum 13:243–246, 1970.

Staab HJ, Anderer FA, Stumpf E, Fischer R: Carcinoembryonic antigen follow-up and selection of patients for second-look operation in management of gastrointestinal carcinoma. J Surg Oncol 10:273–282, 1978.

Stimson WH: Transplantation—nature's success. Lancet 1:684, 1972.

Stimson WH: Variations in the level of pregnancy-associated alpha-macroglobulin in patients with cancer. J Clin Pathol 28:868–871, 1975a.

Stimson WH: Variations in the serum concentration of a human pregnancy-associated alpha-macroglobulin during pregnancy and after delivery. J Reprod Fertil 43:579–582, 1975b.

Stimson WH, Blackstock JC: Synthesis of a pregnancy-associated alpha-macroglobulin by human leucocytes. Experientia 31:371–373, 1975.

Talley RW, Block MA, Ormond RS: Natural history of recurrent colon cancer (Abstract). Ninth International Cancer Congress, Tokyo, 1966, p. 515.

Taylor RN, Fulford KM, Huong AY: Results of a nationwide proficiency test for carcinoembryonic antigen. J Clin Microbiol 5:433–438, 1977.

Thompson DE, Jacob LW: Analysis of screening strategies for colorectal cancer: an extension of the model. Michigan Cancer Foundation Workshop, Detroit, Michigan, May 1977.

Voyles CR, Richardson JD, Bland KI, et al: Emergency abdominal wall reconstruction with polypropylene mesh: short-term benefits versus long-term complications. Ann Surg 194:219–223, 1981.

Waggoner CM, Spratt JS Jr: Prognostic significance of radiographic ureteropathy before and after irradiation therapy for carcinoma of the cervix uteri. Am J Obstet Gynecol 105:1197–1200, 1969.

Wagner HM: Principles of operations research with applications to managerial decisions. Englewood Cliffs, NJ, Prentice-Hall, 1974, p. 364.

Wanebo HJ: Are carcinoembryonic antigen levels of value in the curative management of colorectal cancer? Surgery 89:290–295, 1981.

Wanebo HJ, Rao B, Pinsky CM, et al: Preoperative carcinoembryonic antigen level as a prognostic indicator in colorectal cancer. N Engl J Med 299:448–451, 1978.

Wangensteen OH, Griffin WO Jr, Lewis FO, Arhelger SWL: The second-look operation in the management of abdominal cancer. *In* Pack G, Ariel I (eds): Treatment of Cancer and Allied Diseases. 2nd ed. Vol. V, New York, Boeber, 1959, pp. 62–74.

Welin S, Youker J, Spratt JS Jr: The rates and patterns of growth of 375 tumors of the large intestine and rectum observed serially by double contrast enema study (Malmö technique). AJR 90:673–687, 1963.

Williams RD, Yurko AA, Kerr G, Zollinger RM: Comparison of anterior and abdominoperineal resections for low pelvic colon and rectal carcinoma. Am J Surg 111:114–119, 1966.

Wood CB, Horne CHW, Towler CM, et al: The value of pregnancy-associated alpha$_2$glycoprotein in patients with colorectal cancer. Br J Surg 65:653–656, 1978a.

Wood CB, Horne CHW, Towler CM, et al: A critical comparison of the value of pregnancy-associated alpha$_2$glycoprotein and carcinoembryonic antigen assays in patients with colorectal cancer. J Clin Pathol 31:1065–1067, 1978b.

Zelas P, Haaga JR, Lavery IC, Fazio VW: The diagnosis by percutaneous biopsy with computer tomography of a recurrence of carcinoma of the rectum in the pelvis. Surg Gynecol Obstet 151:525–527, 1980.

FIVE

Radiology of Neoplastic Colon Disease

R. E. Miller, M.D.

Examination of the colon in its entirety is accomplished best and most economically by roentgenology. Ancillary methods of examination are sigmoidoscopy, colonoscopy, arteriography, and scintigraphy.

Two methods of roentgenographic examination of the colon are most commonly used: In one, a full column of low-density barium sulfate suspension (about 2000 ml) is used to fill the colon, and in the other, the double contrast enema study, a small quantity (about 250 ml) of a high-density barium sulfate suspension is used to coat the mucosa, after which the colon is filled and distended by insufflation with air. Both types of barium enema studies are highly accurate when properly performed and tailored to answer specific questions raised by the referring physician.

The single most important aspect of the colon examination is assumption by the examiner of complete responsibility—moral, legal, and technical—for the preparation of the patient, the technique of the examination, and the interpretation of the results.

Contraindications to the examination must be carefully considered. These include suspected perforation of the colon, toxic megacolon, biopsy of the colon after rigid sigmoidoscopy, or polypectomy by colonoscopy. However, the examination can be performed after a superficial mucosal biopsy or biopsy of a large exophytic lesion using the flexible fiberoptic endoscope. Biopsy through the rigid sigmoidoscope may be a deep biopsy through the muscularis mucosae. Therefore, after the procedure, a waiting period of 6 to 7 days should elapse before a barium enema is performed (Harned et al., 1982; Maglinte et al., 1982). It is the responsibility of the endoscopist to inform the radiologist if biopsy has been done so that he will cancel the barium enema examination. Recent studies show that barium enemas can be performed on the same day as endoscopy without significant diagnostic interference, provided that *no* deep biopsy has been made (Lappas et al., in press). Barium examinations also are contraindicated if there is definite evidence of *acute* diverticulitis or other *acute* inflammatory bowel disease. Barium enemas should be delayed for a period of 10 to 14 days for medical management to quiet the inflammation.

The radiologist must assume the major responsibility for finding early lesions. He has the tools at hand; what he must now do is assume the responsibility for proper preparation and technique. He can no longer delegate this to some well-meaning, but perhaps ill-informed, referring physician. The radiologist does not do this for angiography or endoscopy, and he must not do this for gastrointestinal examinations. Most missed lesions in the colon are due to poor preparation, faulty technique, and inadequate attention to detail rather than to an inherent invisibility of a lesion.

PREPARATION FOR EXAMINATION

It is a primary requirement that the colon be well prepared for all colon examinations except in emergencies. Fecal matter simulating polyps will be seen in any type of examination if the colon is not clean. A combination of diet, laxatives, and enemas must be used for successful cleansing.

The patient is put on a low residue or clear liquid diet on the day before the examination and for 2 to 3 days, if possible, preceding the study. The recently introduced Ensure* liquid diet for colon preparation may be substituted for the "clear liquid" diet. The Ensure diet is nutritionally complete and can be given for more than 1 day.

Two laxatives should be taken the day before the examination. The administration of 2 oz (60 ml) of castor oil at noon or shortly thereafter plus 2.5 oz (75 ml) of X-Prep liquid† at 4:00 P.M. is my preference and is usually reliable. In certain instances, such as if a patient is diabetic, I sometimes substitute 10 oz (300 ml) of magnesium citrate or 20 gm of magnesium sulfate for one or the other of these cathartics. But magnesium salts must be avoided in patients with renal disease. Twenty mg of bisacodyl (4 tabs) can also be substituted for *one* of the cathartics. A large volume of oral liquids also must be given to assist in an effective purge. I urge the consumption of a full 8 oz glass of clear liquid each hour for 8 hours on the day preceding the examination. This totals about 2 l.

In addition to laxatives, a single 2000-ml tap water enema is given in the x-ray department on the morning of the study (Miller, 1975a). This combination has proved as effective as any method I have tried for obtaining a clean colon. One carefully done 2000-ml enema is far better and less traumatic than the administration of 15 to 20 "enemas until clear." The patient must be given not only precise, *written* instructions concerning the cathartics and the necessity for a clear liquid diet and fluid intake the day before examination but also reasons for following the instructions closely. I do this by giving each patient a printed pamphlet written and furnished by the radiology department. The patient must also be given instructions and encouragement just before and during administration of the cleansing enema (Miller, 1975a).

Good evacuation usually follows the 2000-ml tap water enema, whereas a 500 to 1000-ml enema may be retained in the rectum and the sigmoid colon. I allow a full 30 minutes for evacuation before giving glucagon (Miller et al., 1974a, 1978). Rarely some water is retained in the colon, but this can be tolerated because of the high radiographic density of the barium suspension, especially in air contrast studies.

The radiologist needs, deserves, and must demand as clean a colon as does the colonoscopist. The latter may give cathartics for 3 nights, a liquid diet for 48 hours, and a high colonic enema 1 to 3 hours before the examination. This combination of all three methods ensures a liquid diarrhea and a clean colon (Marks, 1978; Shinya, 1974). If the attending physician resists using the radiology department's standard preparation, insisting on a 1 day preparation, I will agree to using the colonoscopist's procedure—but nothing less. I refuse to do poor radiology and poor medicine. I am personally aware of several malpractice cases in which the problem of missed tumors resulted from inadequate preparation. In each instance, the attending physician and radiologist were *both* held accountable, in spite of strenuous efforts of each one to blame the other!

DRUGS

During barium enema examinations, when the colon does not fill properly because of muscle spasm or for other reasons, anticholinergic drugs are often administered. In 1958, Welin (1953, 1967) recommended that, with few exceptions, these drugs be given routinely to patients before air contrast studies of the colon. The anticholinergic purportedly reduced smooth muscle spasm and prevented vasovagal reflex, allowing the radiologist to accomplish a more detailed and complete examination with less discomfort to the patient (Miller, 1974). However, adverse effects (Ferrucci and Benedict, 1971; Friedland, 1973; Gelfand and Moskowitz, 1970; Miller and Lehman, 1972; Miller et al., 1973; Miller et al., 1974b) of propantheline bromide or atropine sulfate in colon examinations may persist long after the examination has been completed. I now routinely use 0.5 to 0.75 mg glucagon IV immediately prior to the examination.

The short action of glucagon and the fact that it provides excellent relaxation and few side effects lead me to agree with Ferrucci and Benedict (1971) that hypotonic examination of the colon is useful in a number of situations. According to these researchers, the indications for a hypotonic barium enema examination are as follows:

*Ensure: Ross Laboratories, Columbus, Ohio.

†Liquid X-Prep: Gray Pharmaceutical Company, affiliate, The Purdue Frederick Company, Norwalk, Connecticut 06856.

1. Lesions with diffuse painful spasm, such as ulcerative or granulomatous colitis or functional disorders.

2. Areas of localized narrowing, e.g., spasm versus constricting lesions, colonic valves or sphincters, or evaluation of strictures in colitis.

3. Diverticular disease, with sigmoid spasm.

4. Decrease in smooth muscle tone for adequate distention during an air contrast study.

5. Functional inability to retain the enema; this is seen especially in aged patients.

Glucagon relaxes the colon and makes the patient more comfortable during barium enema examination in the situations just listed. All the preceding occur in patients with neoplastic disease of the colon. Glucagon is better than atropine sulfate as a hypotonic agent because it produces better relaxation with fewer side effects. I believe that glucagon should be used in patients who have any of the indications previously described. These indications occur more commonly in older patients and in those who have neoplastic disease. It cannot be anticipated in advance who will require glucagon. Therefore, I routinely use it in all patients over 40 years of age and in any patients when searching for neoplastic disease. Spasm can easily mimic carcinoma.

EQUIPMENT

The image-intensified fluoroscope with automatic collimation and photo-timed spot filming devices are mandatory for these examinations. It is important that these instruments have high ratio 12:1 or 6:1 crisscross grids in the spot film device for either conventional or 100 mm spot films (Hayt et al., 1969). I also use and recommend a 12:1 linear grid for tabletop Bucky films and a 6:1 crisscross aluminum interspaced grid for the lateral decubitus apparatus that can be attached to any fluoroscopic table for lateral decubitus films (Miller, 1970). This device permits decubitus films to be made easily in a few seconds. Short exposures are desirable, and therefore, the generator should be capable of delivering exposure in the 120 kVp or higher range, with high milliamperage output to reduce the time of exposure.

I also prefer a disposable plastic bag, tubing, and tip, with short large bore 0.5 in. (1.25 cm) internal diameter tubing and a flexible enema tip.* Our recently reported rapid, low radiation, and lower cost "seven pump" method for pneumocolon examinations has now become routine in many hospitals (Maglinte and Miller, 1983).

*Enema tips and Liquid Polibar: E-Z-EM Company, 7 Portland Avenue, Westbury, New York 11590.

PLAIN FILMS OF THE ABDOMEN

Preliminary films of the abdomen are most useful in examination of the colon. Certainly this is a part of the usual examination of the acute abdomen prior to any emergency colon examination. Calcifications and unusual air or fluid collections as well as fluid-filled loops, fecal collections in the colon, and contrast material remaining in the stomach or bowel from previous examinations may be noted. This easily solves many problems that can arise either during fluoroscopy or after the roentgenograms are developed. If preliminary films are not available for comparison, residual contrast material can cause great confusion in determining whether fistulas or other lesions exist. Frequently films taken shortly before examination in an acute abdominal series or with excretory pyelograms may be used for comparison. With proper equipment, preliminary spot films may be substituted for the usual overhead radiograms. I agree with Margulis (1973) that the advantages of a permanent record over the memorized impressions of even an expert fluoroscopist are so obvious that they need no further discussion.

EVALUATION AND CHOICE OF RADIOGRAPHIC METHOD

The diagnostic yield in radiographic colon examinations depends primarily on a reliable technique. Although human factors play an important role in all x-ray examinations, the efforts of a competent examiner may be wasted if he does not know and use the best available techniques. Because a high percentage of malignant lesions found in the colon are operable and resection of early lesions usually means cure, technique in finding a tumor becomes extremely important. Selected studies report an 81 percent 5-year survival rate after surgery of localized disease (Turnbull, 1975). Roentgenologic techniques to detect colon cancer are limited to recognition of macroscopic disease, but roentgenograms can even detect lesions that measure only a few mm in diameter (Welin, 1953; Carlile, 1967; Miller, 1974b; Miller and Lehman, 1976). Currently a 4- to 5-mm tumor in any part of the colon from the anus to the appendix is detectable. This is the present limit in diagnostic roentgenology for colon carcinoma, and this limit is also the goal toward which the radiologist should continually aspire (Miller, 1974b; Sherman, 1960). Advanced radiologic technique also can be used to examine the entire colon through very narrow constrictions (Fig. 5–1). The examination of the entire colon is mandatory to detect synchronous carcinomas or other co-existent lesions. Synchronous carcinomas occur in approximately 4 to 7 percent of patients who have carcinoma of the colon (Ekelund and Pihl, 1974; McGregor and Bacon, 1958; Moertel et al., 1958; Peabody and Smithwick, 1961; Schottenfeld et al., 1969). I do not believe it is good medicine to take out one carcinoma and leave behind another when both can be removed at the same time.

At the very least, there is a high risk group of patients that should have an air contrast colon examination as the primary examination. This group includes patients with any of the following characteristics:

(1) Rectal bleeding for any reason or a history of bleeding.

(2) Polyps on proctoscopic examination.

(3) A previous history of polyps or carcinoma.

(4) A strong family history of polyps or carcinoma (this includes familial polyposis, Peutz-Jeghers syndrome, Gardner's syndrome, and Turcot syndrome).

(5) Patient over 40 years of age.

(6) A change in bowel habits, weight loss, unexplained anemia, previous ureterosigmoid anastomosis, long-standing (10 years) inflammatory bowel disease, Hemoccult-positive

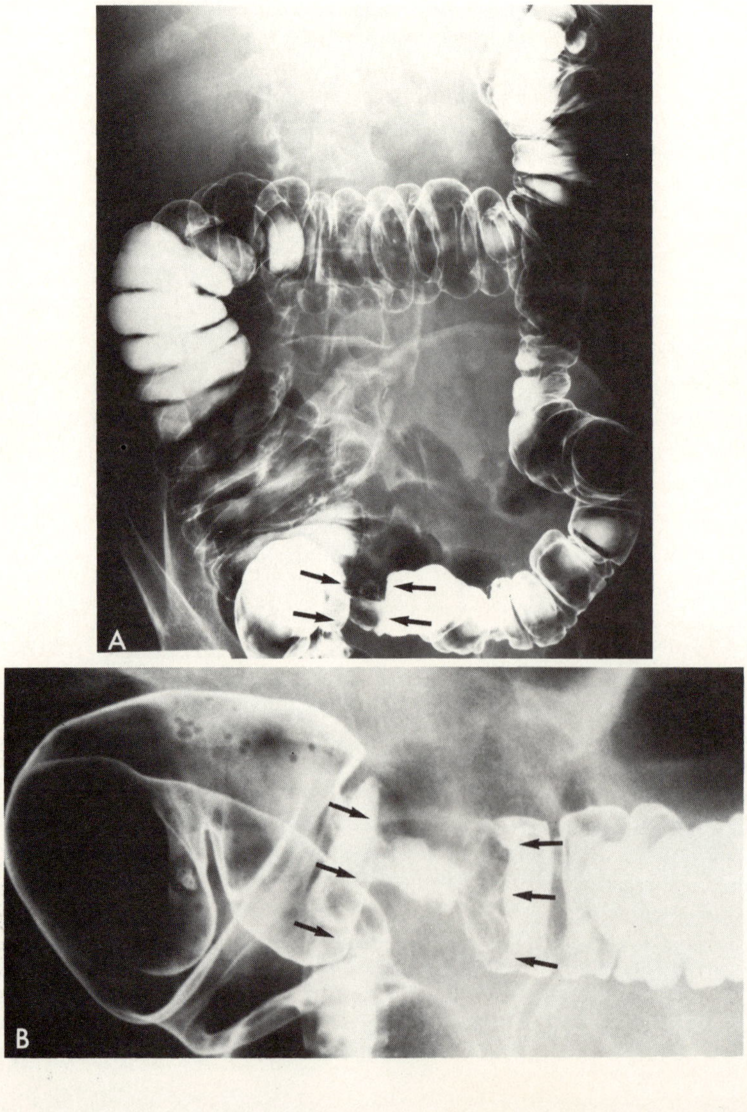

Figure 5–1. *A,* There is a constricting adenocarcinoma of the rectosigmoid colon. Only 250 ml of barium were used to coat the entire colon despite the constricting lesion. *B,* Spot films of same patient as in Figure 5–1*A*, showing constricting adenocarcinoma of the sigmoid.

stools, or other signs, on the basis of which the clinician or radiologist should have a high index of suspicion for carcinoma (Haney and McGarity, 1971; Preissing et al., 1974; Whitaker et al., 1971).

Carcinomas

Carcinomas in the gastrointestinal tract are polypoid, ulcerative, or infiltrative. They may be small, large, ragged, smooth, localized, multiple, annular, or stenosing. Special types of adenocarcinoma are mucoid, colloid, scirrhous, and villous. These tumors cannot be differentiated from the usual adenocarcinoma by roentgenologic examination. However, the scirrhous carcinoma occurring in ulcerative colitis and the villous adenoma are exceptions. Both of these have different roentgenologic characteristics. The mucinous carcinoma may have radiologically visible calcifications.

Early lesions are small, elevated, buttonlike, polypoid masses (Robbins, 1967). For a long time the lesions remain superficial and are in small areas of cancerous transformation that are asymptomatic. It is for these reasons that lesions must be found early. However, they cannot be differentiated from adenomatous polyps either by colonoscopy or by radiography (Kobayashi et al., 1974). This can only be done by adequate biopsy. In early scirrhous carcinoma, the infiltrative carcinoma produces no narrowing or obvious stiffening of the walls of the colon and is confined at first to one side of the colonic lumen. As the lesion progresses, the infiltrate spreads circumferentially as well as longitudinally. Then the lumen narrows. Eventually a stenotic lesion of about 10 to 30 cm in length, with a lumen of 1 to 3 cm in diameter, develops.

Scirrhous carcinoma constitutes about one third of the tumors occurring in ulcerative colitis (McQueeney et al., 1967). In ulcerative colitis, the carcinomatous change is often difficult and sometimes impossible to differentiate from a long, benign stricture. In most instances, the neoplasm does not appear in the first 10 years, but becomes increasingly frequent in people who have had the disease 10 years or longer (McMillan et al., 1968). Therefore, all strictures in patients with a history of ulcerative colitis for 10 years are suspect, and the abnormal tissue should be resected or biopsied through the colonoscope. Site and extent of strictures are detected most readily by radiology.

Occasionally, calcifications in adenocarcinoma of the colon are seen on plain films along the course of the colon. Calcifications will also appear in the metastatic lesions to lymph nodes, the liver, or the peritoneal cavity. All recorded cases of calcification are from mucoid carcinomas (Fred et al., 1964; Zboralske and Amberry, 1962). Calcifications can also occur in hemangiomas of the colon, but these have a characteristic round rim with radiolucent centers similar to phleboliths that are seen in the pelvis.

Villous adenomas are papillary tumors consisting of long slender projections of mucosa called fronds. They occur anywhere in the colon, but are usually found in the rectum. The lesions are sessile, bulky, and soft and are easily missed by palpation. They show linear streaks on roentgenograms, which are produced by barium lodged between fronds and have been likened to a barium-soaked sponge. Some villous adenomas, especially right-sided, do not have a spongelike appearance, and without an electrolyte imbalance, they cannot be distinguished from other masses (Tung and Goldman, 1970).

Endometriosis

Endometrial tissue sometimes invades and deforms the colon. Symptoms are exaggerated during menstruation, and with this exacerbation, fibrosis is produced. The sigmoid colon and rectosigmoid junction above the reflection of the peritoneum at the level of the third sacral segment is the usual site of this tumor. On the lateral view, the tumor causes a sharply defined indentation on the anterior wall of the rectosigmoid junction (Fig. 5–2). This latter pattern is expected because the tumor invades the cul-de-sac. The indentation may be smooth or have thornlike edges.

Sarcomas

Sarcomas of the colon are usually lymphosarcoma, reticulum cell sarcoma, and leiomyosarcoma. They can occur anywhere in the colon. Some of them ulcerate and form a large irregular ulcer surrounded by thick rolled-up margins.

Pseudotumors

Pseudotumors are caused by pressure, external masses, or adhesions and may mimic

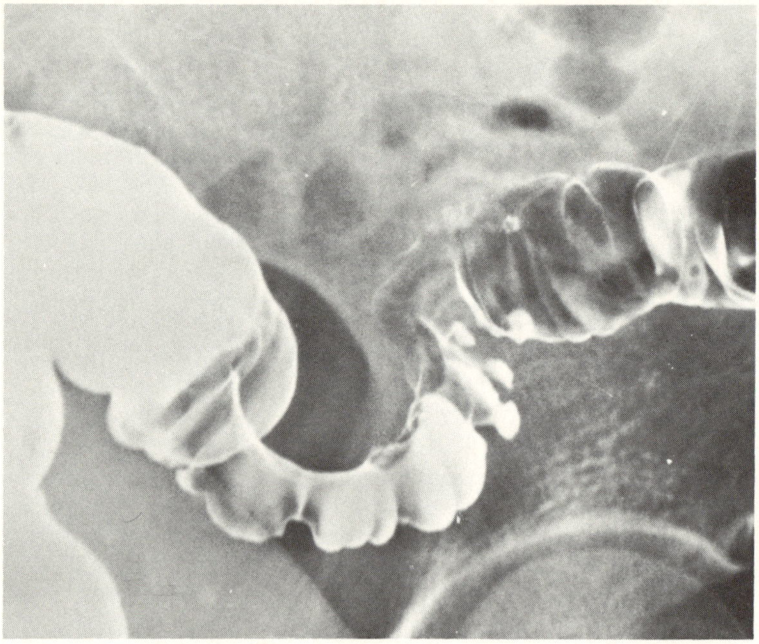

Figure 5–2. Generally smooth but slightly irregular indentation of the rectosigmoid colon from endometriosis, but this could be mistaken for an abscess from diverticulitis or other forms of tumor.

carcinoma. They can be differentiated from colonic lesions by distending the colon and especially the cecum (the most common site of pseudotumors) with air after barium has been administered. Distention makes diagnosis possible. As the cecum distends, the walls balloon out and become smooth, and the pseudotumor "disappears" (Matter and Rotke, 1969).

TECHNIQUES OF RADIOGRAPHIC CONTRAST EVALUATION OF THE COLON

Full Column Techniques

I prefer full column techniques for *unprepared emergency* examinations for *bowel obstruction*, reduction of an intussusception, or volvulus, all of which may occur from neoplastic disease. I use 15 or 20 percent weight/volume barium sulfate with 110 kVp single-phase units or 100 kVp three-phase equipment. This is optimal for the average patient (27.5 mm Al 1/20 value layer). In suspected abscess or fistula from perforated diverticula or neoplasm below the peritoneal reflection, a water-soluble contrast material such as Hypaque diluted 3:1 may be used. This special type of examination should be evaluated and approached most carefully. If there is suspected perforation above the peritoneal reflection, and certainly if any pneumoperitoneum is present, enemas should not be done at all (Miller, 1973a, 1973b).

Water enemas may be used for diagnosis of lipomas, but I prefer air contrast techniques with compression to show change in the shape of the lesion (Fig. 5–3). The more modern computed axial tomography (CAT) scan has made the water enema obsolete.

With full column techniques, using phantoms and human volunteers, Miller (1975b) has shown that 1-cm tumors in a 10-cm diameter colon or rectum cannot be seen in any patient of 29-cm thickness with any equipment at any energy level. These tumors will also be missed in noncompressible colon segments in patients over 21 cm in thickness. These noncompressible areas from overlying skeletal structures are usually the hepatic and splenic flexures, the cecum, the rectosigmoid colon, and the rectum. Unfortunately, these areas are frequently the sites of neoplasms. Recently, Gilbertsen and associates (1979) showed that the (single contrast) barium enema misses 35 percent of all colon carcinomas and 42 percent of early (Dukes' A and B) potentially curable carcinomas! Recently, Thorpe, Grayson, and Wingfield (1981) concluded that the air contrast enema detected 96 percent of Dukes' C and D lesions and 91 percent of Dukes' A and B lesions in proven carcinoma of the colon. Unless there is complete obstruction, the full column technique is obsolete in the search for neoplasm of the entire colon.

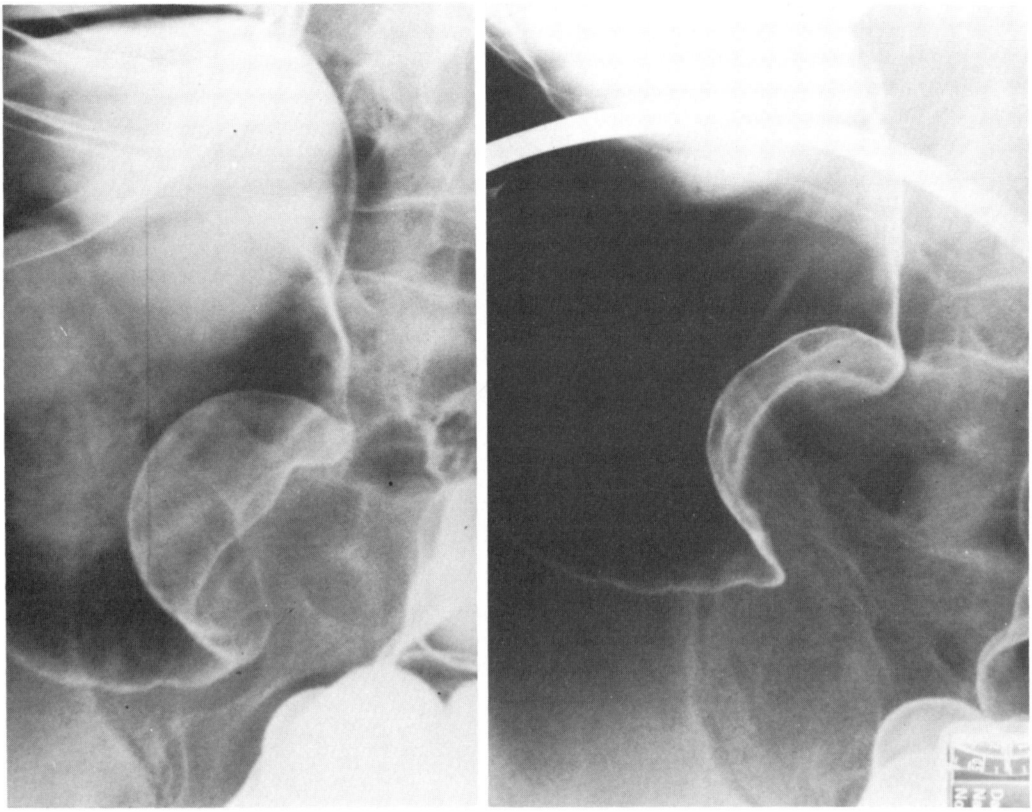

Figure 5–3. Smooth round lesion of the cecum showing deformity on compression. The lesion was a benign lipoma.

Air Contrast Techniques

To achieve adequate air contrast studies, five requirements must be fulfilled, all of which are attainable:

1. A clean colon (adequate preparation).
2. A suitable barium suspension that will coat well and not bubble or "flake out."
3. Adequate insufflation of the bowel.
4. Drainage of excess barium from the rectum.
5. An adequate number of films with good radiologic technique.

Barium Suspension

I use a liquid ready-to-use barium suspension for air contrast colon examinations (HD-85* or Liquid Polibar†). This assures quality control.

*HD-85 Barium: Lafayette Pharmacal Company, P. O. Box 4499, Lafayette, Indiana 47902.

†Enema tips and Liquid Polibar: E-Z-EM Company, 7 Portland Avenue, Westbury, New York 11590.

Air Insufflation

Adequate insufflation adds greatly to the visibility of lesions but adds little to patient discomfort after bowel relaxation with 0.5 to 0.75 mg of glucagon IV. A total of 2500 cc or more of air usually is necessary in adults. This equals 60 or more full compressions of a sphygmomanometer bulb. Adequate insufflation is routinely assured using the seven pump method (Miller and Maglinte, 1982) (Fig. 5–4).

Drainage

Excellent demonstration of the rectum and distal sigmoid lesions is one of the greatest advantages of good air contrast studies. This simply requires drainage of excess barium through the enema tip before or after air instillation; there should be a short final check just before film exposure to make sure there is no excess barium, which would hide obvious lesions. Drainage is achieved by placing the enema bag between the patient's legs on the table top and releasing the tubing clamp. This

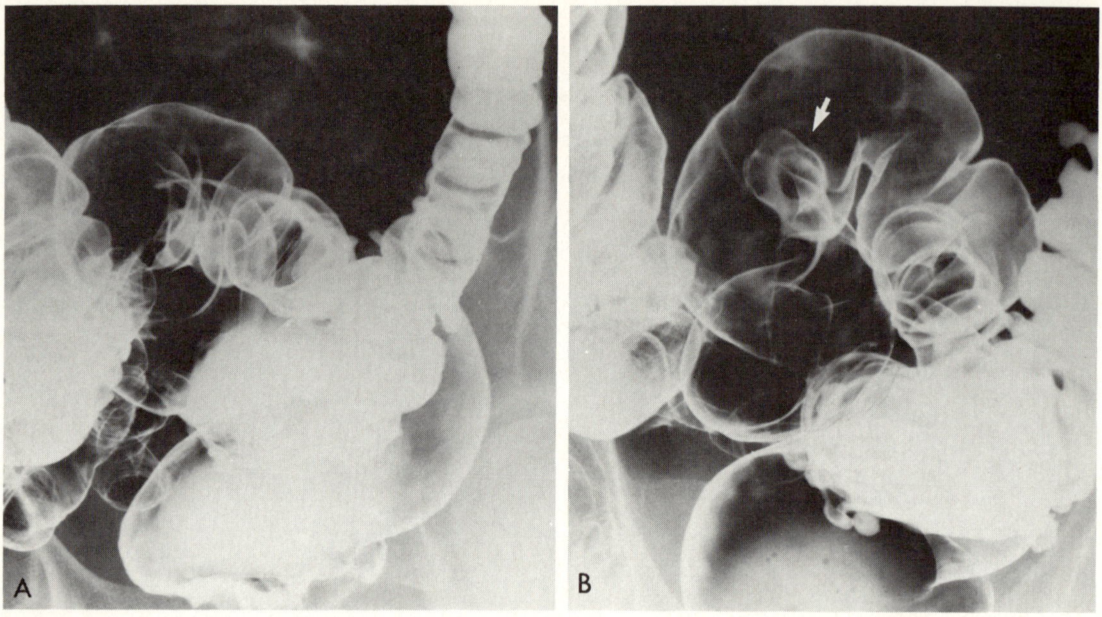

Figure 5–4. *A,* Radiograph of the rectosigmoid colon shows no lesion because of the lack of distention, *B,* Because the colon is now distended with air and the rectosigmoid lifted out of the pelvis, the lesion is shown to good advantage (a polyp in the rectosigmoid colon).

sometimes is helped by elevating the head of the fluoroscopic table (Miller and Peterson, 1978). Evacuation of the rectum is observed and controlled by fluoroscopy. Some air also may escape, but this is easily reinstilled, especially when using the Miller air tip* (Miller, 1969). This tip allows complete control of barium, air, and rectal drainage at any point during the examination. Since the tubing for instilling the air extends to the end of the enema tip, instillation of air does not force residual barium in the enema tubing back into the patient.

Adequate radiograms in sufficient number are necessary to obtain reliable information on all segments of the colon. In air contrast barium enema examinations, as opposed to conventional barium enema examination, the barium should be instilled with the patient in the prone or left lateral position. Angled films of the rectosigmoid should be taken early in the examination, as is prescribed in the seven pump method (Miller and Maglinte, 1982).

DETAILS OF THE COLON EXAMINATION

Before the examination, the radiologist briefly explains the procedure to the patient and slowly injects 0.5 to 0.75 mg glucagon IV. Using a Miller air tip, insert the rectal tube in the left lateral position and instill a high-density, high-viscosity barium mixture (HD-85 or Liquid Polibar). In the average patient, no more than 250 ml of barium are used (Fig. 5–5). If the scout film shows a low-lying transverse colon, an extra "loop" at the flexures (high or subdiaphragmatic flexural gas shadows), or a redundant sigmoid, an additional 50 ml of contrast are given. A one ft (30.5 cm) tubing enema bag is used, and the entire (measured) amount is gently squeezed into the rectum. The table may be tilted in a slight (15 degrees) Trendelenburg position to aid in increasing flow. As soon as the entire volume of contrast material has been introduced, the barium tube is clamped and the table brought to a horizontal position. Air is pumped into the colon in the following seven position sequence, one "pump" consisting of a slow full squeeze on a regular sphygmomanometer bulb: (1) seven pumps in the left lateral position; (2) seven pumps (left anterior oblique position); (3) seven pumps (prone position); (4) seven pumps (right anterior oblique position); (5) seven pumps (right lateral position); (6) seven pumps (right posterior oblique position); and (7) seven pumps (supine position) (Fig. 5–6).

With the patient in a slight 15- to 20-degree oblique position, 30-degree angled views of

*Enema tips and Liquid Polibar: E-Z-EM Company, 7 Portland Avenue, Westbury, New York 11590.

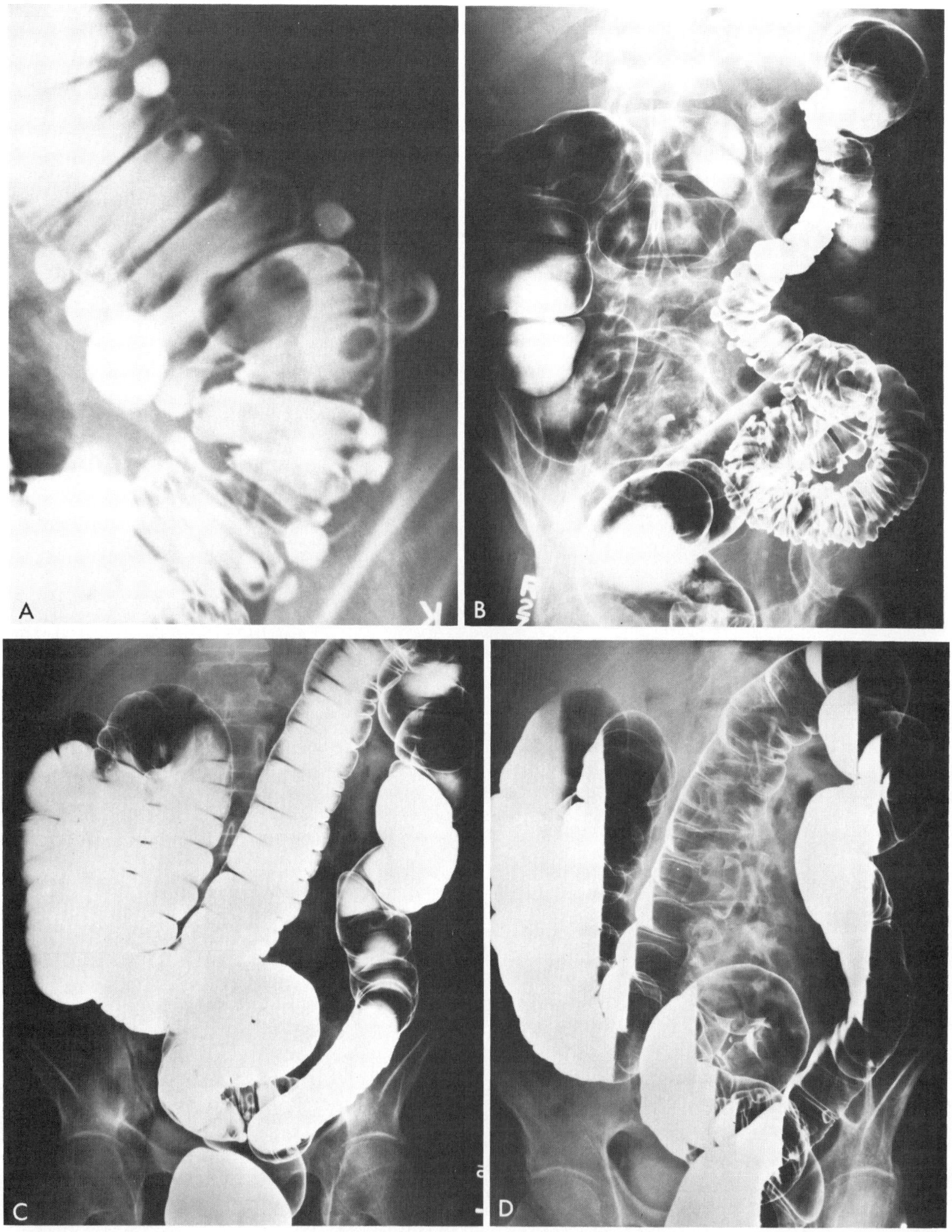

Figure 5–5. *A,* There is a polyp lying in the barium pool of the rectosigmoid colon, which contains numerous diverticula. The diagnosis is easily made because there is adequate distention and there is not too much barium in the involved segment. *B,* This patient has an extensive area of diverticulosis, but the entire colon and cecum are well coated. Only 250 ml of barium sulfate suspension were used. *C,* This supine view shows the result of too much barium, which obviously can hide lesions. *D,* Lateral decubitus view of same patient as in Figure 5–5*C*, again showing that too much barium can hide lesions. Five hundred ml or more of barium were used.

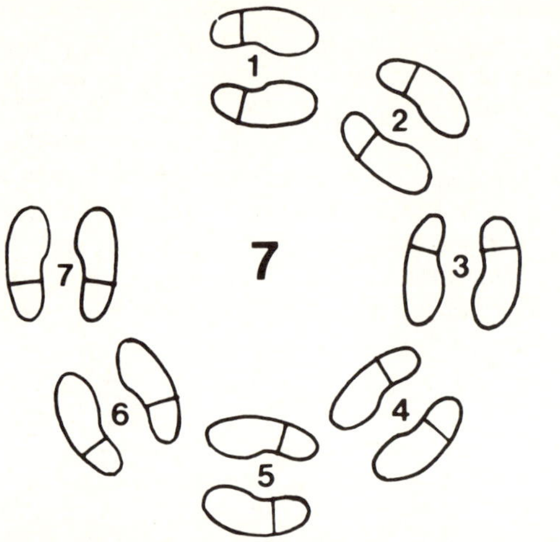

Figure 5–6. After the instillation of 250 ml of barium sulfate suspension, the patient is positioned in these seven positions shown and given seven slow full pumps of air from a sphygmomanometer bulb, in each position.

the sigmoid in the supine and prone projections are then obtained with the overhead tube. These two views ensure unobstructed views of the sigmoid before the right colon is fully distended and in the event that barium subsequently refluxes into the distal ileum. The table is then elevated with the patient prone, and the rectum and lower sigmoid are drained (Miller and Peterson, 1978). This maneuver also brings more barium into the cecum. After drainage, the table is brought horizontal again with the patient prone, and additional air instilled. Seven pumps with the patient prone and seven pumps with the patient in the left lateral position are repeated before fluoroscopy is started.

Brief fluoroscopy is used to see that barium is in the cecum and that there is adequate distention. Rarely is additional positioning needed at this time to place barium in the cecum. However, using fluoroscopic guidance, additional air often is given at this time, with the patient in the prone position, until adequate distention is achieved.

If needed, additional drainage of the rectum can be done at this time simply by placing the enema bag on the table between the patient's legs and releasing the clamp. After such drainage, additional air is instilled to distend the rectum and sigmoid. The entire procedure usually takes a total of 62 to 70 pumps. The patient is then slowly rotated a full 360 degrees and brought to the supine position. Spot filming and overhead radiography are then begun. Routine films for a satisfactory examination are obtained using conventional overhead units (Peterson and Miller, 1978).

In a small percentage of patients, barium will not have traversed to the cecum, and the following procedure is used to place barium in the cecum (Miller, 1979). The procedure consists of tilting or turning the patient and guiding the head of the barium pool much as one maneuvers a ball through a maze. This has been called the maze maneuver (Fig. 5–7). A low-lying transverse colon, redundant sigmoid,

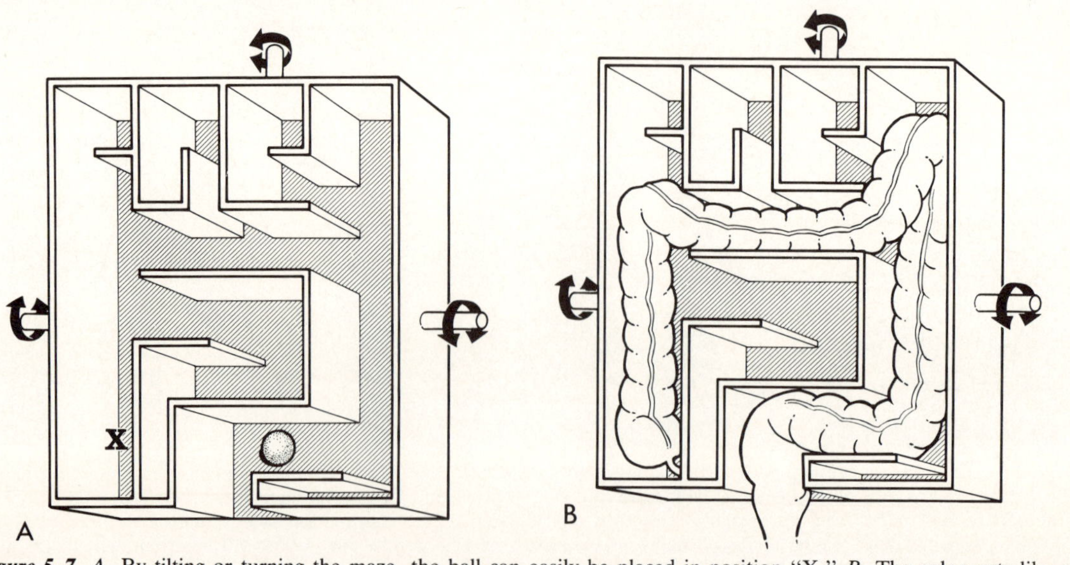

Figure 5–7. *A,* By tilting or turning the maze, the ball can easily be placed in position "X." *B,* The colon acts like a maze. If the colon is distended, the head of the barium pool can be maneuvered like a ball in a maze to place barium in the cecum if the colon is distended.

or an extra loop at the flexures are the usual circumstances requiring the additional procedure. Only a few minutes of additional fluoroscopy are required and would be needed also in these patients when using the conventional fluoroscopically guided barium and air insufflation methods to get the barium to the cecum.

The amount of barium is measured by using a common glass kitchen measuring cup. Only 250 ml are placed in the bag. Accurate measuring of the barium results in savings in the cost of contrast material and prevents excess barium in the colon that can obscure small lesions. The bag with 1-ft (3.0-cm) tubing is tied, taped, or strapped to the patient's inner thigh. This makes it easy for the patient to turn, and also hold, without disturbing the inserted enema tip even in the standing position. The tape is secured to the enema apparatus where the large 0.5-inch (1.3-cm) tubing enters the enema bag, and care is taken not to kink or collapse the enema tubing. After first checking the enema tip position and connections, all the material from the bag is gently squeezed into the patient without fluoroscopy, and the sequence of steps outlined previously is then performed entirely without fluoroscopy. Only after the overhead oblique angled views of the sigmoid are exposed, the rectum drained, the table returned to the horizontal position, and the additional 14 pumps of air administered is fluoroscopy started. This is to be sure that the barium is in the cecum, the rectum is properly drained, and the colon is well distended. As with other techniques, ease of examination improves with experience.

The examination is terminated after the radiographs have been checked by the supervising radiologist. He must be available to take fluoroscopic spot films or refill and fluoroscopically examine the colon when the rare need arises.

Some physicians may object to depending on a method that primarily uses films for diagnosis. I do not deny the value of palpation, compression, and various positioning under fluoroscopy (Schwartz, 1982). I simply do not believe these procedures are needed first in screening the asymptomatic patient who is at high risk for carcinoma and who has blood in his stools, a positive Hemoccult test, or a positive family history. I depend on compression and special positioning procedures after the initial films are looked at carefully.

Obviously, when this radiographic procedure is used, patients must be carefully selected. One cannot do this procedure "blind" when fistulas or partial obstruction, post colon resection, volvulus, or megacolon are suspected. The radiologist must screen all requests for the procedure and be immediately available at all times during the filming procedure. He must determine when to undertake additional fluoroscopic examination. With this sort of radiologic supervision and participation (even when barium does not initially reach the cecum), we have not failed to have a diagnostically complete examination in the last 3 years.

This method takes into account the anatomic positions of the various segments of colon, the role of gravity, and the time needed in each position (Fig. 5–8). I have found this easy to teach by using the number "7." Seven pumps and seven positions are easily remembered. Two additional pumps of seven with the patient in the prone and left lateral positions are also needed before final evaluation under fluoroscopy. A fast double contrast barium enema with optimal coating and distention can be obtained in most patients by following this easily remembered, uncomplicated method.

This is a reliable technique for screening the uncomplicated, relatively asymptomatic patient who is at high risk for colon carcinoma (Miller and Lehman, 1976). I believe this method has a place in busy radiology departments. Obviously, care must be used in selecting patients. This dependable method produces high-quality double contrast colon radiographs and can reduce examination time, cost, and patient radiation. The time saved can be used by the radiologist to discover subtle changes and find curable colon carcinoma at an earlier stage (Kelvin et al., 1981).

Air in front of the barium should cause no concern because this lifts the ileocecal valve and prevents barium from entering the terminal ileum. When the colon is distended with air, accordionlike folds also are straightened and the barium flows easily and quickly. The patient is not sent to the toilet for evacuation before either instillation of air or completion of the study. Standing upright and then sitting and straining during defecation might force barium into the terminal ileum and ruin an otherwise competent study. The proper procedure is to instill more air.

There are a minimum number of films that should be obtained.

1. Posteroanterior (PA) view to include the rectum-perpendicular central ray.
2. Fifteen-degree right anterior oblique (RAO) view with 35-degree caudad central ray.
3. Right lateral view—25 × 30 cm film.

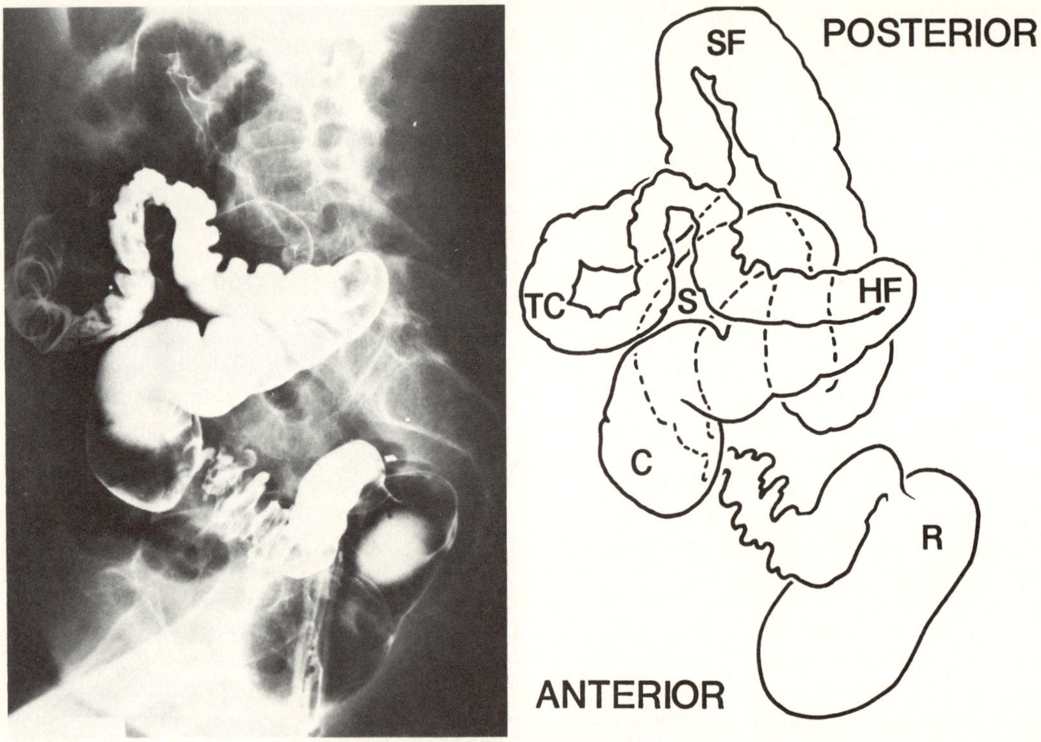

Figure 5–8. Schematic drawing of a lateral radiograph showing that the rectum (R), hepatic flexure (HF), and splenic flexure (SF) lie in a posterior position in the abdomen. It also shows that the transverse colon (TC), sigmoid (S), and cecum (C) lie anteriorly. This anatomic information helps the colonoscopist to position the tip of the colonoscope by palpation and the radiologist to position barium with the aid of gravity.

4. Twenty-degree right posterior oblique (RPO) view to include descending and splenic flexures.

5. Forty-five-degree left posterior oblique (LPO) view with perpendicular central ray.

6. Fifteen-degree (LPO) view with 35-degree cephalad central ray.

7. Right lateral decubitus view to include rectum.

8. Left lateral decubitus view to include rectum.

9. Supine compression spot film of cecum (often in some degree of obliquity and in Trendelenburg).

10. Upright compression spot films of flexures and transverse colon. (Occasionally these cannot be made with the patient in a completely upright position, but the patient should be made as erect as possible.)

The necessity for high-quality decubitus films must be emphasized. With the technical modifications first described by Miller (1970), this is an easily accomplished task. However, it should be obvious that any of the "overhead" films described previously may be taken on spot films or remote-control apparatus if appropriate equipment for beam angulation and direction is available. The preceding system can be done on the most simple radiographic fluoroscopic units.

Some colon anatomy can be adequately demonstrated on two or three views, but the large majority of patients can be well evaluated by only a minimum of eight overhead and four spot radiographs. Occasionally, redundancy and anatomic variations will be encountered, and then, even this number of films will not totally evaluate a given segment of the colon. The views described not only represent a reduction in the number of films originally advocated by Peterson and Miller (1978); they also result in an even more precise examination. Any further reduction will result in a compromised examination.

Critical Initial Review of Radiograms

The radiograms must be evaluated carefully by the radiologist before the patient leaves the department in case further overhead or spot films are required to evaluate suspicious or frankly abnormal areas. The pliability of the liquid ready-to-use barium preparation allows a thorough radiographic examination without haste.

COMMENT

Obviously, it takes a little effort, some know-how, and the desire on the part of the examiner to develop a reliable and consistent air contrast technique. I have outlined one such technique previously. Are the results of high-quality air contrast studies worth these efforts? The facts, not opinions, are as follows:

In a series of 182 patients having both barium enemas and colonoscopy, Williams and associates (1974a) reported that the regular barium enema examinations missed 43 percent more tumors than the air contrast examinations. He also showed that the air contrast technique revealed 98 percent of all tumors over 1 cm. Theoni and Menuck (1977), two gastrointestinal radiologists, found a 45.2 percent error rate with the single contrast dilute barium high kV technique; this is a 33.4 percent higher error rate than that with the air contrast technique. I believe that these percentages are significant. To date, no other examination has been proved to give such precise information on the *entire* colon as does the air contrast procedure. In addition, inflammatory lesions in the mucosa will show up earlier and in greater detail with air contrast studies (Laufer et al., 1978; Laufer, 1975; Welin and Brahme, 1961).

Again, as mentioned previously, at the very least, that group of patients at high risk for colon carcinoma should have an air contrast colon examination as the primary examination.

THE BARIUM ENEMA AND ENDOSCOPY

Proctosigmoidoscopy and the barium enema have historically been extremely valuable diagnostic tools in the study of colon disease. Results of barium enema studies are far superior to those using sigmoidoscopy. However, proctosigmoidoscopy can be used to directly examine areas that are difficult to evaluate radiologically (rectum and rectosigmoid). Therefore, the two techniques are obviously complementary. Current evidence also shows that colonoscopy and the double contrast barium enema are also complementary. Each technique has its distinct advantages and disadvantages. The modern clinician must be fully aware of the relative merits of each method in order to utilize them effectively.

Colonoscopy has limitations (Marks, 1974; Williams et al., 1974b; Stevenson, 1980). The colonoscope is unable to make extremely acute bends, and lesions may not be reached. Blind areas occur at sharp angles, acute bends, flexures, or folds in the colon. The blind areas encountered most frequently are in the rectosigmoid colon, in the splenic and hepatic flexures, and near the ileocecal valve. Fixation and constriction of the colon from adhesions, inflammation, neoplasms, and diverticula limit colonoscopy (Fig. 5–9). Although success rates vary with the skill of the examiner, the entire colon will not be examined in about 43 percent of colonoscopies (Stevenson, 1980; Gaisford, 1974; Sakai, 1974; Gelfand, 1979). However, the examination of the entire colon is mandatory to detect synchronous carcinomas (4 to 7 percent) or other co-existent lesions (Gelfand et al., 1979; Ekelund and Pihl, 1974; Peabody and Smithwick, 1961).

The barium enema study is often superior to other methods for localizing a lesion prior to surgery. Measurements from the colonoscope cannot be transferred to the patient at laparotomy because of "bowing" and "telescoping" of the colon on the colonoscope.

The advantages of colonoscopy relate to the detection of mucosal change, polyps, and vas-

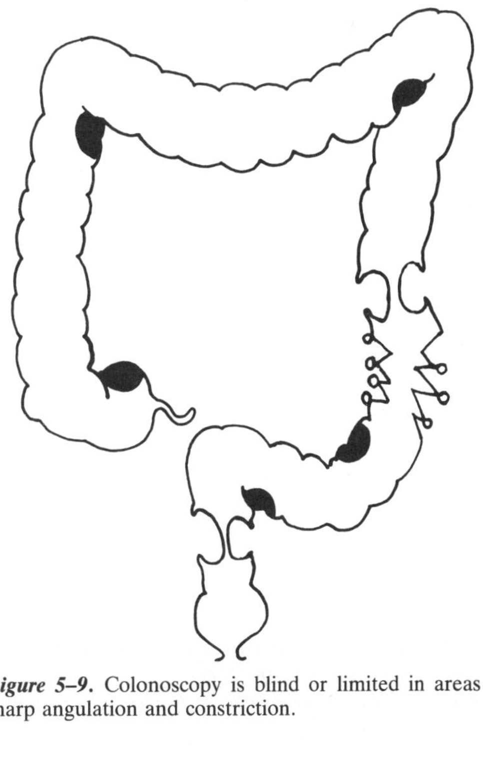

Figure 5–9. Colonoscopy is blind or limited in areas of sharp angulation and constriction.

cular lesions too subtle for barium enema study and to the provision of biopsy material. Williams and associates (1974b) reported that only 18 percent of colonoscopically diagnosed polyps of less than 1 cm were seen by conventional single contrast barium enemas, although 78 percent of such polyps were seen by air contrast examinations. Similarly, Miller (1974b) confirmed that 40 percent more colon polyps were seen by air contrast enemas than by conventional single contrast enemas. Williams and co-workers (1974b) also reported that the air contrast barium enema identified a very respectable 98 percent of colonoscopically diagnosed polyps greater than 1 cm.

H. G. Wells said that it takes 50 to 100 years from the time of the perception that something ought to be done until a serious attempt is made to do it. In the detection of neoplasms and especially curable colon cancer, we clearly do not have and cannot afford that amount of time! In the majority of cases, if the colonoscopist does not have a good air contrast barium enema study for guidance before colonoscopy, it is the endoscopist's own fault.

Colonoscopy has a distinct advantage over air contrast enema study in the diagnosis of small polyps and a small, but important, advantage in the detection of larger polyps. Occasionally, the air contrast enema will not detect a large polyp, but even a 4-cm malignant neoplasm of the cecum has been missed at endoscopy (Miller, 1975b; Saunders and MacEwen, 1971; Wolf et al., 1975). Therefore, colonoscopy and air contrast barium enemas are complementary examinations.

Of 94 cases of polypoid colonic lesions studied in our department and by our endoscopic and radiologic colleagues, endoscopy failed to identify any of these lesions on first examination, even though the endoscope was at or beyond the site of the lesion (Fig. 5–10). Twenty-five of the lesions were carcinoma. Most undetected lesions ranged from 0.5 to 1.5 cm in diameter. Histologic proof of each lesion was obtained by repeat endoscopy with biopsy, polypectomy, or surgery.

An incomplete examination obviously accounts for failure to identify colonic lesions by colonoscopy in many cases. Also, the operator may miss a lesion just as the radiologist may fail to see a lesion at fluoroscopic examination or on film. The problem is that if the endoscopist reaches or passes the area in question and does not see a lesion, an endoscopy report of "normal" cannot be checked. The fluoroscopist's radiographs can be reviewed. Most endoscopists do not think it practical during each colonoscopic examination to obtain a set of photographs of all areas of the colon for subsequent review whether or not lesions are seen. Therefore, a "normal" report must be interpreted within the limitations of the procedure. Failure to appreciate these limitations can result in inappropriate patient management. Colonoscopy should remain identified by the air contrast barium enema.

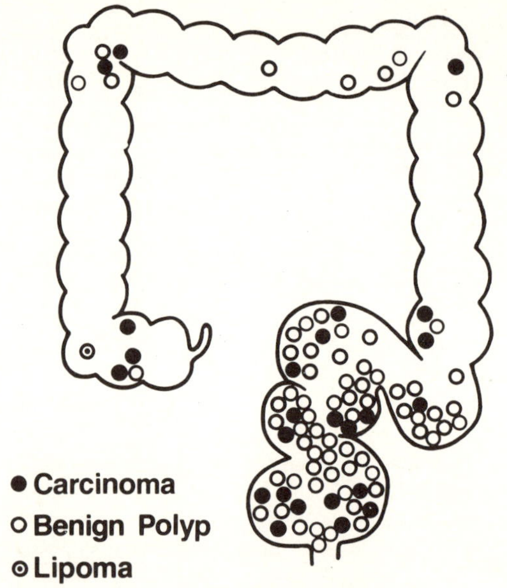

Figure 5–10. Ninety-four lesions missed by endoscopy, even though the endoscopist was at or beyond the site of the lesion.

The greatest assets of colonoscopy are those of combined biopsy or polypectomy. With minimal additional time, cost, and patient risk, lesions can be biopsied or polypoid lesions removed by electrocautery (Figs. 5–11 and 5–12). When following changes in polyp size, polypectomy subsequently spares the patient the time, cost, and radiation exposure of annual repeat barium enemas. After complete polypectomy, a repeat air contrast barium enema or colonoscopy is suggested for the first year following treatment and then alternately repeated every 3 years if no new polyps are found. Such a program combined with annual clinical follow-up and proctosigmoidoscopy avoids both unnecessary colonoscopies and barium enemas (Williams et al., 1974b). After resection for carcinoma, a rational approach is to obtain a baseline air contrast colon examination, and then follow the patient yearly, alternating between colonoscopic and pneumocolon examinations (Fig. 5–13).

Despite the assets of colonoscopy, most co-

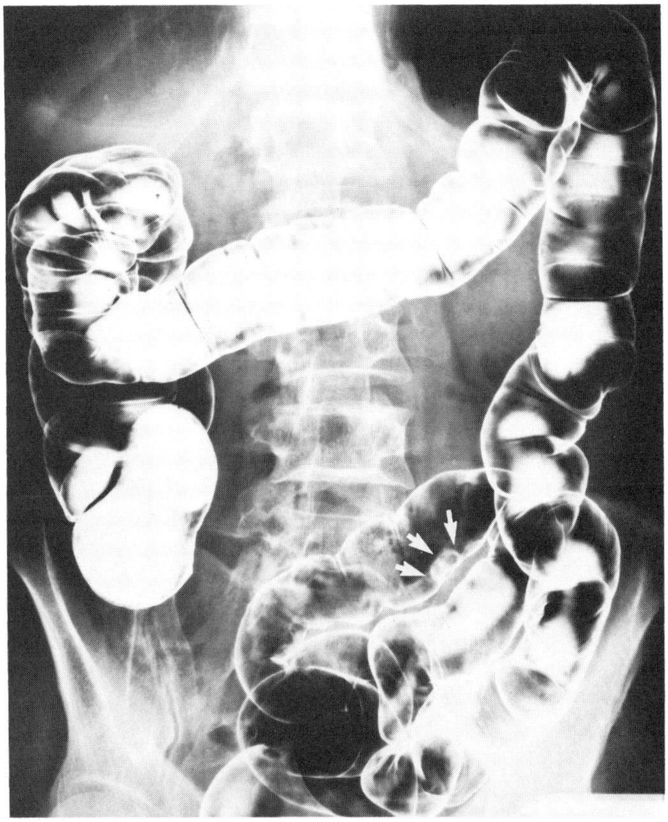

Figure 5–11. Small sessile polyp in the rectosigmoid colon is well demonstrated with only 250 ml of barium sulfate. Note that there is adequate barium in the ascending colon and cecum even in this relatively redundant colon.

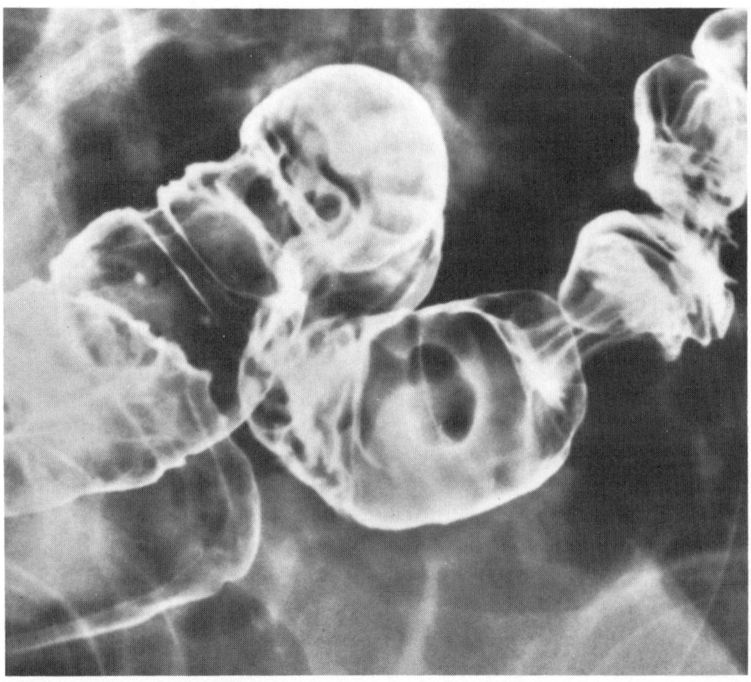

Figure 5–12. Small polyp with a stalk is seen in the barium pool of the rectosigmoid colon.

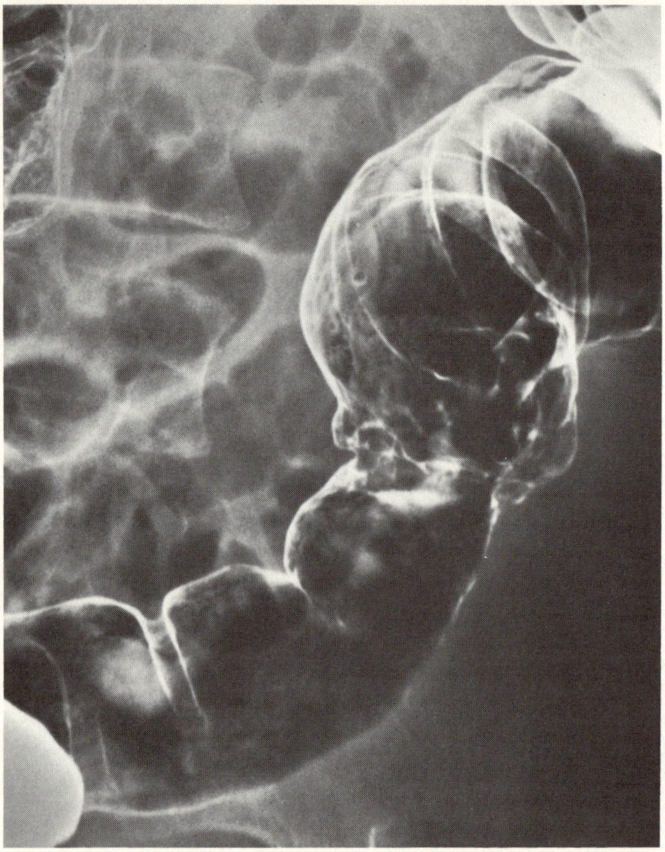

Figure 5–13. There is irregularity of the anastomotic site, showing recurrent adenocarcinoma from previously resected carcinoma of the colon.

lonoscopists agree that the air contrast barium enema and proctosigmoidoscopy should remain the primary examinations for patients with suspected colonic disease. Recent studies showing a changing site distribution of carcinoma emphasize the need for an accurate and inexpensive technique to evaluate the entire colon. That data also suggests that the barium pneumocolon examination should be included in the screening of high-risk patients (Maglinte et al., 1983). Wolff and Shinya (1974) believe that "colonoscopy serves as a background procedure to the contrast enema." Errors in interpretation of barium enema roentgenograms are more common than failure of the air contrast technique itself (Kelvin et al., 1981). If anything, radiologists tend to slightly "underread" air contrast studies. With cooperative feedback, the colonoscopists' findings make a careful review of the x-ray films an enlightening and beneficial learning experience for both the radiologist and colonoscopist (Miller and Lehman, 1978, 1976).

OTHER METHODS USEFUL IN MANAGEMENT OF COLONIC NEOPLASIA

Angiography

Currently colonic angiography is the usual procedure of choice to detect colonic vascular malformations. It also is useful in locating an active bleeding site and treating colonic hemorrhage either by drug infusion or embolization. However, the patient must be bleeding at a rate of 0.5 ml per minute for angiography to be useful. If the rate is less than this, the angiogram fails to detect the bleeding site. Even if a vascular malformation is detected, one does not always know whether that lesion is responsible for the bleeding. A good alternative is to use radiopharmaceuticals that are capable of detecting bleeding rates of 0.05 to 0.1 ml per minute. If the bleeding site is found by radiopharmaceuticals, selective diagnostic angiography can be followed by therapeutic angiographic intervention (Alavi, 1977, 1980).

Computed Tomography

Computed tomography (CT) is not a procedure for initial diagnosis of colonic neoplasia. It is, however, useful in patients with suspected recurrent rectal carcinoma. It plays a very important role in the pretherapy staging of colorectal neoplasms. It does this by its ability to define the intramural and extramural extent of a colonic mass. CT has proved to be accurate in determining the extent of involvement of viscera adjacent to colonic neoplasms (Ellert and Kreel, 1980; Husband et al., 1980; Mayes and Zornoza, 1980). Examiners using CT can also get information from sections of the entire abdomen and pelvis on the integrity or invasion of neoplasms into adjacent organs and retroperitoneal lymph nodes.

Colonic neoplasms have been classified into four stages using CT:

Stage I. Intraluminal mass without colon wall thickening.

Stage II. Colon wall thicker than 1 cm but no extension of the tumor into adjacent organs.

Stage III. (A) Extension of the tumor into adjacent organs but not extending to the pelvic sidewalls. (B) Extension of the tumor to pelvic sidewalls.

Stage IV. Any stage tumor with distant metastatic disease.

CT is apparently a reliable method for determining the stage of primary rectosigmoid tumors (Thoeni et al., 1981) and for detecting recurrent rectosigmoid carcinoma after surgical therapy (Ellert and Kreel, 1980; Husband et al., 1980; Mayes and Zornoza, 1980). Thoeni and associates (1981) reported CT has a 95 percent rate of accuracy in determining the *extent* of primary rectal and rectosigmoid carcinomas. They found CT invaluable in planning appropriate radiation therapy. Furthermore, Moss and co-workers (1981) reported that CT has a 95 percent rate of accuracy in detecting or excluding *recurrent* rectal carcinoma (Ellert and Kreel, 1980).

The difficulty in using CT is distinguishing postoperative or radiation-induced fibrous tissue from recurrent neoplasm. Some therefore have recommended that a baseline CT of the pelvis should be done 2 to 3 months following surgery or at the completion of radiotherapy. It can then be done every 6 months for 2 years. This is because 50 percent of the local recurrences occur in the first postoperative year, and 80 percent of all recurrences occur within 2 years. Of the local recurrences, 92 percent are contiguous to the surgical anastomosis. Furthermore, 44 percent to 60 percent of patients with a recurrent carcinoma have only local recurrences (Cass et al., 1976; Gilbert, 1978; Hoth and Petucci, 1976).

Although it has been reported that CT is capable of detecting recurrent tumors only 1 to 3 cm in size, most cases have been found to be greater than 5 cm in diameter (Ellert and Kreel, 1980; Husband et al., 1980; Mayes and Zornoza, 1980; Thoeni et al., 1981; Moss et al., 1981). It should be obvious then that CT scans are not the tool to use to initially find small neoplasms of the colon. If it is not possible to distinguish between fibrosis and a tumor by imaging, other approaches can be used. If early recurrence is suspected, one can repeat the CT scan 1 to 2 months after the baseline examination in order to determine if there has been a change or increase in the mass, or one can perform a thin needle biopsy of the mass under CT guidance.

Thin needle biopsy using CT guidance is a procedure exhibiting high accuracy, low morbidity, and ease of performance (Coel and Niwayama, 1978; Ferrucci and Wittenberg, 1978; Haaga and Alfidi, 1976; Jaques et al., 1978). The procedure in most instances provides a rapid, clear-cut diagnosis and is almost painless. Generally the diagnosis of fibrosis or recurrent carcinoma can be made with a high degree of accuracy.

Ultrasonography

Ultrasonography has not been extremely valuable or widely employed for evaluation of the colon because of the colon's gas-containing nature. Rubin and associates (1978) reported that ultrasonography has the ability to show the retrovesical anatomy, the rectosigmoid region, the posterior aspect of the bladder, and the rectouterine spaces following a water enema. However, I believe CT is the method of choice.

Ultrasonography is most valuable in evaluating patients with a suspected pericolonic abscess. Abscesses are easily detected, and treatment can be followed by ultrasonography (Doust and Doust, 1976; Korobkin et al., 1978). Ultrasonography, like CT, can be used as a guide for percutaneous biopsy and may also be used for catheter drainage of abscesses affecting the colon (Gronvall et al., 1977).

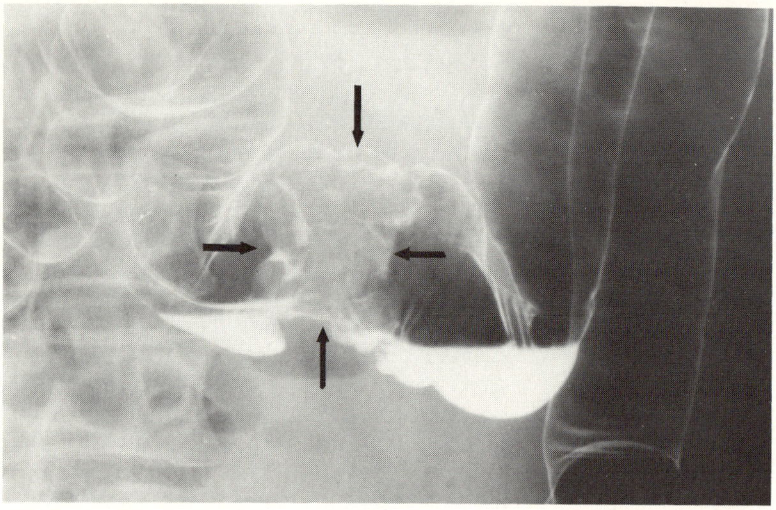

Figure 5–14. Superficial but large adenocarcinoma of the transverse colon. This would be missed on the usual full column enema examination, but is easily seen on the air contrast study. The patient had two previous full column enema studies, and the tumor was missed both times. The continued presence of blood in his stool resulted in a change in diagnostic technique which resulted in the diagnosis. This patient is alive and well 18 years after resection.

Nuclear Medicine

Gallium-67 (^{67}Ga) and technetium-99m DTPA (^{99m}Tc-DTPA) have been widely employed in the detection of inflammatory processes and tumors of the colon (Hoffer, 1980; Kadir and Strauss, 1979; Pechman et al., 1978; Shimshak et al., 1978). Each of these isotopes has a normal colonic excretion, and therefore the colon must be extremely clean. With gallium injection, the delay in interpreting the images may be too great, and CT or ultrasonography have for the most part become the preferred techniques to detect abscesses in acutely ill patients (Korobkin et al., 1978; Shimshak et al., 1978). Often the radionuclide images are not sufficient for precise preoperative localization, and commonly, other imaging techniques must be employed prior to surgery. However, the radionuclide diagnostic procedure is becoming the procedure of choice for detecting gastrointestinal bleeding sites.

SUMMARY

All scientific evidence to date reveals that good air contrast studies are superior to full column or so-called combined techniques for detecting superficial and small tumors in the entire colon in those patients at high risk for carcinoma (Fig. 5–14). The scientific evidence, imperfect as it may be, is substantial (Miller, 1975b; Thoeni and Menuck, 1977; Williams et al., 1974a; Miller, 1978; Miller, 1977). Radiologic examination complements other types of studies and should precede colonoscopic examination.

What Leo Rigler, M.D., emphasized about lung cancer applies equally to neoplasms of the colon: "No matter how great or sophisticated our mental ability and our tools are in differential diagnosis, it is all in vain if we do not find the lesion" (Rigler, 1975; Miller, 1975). We can and must find the 35 percent of all cancers and 42 percent of early potentially curable (Dukes' A and B) carcinomas that currently are missed on the initial colon examination (Gilbertsen et al., 1979). Not to find the lesion is the irrevocable error. The highly variable appearances and the details of roentgenographic interpretation of colon neoplasms are more fully described in the textbook by Miller and Skucas (1983).

References

Alavi A: Scintigraphic demonstration of acute gastrointestinal bleeding. Gastrointest Radiol 5:205, 1980.

Alavi A, Dann RW, Baum S, et al: Scintigraphic detection of acute gastrointestinal bleeding. Radiology 124:753, 1977.

Carlile T: The roentgenologic diagnosis of carcinoma of the colon. *In:* Cancer of the gastrointestinal tract. Chicago, Year Book Medical Publishers, 1967, pp. 187–211.

Cass AW, Million AR, Pfaff WW: Patterns of recurrence following surgery alone for adenocarcinoma of the colon and rectum. Cancer 37:2861, 1976.

Coel MN, Niwayama G: Safety of percutaneous fine-needle pancreatic biopsy: A porcine model. Invest Radiol 13:547, 1978.

Doust BD, Doust VL: Ultrasonic diagnosis of abdominal abscess. Am J Dig Dis 21:569, 1976.

Ekelund GR, Pihl B: Multiple carcinomas of the colon and rectum. Cancer 33:1620, 1974.

Ellert J, Kreel L: The value of CT in malignant colonic tumors. CT 4:225, 1980.

Ferrucci JT Jr, Benedict KT Jr: Anticholinergic-aided study of the gastrointestinal tract. Radiol Clin North Am 9:23, 1971.

Ferrucci JT Jr, Wittenberg J: CT biopsy of abdominal tumors: Aids for lesion localization. Radiology 129:739, 1978.

Fred H, Eiband JM, Collins LC: Calcifications in intra-abdominal and retroperitoneal metastases. AJR 91:138, 1964.

Friedland G: Colon preparation. *In:* Detection of Colon Lesions, First Standardization Conference 1969. Chicago, American College of Radiology, 1973, p. 107.

Gaisford W: Fiberendoscopy of the cecum and terminal ileum. Gastrointest Endosc 21:13, 1974.

Gelfand DW, Moskowitz M: Massive gastric dilatation complicating hypotonic duodenography. A report of three cases. Radiology 97:637, 1970.

Gelfand D, Wu W, Ott D: The extent of successful colonoscopy and its implication for the radiologist. Gastrointest Radiol 4:75, 1979.

Gilbert SG: Symptomatic local tumor failure following abdominoperineal resection. Int J Radiat Oncol Biol Phys 4:801, 1978.

Gilbertsen VA, Williams SE, Schuman L, McHugh R: Colonoscopy in the detection of carcinoma of the intestine. Surg Gynecol Obstet 149:877, 1979.

Gronvall J, Gronvall S, Hegedus V: Ultrasonic-guided drainage of fluid-containing masses using angiographic catheterization techniques. AJR 129:997, 1977.

Haaga JR, Alfidi RJ: Precise biopsy localization by computed tomography. Radiology 118:603, 1976.

Haney MJ, McGarity WE: Ureterosigmoidostomy and neoplasms of the colon. JAMA 103:69, 1971.

Harned RK, Consigny PM, Cooper NB, et al.: Barium enema examination following biopsy of the rectum or colon. Radiology 145:11, 1982.

Hayt DB, Simon DF, Collica CJ: Grid choice in high kilovoltage 70 mm. radiographic spot filming. Radiology 93:135, 1969.

Hoffer PB: Gallium imaging of the abdomen. *In* Alavi A, Arger PH (eds.): Multiple Imaging Procedures, Vol. 3. New York, Grune & Stratton, 1980.

Hoth DF, Petucci PE: Natural history and staging of colon cancer. Semin Oncol 3:331, 1976.

Husband JE, Hodson NJ, Parsons CA: The use of computed tomography in recurrent rectal tumors. Radiology 134:677, 1980.

Jaques PF, Stabb E, Richey W, et al: CT-assisted pelvic and abdominal aspiration biopsies in gynecological malignancy. Radiology 128:651, 1978.

Kadir S, Strauss W: Evaluation of inflammatory bowel disease with 99mTc-DTPA. Radiology 130:443, 1979.

Kelvin FM, Gardiner R, Vas W, Stevenson GW: Colorectal carcinoma missed on double contrast barium study: A problem in perception. AJR 137:307, 1981.

Kobayashi S, Mizuno H, Kasugai T: Early colonic cancer presenting as a pedunculated polyp. Gastrointest Endosc 20:118, 1974.

Korobkin M, Callen PW, Filly RA, et al: Comparison of computed tomography, ultrasonography and gallium-67 scanning in the evaluation of suspected abdominal abscess. Radiology 129:89, 1978.

Lappas JC, Miller RE, Lehman GA, et al: Post endoscopy barium enemas: Facts versus fiction. Radiology (In press).

Laufer I: The radiologic demonstration of early changes in ulcerative colitis by double contrast technique. J Can Assoc Radiol 26:116, 1975.

Laufer I, Mullens JE, Hamilton J: Correlation of endoscopy and double contrast radiography in the early stages of ulcerative and granulomatous colitis. Radiology 118:1, 1976.

McGregor RA, Bacon HE: Multiple cancers in colon surgery. Surgery 44:828, 1958.

McMillan WO Jr, Garbutt JT, Ruffin JM: Problem of cancer in ulcerative colitis. South Med J 61:526, 1968.

McQueeney AJ, Olson RW, Medwid A: Primary scirrhous carcinoma of the colon. AJR 101:306, 1967.

Maglinte DDT, Keller KJ, Miller RE, Chernish SM: Colon and rectal carcinoma: Spatial distribution and detection. Radiology 147:669, 1983.

Maglinte DDT, Miller RE: Simplified barium pneumocolon examination. Applied Radiology 12:93, 1983.

Maglinte DDT, Strong RC, Strate RW, et al: Barium enema after colorectal biopsies: Experimental data. AJR 139:693, 1982.

Margulis AR: Examination of the colon. *In* Margulis AR, Burhenne HJ (eds.): Alimentary Tract Roentgenology, Vol. 2, 2nd ed. St. Louis, CV Mosby Company, 1973, pp. 923–924.

Marks G: Flexible fiberoptic colonoscopy: A guide for its use in the management of diseases of the colon. JAMA 228:1411, 1974a.

Matter B, Rotke KH: Pseudotumors—radiographic findings in the colon. Radiol Diagn 10:573, 1969.

Mayes GB, Zornoza J: Computed tomography of colon carcinoma. AJR 135:43, 1980.

Miller RE: A new enema tip. Radiology 92:1492, 1969.

Miller RE: Simple apparatus for decubitus films with horizontal beam. Radiology 97:682, 1970.

Miller RE: The technical approach to the acute abdomen. Semin Roentgen 8:267, 1973a.

Miller RE: The radiological evaluation of intra-peritoneal gas (pneumoperitoneum). *In* Wang Y (ed): Critical Reviews in Clinical Radiology and Nuclear Medicine, Vol. 4. Cleveland, Chemical Rubber Company Press, 1973b, p. 61.

Miller RE: Shock following saline barium enema in elderly patient. JAMA 228:1169, 1974a.

Miller RE: Detection of colon carcinoma and the barium enema. JAMA 230:1195, 1974b.

Miller RE: The cleansing enema. Radiology 117:482, 1975a.

Miller RE: Examination of the colon. Curr Probl Diagn Radiol 5:3, 1975b.

Miller RE: The barium enema as a cancer detection procedure: Its use and abuse. *In* Radiologic and Other Biophysical Methods in Tumor Diagnosis. Chicago, Year Book Medical Publishers, 1975c, p. 277.

Miller RE: The barium enema in the high risk carcinoma patient. (Letter). Radiology 123:813, 1977.

Miller RE: The barium enema versus endoscopy. Gastrointest Endosc 28:40–41, 1982.

Miller RE: The barium enema in the high risk carcinoma patient—Epilogue. (Letter). Radiology 127:271, 1978.

Miller RE: Solution for the "air block" problem during fluoroscopy. AJR 132:1020, 1979.

Miller RE, Chernish SM, Brunelle RL, Rosenak BD: Double blind roentgenographic study of dose response to I.V. glucagon for hypotonic duodenography. Radiology 127:55, 1978.

Miller RE, Chernish SM, Rosenak BD, Rodda B: Hypotonic duodenography with glucagon. Radiology 108:35, 1973.

Miller RE, Chernish SM, Skucas J, et al: Hypotonic colon examination with glucagon. Radiology 113:555, 1974a.

Miller RE, Chernish SM, Skucas J, et al: Hypotonic roentgenography with glucagon. AJR 121:264, 1974b.

Miller RE, Lehman G: Localization of small bowel hemorrhage: Complete reflux small bowel examination. Am J Dig Dis 107:1019, 1972.

Miller RE, Lehman G: The barium enema: Is it obsolete? JAMA 235:2842, 1976.

Miller RE, Lehman G: Polypoid colonic lesions undetected by endoscopy. Radiology 129:295, 1978.

Miller RE, Maglinte DDT: Barium pneumocolon: Technologist-performed "7 pump" method. AJR 139:1230, 1982.

Miller RE, Peterson GH: Drainage of the rectum: A simple maneuver to improve the accuracy of colon examinations. Radiology 128:506, 1978.

Miller RE, Skucas J: The Radiological Examination of the Colon: Practical Diagnosis. Hingham, MA, Martinus Nijhoff Publishers, 1983.

Moertel CG, Bargen JA, Dockerty MB: Multiple carcinomas of the large intestine. Gastroenterology 34:85, 1958.

Moss AA, Thoeni RF, Schyder P, et al: Value of computed tomography in the detection and staging of recurrent rectal carcinomas. J Comput Assist Tomogr 5:870, 1981.

Peabody CN, Smithwick RH: Practical implications of multiple tumors of the colon and rectum. N Engl J Med 264:853, 1961.

Pechman R, Tetalman M, Antonmattei S, et al: Diagnostic significance of persistent colonic gallium activity: Scintigraphic activity. Radiology 128:691, 1978.

Peterson GH, Miller RE: The barium enema: A reassessment looking toward perfection. Radiology 128:315, 1978.

Preissig RS, Barry WF Jr, Lester RG: The increased incidence of carcinoma of the colon following ureterosigmoidostomy. AJA 121:806, 1974.

Rigler L: Peripheral carcinoma of the lung: Incidence, possibilities for survival, methods of detection, identification. *In* Radiologic and Other Biophysical Methods in Tumor Diagnosis. Chicago, Year Book Medical Publishers, 1975, p. 23.

Robbins SL: Pathology. Philadelphia, WB Saunders Company, 1967.

Rubin C, Kurtz AB, Goldberg BB: Water enema: New ultrasound technique in defining pelvic anatomy. JCU 6:28, 1978.

Sakai Y: Further progress in colonoscopy. Gastrointest Endosc 20:143, 1974.

Saunders CG, MacEwen DW: Delay in diagnosis of colonic cancer: A continuing challenge. Radiology 101:207, 1971.

Schottenfeld D, Berg JW, Vitsky B: Incidence of multiple primary cancers. II. Index cancers arising in the stomach and lower digestive system. J Nat Cancer Inst 43:77, 1969.

Schwartz SS: Missed colorectal carcinoma on barium enema studies. AJR 138:368, 1982.

Sherman RS: The roentgenologist as a consultant. Radiology 75:293, 1960.

Shimshak R, Korobkin M, Hoffer PB: Complementary role of gallium citrate imaging and computed tomography in the evaluation of suspected abdominal infection. J Nucl Med 19:262, 1978.

Shinya H: Fiberoptic colonoscopy for diagnosis and treatment of colonic disease. *In* Najarian JS (ed): Surgery of the Gastrointestinal Tract. New York, Intercontinental Medical Book Corporation, 1974, pp. 455–462.

Stevenson GW: Who needs radiology? Gastrointest Endosc 26:119, 1980.

Thoeni RF, Menuck L: Comparison of barium enema and colonoscopy in the detection of small colonic polyps. Radiology 124:621, 1977.

Thoeni RF, Moss AA, Schnyder P, Margulis AR: Detection and staging of primary rectal and rectosigmoid cancer by computed tomography. Radiology 141:35, 1981.

Thorpe CD, Grayson DJ Jr, Wingfield PB: Detection of carcinoma of the colon and rectum by air contrast enema. Surg Gynecol Obstet 152:307, 1981.

Tung CHK, Goldman H: The incidence and significance of villous changes in adenomatous polyps. Am J Clin Pathol 53:21, 1970.

Turnbull RB, JR: The no-touch isolation technique of resection. JAMA 231:1181, 1975.

Welin S: Modern trends in diagnostic roentgenology of the colon. Br J Radiol 31:453, 1953.

Welin S: Results of the Malmö technique of colon examination. JAMA 199:369, 1967.

Welin S, Brahme F: The double contrast method in ulcerative colitis. Acta Radiol 55:257, 1961.

Whitaker RH, Pugh RCB, Dow D: Colonic tumors following ureterosigmoidostomy. Br J Urol 43:562, 1971.

Williams CB, Hunt RH, Loose H, et al: Colonoscopy in the management of colon polyps. Br J Surg 61:673, 1974a.

Williams CB, Hunt RH, Loose H, et al: Colonoscopy in the management of colon polyps. Br J Surg 61:673, 1974b.

Wolff W, Shinya H: Modern endoscopy of the alimentary tract. Curr Probl Surg 1:30, 1974.

Wolff WI, Shinya H, Geffen A, et al: Comparison of colonoscopy and the contrast enema in 500 patients with colorectal disease. Am J Surg 129:181, 1975.

Zboralske F, Amberry J: Calcified mucinous adenocarcinoma of the colon. Am J Gastroenterol 38:675, 1962.

SIX

Flexible Endoscopic Examinations and Treatment

J. S. Spratt, M.D.,
T. Leake, R.N.,
C. O. Knutson, M.D.

The state of the art of flexible colonoscopic examinations in Louisville was recently studied (Knutson and Max, 1979). The results of 662 therapeutic and diagnostic colonoscopic examinations were reviewed to assess the morbidity, clinical benefit, and diagnostic accuracy of the procedure and the indications for it. The role of the flexible endoscope in detecting and excising (transendoscopically) small, occult, invasive cancers was emphasized. Overall, the frequency of detecting occult lesions (19 percent), the ability to clarify questionable radiographic findings (89 percent), and a substantial reduction in laparotomy-colotomy procedures required for removal of colonic polyps (88 percent), along with a low morbidity (3 percent) and low rate of false-negative findings (1 percent), established colonoscopy as one of the more promising advances in the management of colonic disease in recent years. Although early experience suggests that small, occult, invasive carcinomas, when properly selected, can be adequately treated by endoscopic excision, larger series and longer follow-up periods are necessary to validate any conclusions regarding the decision to manage these lesions conservatively. Cancers beginning as invasive ulcers will rarely be candidates for transendoscopic ablation.

Colonoscopy, with its ability to visualize the entire colon interior directly, must be placed in perspective with the traditional radiographic diagnostic techniques (Sivak et al., 1974; Miller 1974; Wolff et al., 1975; Coller et al., 1976). The therapeutic ability to remove polypoid lesions of the proximal colon has greatly reduced the need for laparotomy (Wolff and Shinya, 1973a, 1973b; Sugarbaker and Vineyard, 1973; Berci et al., 1973; Knutson et al., 1974; Wolff et al., 1975; Christie, 1976a). Flexible fiberoptic colonoscopy was introduced in this country by Wolff and Shinya (1971, 1972), who, along with other investigators, have identified an increasing number of appropriate clinical applications (Williams and Muto, 1972; Waye, 1972; Gaisford, 1972; Teague et al., 1973; Sugarbaker et al., 1974; Schmitt et al., 1975; Overholt, 1975; Christie, 1976b; Max and Knutson, 1978). They also determined the overall safety of the procedure (Goldhaber et al., 1974; Ragins et al., 1974; Berci et al., 1974; Rogers et al., 1975; Geenen et al., 1975; Smith and Nivatvongs, 1975; Meyers and Gharhremani, 1975). Assessment of the impact colonoscopy has had on the diagnosis and treatment of colonic disorders requires periodic critical review of the beneficial clinical yield and indications for performing this procedure. Experience has allowed continuing refinement of criteria for the appropriate and effective use of endoscopy. In time, controlled trials may be required to verify optimum strategies for its use.

Knutson and Max (1979) reviewed a total of 662 consecutive patients managed by diagnostic or therapeutic colonoscopy. A two-day mechanical colon-cleansing preceded the examinations (Table 6–1).

Premedications included atropine sulfate (0.6 mg), diazepam (10 to 20 mg), and meperidine hydrochloride (50 to 75 mg), which were given as intramuscular injections 1 hour before

Table 6–1. **BOWEL PREPARATION FOR COLONOSCOPY**

Prior to Hospital Registration (At Home)
- Day 1
  - Clear liquids
  - Castor oil, 60 ml at 8 AM
  - Bisacodyl tablets, 20 mg at 8 AM
- Day 2
  - Clear liquids
  - Bisacodyl tablets, 20 mg at 8 AM
  - Two 1,000-ml tap water enemas at bedtime

Following Hospital Registration
- Day 3
  - Nothing by mouth
  - 1,000-ml normal saline water enemas until clear

*From Knutson CO, Max MH: Diagnostic and therapeutic colonoscopy. A critical review of 662 examinations. Arch Surg 114:430–435, 1979. Copyright 1979, American Medical Association.

the procedure. Satisfactory systemic analgesia during the procedure was almost routinely achieved with single, intravenous injections of 5 to 10 mg of diazepam. The Olympus CF-MB2 (110 cm), TCF-2L (160 cm), or CF-LB2 (186 cm) colonoscope was used in conjunction with the CLX light source. Although fluoroscopy was not required routinely, all examinations were performed in the radiology department with fluoroscopic and television monitoring equipment available. With the patient lying in the left lateral position, adequate fluoroscopic views were possible for both scope position and sigmoid splinting, without requiring a change in the patient's position. The average procedure time was 20 ±10 minutes.

A wide variety of flexible fiberoptic endoscopes are available from various manufacturers. The mechanical components of all are essentially the same. Adapters are available

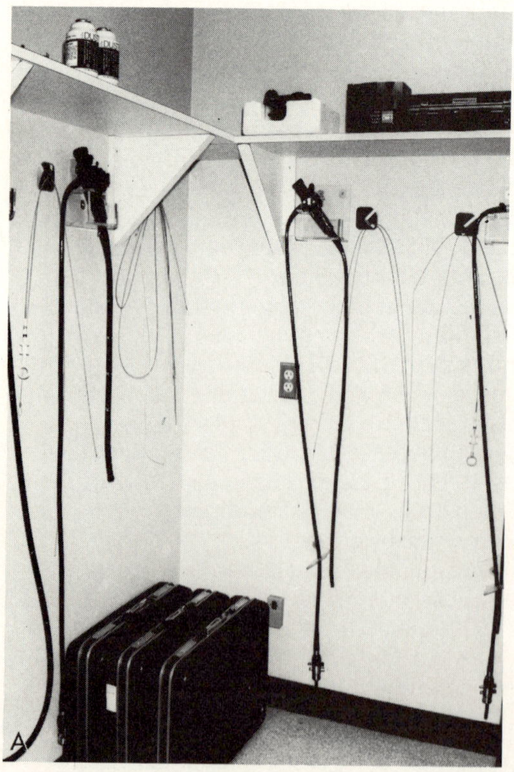

A

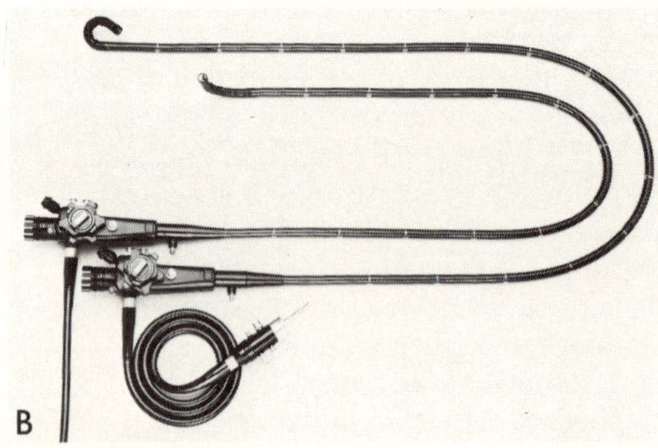

B

Figure 6–1. Endoscopes and cabinet with accessories. *A,* For upper gastrointestinal panendoscopy in adults, a forward viewing instrument is routinely used. For pediatric patients and debilitated adults, a smaller caliber instrument is available. It can also serve as a backup should the standard endoscope be out for repair. For endoscopic retrograde cholangiopancreatography, a side viewing instrument is, of course, essential. *B,* For lower intestinal examinations, the 180-cm colonoscope is the instrument of choice because of the desirability of doing total colonoscopy (to the cecum). The flexible 60-cm sigmoidoscope is also gaining popularity over the rigid sigmoidoscope owing to several factors such as increased patient acceptance and greater diagnostic capabilities. Obviously the medium-length colonoscopes can be used as well. (Photographs courtesy of Kosair-Children's Hospital.)

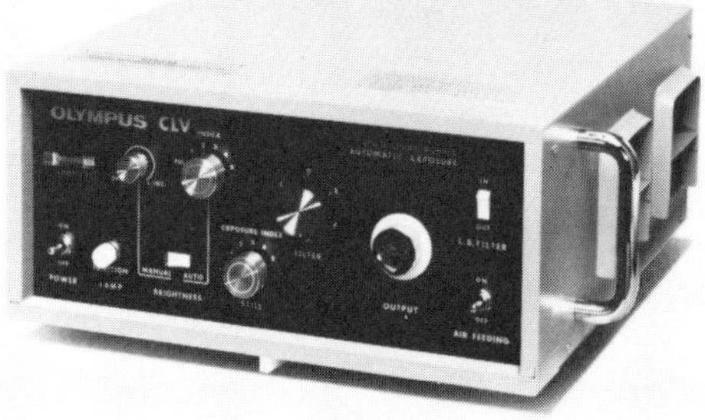

A

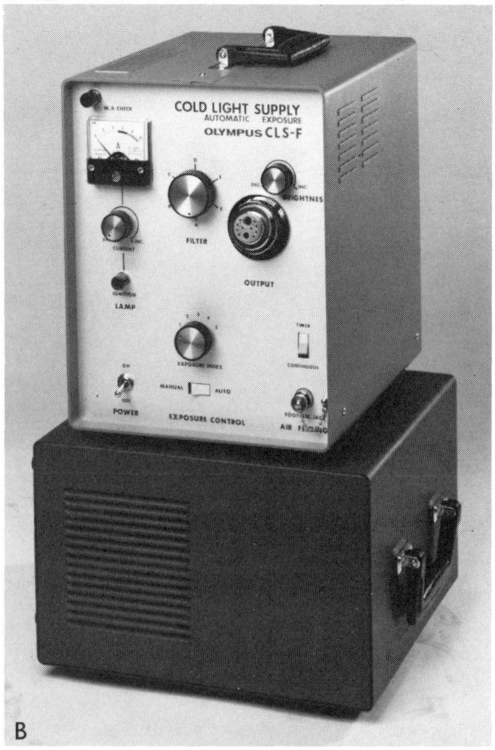

Figure 6–2. *A* and *B*, Light sources. Since the trend is toward the use of smaller caliber endoscopes with thinner light bundles, an even more basic tool for successful endoscopic procedures is a light source that produces adequate illumination. Cinephotography and color television monitoring can be accomplished with the light sources available currently. (Photograph courtesy of Olympus Corporation.)

for the interchange of accessories, but, in general, each endoscope works best with its own accessories.

The basic instruments for both rigid and flexible endoscopic examinations are illustrated in Figures 6–1 to 6–8.

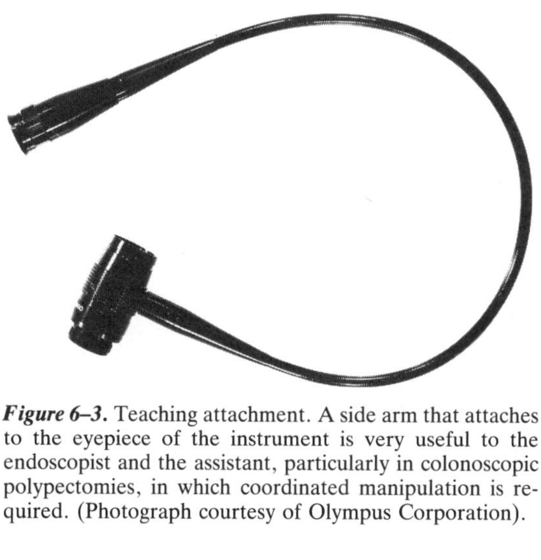

Figure 6–3. Teaching attachment. A side arm that attaches to the eyepiece of the instrument is very useful to the endoscopist and the assistant, particularly in colonoscopic polypectomies, in which coordinated manipulation is required. (Photograph courtesy of Olympus Corporation).

CARE AND MAINTENANCE OF EQUIPMENT

Endoscopes are very delicate instruments and must be maintained in a careful, methodical manner by an experienced person. The Society of Gastrointestinal Assistants offers a biannual course in the care and maintenance of endoscopic equipment. The life expectancy of flexible endoscopes and accessories is greatly enhanced by proper handling and maintenance.

RIGID INSTRUMENTATION

The rigid sigmoidoscope and the anoscope, which have been traditionally used for diagnostic purposes, still serve a useful function in the field of endoscopy.

In actively bleeding patients, the rigid sigmoidoscope provides a better irrigation and suction system than the flexible endoscope and should be employed. The flexible scope has an easily clogged suction system. Cost to the patients is less as well. The diagnostic and, occasionally, therapeutic capability of the an-

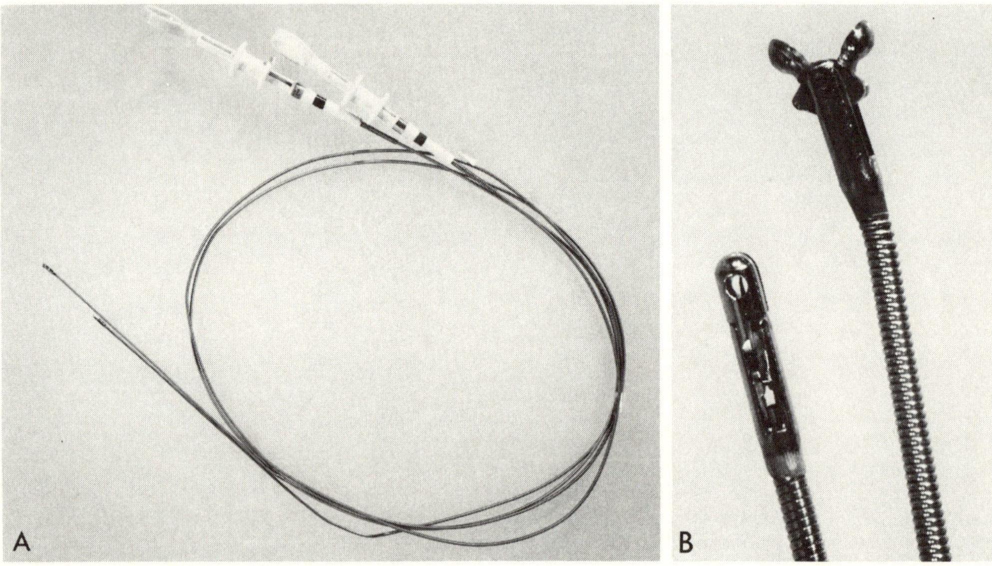

Figure 6–4. *A* and *B,* Biopsy forceps. A metal wire with two cups of varying sizes (2 to 3 mm) and shapes is used to extract tissue for examination. Excessive bleeding or perforation is highly unlikely unless there is a blood dyscrasia or unusual thinning of the wall of the organ. In addition, an electrocoagulating forceps is available for use when warranted. (Photographs courtesy Norton Hospital.)

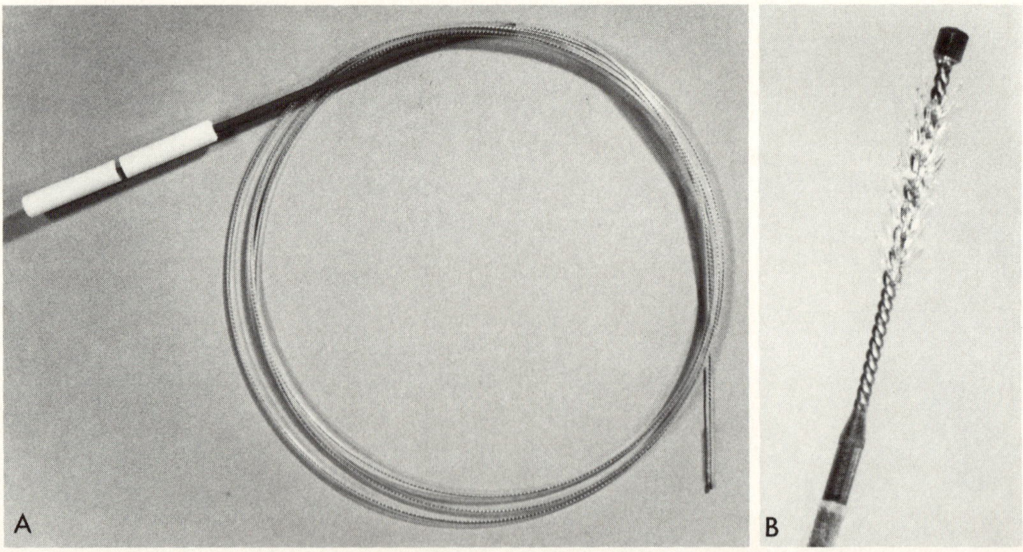

Figure 6–5. *A* and *B,* Cytology brushes. Teflon-sheathed brushes are used to provide tissue fragments to be examined for evidence of malignant cells. Generally, the brushes are of little value in colonoscopic examinations. (Photographs courtesy Norton Hospital.)

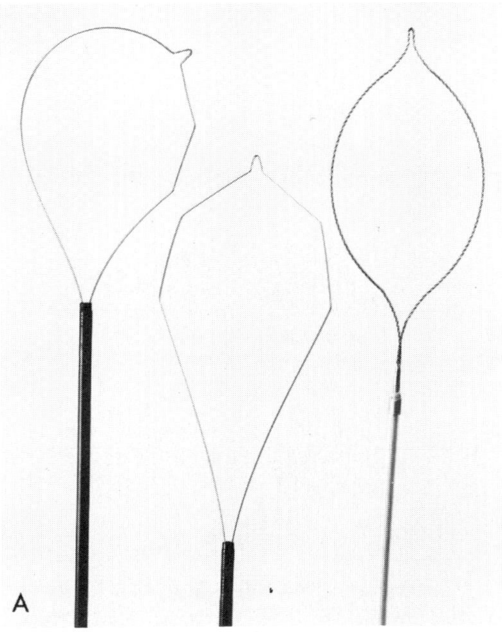

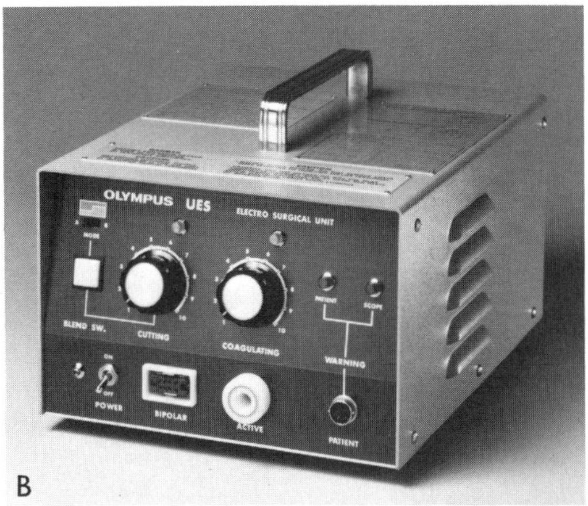

Figure 6–6. *A* and *B,* Snares and electrocautery unit. Single or braided wire Teflon-sheathed snares are used for polypectomies. The choice of a snare wire depends on the size of the polyp and its stalk, the location of the polyp, and the type of electrocautery unit used. (Photograph courtesy of Olympus Corporation.)

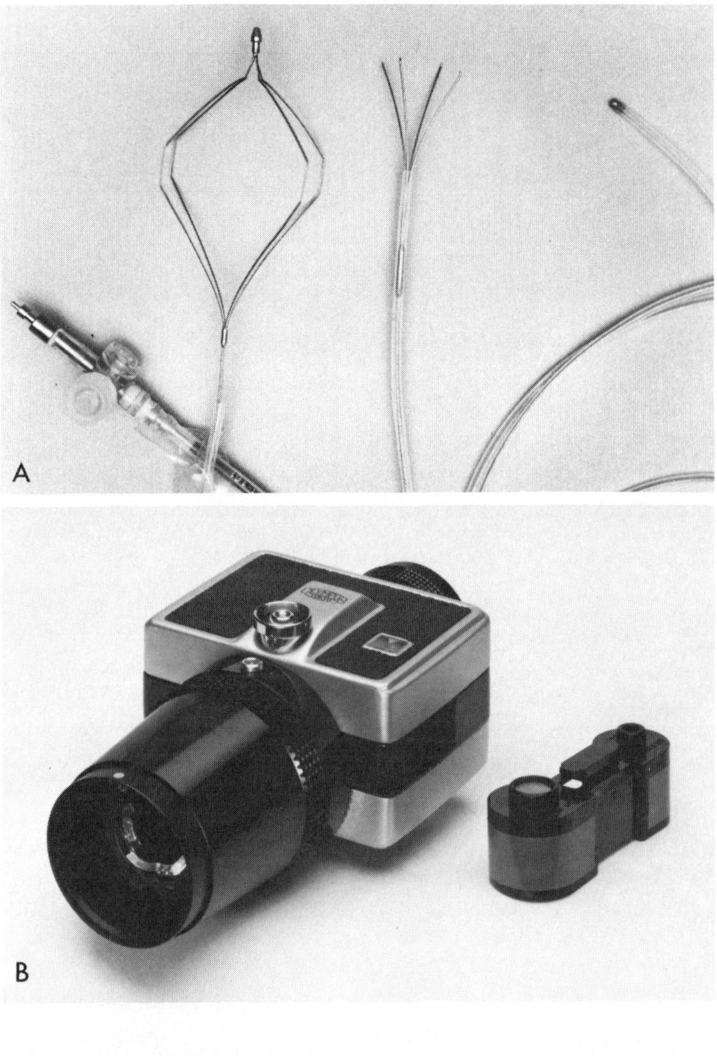

Figure 6–7. *A* and *B,* Other accessories. Grasping forceps, basket forceps, measuring catheters, and injection catheters are all designed to facilitate procedures, such as polypectomies and foreign body retrieval. Several types of cameras are available for documentation purposes. (Photograph of camera courtesy of Olympus Corporation. Photograph of forceps and catheters courtesy of Norton Hospital.)

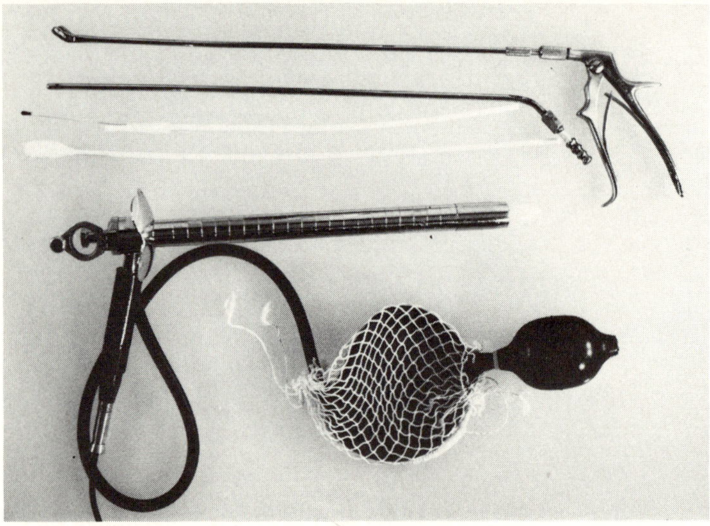

Figure 6–8. Rigid sigmoidoscope and accessories. The rigid sigmoidoscope, traditionally used for diagnostic purposes, still serves a useful function in the field of endoscopy. In actively bleeding patients, the rigid sigmoidoscope should be employed because of its superior irrigation and suction systems. (Photograph courtesy of Norton Hospital.)

oscope is obviously limited to low-lying rectal and anal lesions. An excellent review of surgical methods using rigid scopes and transabdominal evaluation and removal of polyps is provided by Welch (1964).

CRITICAL CHARACTERISTICS OF FLEXIBLE ENDOSCOPES

The ultimate goal of colonoscopy can be defined simply as the consistent ability to examine the entire colon with visual accuracy, speed, and safety while minimizing patient discomfort and inherent "blind" areas in the colon. Currently, there are over 20 different colonoscope and sigmoidoscope models produced by four major medical fiberscope manufacturers (Olympus, American Cystoscopy Manufacturer Inc. [ACMI], Fujinon, and Pentax). Generally speaking, all the currently available fiberscope models have tips that flex; insertion tubes that passively bend; internal channels for sucking, blowing, and washing; and channels for passing instruments. These delicate instruments frequently break down and are exceedingly expensive. They all provide accessories for excising, incising, retrieving, coagulating, brushing, grasping, and photographing. Although endoscopes are similar, the individual manufacturer's specifications may be significantly different. These specifications are the true determinants of an individual instrument's capability and capacity for achieving the ultimate endoscopic goal. Each of the critical characteristics deserves specific comments.

Length. The minimum scope length essential for consistent, total colonoscopic examinations varies depending on the skill of the endoscopist. However, general consensus suggests a minimum scope length of 1500 mm. In most instances, this is sufficient to routinely evaluate the cecum. In addition, if purchase cost is a critical consideration, a long colonoscope can do everything that a short flexible colonoscope can, eliminating the need to purchase the shorter instrument.

Diameter. The actual diameter of the scope tip, or insertion tube, is not critical. On the basis of actual experience, there appears to be a definite advantage in the use of endoscopes constructed with a two-stage insertion tube stiffness because of the ease with which they can be passed to the cecum. This design has virtually eliminated the need for splinting the sigmoid colon with an external device.

Biopsy-Channel Diameter. The diameter of the biopsy channel should be as large as possible for several reasons: (1) It accepts the largest available forceps, thereby allowing larger biopsies and increasing diagnostic accuracy. (2) Adequate suction capability can be maintained with the instrument in the working channel. (3) The ease of passing instruments through the working channel is not impaired even deep within the colon, with the endoscope curved and with the tip flexed 180 degrees.

Angle of Forward View. A wide forward viewing angle minimizes "blind" areas (1) behind the haustral ridges and (2) at acute angles within the colon, such as the hepatic or splenic flexures. A 100-degree forward viewing angle is a reasonable minimum standard.

Table 6–2. **CRITICAL ENDOSCOPE CHARACTERISTICS**

Characteristics	Suggested Minimal Specifications
Length (mm)	1500.0
Diameter	Two stage
Biopsy channel diameter (mm)	3.7
Angle of forward view (°)	100
Bending angles	
Vertical (°)	360
Horizontal (°)	320
Auto exposure system	Yes
Low breakdown rate and high reliability	Varies with design, quality, back-up units, and back-up services.

Bending Angles. Ideally, a 360-degree tip flexion arc in both the vertical and horizontal planes provides maximum ability to negotiate acute angles within the colon, especially in nonmobile segments. However, few nonnegotiable situations will be encountered if the scope has a 360-degree tip flexion arc in at least one of the two planes of motion.

Auto Exposure. Auto exposure consistently provides well-exposed pictures without the need of operator intervention.

The previously discussed critical endoscope characteristics and suggested minimum acceptable specifications for general, total colonoscopic examinations are outlined in Table 6–2.

In addition to the previous considerations, an endoscope design that enables the endoscopist's left hand to hold the scope head, operate the air and water and suction valves as well as the vertical plane flexion control while the right hand remains free for insertion tube manipulation and horizontal flexion control allows more rapid, smooth *perceptive* total colonoscopic examinations. This "eye/hand" coordination of *one* operator is one of the more subtle considerations prerequisite to improving "total colonoscopy" success rate. It is extremely difficult for the authors of this chapter to understand the logic of a "two-operator" colonoscopic examination wherein an assistant advances the scope while the endoscopist views the colon lumen and operates the endoscope control head. Examination speed, the distance that the scope can be advanced, and the amount of colon lumen visualized are greatly enhanced by the perception acquired with the "eye/hand" coordination of a single operator. Also, patient discomfort is minimized.

ENDOSCOPIC EXAMINATION

In the study by Knutson and Max (1979), routine oral alimentation was resumed 1 to 2 hours following the procedure except when an intraendoscopic complication occurred or a lesion that appeared to be malignant dictated otherwise. Outpatients were released to home care following a short period of convalescence.

Endoscopic visualization of the area of colon pathology was possible in 601 of the 662 patients (91 percent), and the cecum was visualized in 271 of 306 attempts (89 percent). In 1977, the most recent year reviewed, for 175 endoscopic examinations performed, the corresponding figures were 96 percent and 95 percent, respectively, perhaps quantifying a learning curve.

No substantial complications were encountered with diagnostic colonoscopy. The only morbidity observed was related to excision or biopsy by way of electrocautery of polypoid colon lesions. Postendoscopic complications associated with total removal or biopsy of 421 lesions were the following: 15 episodes of bleeding (2 percent), with four requiring transfusions (0.6 percent); two colon perforations (0.3 percent); and one episode of fever (0.2 percent), which persisted for 36 hours without other clinical manifestations.

Colonoscopic examinations were carried out on 514 patients with either radiographic interpretations of definite lesions or totally negative barium contrast enema results. This permitted a comparison of diagnostic accuracy (Table 6–3). The overall accuracy rates of the barium

Table 6–3. **COMPARISON OF ACCURACY OF COLONOSCOPY AND BARIUM CONTRAST ENEMA***

Accuracy	Barium Contrast Enema (%)	Colonoscopy (%)
True-positive	169 (33)	269 (52)
True-positive†	54 (10)	—
False-positive	60 (12)	—
True-negative	120 (23)	180 (35)
False-negative‡	50 (10)	4 (1)
Indeterminate§	61 (12)	61 (12)
Total	514	514

*From Knutson CO, Max MH: Diagnostic and therapeutic colonoscopy. A critical review of 662 examinations. Arch Surg 114:430–435, 1979. Copyright 1979, American Medical Association.

†All colon lesions present were not seen on x-ray study.

‡False-negative results of barium enemas confirmed by air contrast enema.

§Includes endoscopic failures (43, 8 percent) and patients without roentgenograms (18, 4 percent).

Table 6–4. **OVERALL ACCURACY RATES OF COLONOSCOPY AND BARIUM CONTRAST ENEMA***

Accuracy	Barium Contrast Enema (%)	Colonoscopy (%)
Accurate	343 (67)	449 (89)
Not accurate	110 (21)	47 (9)†
Indeterminate	61 (12)‡	18 (4)

*From Knutson CO, Max MH: Diagnostic and therapeutic colonoscopy. A critical review of 662 examinations. Arch Surg 114:430–435, 1979. Copyright 1979, American Medical Association.

†Includes endoscopic false-negative examination results and failures.

‡Patients without roentgenograms and endoscopic failures.

contrast enema and colonoscopic studies were 67 percent and 89 percent, respectively (Table 6–4).

A total of 421 polypoid lesions were visualized endoscopically in 281 patients; of these, 407 were either totally excised (375 lesions) or underwent biopsy (32 lesions) with the electrocautery wire snare. Histologically, 320 lesions (76 percent) were benign and 30 (9 percent) were malignant. In the remaining 62 cases (15 percent), no tissue was recovered for microscopic evaluation. However, only 13 lesions (3 percent) were unintentionally lost (Table 6–5). No attempt was made to recover the 35 lesions (8 percent) that were less than 0.5 cm in diameter; 14 lesions (4 percent) were either visualized without an attempt to remove them, or for technical reasons could not be removed because the endoscope could not be passed to the location of the radiographically observed lesions (Table 6–6).

Rectal blood loss of undetermined origin was the indication for colonoscopy in 141 patients. The cecum was visualized in 123 examinations (87 percent). Thirty-three unsuspected lesions were discovered in 30 patients (21 percent). Twenty-nine of the lesions were benign, and three of these were between 2 and 3 cm in diameter; the remaining four lesions were malignant (3 percent).

A nondiagnostic radiographic examination suggestive of a colon abnormality was the indication for 115 endoscopic examinations. Endoscopically, the colonic area in question was visualized in 102 patients (89 percent). Colon disease was definitely excluded as a diagnosis in 71 patients (62 percent). In the remaining 31 patients (27 percent), a pathologic state, including eight cancers (7 percent), was confirmed.

Follow-up colonoscopic examinations were performed on 33 patients 3 to 4 years after previous endoscopic polypectomy. New benign polyps were detected in 11 patients (33 percent); however, none of these patients had colon cancer.

Following negative findings from barium contrast enemas, colonoscopic examinations were performed on 38 patients for a variety of vague colonic complaints. Indications for the procedure included colic-type abdominal pain, chronic diarrhea, increasing constipation, and rectal mucous discharge. Four patients were found to have small benign polyps, but none of these examinations provided information that could explain the patients' symptoms.

The remaining 54 colonoscopic examinations were performed for a variety of other reasons. Nine procedures were to confirm an estab-

Table 6–5. **HISTOLOGIC RESULTS OF 421 COLONOSCOPIC POLYPECTOMIES***

Benign	
Adenomas	290
Lipomas	13
Villous tumors	9
Hyperplastic polyps	8
Subtotal	320 (76%)
Malignant	
In situ	4
Invasive	35
Subtotal	39 (39%)
No Tissue Recovered	62 (15%)
Total	421

*From Knutson CO, Max MH: Diagnostic and therapeutic colonoscopy. A critical review of 662 examinations. Arch Surg 114:430–435, 1979. Copyright 1979, American Medical Association.

Table 6–6. **RESULTS OF COLONOSCOPIC POLYPECTOMY OF 421 POLYPOID LESIONS***

Procedure	Status of Polyp	No. of Polyps (%)
Total excision	Recovered	327 (78)
Total excision	Lost	13 (3)
Total excision	No attempt to recover	35 (8)
Biopsy	Recovered	32 (7)
Biopsy	Lost	0
Visualization only	No attempt to recover	3 (1)
Could not reach with endoscope	Not removed	11 (3)

*From Knutson CO, Max MH: Diagnostic and therapeutic colonoscopy. A critical review of 662 examinations. Arch Surg 114:430–435, 1979. Copyright 1979, American Medical Association.

lished radiographic diagnosis, two of which turned out to be false-positive findings from barium contrast enema studies. The motivation for the remaining 45 procedures was either a search for synchronous or metachronous carcinomas or a search for carcinomas in patients with chronic ulcerative colitis. Five patients had benign lesions that were not seen on barium contrast examination; no cancers were detected.

Of 54 patients who had carcinomas examined endoscopically, 12 (22 percent) had truly occult lesions not previously detected by radiographic contrast studies. Nineteen patients underwent endoscopic excision of polyps, which, when microscopically examined, were superficial (in situ) or invasive cancers. Histologically, the margin between tumor cells and excised surface was adequate in nine lesions (47 percent), questionable in four (21 percent), and inadequate in the remaining six lesions (32 percent). The nine patients with lesions that had adequate tissue margins did not undergo additional operative therapy. Histologically, four of these lesions were in situ, three were invasive, and the remaining two were polypoid carcinomas. Close follow-up of these patients has shown no recurrent disease. However, insufficient time has elapsed to allow for lead-time bias. One additional patient with a 0.9-cm carcinoid tumor of the rectosigmoid part of the colon and a histologically questionable margin underwent no additional operation. This patient has been observed for 2 years without evidence of recurrent disease. The remaining three patients with lesions excised with questionably adequate margins and six patients with inadequately excised lesions underwent definitive colon resection. All nine of the resected colon specimens were examined histologically. Residual cancer was found at the site of endoscopic excision in three patients, and regional lymph nodes were positive for metastatic disease in one patient.

Excluding all patients with questionable radiographic findings and those without pre-endoscopic roentgenograms, 100 of the remaining 514 patients (19 percent) had truly occult lesions detected by endoscopy that were not previously observed by barium contrast enema study. Eighty-eight lesions were benign (17 percent), and 12 were malignant (2 percent). Fifty-three of the occult lesions (53 percent) were less than 1 cm in diameter, whereas 39 lesions (39 percent) were between 1 and 2 cm in diameter. The remaining eight lesions (8 percent) were between 2 and 3 cm in diameter (Table 6–7).

Table 6–7. **SIZES OF 100 OCCULT LESIONS MISSED BY BARIUM ENEMA STUDY***

Size (cm)	No. of Lesions (%)
< 0.5	6 (6)
0.5–0.9	47 (47)
1.0–1.4	23 (23)
1.5–1.9	16 (16)
2.0–2.4	3 (3)
2.5–2.9	5 (5)
≥ 3.0	0

*From Knutson CO, Max MH: Diagnostic and therapeutic colonoscopy. A critical review of 662 examinations. Arch Surg 114:430–435, 1979. Copyright 1979, American Medical Association.

In the visualization of the entire colonic lumen, the endoscope has an important place in the diagnosis and treatment of colonic disorders. It requires considerable expertise to realize the endoscope's potential. The danger of morbidity is real; however, when performed by experienced examiners, the incidence of significant morbidity has been minimal. Rogers and associates (1975) compiled the combined morbidity and mortality for colonoscopy and polypectomy from most major series. This review of 32,881 diagnostic colonoscopic examinations revealed a 0.23 percent (range, 0 percent to 0.8 percent) incidence of colon perforation and a 0.01 percent mortality. Endoscopic excision of 7955 colon polyps was associated with a 1.7 percent (range, 0.2 percent to 6.1 percent) incidence of postendoscopic hemorrhage, a 0.3 percent (range, 0 percent to 0.7 percent) perforation rate, and only one death in the entire composite series. Other isolated, unusual complications have also been reported (Rogers et al., 1975; Meyers and Gharhremani, 1975; Livstone and Kerstein, 1976; Ragins et al., 1974; Smith and Nivatvongs, 1975; Bond and Levitt, 1975). However, experience and attention to appropriate indications, contraindications, patient medication, and procedural technical details make the probability of these types of complications low.

Accuracy of Endoscopic Examination

By comparison, accuracy of routine barium contrast enema examination varies with the methodology, as stressed in Chapter Five. The incidence of false-negative contrast examination findings may well be in excess of 10 percent. Less well known is the incidence of false-positive routine barium contrast enema findings (Schmitt et al., 1975). This incidence definitely varies in different radiology departments. In a previous review, barium contrast enema studies of 250 patients revealed definite colon lesions; 17 percent of the examination results were false-positive. The overall inaccuracy of the routine barium contrast enema study approaches 30 percent (see Table 6–4). Certainly the accuracy of the double-contrast barium enema study was superior to that of the routine barium study (Miller, 1974) (see Chapter Five). However, a continuing controversy among radiologists regarding this subject has prevented routine use of the former study. Also, in our opinion, many of the false-positive results of routine barium contrast enemas could be eliminated with a two-day bowel preparation. This issue is discussed more fully in Chapter Five.

In this series, a comparison of diagnostic accuracy of the barium contrast enema and colonoscopic studies was possible in 514 patients with results of barium enema studies that were either definitely positive or totally negative. Patients with questionable radiographic findings and patients who were intentionally prepared for endoscopy without pre-endoscopic barium contrast studies were excluded from this analysis. There were 61 indeterminate cases—18 patients without available radiographic studies and 43 patients who were considered endoscopic failures (see Table 6–3). In determining the overall accuracy for each diagnostic modality, all 61 indeterminate cases were excluded from the barium contrast enema accuracy calculation, whereas the 43 endoscopic failures were placed in the inaccurate endoscopic group (see Table 6–4). In addition, barium contrast studies that detected some, but not all, of the colonic lesions present (true-positive-plus) were considered with roentgenographically accurate studies. Therefore, the comparative accuracy percentages reflect the endoscopic failures as inaccurate endoscopic examinations and the partially accurate contrast studies as accurate radiographic examinations. Thus, even though the resulting bias actually favors the radiographic study, the diagnostic accuracy of colonoscopy is superior.

If accuracy is the only consideration, an obvious conclusion from this analysis could be that there is a need for more colonoscopy and fewer barium enema studies. However, in patients 50 years of age or older, an endoscopic examination that fails to visualize the cecum is no better than a poor routine barium enema study. Evidence suggests that total colonoscopy is preferable in this age group (Coller et al., 1976; Williams and Muto, 1972). In a study by Knutson and associates (1978) three patients over the age of 50 years developed clinical colon cancer proximal to the colonoscopic examination end point. In experienced hands, the incidence of failure to visualize the cecum ranges from 5 percent to 10 percent, and that area must be examined by other means. Therefore, the two studies are complementary and should not be competitive. Obviously, there are certain aspects of the barium enema study that could improve the diagnostic yield (Miller, 1974), and it is to be hoped that evolving data will provide a basis for initiating improvements. The barium contrast enema is universally available, has minimal potential for morbidity, has excellent patient acceptance, and is less expensive than colonoscopy. All factors considered, we believe that even with the improved diagnostic accuracy and added advantages of biopsy and excision that colonoscopy provides, in most situations a well-executed barium enema should still be the primary initial diagnostic modality for detecting abnormalities of the colon.

Clarification of Radiologic Findings

One of the major indications for diagnostic colonoscopy is gross or microscopic rectal blood loss that is unexplained by routine studies, including barium contrast radiography. In Knutson's (1979) series, 33 unsuspected lesions were found in 21 percent of patients examined for that indication. Of these lesions, four (3 percent) were occult carcinomas. Also, three of the benign lesions were greater than 2 cm in diameter. These findings are consistent with reports of other investigators.

Clarification of questionable radiographic findings remains one of the most common indications for colonoscopy and was possible in 89 percent of patients examined. The verification of eight carcinomas (7 percent), although they were not considered occult lesions, avoided delays in appropriate therapy. Effective endoscopic differentiation between colon carcinoma and the benign inflammatory changes associated with diverticular disease has been previously reported by Sugarbaker and associates (1974). Max and Knutson (1978) also found this helpful in 26 similar cases.

The indications for the remaining 92 colonoscopic examinations were based on negative barium contrast enema studies and persistent complaints relative to the colon, confirmation of established radiographic lesions, or the presence of colonic disease in high-risk patients. The endoscopic yield was low; no firm conclusions were justified. However, even with two endoscopically proved false-positive x-ray film results, documentation of established radiographic lesions appears to have questionable value and probably is only justifiable in selected situations.

Knutson and Max (1979) detected endoscopically 88 (17 percent) benign and 12 (2 percent) malignant lesions missed by barium contrast enema studies in 100 patients. These patients represented a subset biased sample, thus precluding generalizations as to the whole population. Defining the role of colonic endoscopic examination as a cost effective screening procedure has yet to be done.

Jesseph, in discussing the report of Knutson and Max (1979), observed that their reported data would have required the examination of 15 patients a week, requiring 5 to 6 hours of work per week. Although this is not an excessive surgical workload, it must be considered by each surgeon when determining his priorities. Practically, as long as the surgeon-endoscopist is appropriately trained and has the prerequisite technical expertise to consistently provide the highest possible quality colonic examinations, the allocation of time is up to the surgeon and the demands for his service.

Flexible colonoscopy is possible, but not recommended, when the colon is actively bleeding. Knutson and Max (1979) properly pointed out that the primary concern is with cancers. In perspective, clinical symptoms and barium enema studies must be used to identify patients in whom colonoscopy will be useful. Jesseph's view was that as a screening procedure, colonoscopy is too expensive. Excellent air contrast barium enema studies should be used to screen and eliminate those in whom colonoscopic examinations are unnecessary.

Jesseph's experience with air contrast colonic examination is covered in Chapter Five. The diagnostic radiology of the colon described in that chapter was performed at the University of Indiana during Jesseph's tenure. Because of the interest and experience of the investigators, the studies were of very high quality with fewer false-positive results than usual. There are no data available for determining the frequency of false-negative studies by either colonoscopic or barium enema examinations.

TREATMENT USING ENDOSCOPY

There is little controversy regarding the advantages of removing benign polyps endoscopically from the proximal part of the colon versus subjecting a patient to formal abdominal operation and colostomy (Wolff et al., 1973a, 1973b, 1973c; Sugarbaker and Vineyard, 1973; Berci et al., 1973; Knutson et al., 1974; Wolff et al., 1975). In Knutson's experience (Knutson and Max, 1979), successful endoscopic examinations were possible in 95 percent of 281 patients, with avoidance of laparotomy and colotomy in 246 patients (88 percent). However, the "lost polyp" still remained a problem inherent in endoscopic removal of polypoid lesions. Twenty-two lesions were excised and unintentionally lost during the endoscopic procedure; nine (41 percent) were recovered with judicious enemas following the procedure. Certainly, when a polyp 1.5 cm or greater in diameter is not recovered, a more stringent follow-up should be undertaken, since greater size is associated with a greater probability that the polyp is cancerous (Grinnell, 1964) (see Chapter Two).

Malignant sessile polyps are still best treated with definitive colon resection. The patient with a malignant, pedunculated polyp presents a more difficult therapeutic problem. Guidelines are evolving for the conservative endoscopic management of such lesions; however, the long-term results of this approach are not yet available (Wolff and Shinya, 1973b; Knutson et al., 1974; Wolff et al., 1975; Christie, 1976; Shinya et al., 1975; Turnbull et al., 1961) (see Chapter Ten).

Because noninvasive (in situ) lesions rarely, if ever, metastasize, most physicians prefer to remove them by endoscopic excision. Following adequate endoscopic excision of pedunculated, invasive carcinomas (malignant penetration through the muscularis mucosae), the decision regarding further intervention depends on the depth of the invasion, lesion diameter, length of margin obtained by the pedicle, and the patient's age and general condition. The possibility of operative mortality associated with a colon resection, determined by recent reviews to be from 4 to 10 percent (Knutson et al., 1978; Polk et al., 1973), must be counterbalanced against the low probability that metastatic lymph nodes are present. Since the older age group is most commonly afflicted with colon cancer, the greater risk of major surgery with increasing age favors nonresection in the elderly. In a retrospective study, Grinnell (1964) observed that no metastatic regional lymph nodes were present with malignant polyps 1.5 cm or less in diameter. However, the incidence of positive regional lymph nodes associated with 3-cm malignant polyps was 23 percent. These data must be weighed in the patient benefit equation in considering conservative versus operative management. Regardless of the adequacy of endoscopic excision, if the patient's general condition permits, definitive surgical resection is favored for pedunculated, polypoid carcinomas (no histologic definable pre-existing adenoma).

The three pedunculated invasive carcinomas in Knutson's (1979) series were less than 2 cm in diameter, and histologic examination disclosed minimal invasive penetration and normal pedicles. Further resections were not done. The decision for conservative treatment in two of the patients was based on the patients' advanced age, histologic evidence of normal pedicles, and pre-existing chronic diseases associated with an increased risk of operative mortality. This risk exceeded the probability of metastatic disease. Too few data and too short a follow-up time existed to allow any final conclusions regarding the permanent control of the cancer in these cases. Definitive colon resections, as recommended by Wolff and Shinya (1971), were performed on three of the four patients in whom adequate excision of a malignant lesion was questionable and the six patients with inadequately excised malignant lesions. Only three of the nine (33 percent) had residual tumor at the excision site, and only one (11 percent) had positive regional lymph nodes. One additional patient reported by Knutson and Max (1979) with a 0.9-cm carcinoid tumor in the rectosigmoid colon had a questionable tumor-free margin and did not have further surgery. This decision for conservative therapy was based on the small size of the carcinoid and the fact that the excision site had been well cauterized. The reported patient was observed for 2 years, with no evidence of recurrent or systemic disease.

Another problem is the patient whose histologic findings suggest, although not with certainty, complete removal. Pathologists are often insecure about analyzing sections from lesions that have been removed with electrocautery. The coagulation artifact is sometimes distorting. In these few situations, colon resection is probably justified.

Jesseph believed all malignant lesions that were invasive should be treated by resection of the involved colon. On the basis of extensive clinical experience with rigid proctosigmoidoscopy at the Cleveland Clinic, Turnbull and associates (1961) established the fact that many small, invasive rectal and rectosigmoid malignant neoplasms could be cured by local excision only. To suggest that small, invasive malignant lesions of the more proximal colon now accessible as lesions in the rectal ampulla could be cured only by local excision is merely an extension of an already established approach published in 1961. A significant percentage of these small proximal bowel cancers are of the nonmetastasizing variant of colorectal adenocarcinoma (see Chapter Ten).

The most difficult decision regarding further surgery involves the group of patients in whom the risk of operative mortality overlaps the risk of residual metastatic disease in the regional lymph nodes. The risk of mortality associated with the endoscopic procedure is minimal. However, with mortality following a colectomy in a patient with no residual disease the death becomes a negative factor against the value of the cancer control system. Selective criteria for the local resection of colon cancers are emerging. However, much greater experience and a longer follow-up period are necessary to validate any conclusions regarding the proper management of these small cancers. For many equivocal points, controlled clinical trials to ascertain the best strategy of intervention may eventually be required. The smallness of the cancers, the slowness of growth, the age of most patients, and the associated risks of both lead-time and length bias in the evaluation of end result benefits require long-term follow-up in the evaluation plan. Reports as that by Lipper and associates (1983) help refine clinical decisions. They reported the outcome of 51 patients who had large bowel polyps removed that on histologic examination contained cancer. Only one finding predicted residual cancer, that was, the presence of cancer at the line of resection. The authors considered that of 23 transabdominal colectomies performed, only one was justified. That one was identifiable by the presence of cancer at the margin of diathermy resection.

Of the remaining 28 patients, all were treated initially by polypectomy alone. One patient developed a Dukes B cancer 9 months later at the same site as the polyp. In this case, also, cancer was present at the diathermy margin at the time of the original polypectomy. Using the authors' criteria for the presence of cancer at the diathermy margin, this case should have been resected earlier.

References

Berci G, Panish J, Morgenstern L: Diagnostic colonoscopy and colonoscopic polypectomy. Arch Surg 106:818–819, 1973.

Berci G, Panish J, Schapiro M, et al: Complications of colonoscopy and polypectomy: report of the South California Society for Gastrointestinal Endoscopy. Gastroenterology 67:584–585, 1974.

Bond JH Jr, Levitt MD: Factors affecting the concentration of combustible gases in the colon during colonoscopy. Gastroenterology 68:1445–1448, 1975.

Christie JP: Fiberoptic colonoscopy: diagnostic value in 250 consecutive patients. South Med J 69:540–549, 1976a.

Christie JP: Which colonic polyps should be excised endoscopically? South Med J 69:1143–1145, 1976b.

Coller JA, Corman ML, Veidenheimer MC: Colonic polypoid disease: need for total colonoscopy. Am J Surg 131:490–494, 1976.

Cooley RN, Agnew CH, Rios G: Diagnostic accuracy of the barium enema study in carcinoma of the colon and rectum. AJR 84:316–331, 1960.

Fenlon JW, Margulis AR: The radiologic diagnosis. JAMA 231:752–755, 1975.

Gaisford WD: Gastrointestinal fiberendoscopy. Am J Surg 124:744–749, 1972.

Geenen JE, Schmitt MG Jr, Wu WC, Hogan WJ: Major complications of colonoscopy: bleeding and perforation. Am J Dig Dis 20:231–235, 1975.

Goldhaber SZ, Bloom BS, Sugarbaker PH, O'Connor NE: Effects of the fiberoptic laparoscope and colonoscope on morbidity and cost. Ann Surg 179:160–162, 1974.

Grinnell RS: The chance of cancer and lymphatic metastases in small colon tumors discovered on x-ray examination. Ann Surg 159:132–138, 1964.

Knutson CO, Fry DE, Barbie RD, Polk HC Jr: Reassessment of intraoperative decisions: Why operations for cancer of the large bowel fail. Ann Surg 187:549–554, 1978.

Knutson CO, Max MH: Diagnostic and therapeutic colonoscopy. A critical review of 662 examinations. Arch Surg 114:430–435, 1979.

Knutson CO, Schrock LG, Polk HC Jr: Polypoid lesions of the proximal colon: comparison of experiences with removal at laparotomy and by colonoscopy. Ann Surg 179:657–662, 1974.

Lipper S, Kahn LB, Ackerman LV: The significance of microscopic invasive cancer in endoscopically removed polyps of the large bowel cancer 52:1691–1699, 1983.

Livstone EM, Kerstein MD: Serosal tears following colonoscopy. Arch Surg 111:88, 1976.

Max MH, Knutson CO: Colonoscopy in patients with inflammatory colonic strictures. Surgery 84:551–555, 1978.

Meyers MA, Gharhremani GG: Complications of fiberoptic endoscopy: II. Colonoscopy. Radiology 115:301–307, 1975.

Miller RE: Detection of colon carcinoma and the barium enema. JAMA 230:1195–1198, 1974.

Overholt BF: Colonoscopy: a review. Gastroenterology 68:1308–1320, 1975.

Polk HC Jr, Ahmad W, Knutson CO: Carcinoma of the colon and rectum. Curr Probl Surg 1:64, 1973.

Ragins H, Shinya H, Wolff WI: The explosive potential of colonic gas during colonoscopic electrosurgical polypectomy. Surg Gynecol Obstet 138:554–556, 1974.

Rogers BH, Silvis SE, Nevel OT, et al: Complications of flexible fiberoptic colonoscopy and polypectomy. Gastrointest Endosc 22:73–77, 1975.

Schmitt MG Jr, Wu WC, Geenen JE, Hogan WJ: Diagnostic colonoscopy: an assessment of the clinical indications. Gastroenterology 69:765–769, 1975.

Shinya H, Wolff WI: Colonoscopic polypectomy: technique and safety. Hosp Pract 10:71–78, 1975.

Sivak MV Jr, Sullivan BH Jr, Weakley FL, Rankin GB: Colonoscopic polypectomy. Am J Dig Dis 19:339–343, 1974.

Smith LE, Nivatvongs S: Complications in colonoscopy. Dis Colon Rectum 18:214–220, 1975.

Sugarbaker PH, Vineyard GC: Fiberoptic colonoscopy: a new look at old problems. Am J Surg 125:429–431, 1973.

Sugarbaker PH, Vineyard GC, Lewicki AM, et al: Colonoscopy in the management of diseases of the colon and rectum. Surg Gynecol Obstet 139:341–349, 1974.

Teague RH, Salmon PR, Read AE: Fibreoptic examination of the colon: a review of 255 cases. Gut 14:139–142, 1973.

Turnbull RB Jr, Hazard JB, O'Halloran A: Occult invasive cancer in polypoid adenomas of the colon and rectum. Dis Colon Rectum 4:111–114, 1961.

Waye JD: Colonoscopy. Surg Clin North Am 52:1013–1024, 1972.

Welch CE: Polypoid Lesions of the Gastrointestinal Tract. Philadelphia, WB Saunders Company, 1964.

Williams C, Muto T: Examination of the whole colon with the fiberoptic colonoscope. Br Med J 3:278–281, 1972.

Wolff WI, Shinya H: Colonofiberoscopy. JAMA 217:1509–1521, 1971.

Wolff WI, Shinya H: Polypectomy via the fiberoptic colonoscope. Removal of neoplasms beyond reach of the sigmoidoscope. N Engl J Med 288:329–332, 1973a.

Wolff WI, Shinya H: Colonofiberscopic management of colonic polyps. Dis Colon Rectum 16:87–93, 1973b.

Wolff WI, Shinya H: A new approach to colonic polyps. Ann Surg 178:367–378, 1973c.

Wolff WI, Shinya H: Endoscopic polypectomy: therapeutic and clinico-pathologic aspects. Cancer 36:683–690, 1975.

Wolff WI, Shinya H, Geffen A, Ozoktay SZ: Colonfiberoscopy. Am J Surg 123:180–184, 1972.

Wolff WI, Shinya H, Geffen A, et al: Comparison of colonoscopy and the contrast enema in five hundred patients with colorectal disease. Am J Surg 129:181–186, 1975.

SEVEN

Preoperative Preparation and Antibiotic Utilization in Operations for Carcinoma of the Colon and Rectum

H. C. Polk, Jr., M.D.,
J. R. Ausobsky, M.B., F.R.C.S.

The treatment of colorectal cancer usually involves extirpation and the results presently obtained from the various procedures utilized represent some of the most positive aspects of current abdominal surgery. However, it is probable that no other types of procedures have higher risks of endogenous perioperative contamination culminating in intraperitoneal or parietal infection, with its attendant sequelae. Prevention of this contamination, together with measures to promote host-defense capacity in the event of contamination, therefore appears to be mandatory before and during these operations. However, during the past 40 years, the most controversial issue in colorectal surgery has concerned the use of preoperative bowel preparation, in particular the use of pre- and perioperative antimicrobial prophylaxis. Preparation of the bowel for surgery necessitates, first, the attainment of an empty viscus by some mechanical method and, second, the use of antimicrobial agents either to sterilize the lumen or to provide protection during surgery. Until a decade ago, major discussion focused on whether to administer antibiotics before and/or during surgery; the confusion arose primarily because of the erroneous design or interpretation of the many experimental and clinical trials undertaken on this subject. Today, however, there has emerged incontrovertible evidence that the use of antibiotics has a definite role before and/or during colorectal operations; therefore, the debate now centers on the most efficacious method of emptying the bowel and, more importantly, on the type, route, and time of administration of antimicrobial substances.

Aside from the administration of antimicrobial agents, the overall supportive care of patients likely to undergo an operation for colon cancer is not significantly different from that of patients undergoing other major surgical procedures. It is also different in the sense that the patients are usually elderly and may or may not have systemic signs and symptoms associated with the secondary effects of neoplastic disease. The emphasis in the supportive care of the patient who is a candidate for elective surgery is therefore like that for many other illnesses. Similarly, patients who present with complications of colorectal cancer such as obstruction, perforation, and bleeding must receive treatment that is standard for other patients presenting with similar complaints. This chapter emphasizes the antimicrobial factor in colorectal surgery but also provides information on material and matters that may be pertinent in the general supportive care of the surgical candidate with colorectal cancer.

Before we discuss the relative merits of the various methods of colorectal preparation, it is important and salutatory to reflect on the fact that, in this time of polypharmacy, the assumptions that colorectal surgery has been made safe and operative mortality has been reduced to very acceptable levels by use of antibiotics are erroneous. This is contrary to the opinion of many.

The senior author and his associates (Polk et al., 1964) showed clearly in a review of patients treated for colorectal cancer over a period of 40 years in the Barnes Hospital that surgical mortality decreased significantly in 1941, coinciding with, and presumably dependent upon, the institution of blood banking facilities, together with improved surgical expertise (Fig. 7–1). By 1946, when antimicrobial bowel preparations were instituted, the hospital mortality rate (up to 30 days from operation) in that institution had stabilized at approximately 6 percent. In order to extend operative mortality data to the present, it is advantageous to examine pooled data. Baum and associates (1981) evaluated retrospectively all properly conducted trials of antibiotic prophylaxis in colon surgery. Twenty-six studies published after 1965 were judged acceptable, i.e., those with random assignment of treatment and control regimens with prospective evaluation of end points, including control regimens utilizing no antibiotics. It is of interest that only 17 of 26 studies reported mortality figures. Between 1965 and 1975, in eight trials reported, the mortality rate was 4.5 percent in treatment patients, and 11.2 percent in the untreated control groups; between 1975 to 1980, in nine studies reported, the mortality rates were 3.4 percent and 8.7 percent, respectively (Table 7–1). We must, therefore, accept that the use of correct antimicrobial prophylaxis does reduce operative mortality significantly ($p < 0.01$, 1965 to 1975). However, considering again the data from the Barnes Hospital (Polk et al., 1964), i.e., a mortality rate of 6 percent before the use of antibiotic bowel preparations, it is obvious that good results can be obtained by careful attention to surgical techniques and asepsis and that the ability to control large bowel flora with antimicrobial agents is not a substitute for these factors.

The other sequelae of intraoperative contamination are infections of the peritoneal cavity and parietal wound. Baum and co-workers (1981) showed that antibiotics administered either enterally or systemically reduced infection rates to 16 percent, compared with 42 percent in untreated controls (see Table 7–1). The conclusions, therefore, are that significant benefits in terms of operative mortality and infection are attendant on the use of antibiotic prophylaxis in colorectal operations, and there is presently no ethical justification for the use of placebo controls in clinical trials (Baum et al., 1981) or omission of appropriate antimicrobial agents in the preparation of the patient for large bowel operations (Condon, 1982). There is still considerable discussion about the optimum method of antimicrobial prophylaxis,

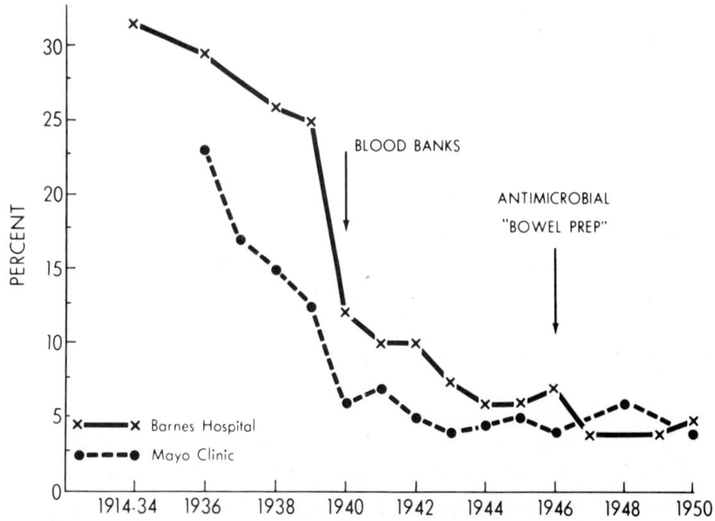

Figure 7–1. Operative mortality for carcinoma of the large bowel. (From Polk HC Jr, Ahmad W, Knutson CO: Carcinoma of the colon and rectum. *In* Ravitch MM, et al (eds): Current Problems in Surgery. Copyright© 1973 by Year Book Medical Publishers, Inc, Chicago. Reproduced with permission.)

Table 7–1. INFECTION AND MORTALITY RATES FOR THE TREATED PATIENTS AND NO-TREATMENT CONTROLS, EXTRAPOLATED FROM ASSESSABLE CLINICAL TRIALS 1965–1980*

Period	No. of Trials†	No. of Patients Control	No. of Patients Treatment	Rate (%) Control	Rate (%) Treatment	Difference Between Rates (± 2 SE)
1965–1975						
Infection	12	387	632	35.7	21.8	13.9 ± 5.8
Mortality	8	267	469	11.2	4.5	6.7 ± 4.4
1976–1980						
Infection	14	475	558	41.9	16.3	25.6 ± 5.6
Mortality	9	390	443	8.7	3.4	5.3 ± 3.4

*From Baum ML, Anish DS, Chalmers TC, et al: A survey of clinical trials of antibiotic prophylaxis in colon surgery: Evidence against further use of no-treatment controls. N Engl J Med 305:795, 1981. Reprinted by permission of the New England Journal of Medicine.

†Only 17 of the 26 trials reported mortality data.

and this will be dealt with in the relevant sections.

It is also important to appreciate that postoperative morbidity and mortality have multifactorial causation and that good surgical technique, strict asepsis with careful avoidance of contamination, and, above all, an empty viscus are of vital importance in the safety of colorectal surgery.

MICROBIOLOGY

Normal Flora

The healthy colon maintains a complex symbiotic relationship with the microflora present in its lumen. Relatively few microorganisms are present in the upper small bowel. This amount increases to approximately 10^8 aerobic and anaerobic bacteria per ml of contents in the distal ileum, this level heralding the initial appearance of fecal anaerobes. In the colon, the concentration of anaerobic nonsporing forms, predominantly *Bacteroides* species, increases to approximately 10^{11} organisms per ml of contents, with aerobic bacteria increasing to 10^8 organisms per ml. *Bacteroides fragilis* is the most common anaerobe isolated, and *Escherichia coli*, the most common aerobe isolated, but in all, the normal colonic microflora comprises some 300 to 500 different types of microorganisms (Gebbers et al., 1981). Other major organisms are aerobic and anaerobic *Lactobacilli* and *Streptococci*, and more minor organisms are *Clostridia, Staphylococci, Proteus,* and *Pseudomonas*. Even in a healthy person there are pathogenic microflora, but they are normally maintained in ecologic equilibrium not only by various interactions with the host but also by complex interactions among the various species of bacteria themselves, which competitively inhibit and suppress potentially pathogenic bacteria and prevent new organisms from spreading to the intestine.

Bacteriology of Postoperative Infections

Microbiologic studies of infected postoperative exudates indicate that most postoperative infections that develop after colorectal operations are polymicrobial in nature, yielding mixed growths of aerobic and anaerobic flora. *Bacteroides fragilis* is the most frequently cultured anaerobe, and it is also the most frequently found microbe (Bartlett et al., 1978). The *Bacteroides* species, *Peptostreptococci* and *Clostridia,* are other common anaerobic pathogens. The most frequently cultured aerobe is *E. coli.* Other varieties of coliform, such as *Klebsiella, Proteus,* and *Pseudomonas*, are also regularly isolated, together with *Streptococcus faecalis* and other species of *Streptococcus*.

In addition to the usual polymicrobial nature of the cultures, it is also notable that virtually all bacteria are endogenous, indicating that this form of contamination is by far the most important source of postoperative sepsis in colorectal surgery.

Significance of Anaerobic Bacteria

Because of improvements in transport and culture media, it is evident that nonsporing anaerobic bacilli, especially *B. fragilis*, are the predominant organisms in the colon and also in postoperative infections (Leigh, 1975). However, there is now a marked difference in opinion as to the significance of these organisms in the pathogenesis of postoperative infections and, particularly, as to the need to administer specific antianaerobic antimicrobial preparations perioperatively in colorectal surgery.

Many surgeons have reported excellent results from including specific antianaerobic antibiotics in their perioperative preparations (Keighley et al., 1976; Lewis et al., 1981; Hanel et al., 1980; Matheson et al., 1978). However, some surgeons report similar effects using only antianaerobic antimicrobial agents (Bjerkeset and Digranes, 1980; Dion et al., 1980).

The authors, however, presently believe that clinical data suggesting an advantage in using combination prophylaxis against both aerobes and anaerobes are somewhat deficient. Experimental and clinical data (Stone et al., 1975; Kelly, 1978) suggest synergy between common intraperitoneal aerobic bacteria implicated in infection and *Bacteroides*, and in a review of therapeutic methods used in proven *Bacteroides* bacteremia, Fry (1979) concluded that appropriate mechanical measures and antibiotics directed against aerobic bacteria are not improved upon by the addition of drugs specific for anaerobes.

One possible theoretic explanation is that aerobic bacteria, by producing metabolites that lower the ambient oxidation reduction potential, create a milieu acceptable to anaerobic organisms, and that by either treatment of aerobes or prevention of their growth, the necessary milieu for anaerobic growth is destroyed. The issue, however, of whether specific antianaerobic antibiotics are required remains a matter of some conjecture, and further experimental and clinical trials are necessary before it can be resolved.

THEORETIC CONSIDERATIONS OF COLORECTAL PREPARATION BEFORE SURGERY

Mechanical Preparation

Preoperative emptying of the colon by some mechanical method remains the cornerstone of effective bowel preparation. An empty bowel is a distinct advantage during surgery, decreasing the risk of fecal contamination of the greater sac and parietal wound and lessening postoperative perianastomotic leakage. In addition, enteral prophylaxis is rendered virtually useless in the presence of gross fecal loading. Rosenberg and associates (1971) noted in their early prospective study that those patients in whom gross fecal loading was present at operation fared substantially worse than their counterparts who received good mechanical preparation. The quality of the preparation was assessed subjectively. Irvin and Goligher (1973) observed a significant decrease in anastomotic dehiscence in patients with a clean colon, from 24 percent to 7 percent.

However, even though thorough mechanical preparation of the colon and rectum results in a decrease in fecal content, the residual colonic bacterial population per ml of contents is only minimally and transiently altered, and the feces remaining are not sterile (Nichols and Condon, 1971); mechanical preparation only is by no means sufficient preparation for colorectal surgery (Editorial, British Medical Journal, 1976).

Several methods of mechanical preparation are presently available (Table 7–2), and these are discussed later. For the purposes of mechanical preparation, all patients with colorectal carcinoma are considered to be part of one of three groups (Herter, 1972). They may be classified as either having (1) no obstruction, (2) partial obstruction, or (3) total or near total obstruction.

Each case must be assessed and prepared on its own merits. In general, patients with no obstruction should present little problem. In those patients with partial obstruction, a more circumspect approach should be adopted, with careful evaluation of progress made to assess the effectiveness of mechanical measures. In those patients with total or near total obstruction, mechanical preparation is both worthless and dangerous. In the latter patients, utilization of defunctioning stomata is required, although "on table" intraoperative irrigation of the bowel, permitting primary anastomosis, may have much to recommend it (Dudley et al., 1980).

Enteral Prophylaxis

Theoretic Trials

Poorly absorbed antimicrobial agents are used preoperatively to reduce colonic bacterial

Table 7–2. METHODS OF MECHANICAL PREPARATION

1. Traditional method—dietary restrictions, purgatives, enemas, retrograde washouts
2. Mannitol
3. Whole gut irrigation (± mannitol)
4. Intraoperative anterograde lavage

flora. Absolute "sterility" of the colon is impossible to achieve; even though optimum antimicrobial therapy produces a 2 to 3 log decrease in bacterial concentration, it regularly leaves bacterial densities of 10^5 to 10^6 organisms per ml of colonic contents. However, by decreasing the number of viable bacteria in the colon, the number present in a contaminating inoculum is also decreased, increasing the likelihood that host defenses will be able to eradicate this primary lodgment.

It has also been shown experimentally in a canine model that the use of intestinal antiseptics protects an anastomosis performed on ischemic bowel (Poth, 1960). It was also shown that, histologically, antibiotic prophylaxis initiated orderly repair of the anastomosis, compared with a marked inflammatory response in untreated controls. The theory behind these events was that antibiotics prevent the formation of a microabscess at the anastomotic suture line by suppressing colonic bacteria. In an unprepared bowel, microabscesses occur, causing local thrombosis of small vessels and infarction, with subsequent necrosis and dehiscence. In the clinical situation, Herter and Slanetz (1967) initially found that the anastomotic "protection" was only given to extraperitoneal anastomoses of low anterior resections, but more recent reports indicate that colorectal anastomoses at any level are less liable to breakdown following enteral antibiotic preparation.

The preceding considerations concerning the mode of action of enteral antimicrobial agents (i.e., their action is solely dependent on their local activity on colonic microflora) have been challenged by other researchers, such as Altemeier (1974), who believed that all positive benefits accrued from enteral prophylaxis derive from systemic absorption of the agents employed, and if absorption was prevented, the effects would be significantly decreased.

Systemic Prophylaxis

In contrast to the somewhat equivocal basis of enteral prophylaxis, systemic prophylaxis by way of antimicrobial agents administered perioperatively is based on sound experimental precepts and clear clinical confirmation.

Data from the work of Miles, Miles, and Burke (1957), amplified by Burke (1961) and by Polk and Miles (1973), indicated that during the first 3 to 4 hours following primary lodgment of infecting bacteria, there was an extensive "kill" by host defenses, which cease to operate following this time, and that the subsequent course of the infection was determined by the number of bacteria surviving. Antibiotics adjuvant to host defenses are only effective if they are present during this time. Extrapolating to the clinical situation, it follows that antibiotic administration should precede contamination so that adequate tissue concentrations of antibiotics will act with host defenses to increase the efficacy of both during the decisive period. By the use of systemic prophylaxis, the consequences of any contamination are minimized, the number of perianastomotic abscesses are reduced, and the results of perianastomotic leakage are mitigated.

There are insufficient data to determine appropriate length of antibiotic administration, although available evidence indicates a short perioperative course provides optimum prophylaxis.

METHODS OF MECHANICAL PREPARATION

Traditional Method

Until recently the most common method of mechanical bowel preparation was by the combined use of purgatives, enemas, and washouts. Various practices are followed, there being no single universal regimen. Preparation may involve dietary restrictions for 2 to 4 days prior to operation, together with daily use of variations of the above triad. Care must be taken during vigorous preparation that metabolic disturbances are not induced, especially in elderly and frail patients.

In the nonobstructed patient, these regimens, if performed properly, will result in effective emptying of gross feces and scybala but not in a reduction of most components of the fecal microflora. Nichols and co-workers (1971), in a study of the microbiologic effects of vigorous preparation found that only coliforms were significantly reduced by this method but that there was essentially no change in the other major bacterial components. The residual feces are still a reservoir of bacteria.

Mannitol

Mannitol, a poorly absorbed carbohydrate that acts as an osmotic cathartic, has recently been shown to be very effective in the mechanical cleansing of the nonobstructed colon

(Newstead and Morgan, 1979; Palmer and Khan, 1979). Approximately one half hour after bolus by oral administration of 500 ml of a 10 percent or 20 percent solution of mannitol, bowel action commences, fecal at first, then becoming watery. By the use of concomitant intravenous fluids to compensate for fecal loss, electrolyte disturbances are minimized. Care must be taken in the elderly patient, and the method is contraindicated if there is any evidence of obstruction. The advantage of this method is that the patient can be prepared on the evening before surgery, thus decreasing duration of hospital stay.

The correct use of the method yields good results, although there may be residual fluid in the cecum and right colon. Keighley and associates (1981) recently have drawn attention to the increase in fecal gas–producing *E. coli* following the use of the mannitol preparation alone, possibly resulting in increased postoperative sepsis when used in conjunction with systemic antibiotics. When mannitol was used in conjunction with neomycin and metronidazole for enteral prophylaxis, extremely effective sterilization of the colonic contents was achieved (Table 7–3). When mannitol is used, there is no need for repeated enemas or passage of a nasogastric tube, and it is generally very well tolerated, especially in the elderly.

Whole Gut Irrigation

Whole gut irrigation, first reported by Hewitt and co-workers (1973), has recently gained popularity. Following passage of a nasogastric lavage tube, irrigation is performed with warm isotonic saline at the rate of 3 to 4 L per hour (Crapp et al., 1975); a total of 12 to 14 L is usually necessary to achieve a clear effluent.

The problems associated with this method are fluid gain and electrolyte disturbances, making the method unsuitable for use in patients with cardiac decompensation. Donovan and co-workers (1980) reported that the method is also somewhat ineffective in preparing the left colon. These authors report improvement in colon cleansing and a decrease in water and electrolyte disturbances by oral administration of 50 gm of mannitol before operation.

Advantages of the method are that it does not involve extensive preoperative preparation, it is fairly rapid, and it can be used judiciously in patients with incomplete obstruction if used with a stool softener (Condon, 1979).

Intraoperative Irrigation

The on table "washout," first described by Muir (1968) and later by Dudley (1980), mechanically prepares the colon by anterograde lavage intraoperatively. This method allows a macroscopically clean colon to be obtained, and it can be used as routine preparation and also as preparation in the totally obstructed patient, allowing immediate left-sided anastomosis to be performed with systemic prophylactic cover. Reports of its use are scarce, but

Table 7–3. **MEAN COUNTS OF COLONIC BACTERIA (log_{10}) AFTER VARIOUS PREPARATIVE REGIMENS***

	Mannitol alone (n = 11)	Mannitol + antibiotic† (n = 11)	Whole bowel irrigation (n = 11)	No preparation (n = 11)
Staphylococcus albus	8×10^2	—	4×10^1	9×10^1
Staphylococcus aureus	—	—	—	—
Streptococcus viridans	7×10^1	—	5×10^2	5×10^1
Streptococcus faecalis	2×10^5	1×10^3	3×10^1	2×10^4
Escherichia coli	8×10^8‡	7×10^1	9×10^5	8×10^7
Klebsiella species	6×10^2	—	8×10^1	9×10^1
Proteus species	6×10^2	—	1×10^2	9×10^2
Pseudomonas aeruginosa	8×10^1	—	5×10^1	—
Bacteroides fragilis	2×10^8	—	5×10^9	7×10^9
Bacteroides melaninogenicus	7×10^2	—	4×10^3	7×10^1
Peptostreptococcus species	7×10^3	—	2×10^3	4×10^1
Clostridium species	2×10^5	7×10^1	6×10^3	9×10^3
Bifidobacterium species	8×10^2	—	4×10^1	9×10^3
Veillonella species	9×10^2	—	2×10^2	—

*From Keighley MRB, Taylor EW, Hares MM, et al: Influence of oral mannitol bowel preparation on colonic microflora and the risk of explosion during endoscopic diathermy. Br J Surg 68:554, 1981. Reproduced with permission.

†Enteral neomycin and metronidazole.

‡P = 0.001 compared with mannitol + antibiotic and whole bowel irrigation.

it may well prove to be a useful alternative method of preparation. It can be combined with the use of intraluminal povidone-iodine, a topical microbicide with a wide antibacterial spectrum, which has been shown to produce a significant reduction in both aerobic and anaerobic colonic bacteria in experimental animals (Jones et al., 1975).

Which Mechanical Preparation?

The choice of preparation will inevitably be based on the surgeon's personal preference. In spite of the efficacy of orthograde irrigation in decreasing colonic fecal content, this method does not avoid postoperative infective complications when used without antimicrobial preparation. Raahave and associates (1981) reported a high rate of abdominal (24 percent) and perineal (75 percent) wound infections when irrigation only was used to prepare patients.

The use of mannitol or whole gut irrigation results in a shorter preoperative hospital stay, and although a combination of mannitol and whole gut irrigation achieves the most effective preparation, mannitol used alone is judged more acceptable by patients and nursing staffs (Minervini et al., 1980).

Clinical Trials

Poorly absorbed oral antibiotics to "sterilize" the colon and rectum before surgery have been commonly used for some 4 decades. Properties that an ideal agent should exhibit include a broad antibacterial spectrum, minimal systemic absorption, minimal toxicity, and rapid action.

Well-recognized general principles of prophylaxis dictate that any regimen should be selected on the basis of safety, antibacterial spectrum, and distribution of kinetics, in that order, and that the agent should be used for as short a time as possible. Selection should also be based on proven efficacy, as judged in well-controlled clinical trials. Until the beginning of the last decade, use of enteral bowel preparation produced inconsistent results, engendered by inadequate appreciation of experimental results and a lack of well-controlled clinical studies. The prolonged use of preoperative oral therapy, together with the use of concomitant systemic antimicrobial agents, often continued well into the postoperative period, was responsible for many adverse effects, such as staphylococcal enterocolitis and the development of resistant hospital microbial populations. It is only relatively recently that properly controlled, randomized prospective clinical trials have demonstrated clearly the effectiveness and safety of certain regimens, as well as determined which agents have the lowest incidence of systemic toxicity and microbial selection pressures.

Washington and colleagues (1974) were first in the United States to report the results of a well-designed prospective double-blind trial of oral antibiotic preparation compared with mechanical cleansing alone. In addition to mechanical preparation, patients undergoing elective colonic surgery were selected randomly to receive either neomycin alone, neomycin and tetracycline, or a placebo. Combined prophylactic agents significantly reduced infective complications, whereas neomycin alone or placebo did not. However, the beneficial effects of this combination of antibiotics may have accrued because of systemic absorption and the activity of tetracycline. Since this report, many trials of oral antimicrobial preparation have included neomycin in combination with various other agents. Combination therapy is used because no single antibiotic of low toxicity is available with an antibacterial spectrum that effectively covers all the colonic microflora.

Clarke and associates (1977) found that neomycin and erythromycin were an effective combination when used in patients who received vigorous mechanical preparation and who were randomly allocated to receive neomycin and erythromycin or placebo in three doses on the final preoperative day. Antibiotic preparation resulted in a significant decrease in wound infections (from 35 percent to 9 percent) and in intra-abdominal infections (from 17 percent to 4 percent) and also resulted in a significantly reduced rate (4 percent) of anastomotic leakage, as compared with that in the placebo group (17 percent). Quantitative microbiology demonstrated a 4 to 6 log decrease in the concentration of both aerobic and anaerobic organisms in the treatment group (Bartlett et al., 1978), indicating a profound impact on colonic microflora, as well as the efficacy of a high dose and short course of prophylaxis. This combination of neomycin plus erythromycin also has been found to be effective by others (Lewis et al., 1978).

Neomycin plus metronidazole has also been shown to be a satisfactory combination. Metronidazole, a nitromidazole, has been extensively investigated with respect to its properties of prophylaxis in colorectal surgery. It has bactericidal effects specific for anaerobes, especially *Bacteroides* species, and is virtually free from side effects. It has, however, been demonstrated to have mutagenic activity in mice (Rustia and Shubi, 1972), but this is dependent on its conversion to nitrometabolites, a phenomenon that has not been shown to occur in humans; despite the very extensive use of metronidazole, there have been no reports of any carcinogenic activity in humans. The use of metronidazole is somewhat contrary to the accepted pure principles of enteral preparation because it is readily absorbed (Bjerkeset and Diagranes, 1980) and, therefore, its concomitant systemic effects will contribute considerably to the efficacy of prophylaxis.

Brass and associates (1978) compared the combination of metronidazole and neomycin with neomycin plus erythromycin oral preparation. The incidence of infectious complications with metronidazole was 5 percent, and with erythromycin, 25 percent; metronidazole was the more effective in reducing colonic anaerobes. The high rate of sepsis with the neomycin plus erythromycin preparation conflicts somewhat with the results reported by Clarke and associates (1977), but a change of the dose and the timing of administration of these agents may have contributed to this discrepancy. Matheson and colleagues (1978) also studied the combination of neomycin and metronidazole and compared it with a placebo in a randomized controlled multicenter trial. The incidence of wound and intra-abdominal sepsis was significantly decreased, to 18 percent in the treatment group, compared with 47 percent in the control group. In addition, septicemia and anastomotic dehiscence were significantly reduced, and there were five deaths in the placebo group, compared with no mortality in the experimental group. Metronidazole has also been used as a single agent enteral preparation. Bjerkeset and Digranes (1980) reported a controlled trial of patients undergoing elective colorectal surgery who were randomly selected to receive either oral metronidazole pre- and postoperatively or a placebo, in addition to mechanical preparation. A significantly lower frequency (16 percent) of wound and perineal sepsis, intra-abdominal complications and septicemia was found in the metronidazole group as compared with the control group (45 percent). Although the use of systemic gentamicin in one dose given immediately preoperatively to all patients makes it difficult to analyze the effects of metronidazole, Willis and associates (1977) also reported a 15 percent rate of morbidity in patients receiving oral metronidazole pre- and postoperatively, compared with a 63 percent rate in the control group; nearly all of the infections in the control group involved anaerobic pathogens. However, all infections in the experimental group were caused by aerobic organisms (in spite of perioperative systemic gentamicin). Taylor and associates (1979) found that there was a 12 percent rate of aerobic infections in the group prepared with metronidazole. It appears that metronidazole is effective in controlling the anaerobic but not the aerobic component of infections when it is used as a single-agent preparation.

Goldring and co-workers (1975) compared one group who had a 3-day preoperative regimen of oral kanamycin and metronidazole with a control group receiving no antibiotics. Both groups had mechanical cleansing with purgatives. The incidence of postoperative infectious morbidity was 8 percent in the kanamycin plus metronidazole group, compared with 44 percent in the control group. This difference is significant. Proud and Chamberlain (1979) also reported this combination to be an effective one. This same combination was studied by the Keighley group (1979). Kanamycin plus metronidazole was administered orally or systemically. Postoperative sepsis occurred in 6.5 percent of the group given systemic perioperative microbial agents and 36 percent in those patients receiving oral prophylaxis. Other somewhat startling findings were that 15 infections in the oral regimen group were caused by organisms resistant to kanamycin. In this group, six patients had *Staphylococcus aureus* overgrowth and another six patients had pseudomembranous colitis. This failure of the oral regimen is explained by the particular regimen utilized. Kanamycin was administered in a low dosage (3 gm/day) for 3 days. Oral aminoglycosides administered for more than 48 hours are associated with the emergence of resistant bacterial strains. Also, metronidazole was stopped 36 hours before operation, thereby facilitating regrowth of anaerobic organisms in the colon. Use of this regimen invalidates the findings in the oral regimen group, but the study proved the efficacy of the intravenous regimen of kanamycin plus metronidazole administered on an optimum schedule perioperatively.

Kanamycin has also been used in conjunction with erythromycin. In a prospective study, Wapnick and associates (1979) randomly selected patients to receive either oral kanamycin and placebo or kanamycin and erythromycin for 2 days preoperatively. This combination antimicrobial preparation significantly decreased wound infections, compared with kanamycin alone, indicating again the need for combination therapy.

The dosage and timing of administration of the preceding regimens are presented in Table 7–4.

SYSTEMIC PROPHYLAXIS

As mentioned earlier in this chapter, the use of systemic perioperative prophylactic antimicrobial agents to prevent the consequences of intraoperative contamination is experimentally well founded, and since the classic work of Polk and Lopez-Mayor in 1969, there has emerged a solid body of clinical evidence pertaining to the efficacy of this type of antibiotic use. During surgery for colorectal carcinoma, the colon is opened under controlled conditions, and it is at this time that contamination may occur. In order to minimize this problem, the mechanical preparation must be as thorough as possible because even if adequate antibiotic levels are present, they will be negated by a massive inoculum. The antimicrobial agent chosen must be safe, must have a

Table 7–4. **STUDIES OF ENTERAL REGIMENS FOR COLORECTAL PREPARATIONS***

Reference	Experimental Preparation(s)	Control Preparation(s)
Washington et al (1974)	Neomycin, 500 mg, and tetracycline, 250 mg; 4 times/day for 2 days preoperatively†‡	Placebo Neomycin, 500 mg 4 times/day for 2 days preoperatively
Clarke et al (1977)	Neomycin and erythromycin base, 1 gm each at 1 PM, 2 PM, and 11 PM on the preoperative day*†‡	Placebo
Lewis et al (1978)	Neomycin and erythromycin base, 1 gm each at 1 PM, 2 PM, and 6 PM on the preoperative day‡	Cephaloridine, 1 gm IV or IM 2 hr preoperatively, then 5 and 12 hr postoperatively‡
Brass et al (1978)	Neomycin, 1 gm 3 times/day for 24 hr preoperatively; metronidazole, 750 mg 3 times/day for 2 days preoperatively; cephalothin, 1 gm IV preoperatively and 5 and 12 hr later†‡	Neomycin and erythromycin base, 1 gm of each 3 times/day for 24 hr preoperatively; cephalothin, 1 gm, IV preoperatively and 5 and 12 hr later‡
Matheson et al (1978)	Neomycin, 1 gm, and metronidazole, 200 mg; 3 times/day for 48 hr preoperatively†‡	Placebo
Bjerkeset and Digranes (1980)	Metronidazole, 2 gm on evening of preoperative day, then 1–2 gm daily for 5 days†	Placebo Gentamicin, 80 mg IM immediately preoperatively
Willis et al (1977)	Metronidazole, 1 gm 24 hr before surgery, then 200 mg every 8 hr until surgery; postoperative metronidazole, 200 mg orally or 1 gm via suppository 3 times/day for 7 days; gentamicin, 80 mg IM immediately preoperatively†	
Taylor et al (1979)	Metronidazole, 400 mg 3 times/day, and thalazole, 2.5 gm 4 times/day, for 4 days preoperatively	Thalazole, 2.5 gm 4 times/day for 4 days postoperatively
Goldring et al (1975)	Kanamycin, 1 gm, and metronidazole, 200 mg; every 6 hr for 3 days†‡	Placebo
Proud and Chamberlain (1979)	Metronidazole, 400 mg, and kanamycin, 600 mg; 4 times/day for 3 preoperative days†‡ Metronidazole, 400 mg, and placebo; 4 times/day for 3 preoperative days†	Placebo
Keighley et al (1979)	Kanamycin, 1 gm, and metronidazole, 500 mg; IV immediately preoperatively and every 12 hr on first postoperative day†‡	Kanamycin, 1 gm 3 times/day for 3 preoperative days, and metronidazole, 1–2 gm/day for 2 days preoperatively, stopping 36 hr before operation
Wapnick et al (1979)	Kanamycin, 1 gm, and erythromycin, 750 mg; every 6 hr for 48 hr before operation‡	Kanamycin, 1 gm, and placebo; every 6 hr for 48 hr before operation

*All studies included mechanical preparation. All antimicrobial agents given orally unless otherwise stated.
†Indicates significant decrease in postoperative morbidity compared with control regimen.
‡Indicates effective regimen.

spectrum of activity against the expected pathogens, and also must achieve adequate bioavailability in the tissues. This ability of parenterally administered agents to penetrate the tissues in sufficient concentrations so that they exceed the minimal inhibitory concentration of the probable contaminating bacteria is an extremely important factor in determining the usefulness of a particular antibiotic. To illustrate this, Figure 7–2 depicts the wound distribution kinetics of three antibiotics in the cephalosporin group, as assayed in our unit (Polk et al., 1980). It can be seen that whereas cefazolin and cephaloridine maintained, for a sufficient period, wound antibiotic levels exceeding minimum inhibitory concentrations of bacteria, cephalothin sodium did not maintain levels consistent with effective antimicrobial activity, disappearing rapidly from the tissues. This factor probably explains the failure of this agent to confer significant protection in terms of decreased infectious morbidity when used as the sole perioperative prophylactic agent in colorectal operations (Condon et al., 1979; Burdon et al., 1977).

Polk and Lopez-Mayor (1969) were the first to report an appropriately designed and assessed clinical trial of a short perioperative course of systemic antibiotic prophylaxis in patients undergoing gastrointestinal surgery. Patients were randomly selected to receive either cephaloridine (1 gm) immediately preoperatively and at 5 and 12 hours thereafter,

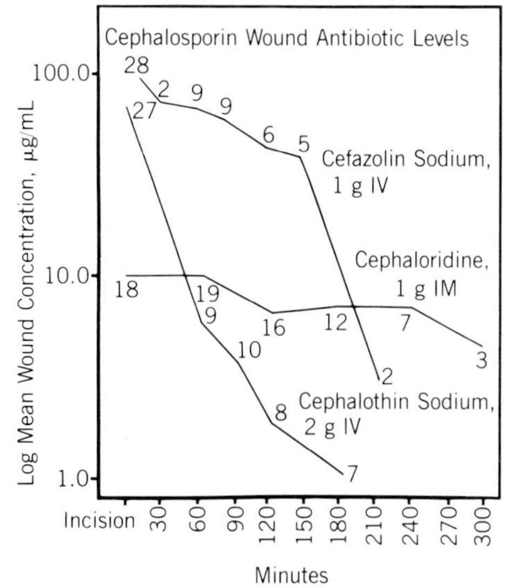

Figure 7–2. Cephalosporin wound antibiotic levels. (From Polk HC Jr, Trachtenberg LS, Finn MP: Antibiotic activity in surgical incisions: The basis for prophylaxis in selected operations. JAMA 244:1353, 1980. Copyright 1980, American Medical Association.)

or a placebo. In the subset of 104 patients undergoing colorectal surgery, none of whom received preparation other than mechanical cleansing of the bowel, there was a significant reduction in postoperative infectious complications in those patients receiving cephaloridine compared with those receiving placebo. Four of 54 (8 percent) patients who were treated with cephaloridine developed sepsis, whereas 15 of 50 (30 percent) of the placebo group developed sepsis.

The fact that cephaloridine is an effective prophylactic agent in colorectal surgery was also shown by Lewis and co-workers (1978), who compared a short perioperative systemic course of this agent with an effective enteral preparation of neomycin and erythromycin. There was no difference in the rates of incidence of infectious complications between either group, 13 percent and 12 percent, respectively.

Many other reports of the use of antimicrobial agents of the cephalosporin group for prophylaxis of colorectal operations have yielded somewhat equivocal results. Condon and associates (1979) carried out a three-arm clinical trial comparing the following methods of colon preparation: (1) oral neomycin plus erythromycin, (2) intravenous cephalothin, and (3) a combination of both regimens. Each regimen also included mechanical cleansing. Those patients receiving only systemic cephalothin fared significantly worse postoperatively, with an incidence of 39 percent of septic complications, compared with their counterparts prepared with oral neomycin plus erythromycin, in whom complications occurred in 6 percent. These findings are similar to those of Burdon and colleagues (1977), who also found that postoperative infections were not altered in the group given intravenous cephalothin perioperatively, as compared with untreated controls. This failure of cephalothin is explained by the biokinetics of the antimicrobial agent (Polk et al., 1980), and this drug's inability to maintain adequate tissue concentrations casts doubt on its continued use as a prophylactic agent.

As stated earlier, Lewis and associates (1978) confirmed that perioperative prophylaxis with systemic cephaloridine constitutes an effective regimen. However, a more recent study by the same unit (Lewis et al., 1981) compared an enteral erythromycin plus metronidazole combination with systemic administration of cephradine, another "first generation" cephalosporin. There were significantly better results with the enteral preparation in terms of infective complications than with the cephradine. Eight percent of those patients prepared with the enteral method developed sepsis, compared with 25 percent in the cephradine group. This apparent failure of cephradine could have been caused by pharmacodynamic factors, rather than by the inadequacy of its bacterial spectrum. Cephradine achieves lower serum levels and has a shorter half-life than cephaloridine; in the preceding study (Lewis et al., 1981), serum levels were not estimated. The investigators postulated that the lack of efficacy was due to an inadequate dose, and are, therefore, repeating this study using high systemic doses of cephradine.

Cefazolin, a first generation cephalosporin, has high tissue levels and a long half-life. Its effectiveness when used as systemic preparation for colorectal resection has been investigated. McDermott and associates (1981) carried out a fully prospective, randomized study comparing the combination of perioperative intramuscular cefazolin and oral metronidazole with the combination of cefazolin and a placebo. There was no significant difference between the groups, there being no complications with the combined regimen and only one wound infection when cefazolin only was used.

The preceding cephalosporin antibiotics, commonly used in prophylaxis, have no in vitro activity against *B. fragilis*. Is this of import with the current trend in surgery increasingly implicating these anaerobic organisms in postoperative complications? McDermott and associates (1981) concluded that although anaerobic organisms greatly outnumber aerobic organisms in the large intestine, chemoprophylaxis can be obtained with an agent effective mainly against aerobes if strict attention is paid to asepsis and surgical techniques. Further evidence of the need to concomitantly provide anaerobic cover in colorectal operations is derived from our unit.

Cefoxitin, a second generation cephalosporin, has an increased gram-negative aerobic spectrum as well as in vitro effectiveness against *B. fragilis*. This agent was evaluated by Fry and Polk (1981) in the prophylaxis of patients undergoing elective gastrointestinal procedures. Two thirds of the patients in the trial underwent a colonic procedure, and in this subset, there was a 12 percent incidence of parietal wound infections. From these data, it did not appear that additional protection was gained by adding coverage against *B. fragilis* to cefoxitin, because infections occurred at rates comparable to those in other series in which cephalosporin antibiotics were used and had no effectiveness against this microbe.

Another second generation cephalosporin that has been submitted for clinical appraisal is cefamandole. This agent does not have antibacteroides activity. Slama and co-workers (1979) have reported its use in a clinical trial that compared patients receiving cephalothin with those receiving cefamandole as perioperative prophylaxis for colorectal operations. Postoperative infection rates were 31 percent with cephalothin and 33 percent with cefamandole, and the authors concluded that neither antibiotic was effective, although there were only 34 cases in their study.

Having considered these somewhat conflicting reports, the question that must be addressed is whether the cephalosporin group of antimicrobial agents provides effective prophylaxis during colorectal surgery. The authors believe that this can certainly be answered affirmatively, provided that the correct agent is used (dependent on the biokinetics of the drug, adequate dosage, and the use of agents whose efficacy has been proved in clinical trials) and that strict attention is paid to preoperative bowel preparation, asepsis, and surgical techniques. The determination of the usefulness of the newer second and third generation cephalosporins in further reducing infective complications following colorectal procedures requires continued investigation.

Several other agents or combinations thereof have been investigated as to their positive attributes in systemic colorectal prophylaxis. Keighley and associates (1976) investigated the effects of intravenous lincomycin on postoperative complications. Patients were randomly selected to receive either lincomycin, 2 doses prior to surgery, followed by a 5-day course, or a placebo. Lincomycin reduced postoperative sepsis from 45 percent to 18 percent in the control group. The trial was extended by Downing and associates (1977) to include patients receiving only perioperative doses of lincomycin in addition to the standard mechanical bowel preparation. In this group, a 23 percent complication rate was recorded; this rate was significantly better than that of the untreated control group, but was statistically equal to that of the 5-day course.

However, postoperative infection rates of 18 to 23 percent are high, and although the lincomycin significantly reduced the number of incidences of anaerobic infection, it had no influence on the number of patients who developed aerobic infection. It would therefore appear that lincomycin given alone systemically is not a fully effective prophylactic agent in colorectal surgery.

Doxycycline, a highly lipophilic tetracycline derivative, is rapidly and almost completely absorbed from the upper small intestine; therefore, even though it is given orally, it can be regarded as exerting only systemic effects. Its antibacterial spectrum includes both nonsporing anaerobes and intestinal aerobes, and it has an affinity for intestinal tissue. In a prospective study by Wetterfors and Hojers (1976), oral doxycycline or a placebo was given preoperatively and once daily for five days postoperatively. The incidence of infectious complications was reduced from 45 percent in the placebo group to 12 percent in the treatment group, the difference being statistically significant. This activity of doxycycline has also been demonstrated when patients were given the drug in a single preoperative intravenous dose (Tornqvist and associates, 1981).

Hanel and co-workers (1980) investigated the combination of clindamycin and cefazolin given in a single preoperative dose either alone or in conjunction with a neomycin plus metronidazole enteral preparation and demonstrated no difference in the incidence of postoperative complications between the two groups. They concluded that the use of single-dose clindamycin and cefazolin was effective prophylaxis.

Metronidazole in combination with trimethoprim plus sulphamethoxazole was found to be an effective single-dose parenteral prophylaxis by Higgins and associates (1980), and metronidazole used alone, administered parenterally in single dose preoperatively, was found by Eykyn and associates (1979) to decrease septic complications from 51 percent in the placebo group to 13 percent in the group given metronidazole.

The systemic regimens evaluated are depicted in greater detail in Table 7–5.

COMBINED SYSTEMIC AND ENTERAL PROPHYLAXIS

Controlled studies of enteral prophylaxis have demonstrated that several regimens are effective. Does the addition of systemically administered antibiotics engender a further reduction in postoperative complications? This issue has only been investigated in a limited number of studies.

Stone and co-workers (1976) assayed the effect of systemic cefazolin used in addition to oral neomycin plus erythromycin preparations for colorectal surgery. Patients receiving the combined oral-systemic regimen had an incidence rate of infectious complications of 8 percent, compared with 22 percent in patients receiving only enteral preparation. However, a 22 percent incidence rate is considerably higher than that usually ascribed to this method of preparation. As stated previously, Hanel and associates (1980) found no benefit when oral neomycin and metronidazole were added to a single dose of clindamycin and cefazolin. Barber and colleagues (1979) measured the benefits conferred by the addition of systemic clindamycin and gentamicin to oral preparation of neomycin and erythromycin. Those patients receiving both enteral and systemic prophylaxis sustained a 7 percent incidence of sepsis, compared with 11 percent in those receiving oral preparation alone. Although these differences are not statistically significant, care must be taken in their evaluation because improvement may indeed be attained but may not be statistically evident because of the smallness of the sample, i.e., a Type II statistical error may be initiated. Finally, Eisenberg (1981) reported that systemic cefamandole given perioperatively, in addition to neomycin plus erythromycin enteral preparation, reduced the postoperative infection rate from 23 per cent in patients given the drug orally to 7 percent in those patients receiving both regimens. However, again, care must be taken in evaluating these results because of the high sepsis rate with the use of neomycin plus erythromycin.

The assessment of the benefits of this type of combination of systemic and oral prophylaxis requires further careful investigation before a definite judgment of its effectiveness can be made.

WOUND AGENTS

The preoperative preparation of the patient with colorectal carcinoma is aimed primarily at the prevention of postoperative infectious morbidity. Intraoperatively, several other ancillary methods may be used, and as they are designed mainly to prevent or minimize the consequences of parietal contamination, they have been loosely termed wound agents.

Wound Protectors

The use of ring drape wound protectors (Cole and Bernard, 1967) to prevent access of

Table 7–5. **STUDIES OF SYSTEMIC ANTIMICROBIAL PROPHYLAXIS FOR COLORECTAL SURGERY***

Reference	Experimental Regimen(s)	Control Regimen(s)
Polk and Lopez-Mayor (1969)	Cephaloridine, 1 gm IV immediately preoperatively, then IM 5 and 12 hr later†‡	Placebo
Lewis et al (1978)	Cephaloridine, 1 gm IV or IM 2 hr preoperatively, then 5 and 12 hr postoperatively‡	Neomycin and erythromycin base, 1 gm each at 1 PM, 2 PM, and 6 PM on the preoperative day‡
Condon et al (1979)	Oral neomycin and erythromycin base, 1 gm of each at 1 PM, 2 PM, and 11 PM on final preoperative day, plus cephalothin, 2 gm IV at 6 PM, 12 PM, and 6 AM preoperatively; 1 gm with anesthesia and thereafter every 6 hr for 48 hr†‡	Placebo plus neomycin and erythromycin base, 1 gm of each at 1 PM, 2 PM, and 11 PM on the final postoperative day†‡
Burdon et al (1977)	Cephalothin sodium, 1 gm IV at commencement of operation and 1 hr later Cephalothin sodium, 2 gm IV as above	Placebo
Lewis et al (1981)	Cephradine, 1 gm IV 1 hr preoperatively, 1 gm postoperatively, and again 6 hr postoperatively	Metronidazole, 750 mg, and erythromycin base, 1 gm; three times on final preoperative day†‡
McDermott et al (1981)	Cefazolin, 1 gm IM 1 hr preoperatively, and metronidazole, 1–2 gm 6 hr preoperatively‡	Cefazolin, 1 gm IM 1 hr preoperatively‡
Fry and Polk (1981)	Cefoxitin, 2 gm IM with premedication and 4 and 8 hr following initial dose‡	
Slama et al (1979)	Cefamandole, 2 gm IV with the premedication in the recovery room, then every 4 hr for 10 more doses	Cephalothin, 2 gm IV with the premedication in the recovery room, then every 4 hr for 10 more doses
Wetterfors and Hojer (1976)	Doxycycline, 200 mg 4–6 hr preoperatively, then 100 mg daily for 5 days†‡	Placebo
Tornqvist et al (1981)	Doxycycline, 200 mg IV 1–1.5 hr preoperatively† Doxycycline, 600 mg IV 1–1.5 hr preoperatively‡	Doxycycline, 600 mg IV postoperatively 2–5 hr after opening colon Doxycycline, 200 mg IV 1–1.5 hr preoperatively and once daily postoperatively for 3 days
Keighley et al (1976); Downing et al (1977)	Lincomycin, 600 mg IV 2 doses preoperatively and 3 times/day for 5 postoperative days† Lincomycin, 600 mg IV immediately preoperatively and 4 and 12 hr postoperatively†	Placebo
Hanel et al (1980)	Clindamycin, 7 mg/kg, and cefazolin sodium, 1 gm; IV immediately preoperatively‡	Metronidazole, 200 mg 4 times/day for 4 days preoperatively; neomycin, 1 gm 3 times/day for 2 days preoperatively Clindamycin, 7 mg/kg, and cefazolin, 1 gm; IV immediately preoperatively‡

*All patients received mechanical preparation.
†Indicates a significant decrease in infectious complications when compared with control or other experimental sets.
‡Indicates effective regimen.

bacteria to the parietal wound is an attractive concept, but controlled trials have not proved its effectiveness. Raahave (1976), by quantitative velvet pad sampling of operative wounds, found that plastic wound drapes used on the alimentary tract in potentially contaminated operations resulted in virtually a 100 percent reduction of the density of enteric bacteria in the wound. However, this decrease in bacterial density was not translated into improved wound infection rates in the clinical studies of Alexander-Williams and associates (1972) and Psaila and associates (1977).

Topical Antiseptics

The development of substances such as povidone-iodine and noxythiolin (*N*-hydroxymethyl-*N'*-methylthiourea) has generated renewed interest in use of antiseptics in surgery, but opinion is diverse as to their usefulness. Experimental work indicated that povidone-iodine, in conjunction with systemic antibiotic prophylaxis, significantly decreased infection rates in heavily contaminated wounds compared with antibiotics alone (Galland, 1982). Gilmore and Sanderson (1975) demonstrated a significant reduction in wound sepsis following colorectal operations by the use of povidone-iodine, but Gray and Lee (1981) and McCluskey (1976) failed to demonstrate similar effectiveness. It appears that lavage of wounds with povidine-iodine is clinically inferior to preoperative antibiotic prophylaxis, but the use has not been adequately evaluated in the clinical setting.

Topical Antibiotics

Advocates of topical antibiotic prophylaxis maintain that it allows direct contact of an antimicrobial substance with the tissues and, therefore, the contaminating inoculum and enables poorly absorbed, more toxic agents to be used in higher local concentrations than can safely be attained by systemic administration.

Virtually all antibiotics have been used for topical prophylaxis, but there are little data indicating an additive effect of enteral or systemic and topical antimicrobial agents in colorectal surgery. Pollock and associates (1978) found that topical cephaloridine reduced wound infection rates in patients who received preoperative enteral preparation who were having high-risk ileocolorectal procedures performed. Stone (1973) demonstrated the efficacy of Neosporin spray in preventing wound sepsis after emergency laparotomy, the patient receiving concomitant systemic antibiotics. This mode of prophylaxis requires further definition, although many surgeons (ourselves included) employ topical prophylaxis in conjunction with other forms of antibiotic colorectal preparation.

GENERAL PATIENT PREPARATION

It is apparent from the foregoing that both the enteral and systemic antimicrobial agents, if used appropriately, are equally effective in decreasing postoperative infective complications in elective operations for colorectal carcinoma when used in conjunction with mechanical cleansing. No clear benefit from either method in terms of reduced infectious morbidity has been determined. In terms of complications attendant upon the use of this antimicrobial prophylaxis, there is, however, a small but definite risk of the development of antibiotic-associated pseudomembranous colitis and staphylococcal overgrowth when the more prolonged enteral preparations are employed. A short perioperative course of systemic antimicrobial agents is unlikely to lead to iatrogenic illness or the emergence of resistant antimicrobial forms. Enteral preparation is also inappropriate when dealing with emergency situations attendant on carcinoma of the large bowel. When providing antibiotic cover for the surgery to remove an obstruction, it is necessary to use systemic agents, and when the operation is performed for perforation of the colon, systemic antibiotics will need to be continued for longer than 5 days.

Our practice is to prepare a patient scheduled for elective surgery mechanically using enemas, and then to use a short perioperative systemic course of an appropriate antimicrobial (a cephalosporin) in conjunction with a wound protector and topical Neosporin spray, if the patient is not involved in a clinical study. The basic issues of which mode of preparation, enteral, systemic, or a combination of the two, should be used together with the questionable need to include specific antianaerobic agents, require further studies to provide complete answers. Progress in this direction will be hindered by the need for large numbers of patients necessary to allow correct statistical analysis of small, but important, decreases in morbidity and mortality when a new, possibly improved, regimen is compared with the best available standard preparation. With regard to the use of specific antianaerobic agents, the evidence suggests that if systemic prophylaxis is utilized, then the addition of those agents is unnecessary, with excellent results being obtained by use of antibiotics without this spectrum of activity, as was discussed earlier in the chapter. However, if a true enteral preparation is used (i.e., one without significant systemic effect), then the addition of specific antianaerobic preparation is necessary to achieve an adequate decrease in the anaerobic population, mainly the decrease of *Bacteroides fragilis*, to prevent subsequent infectious complications due to this organism.

A list of preparations presently known to be effective in colorectal prophylaxis is included (Table 7–6).

In the general preparation of the patient, the physician needs to focus on blood volume and hemoglobin concentration, general and nutritional status, and the presence of associated illnesses.

The colon cancer patient is often anemic, and this anemia may require a high cardiac output to provide tissue oxygenation and may predispose a patient with a relatively sound cardiovascular system to congestive failure. This congestive failure is one of the cardiovascular complications most easily treated, and it tends to revert to normal with restoration of hemoglobin concentration to a near-normal range. In general, the correction of an anemia that has been acquired over many months should be accomplished over several days. The administration of more than a single unit of blood per day in preparation for an elective operation, even when packed red blood cells are used, requires that the patient excrete a certain amount of an involuntarily expanded plasma volume. Congestive heart failure can complicate this process, and the use of careful timing and packed red blood cells is often recommended when correction of an operation is of major concern. Assessment of cardiovascular status is a subject of any number of monographs and descriptions, and I (H. C. P.) have reviewed this subject in some detail in one of the major surgical textbooks (Polk, 1977). The most serious problem with this cardiorespiratory disease is that often there are no clues that such disease exists. One must recall that many myocardial infarctions are silent, and particular attention must be paid both to the patient history and objective assessment of the cardiorespiratory system, which includes an electrocardiogram, a chest film, and assessment of arterial blood gases. Once again, optimization of cardiorespiratory function may require careful preoperative support and preparation, including establishment, as noted previously, of an ideal hemoglobin concentration and even the occasional use of antibiotics to clear superimposed pulmonary infection. The critical goal is to bring the patient to the operative procedure in optimal condition and to accomplish this with respect for and full acknowledgement of the chronic debilitating effects of progressive disease and other organ systems.

The assessment of the cardiorespiratory system is a primary factor in reaching a determination of operative risk, a subject of great concern to both the patient and physician facing a major operation for the treatment of colorectal noeplasms. It is essential that the patient's operation be specifically tailored for the extent and location of the cancer, with full respect for any extra-abdominal limitations im-

Table 7–6. **EFFECTIVE REGIMENS FOR COLORECTAL PROPHYLAXIS**

Effective Antimicrobial Preparations*	Incompletely Effective Preparations
Oral	*Oral*
Neomycin + erythromycin base	Neomycin
Metronidazole + erythromycin base	Metronidazole
Doxycycline	Neomycin + sulfonamide
Neomycin + tetracycline	Metronidazole + sulfonamide
Kanamycin + erythromycin	
Neomycin + metronidazole	
Kanamycin + metronidazole	
Systemic	*Systemic*
Cephaloridine	Cephalothin
Cefazolin	Cephradine
Cefoxitin	Cefamandole
Doxycycline	Lincomycin
Clindamycin + cefazolin	Metronidazole
Cotrimoxazole + metronidazole	
Kanamycin + metronidazole	

*Effective preparation assumes optimum dose and timing of administration.

posed by the patient's inability to withstand a procedure which would otherwise be warranted.

It is impossible in these times to review the supportive care of any surgical patient without a specific note about nutritional support. A careful dietary and nutritional history must be taken and if the patient has sustained a significant weight loss (i.e., ≥ 10 percent of his lean body mass), it must be decided whether the patient would best be served by being rid of the debilitating disease process (i.e., the cancer itself), with postoperative restitution of normal nutrition, or whether surgery should be postponed, often at length until there is evidence of restoration of body weight, lean body mass, and other laboratory parameters compatible with and indicative of good nutrition.

It is hard to overestimate the importance of nutrition, and it is appropriate that it has become an area of concern to surgeons. On the other hand, parenteral hyperalimentation is not a prerequisite of every patient who is over the age of 40 or about to undergo surgery that may last more than half an hour. The physician must use judicious measurements (just as he does in assessing cardiorespiratory parameters) in determining the nutritional status of the patient and making an election for the ideal method and time of reconstitution.

There are numerous other problems that occasionally surface in the preparation and assessment of the patient about to undergo operation for cancer of the colon or rectum or both. However, the foregoing problems are the most significant both in terms of their immediate effects on the patient and in terms of their frequency.

SUMMARY

Standard surgical practice requires that patients undergoing surgery for carcinoma of the colon and rectum be prepared for operation by effective mechanical cleansing and the use of antimicrobial agents to either decrease the colonic microbial flora or minimize the consequences of contamination by these organisms. The use of enteral or systemic antimicrobial agents in no way obviates the pursuit of continued excellence in mechanical preparation, asepsis, or surgical techniques.

The optimum use of either method of administration decreases infectious morbidity to rates of 7 to 9 percent.

The overall assessment and support of the patient with respect to noninfectious matters is much like those of patients undergoing operations for other illnesses. The specific concern with cardiorespiratory function, because of the patient's age, is highly justified, and attention to maximum concentrations of hemoglobin and the attainment of an optimal nutritional state are part of a complete program to allow the optimum support of the individual patient.

References

Alexander-Williams J, Oates GD, Brown PP, et al: Abdominal wound infections and plastic wound guards. Br J Surg 59:142, 1972.

Altemeier WA, in the discussion of Washington JA, Dearing WH, Judd ES, et al: Effect of preoperative antibiotic regimen in development of infection after intestinal surgery. Ann Surg 180:572, 1974.

Barber MS, Hirschberg BC, Rice CL, et al: Parenteral antibiotics in elective colon surgery? A prospective, controlled clinical study. Surgery 86:23, 1979.

Bartlett JG, Condon RE, Gorbach SL, et al: Veterans Administration Cooperative Study on Bowel Preparation for Elective Colorectal Operations: impact of oral antibiotic regimens on colonic flora, wound irrigation cultures and bacteriology of septic complications. Ann Surg 188:249, 1978.

Baum ML, Anish DS, Chalmers TC, et al: A survey of clinical trials of antibiotic prophylaxis in colon surgery: Evidence against further use of no-treatment controls. N Engl J Med 305:795, 1981.

Bjerkeset T, Digranes A: Systemic prophylaxis with metronidazole (Flagyl) in elective surgery of the colon and rectum. Surgery 87:560, 1980.

Brass C, Richards GK, Ruedy J, et al: The effect of metronidazole on the incidence of postoperative wound infection in elective colon surgery. Am J Surg 135:91, 1978.

Burdon JGW, Morris PJ, Hunt P, et al: A trial of cephalothin sodium in colon surgery to prevent wound infection. Arch Surg 112:1169, 1977.

Burke JF: The effective period of preventive antibiotic action in experimental incisions and dermal lesions. Surgery 50:161, 1961

Clarke JS, Condon RE, Bartlett JG, et al: Preoperative oral antibiotics reduce septic complications of colon operations: Results of prospective, randomized, double-blind clinical study. Ann Surg 186:251, 1977.

Cole WR, Bernard HR: Wound isolation in the prevention of postoperative wound infection. Surg Gynecol Obstet 125:257, 1967.

Condon RE: Preparation of the bowel for colon and rectal operations. J Surg Prac 8:10, 1979.

Condon RE: Bowel preparation for colorectal operations. Arch Surg 117:265, 1982.

Condon RE, Bartlett JG, Nichols RL, et al: Preoperative prophylactic cephalothin fails to control septic complications of colorectal operations: Results of controlled clinical trials. Am J Surg 137:68, 1979.

Crapp AR, Powis SJA, Tillotson P, et al: Preparation of the bowel by whole-gut irrigation. Lancet 2:1239, 1975.

Dion YM, Richards GK, Prentis JJ, et al: The influence of oral versus parenteral preoperative metronidazole on sepsis following colon surgery. Ann Surg 192:221, 1980.

Donovan IA, Arabi Y, Keighley MRB, et al: Modification

of the physiological disturbances produced by whole gut irrigation by preliminary mannitol administration. Br J Surg 67:138, 1980.

Downing R, McLeish AR, Burdon DW, et al: Duration of systemic prophylactic antibiotic cover against anaerobic sepsis in intestinal surgery. Dis Colon Rectum 20:401, 1977.

Dudley HAF, Radcliffe AG, McGeehan D: Intraoperative irrigation of the colon to permit primary anastomosis. Br J Surg 67:80, 1980.

Editorial. Preventing infection at the operation site. Br Med J 2:773, 1976.

Eisenberg HW: The use of new antibiotics in colorectal surgery. Am J Proctol Gastroenterol Colon Rectal Surg 32:9, 1981.

Eykyn SJ, Jackson BT, Lockhart-Mummery HE, et al: Prophylactic intravenous metronidazole in elective colorectal surgery. Lancet 2:761, 1979.

Fry DE, Garrison RN, Polk HC Jr: Clinical implications in bacteroides bacteremia. Surg Gynecol Obstet 149:189, 1979.

Fry DE, Polk HC Jr: The use of cefoxitin in systemic antibiotic prophylaxis. Aktuel Probleme in Chir Orthop 19:77, 1981.

Galland RB, Heine KJ, Trachtenberg LS, Polk HC Jr: Reduction of surgical wound infection rates in contaminated wounds treated with antiseptics combined with systemic antibiotics: An experimental study. Surgery 91:329, 1982.

Gebbers JO, Laissug JA, Otto HF: Modern aspects of the functional morphology of the colon. Coloproctology 3:211, 1981.

Gilmore OJA, Sanderson PJ: Prophylactic interparietal povidone-iodine in abdominal surgery. Br J Surg 62:792, 1975.

Goldring J, McNaught W, Scott A, et al: Prophylactic oral antimicrobial agents in elective colonic surgery. Lancet 2:997, 1975.

Gray JG, Lee JR: The effect of topical povidone iodine on wound infection following abdominal surgery. Br J Surg 68:310, 1981.

Hanel KC, King DW, McAllister ET, et al: Single-dose parenteral antibiotics as prophylaxis against wound infections in colonic operations. Dis Colon Rectum 23:98, 1980.

Herter FP: Preparation of the bowel for surgery. Surg Clin North Am 52:859, 1972.

Herter FP, Slanetz CA: Influence of antibiotic preparation of the bowel on complications after colon resection. Am J Surg 113:165, 1967.

Hewitt J, Rigby J, Reeve J, et al: Whole gut irrigation in preparation for large-bowel surgery. Lancet 2:337, 1973.

Higgins AF, Lewis A, Noone P, et al: Single and multiple dose cotrimoxazole and metronidazole in colorectal surgery. Br J Surg 67:90, 1980.

Irvin TT, Goligher JC: Etiology of disruption of intestinal anastomoses. Br J Surg 60:461, 1973.

Jones FE, DeCosse JJ, Condon RE: Experimental evaluation of "instant" preparation of the colon with povidone-iodine. Surg Clin North Am 55:1343, 1975.

Keighley MRB, Arabi Y, Alexander-Williams J, et al: Comparison between systemic and oral antimicrobial prophylaxis in colorectal surgery. Lancet 1:894, 1979.

Keighley MRB, Crapp AR, Burdon DW, et al: Prophylaxis against anaerobic sepsis in bowel surgery. Br J Surg 63:538, 1976.

Keighley MRB, Taylor EW, Hares MM, et al: Influence of oral mannitol bowel preparation on colonic microflora and the risks of explosion during endoscopic diathermy. Br J Surg 68:554, 1981.

Kelly MJ: Pathogenic synergy between *Escherichia coli* and *Bacteroides fragilis* in a guinea-pig wound model. Br J Surg 65:813, 1978.

Leigh DA: Wound infections due to *Bacteroides fragilis* following intestinal surgery. Br J Surg 62:375, 1975.

Lewis RT, Allan CM, Goodall RG, et al: Antibiotics in surgery of the colon. Can J Surg 21:339, 1978.

Lewis RT, Allan CM, Goodall RG, et al: Preventing anaerobic infection in surgery of the colon. Can J Surg 24:139, 1981.

McCluskey B: A prospective trial of povidone iodine solution in the prevention of wound sepsis. Aust NZ J Surg 46:254, 1976.

McDermott FT, Polglase AL, Johnson WR, et al: Prevention of wound infection in elective colorectal resections by preoperative cephazolin with and without metronidazole. Aust NZ J Surg 51:351, 1981.

Matheson DM, Arabi Y, Baxter-Smith D, et al: Randomized multicentre trial of oral bowel preparation and antimicrobials for elective colorectal operations. Br J Surg 65:597, 1978.

Miles AA, Miles EM, Burke J: The value and duration of defense reactions of the skin to the primary lodgment of bacteria. Br J Exp Pathol 38:79, 1957.

Minervini S, Alexander-Williams J, Donovan IA, et al: Comparison of three methods of whole bowel irrigation. Am J Surg 140:400, 1980.

Muir EG: Safety in colonic resection. Proc R Soc Med 61:401, 1968.

Newstead GL, Morgan BP: Bowel preparation with mannitol. Med J Aust 2:582, 1979.

Nichols RL, Condon RE: Preoperative preparation of the colon. Surg Gynecol Obstet 132:323, 1971.

Nichols RL, Gorbach SL, Condon RE: Alterations of intestinal microflora following preoperative mechanical preparation of the colon. Dis Colon Rectum 14:123, 1971.

Palmer KR, Khan AN: Oral mannitol: A simple and effective bowel preparation for barium enema. Br Med J 2:1038, 1979.

Polk HC Jr: Principles of preoperative preparation of the surgical patient. *In* Sabiston D (ed): Davis-Christopher Textbook of Surgery. Philadelphia, WB Saunders Company, 1977, p 119.

Polk HC Jr, Lopez-Mayor JF: Postoperative wound infection. A prospective study of determinant factors and prevention. Surgery 66:97, 1969.

Polk HC Jr, Miles AA: The decisive period in primary infection of muscle by *Escherichia coli*. Br J Exp Pathol 54:99, 1973.

Polk HC Jr, Spratt JS Jr, Bennett D, et al: Surgical mortality and survival from colonic carcinoma. Arch Surg 89:16, 1964.

Polk HC Jr, Trachtenberg LS, Finn MP: Antibiotic activity in surgical incisions: The basis for prophylaxis in selected operations. JAMA 244:1353, 1980.

Pollock AV, Froome K, Evans M: The bacteriology of primary wound sepsis in potentially contaminated abdominal operations: The effect of irrigation, povidone-iodine and cephaloridine on the sepsis rate assessed in a clinical trial. Br J Surg 65:76, 1978.

Poth EJ: The role of intestinal antisepsis in the preoperative preparation of the colon. Surgery 47:1018, 1960.

Proud G, Chamberlain J: Antimicrobial prophylaxis in elective colonic surgery. Lancet 2:1017, 1979.

Psaila JV, Wheeler MH, Crosby DL: The role of plastic wound drapes in the prevention of wound infection following abdominal surgery. Br J Surg 64:729, 1977.

Raahave D: Effect of plastic skin and wound drapes on the density of bacteria in operation wounds. Br J Surg 63:421, 1976.

Raahave D, Hansen OH, Carstensen HE, et al: Septic

wound complications after whole bowel irrigation before colorectal operations. Acta Chir Scand 147:215, 1981.
Rosenberg IL, Graham NG, DeDombal FT, et al: Preparation of the intestine in patients undergoing major large bowel surgery, mainly for neoplasms of the colon and rectum. Br J Surg 58:266, 1971.
Rustia M, Shubi P: Induction of lung tumors and malignant lymphomas in mice by metronidazole. J Natl Cancer Inst 48:721, 1972.
Slama TG, Carey LC, Fass RJ: Comparative efficacy of prophylactic cephalothin and cefamandole for elective colon surgery. Results of prospective, randomized, double-blind study. Am J Surg 137:593, 1979.
Stone HH, Hester TR: Incisional and peritoneal infection after emergency celiotomy. Ann Surg 177:669, 1973.
Stone HH, Hooper A, Kolb LD, et al: Antibiotic prophylaxis in gastric, biliary, and colonic surgery. Ann Surg 184:443, 1976.
Stone HH, Kolb LD, Geheber CE: Incidence and significance of intraperitoneal anaerobic bacteria. Ann Surg 181:705, 1975.
Taylor SA, Cawdery HM, Smith J: The use of metronidazole in the preparation of the bowel for surgery. Br J Surg 66:191, 1979.
Tornqvist A, Ekelund, A, Forsgren A, et al: Single dose doxycycline prophylaxis and peroperative bacteriological culture in elective colorectal surgery. Br J Surg 68:565, 1981.
Wapnick S, Guinto R, Reizis I, et al: Reduction of postoperative infection in elective colon surgery with preoperative administration of kanamycin and erythromycin. Surgery 85:317, 1979.
Washington JA II, Dearing WH, Judd ES, et al: Effect of preoperative antibiotic regimen on development of infection after intestinal surgery. Prospective, randomized, double-blind study. Ann Surg 180:567, 1974.
Wetterfors J, Hojer H: Systemic prophylaxis with doxycycline in surgery of colon and rectum. Scand J Infect Dis 9(Suppl):94, 1976.
Willis AT, Ferguson JR, Jones PH, et al: Metronidazole in prevention and treatment of bacteroides infections in elective colonic surgery. Br Med J 1:607, 1977.

EIGHT

Carcinomas and Precancerous Dermatoses of the Anus and Perianal Area

J. S. Spratt, M.D.

The purpose of this chapter is to review the subject of epithelial neoplasms of the anus and perianal area and discuss their surgical management. Considering the large number of lower gastrointestinal tumors seen annually, carcinomas of the anus occur infrequently. In a review of 6000 cases from Memorial Hospital, Stearns and Quan (1970) reported that, as a group, cancer of the anus represented 3.9 percent of the malignant lesions in the terminal 18 cm of the colon and about 2 percent of all carcinomas involving the lower bowel. They represented between 1 to 3 percent of all lower gastrointestinal carcinomas, with the squamous cell variety being the most prevalent. An association between anal carcinoma and benign anorectal lesions is frequently observed, although there is no epidemiologic proof of a cause-and-effect relationship. Biopsy is necessary to differentiate benign from malignant lesions. Bleeding, pain, and the presence of a rectal mass are the most frequent presenting symptoms. Anatomic location, tumor size, depth of invasion, general patient status, and presence or absence of clinical metastases are the prime determinants in planning therapy. The results of local excision and abdominoperineal resection cannot be directly compared in terms of 5-year survival because each method is used to treat different diseases. Despite the fact that abdominoperineal resection is the treatment of choice for more advanced disease, the incidence of local recurrence following abdominoperineal resection is lower than that for local excision. This must be partially attributable to the nonrandom selection of treatment.

Cancer of the anus is classified according to the tumor cell's ability to manufacture keratin (Sawyers, 1977). There are two major histologic categories: (1) the nonkeratinizing group, which includes basaloid or cloacogenic transitional cell carcinoma, Bowen's disease, Paget's extramammary disease, and basal cell carcinoma, and (2) the keratinizing group, of which epidermoid or squamous cell carcinoma is the sole member. In a 20-year review of the Connecticut Tumor Registry, Beahrs and Wilson (1976) found that squamous cell and basal cell carcinomas made up approximately two thirds of all anal carcinomas reported. Other investigators have reported that squamous cell carcinoma alone accounts for betweeen 80 and 90 percent of the total (Sawyers, 1977). Regardless of the exact figure, the occurrence of the nonkeratinizing type of cancer is infrequent. The other infrequent type of anal cancer is melanoma.

Although the cause of anal carcinoma is unknown, there often exists an association with several common anorectal lesions. In 1973, O'Grady and associates reported that fistula in ano, anal fissure, leukoplakia, hemorrhoids, abscess, and certain venereal diseases (lym-

Table 8–1. ASSOCIATED LESIONS—CONCURRENT OR ANTEDATING TUMOR DIAGNOSIS*

Reference	No. of Patients	Fistula	Fissure	Leukoplakia	Hemorrhoids	Abscess	V.D.
O'Grady et al (1973)	28	1	2	1	10	2	3
Cortese (1975)	43	—†	1	—	10	—	2
Brennan and Stewart (1972)	39	4	3	—	3	3	6
Beahrs and Wilson (1976)	113	8	3	10	47	—	3

*Courtesy of Robert J. Bean (personal communication, 1980)
†— = Not reported.

phogranuloma and condylomata) were favorable sites for the occurrence of anal cancer (Table 8–1). In 1975, Cortese suggested that recognition of the malignancy is of prime importance and outlined general guidelines to be followed when these seemingly benign conditions are present: (1) All suspicious visible or palpable anal lesions should be biopsied. (2) Attention should be directed to chronic as well as newly appearing lesions. (3) Patients must be adequately followed for recurrence. In addition, it is essential that all tissue removed from this region be sent for histopathologic examination. Specifically referred to are generally benign problems, such as fissures, hemorrhoids, and anal tags. Stearns and Quan (1970) emphasized that in nearly one third of the 234 patients they reviewed with proven malignancy, an earlier mistaken clinical diagnosis of a benign inflammatory condition had been made. The possibility is always present that an associated cancer may exist with any chronic anorectal lesion, and histopathologic evaluation is essential.

The mean age at first presentation of anal cancer is 57.7 years, with a female to male ratio of approximately 1.7:1 (Table 8–2).

Signs and symptoms of the cancers, including bleeding, pain, constipation, diarrhea, tenesmus, rectal mass, fullness in the rectum, weight loss, and inguinal mass (Table 8–3), are not specific and often occur with benign disorders. Because these symptoms are familiar to many patients, many authors believe that patient denial is the primary factor in diagnostic delay. This belief, which has been popular for many years, may in fact be erroneous. As has been observed, "The consistent first diagnosis of cancers whose mass is log normally distributed would suggest that a system for early diagnosis based on response of the patient to symptoms may be a fictitious concept" (Spratt, 1969). Any patient's response to the presence of a cancer is similar to the neurophysiologic response to any stimulus. Response is a function of the magnitude of the stimulus, and these magnitudes (or tumor sizes) considered collectively form log

Table 8–2. AGE AND SEX DISTRIBUTION OF ANAL CANCER*

References	No. of Patients	Mean Age (years)	Range (years)	Males	Females
Christiansen and Vitturp (1975)	29	64	40–80	9	20
Golden and Horsley (1976)	26	57	30–75	18	8
Cortese (1975)	38	61	33–90	—	—
Beahrs and Wilson (1976)	113	56	27–81	37	76
Welch and Malt (1977)	53	—†	29–96	17	36
Stearns and Quan (1970)	234	56	24–87	74	135
Dillard et al (1963)	79	61	—	32	47
Brennan and Stewart (1972)	39	—	29–65	19	20
Total	611	57.7	24–96	206	342

*Courtesy of Robert J. Bean (personal communication, 1980).
†— = Not reported.

Table 8–3. **SIGNS AND SYMPTOMS OF CARCINOMA OF THE ANUS AND PERIANAL AREA***

	References				
Signs and Symptoms	*Brennan and Stewart (1972)*	*Sawyers (1977)*	*Beahrs and Wilson (1976)*	*Stearns and Quan (1970)*	*Christiansen and Vitturp (1975)*
Bleeding	43.5%	72%	44.2%	49.6%	62.1%
Pain	38.4%	50%	36.3%	50.0%	55.2
Constipation	7.7%	—†	9.7%	26.1%	—
Diarrhea	7.7%	4%	4.4%	1.2%	10.3%
Rectal fullness	—	16%	—	—	—
Weight loss	12.8%	14%	—	—	—
Rectal mass	35.8%	—	23.9%	7.3%	—
Tenesmus	5.1%	20%	—	—	—

*Courtesy of Robert J. Bean (personal communication, 1980)
†— = Not reported.

normal frequency distributions. No proof exists that smaller lesions will prompt the patient to see a physician sooner as a result of patient education. Patient "compliance" may simply be attributable to the variance in response to the size of the cancer and be determined by individual variance in response to the magnitude of stimuli.

Evaluation of a patient with anorectal complaints suggestive of carcinoma should include direct visualization of the anus and perianal skin with the buttocks spread, anal and proctoscopic visualization, digital palpation, barium enema study, and palpation of the abdomen and groin. Histologic identification of the lesion should then be assured with a representative biopsy.

Once the diagnosis of epidermoid carcinoma of the anus has been made, guidelines can be followed to help in selecting the most effective treatment. These include the histopathologic assessment from biopsy, the size of the lesion, the depth of invasion, the anatomic location with respect to the pectinate line, the patient's

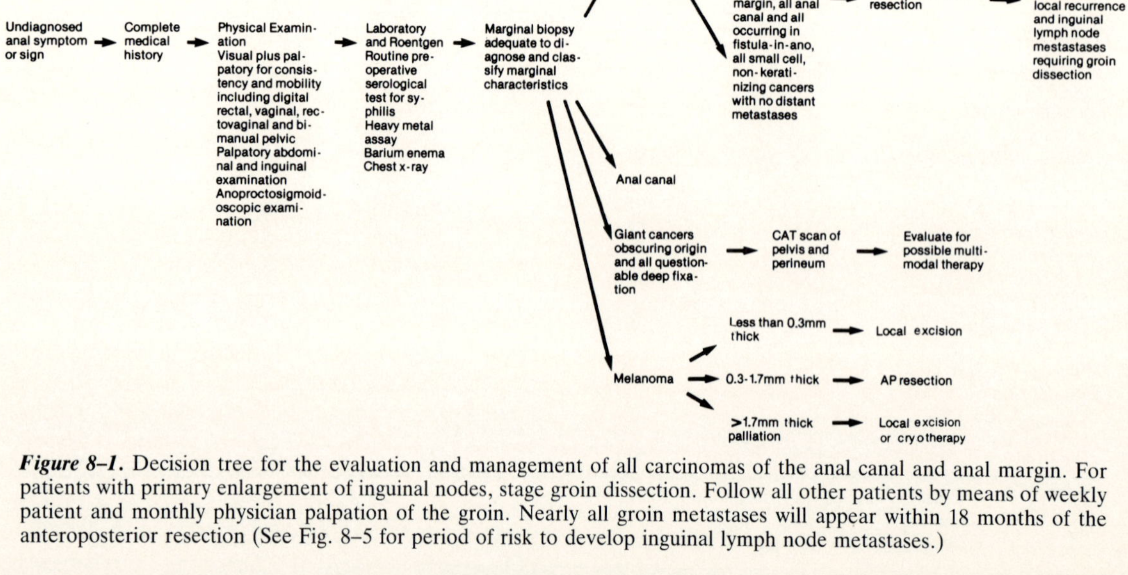

Figure 8–1. Decision tree for the evaluation and management of all carcinomas of the anal canal and anal margin. For patients with primary enlargement of inguinal nodes, stage groin dissection. Follow all other patients by means of weekly patient and monthly physician palpation of the groin. Nearly all groin metastases will appear within 18 months of the anteroposterior resection (See Fig. 8–5 for period of risk to develop inguinal lymph node metastases.)

Table 8–4. FIVE-YEAR SURVIVAL RATES BY TREATMENT*

Reference	Local Excision	Abdominoperineal Resection	Abdominoperineal Resection plus Inguinal Lymph Node Dissection
Stearns (1970)	20/30	34/59	2/14
Sawyers (1977)	3/4	17/33	0/5
Golden and Horsley (1976)	2/2	14/19	—†
Brennan and Stewart (1972)	2/3	6/16	0/2
Dillard et al (1963)	4/14	27/46	2/5
Kuehn et al (1968)	20/26	39/83	0/11
Cortese (1975)	3/7	6/9	3/8
Beahrs and Wilson (1976)	8/10	27/47	—
Total	62/96 (64.6%)	170/312 (54.5%)	7/45 (15.6%)

*Courtesy of Robert J. Bean (personal communication, 1980).
†— = Not reported.

general status, and the presence or absence of clinical metastasis.

The anus can be divided into two anatomically distinct areas according to its efferent lymphatic drainage. In the area above and including the pectinate line, lymph passes predominantly into perirectal and mesenteric lymph nodes. This portion is referred to as the anal canal. The anal margin, below the pectinate line, is drained by superficial lymphatic channels terminating in inguinal lymph nodes.

Dillard and associates (1963), in a review of 79 cases from the Ellis Fischel State Cancer Hospital and Barnes Hospital, showed an increase in absolute 5-year survival for patients with tumors of lower pathologic grade and smaller surface area (less than 4 cm^2). Patients with absence of clinical metastases demonstrated a similar tendency in the same study.

A decision tree (Fig. 8–1) is presented as a guide to the appropriate selection of treatment. This represents a compilation of many views and expresses no one author's bias. Radiotherapy and chemotherapy as primary modalities have been excluded because this discussion deals with surgical management. Chapter Nineteen should be seen regarding the role or potential role of radiotherapy in primary management. Comments on chemotherapy are presented later in this chapter and in Chapter Eighteen.

Table 8–4 shows the effects of each mode of therapy on 5-year survival. These results, however, cannot be directly compared because they represent the application of multiple types of therapy at various stages of the disease, and there was no randomization in case selection.

The incidence of local recurrence following abdominoperineal resection and local excision is shown in Table 8–5. Despite the fact that local excision is the treatment modality most often chosen for minimal disease, local recurrence with this form of less radical therapy is well documented by the authors cited in Table 8–5. When it occurs, abdominoperineal resection or a multimodal therapy should be considered.

Table 8–5. INCIDENCE OF LOCAL RECURRENCE FOLLOWING LOCAL EXCISION AND ABDOMINOPERINEAL RESECTION*

Reference	Local Excision	Abdominoperineal Resection
Cortese (1975)	3/7	3/8
Golden and Horsley (1976)	0/2	4/19
Beahrs and Wilson (1976)	4/10	10/47
Total	7/19 (36.8%)	17/64 (26.6%)

*Courtesy of Robert J. Bean (personal communication, 1980).

NONKERATINIZING EPIDERMOID CARCINOMAS

The nonkeratinizing epidermoid carcinomas of the anus are composed of those cancers that have variously been classified as cloacogenic, basaloid, basal cell, adenoacanthoma, mucoepidermoid, and transitional (Grinvalsky and Helwig, 1956). The composite name cloacogenic was recommended to describe neoplasms arising from that transitional epithelium that is a remnant of the cloacal membrane. Mixture of cellular type is not uncommon. After reviewing the available data on all anal carcinomas and carcinomas of the rectum, Sink and associates (1978) concluded that from 2 to 3.2 percent of the anal and perianal cancers are cloacogenic.

The histologic uniqueness of this region of carcinoma origin arises from the embryology of the cloacal membrane. The cloacal membrane is an area where ectoderm and endoderm come into apposition with no interposed mesoderm. The cloaca is the termination of the hindgut, receiving the allantois ventrally and the mesonephric duct laterally. The cloaca becomes divided by the urorectal septum that develops between the hindgut and the allantois. Growth of the urorectal septum effects an infolding of the lateral walls of the cloaca, ultimately dividing the cloaca into the rectum and upper anal canal dorsally and the urogenital sinus ventrally. Fusion of the urorectal septum results in a division of the cloacal membrane into a dorsal anal and a ventral urogenital membrane.

The anal pit forms next, and the anal membrane normally ruptures during the seventh week of embryogenesis, forming a patent anal canal. Thus, the upper two thirds of the anal canal are derived from the hindgut and the lower one third from the anal pit. The transitional zone, ranging from 0.3 to 1.2 cm in length, is where cloacogenic cancers arise.

The cancers arising in this region have been given a variety of names (Sink et al., 1978), including basosquamous, cylindroma, and small cell cancers, as well as others already mentioned. Only two subdivisions of cloacogenic cancer are of prognostic significance: (1) poorly differentiated small cell cancers and (2) large cell cancers that may show predominance of squamous, transitional, or mixed patterns. The small cell type, with more mitoses, has a poorer prognosis. It metastasizes earlier and is associated with a shorter clinical course (Sink et al., 1978).

Cloacogenic cancers have been reported in both males and females, who range in age from 29 to 89 years. The symptoms are consistent with a neoplasm of the region and none is specific, i.e., bleeding, mass, change in bowel habits, and pain. Other symptoms reported include recurrent abscesses, mucous discharge, pruritus, and weakness. If there are suspicious and persistent problems in this area, a biopsy should be carried out. The net accumulative 5-year survival rate averages 50 percent but varies with some of the prognostic factors indicated.

The etiology of cloacogenic cancers is not known. Associations with other conditions do not establish causality. This even applies to anecdotal observations such as the occasional discovery of these neoplasms in homosexual men who engage regularly in anal intercourse (Cooper et al., 1979; Daling et al., 1982).

The methods and results of treatment of cloacogenic cancers have been recently reviewed by Sink and associates (1978) and Svenson and Montague (1980). From April 1958 through July 1976, Svenson and Montague treated, with curative intent, 23 patients with transitional cloacogenic carcinoma of the anus by abdominoperineal resection alone (15 patients), combination abdominoperineal resection and irradiation (six patients), and irradiation alone (two patients). None of these patients had been previously treated or had distant metastases at the time of presentation. Surgery alone failed to control local or pelvic disease in one of six patients with negative nodes (with a tumor greater than 2 cm in diameter) and in six of nine patients with positive nodes. No local or pelvic disease occurred in patients treated with irradiation alone or preoperative or postoperative irradiation in this small series.

Sink and co-workers (1978) reported a series in which a wide variety of surgical procedures and radiotherapeutic modalities had been used in the initial treatment of cloacogenic carcinomas. The most widely used treatment was abdominoperineal resection, with wide excision of perineal skin and soft tissue. A posterior colpectomy was included if vaginal involvement was present. No increase in survival was demonstrated, however, with colpectomy in the absence of vaginal involvement.

For those patients with clinical evidence of inguinal nodal metastasis, groin dissection as a staged procedure was done if there was no evidence of dissemination elsewhere.

Radiotherapy had been used by some groups both as an adjuvant to surgery and as treatment for nonoperable lesions. The responsiveness of the tumor to radiation was nonconclusive in several studies (Klotz et al., 1967; Lone et al., 1960; Pang and Morson, 1967). Other groups, however, report favorable results with adjuvant radiation therapy (Cullen et al., 1966; Kheir et al., 1972; Nigro et al., 1974).

Recurrent cancer in the pelvic or perineal area was treated surgically and by radiotherapy, with both modalities having equally poor results. In the treatment of distant metastases, 5-fluorouracil was also ineffective (Kheir et al., 1972). A favorable response of some liver metastases has been reported with the combination of radiation and chemotherapy (Nigro et al., 1974).

In most series, the overall 5-year survival rate was reported to be 47 to 50 percent (Grodsky, 1969; Kheir et al., 1972; Klotz et al., 1967). Factors associated with an unfavorable prognosis include tumor size greater than 2 cm in greatest dimension, age less than 40 years or greater than 70 years, poor differentiation of the tumor cells, and large amounts of fibroblastic activity within the tumor. Intense inflammatory response of tissues surrounding the tumor is associated with a favorable response. As with other malignancies, increased depth of invasion, lymphatic and vascular invasion, and nodal or distant metastasis are associated with a poor prognosis (Klotz et al., 1967).

In conclusion, transitional cell cloacogenic carcinoma arises from the remnant of the cloacal membrane and accounts for 2 to 3 percent of all anorectal neoplasms. Although usually occurring below or at the pectinate line, cloacogenic tumors can occur higher in the rectum, originating in anal ducts. Abdominoperineal resection with wide excision of perineal skin and soft tissue is the most widely used treatment. The overall 5-year survival rate is 50 percent. However, with increased depth of invasion, lymphatic and vascular invasion, and nodal or distant metastasis, the prognosis is poor. The many presentations of cloacogenic transitional cell carcinoma make clinical diagnosis difficult. Any nodule, chronic ulcer, or indurated fissure arising near the pectinate line should be biopsied. The physician should be suspicious when nontender, intramural masses occur in the anorectal region and when biopsies taken in this area reveal unusual cell types.

A recent review of a series of 188 carcinomas of the anal canal was large enough to strengthen the significance of conclusions from many smaller studies (Boman et al, 1983). Thirteen patients with superficially invasive squamous cell carcinoma ($\leq$ 2 cm) were treated successfully by local excision only. In only one case did the cancer recur locally, and this recurrence was controlled with an abdominoperineal resection. In all, these squamous cell cancers were mainly local, with only 20 per cent developing regional lymph node metastases and only 2 per cent developing distant spread.

Only 13 patients had cancer of the small cell variety, with only one of seven treated by surgical resection surviving 5 years. The authors concluded that small cell cancer should be regarded as a systemic disease.

Predominantly, recurrences after resection of both squamous cell carcinomas and nonkeratinizing basaloid neoplasms were still confined to the pelvis (80 per cent and 60 per cent, respectively).

MELANOMA OF THE ANUS

Melanomas of the anus and perianal region have been reported in several series; because of the infrequency of these cancers, considerable periods of time were required to accumulate meaningful data. Of the entire series of 230 melanomas of all sites seen at the Ellis Fischel State Cancer Hospital from 1940 to 1969, there was only one perianal melanoma. There was one other melanoma on the buttock and one on the genitals (Knutson et al., 1971).

More recent reviews of cases accumulating over long time periods have been reported (Abbas et al., 1980; Boey et al., 1981; Bolivar et al., 1982; Chiu et al., 1980; Wanebo et al., 1981). Survival in all was related to the stage of the tumor at the time of diagnosis. The advanced size of many melanomas at diagnosis together with the absence of classic dermatologic layers in anal and perianal skin makes classifications by layer of penetration of doubtful value. However, measuring the thickness of melanoma from the surface of the epithelium to the point of deepest penetration may be helpful. In 1977, Quinn and Selah reported no 5-year survivors among patients with anal melanoma measuring more than 1.7 mm thick. Wanebo and associates (1981b) concluded that an abdominoperineal resection might be justified for any anorectal melanoma measuring less than 3 mm in thickness.

Recurrence data suggest that most patients will have a recurrence and that they will die from that recurrence within 2 years. In the series at the Ellis Fischel State Cancer Hospital, no patients manifested a recurrence after 2 years, although some lived longer than 24 months. The period of risk for recurrence is the first 24 postresection months. A satisfactory treatment for a recurrence has yet to be defined.

Mode of manifestation, location in the anus, and tumor size have not been shown to correlate with prognosis. Only patients who had distant disease when first seen could be identified as having a distinctly worse prognosis.

Review of the surgical approach to melanoma reveals little consistency. The surgical experience suggests that radical surgical excision is indicated. Indeed, no patients survived without it (Chiu et al., 1980). Prophylactic inguinal node dissection is of unproven value.

Wanebo and co-workers (1981b) noted that primary malignant melanoma of the anorectum is a rare and virulent malignancy associated with an extremely poor prognosis in spite of aggressive initial therapy. Fifty-one patients with this disease were treated at Memorial Sloan-Kettering Cancer Center during the last 50 years and only six (12 percent) survived 5 years. Wanebo and co-workers (1981a) reviewed in detail 36 of the patients treated since 1950. In this group there was a female predominance (21 females, 15 males), and median age was in the 6th decade (range 27 to 75 years). Common presenting symptoms were pain, bleeding, mass, or "hemorrhoids" of 1 to 12 months' duration. In two thirds of the cases, a radical surgical approach was attempted. Other therapy included local excision alone or combined with groin dissection, local excision followed by delayed rectal resection, and local tumor destruction by cryosurgery or fulguration. Mean survival was 21.5 months. Three patients had palliative treatment only with radiation therapy. Histopathologic study of 30 lesions showed that two thirds were bulky or polypoid lesions and two thirds showed junctional changes. The poor prognosis for primary anorectal melanoma was directly related to tumor size and thickness. Although all four of the 5-year survivors had radical surgery, the three whose tumors could be measured had superficial lesions. In general, curative efforts by radical surgery were no more effective than local treatment by excision or cryosurgery. One patient, however, did have a thin lesion but also had nodal metastases and survived over 5 years after radical surgery. Although these data suggest that radical resection may cure patients with lesions thinner than 3 mm, it does not exclude the possibility that local excision might also be curative. For larger lesions that have not been cured by radical surgery, more conservative local approaches by excision or cryotherapy might be the optimum way of achieving local palliation.

In 1981, Boey and associates emphasized the biologic vagaries of anal malignant melanoma, illustrated by four cases in Chinese patients. All four died within 5 years. Their poor prognosis supported the value of preoperative studies to detect clinically occult metastases and reduce the need for noncurative radical surgery. This suggestion presupposes all metastases are discoverable and that no palliative value comes from the surgical operation even in the absence of cure. Boey and associates (1981) emphasized that many patients already had disseminated disease at the time of diagnosis, and local excision of the tumor provided acceptable palliation. For localized disease, abdominoperineal resection prevents local recurrence and removes the mesenteric nodes, which are frequently involved. Palpable inguinal nodes necessitated therapeutic groin dissection, but prophylactic or elective inguinal resection was performed only when nodes with metastases were found at laparotomy. Pelvic lymphadenectomy was performed in conjunction with abdominoperineal resection. The efficacy of chemotherapy for anorectal melanoma remained uncertain to these reviewers.

Other points on the behavior of melanomas merit re-emphasizing. First, in 1971, Knutson and associates looked at the association of 54 clinical and pathologic variables in seeking characteristics that might be associated significantly with a propensity to metastasize or not metastasize. Only two variables were significant—melanomas in males were more likely to metastasize than those in females. The second variable was the color of the lesion. Actually, by chance alone two of 54 variables might show a significant association by this method of testing.

These cases were reviewed before the classification systems of Clark and Breslow became popular (Clark et al., 1969; Breslow, 1975). However, pathologic slides of 160 of the 230 cases showed that 27 lesions had not penetrated below the papillary dermis, and these melanomas were classified as "superficial." The resulting life tables are shown in Figure 8–2.

As Figure 8–2 very strikingly demonstrates, the accumulative survival curves are almost parallel after a period of time. The lead time of the invasive lesions over the superficial lesions in the curves is 11.5 to 14 months. In the fifth year this increased to 30 months and, from the sixth year on, is not measurable. This strongly suggests that a major difference in survival between patients with melanomas whose deep margin is superficial to the papillary dermis and those with melanomas that have invaded more deeply is due to a minimum lead time bias of 12 to 14 months. This bias could be longer among those who survive more than 14 months.

An explanation of this variation and many of the other "biologic vagaries" of melanoma

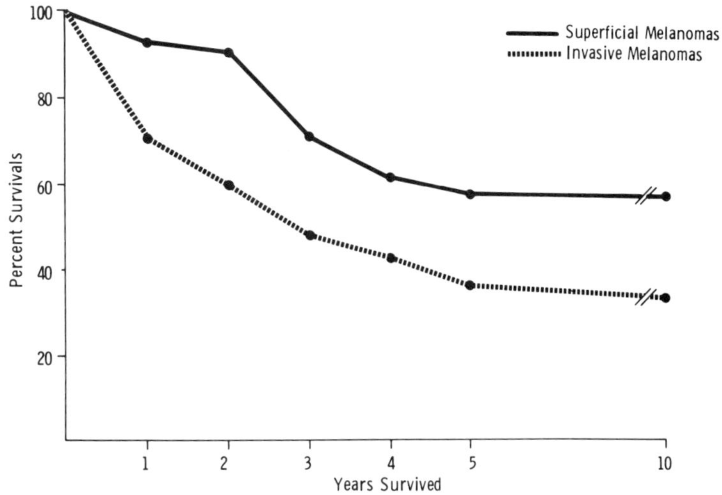

Figure 8–2. Age-adjusted survival curves for 160 melanomas, determined by the depth of invasion. (From Knutson CO, Hori JM, Spratt JS Jr: Monograph on Melanoma. Current Problems in Surgery, December 1971. Copyright © 1971 by Year Book Medical Publishers, Inc., Chicago. Reproduced with permission.)

may lie in the extreme variations in growth rates. Among 32 pulmonary metastases from melanoma, the actual doubling time was 43 days (log mean), with a 95 percent confidence range from 7 to 141 days. This is equivalent to a net increase of 27 new melanoma cells per 1000 existing cells per day, with a 95 percent confidence range of 0 to 63. The frequency distribution of these doubling times is shown in Figure 8–3.

A striking observation on the growth of these melanomas was that random variation in growth rate occurred naturally. All pulmonary metastases were observed for a total of 5028 days. The metastases were undergoing periods of spontaneous (although temporary) regression in size for 516 of these days. *No* form of treatment was being given for 395 of these days. In other words, melanomas were undergoing periods of spontaneous regression in size 8 percent of the time of observation. When the melanomas were being treated with chemotherapy, regression recurred only 2.4 percent of the time. Spratt and Spratt (1964) had previously reported that pulmonary metastases from melanoma grow faster than do most other metastases but still show a wide variance in rates. The biologic vagaries of melanoma can largely be explained by the extreme variance in growth rates. Solely on the basis of estimates derived from observed growth rates of in vivo melanomas, an uncured melanoma might take 280 days (95 percent confidence) to 160 days (99 percent confidence) from the inception of the melanoma to the death of the individual. However, the slower growing melanomas might require 5640 days (15.5 years) to follow the same course, with a 95 percent confidence or 11,800 days (32.3 years), with 99 percent confidence. To determine whether such extreme variance is true of anal melanomas would require much more data than has been reported in the literature, with long-term follow-up (Spratt and Spratt, 1964). A possible example of this variance is provided by Probstein (1957, 1983). A melanoma of the anus was treated by simple local excision at the suggestion of Dr. Carl Moyer. It never recurred locally or in regional lymph nodes. Seven years later, the patient developed hepatic metastases and died as a result of them. She had long survivorship with minimal treatment, suggesting that the cancer had a very slow growth rate.

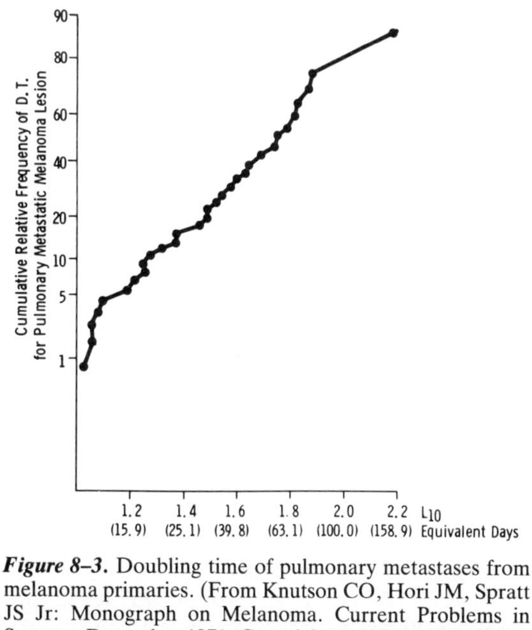

Figure 8–3. Doubling time of pulmonary metastases from melanoma primaries. (From Knutson CO, Hori JM, Spratt JS Jr: Monograph on Melanoma. Current Problems in Surgery, December 1971. Copyright © 1971 by Year Book Medical Publishers, Inc., Chicago. Reproduced with permission.)

SQUAMOUS CANCERS IN PILONIDAL SINUSES

Rarely, both epidermoid and basal cell cancers have been reported in long-standing pilonidal sinuses. Gupta and associates (1981) reviewed the world literature on this subject (beginning with Wolff in 1900), summarized 24 documented cases in the literature, and added a case of their own. In their study, patient ages ranged from 18 to 86 years, and the duration of the pilonidal sinuses was also quite variable, ranging from 1 month to 62 years. The conversion rate of these sinuses to cancer has to be exceedingly low. There were no cancers reported among 86,333 pilonidal sinuses excised among troops in World War II (Denning et al., 1954).

McAnally and Dockerty (1949) reviewed the conversion rates of several types of chronic fistulas—osteomyelitic sinuses, 0.23 percent; fistula in ano, 0.1 percent; empyemic sinuses, 0.7 percent. The prevalence of pilonidal sinus conversion is even lower (Cleveland and Green, 1964).

Actually, these are all accumulative rates. The incidence should be calculated correctly by placing the number of confirmed cancers in pilonidal sinuses in the numerator and the number of person-years of pilonidal sinus duration in the cohort population in the denominator. Adjustment for age would be required to ascertain the age-specific rate of cancer conversion per person-year of life. This type of calculation has never been done and might even be considered a rather pedantic high-cost study. It is important to obtain a histologic evaluation of any chronic sinus, particularly if it exhibits change.

The results of treating cancers in pilonidal sinuses are not unfavorable. About two thirds of the reported cases have been amenable to control by wide local excision. Regional lymph node metastases were infrequent and were associated with a poor prognosis. Prophylactic node dissection could not be justified in Gupta and associates' (1981) data.

PRECANCEROUS DERMATOSES

Bowen's disease, a precancerous dermatosis, occurs in the anal and perianal areas. It may mimic a wide array of chronic minor skin irritations. It is significant that Bowen's disease is a slowly growing intraepidermal squamous cell cancer that only very rarely invades or metastasizes. The confirmatory diagnosis is made only on biopsy, but it should be suspected in any chronic, irritated area of epidermis in the perianal area. It is occasionally found when perianal tissue is removed for other problems. It is cured by local excision with adequate margins (confirmed histologically). Only the involved skin or mucosa needs to be removed and never the deeper tissues.

A collateral consideration with Bowen's disease is its frequent association with visceral cancers. In a series of 12 cases with Bowen's disease, seven persons either had had a systemic or cutaneous cancer or developed one after the diagnosis of Bowen's disease. When Bowen's disease is discovered, a careful evaluation for primary cancers at other sites is indicated (Strauss and Fazio, 1979).

Carcinomatous change with invasion has been reported in conjunction with condyloma acuminatum. When this condition is suspected, the diagnosis needs to be unequivocally confirmed by biopsy, and then treatment should be carried out as the characteristics of the cancer dictate (Prasad and Abcarian, 1980).

ROLE OF ILIOINGUINAL LYMPH NODE DISSECTION IN THE MANAGEMENT OF ANAL CARCINOMAS

The role of ilioinguinal lymph node dissection in the management of anal carcinomas is commented on by many authors. In general, these comments are to a degree anecdotal and historical, since no controlled clinical trial has ever been done to establish, in a rigid scientific sense, the role of prophylactic groin dissection. Considering the relative infrequency and variegated nature of the studied cancers and the even less frequent involvement of inguinal lymph nodes with metastases, the probability is low that any controlled clinical trial will ever be completed. However, a great deal is known about the natural history of untreated inguinal metastases. There is considerable support for the selected use of groin dissections, since a great deal of knowledge on low morbidity techniques for doing the operation exists.

The author's studies of ilioinguinal lymph node dissections for all types of neoplasms have been published as a monograph (Spratt et al., 1965). Selected information from that monograph is stressed in this chapter.

Figure 8–4 shows the status that untreated inguinal lymph nodes metastatic from an epidermoid carcinoma of the anus may reach.

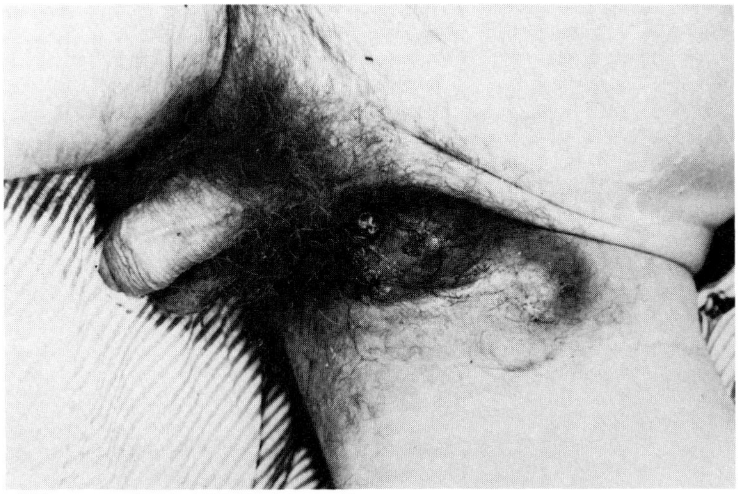

Figure 8–4. Inguinal metastases from an epidermoid carcinoma of the anus that has reached a stage too far advanced to be resectable by means of groin dissection. (From Spratt JS Jr, Shieber W, Dillard BM: Anatomy and Surgical Technique of Groin Dissection. St Louis, CV Mosby Company, 1965.)

The clear relationship existing between the surface area of squamous cell cancers of the anus and both the mesenteric and inguinal lymph nodes is shown in Table 8–6.

The end results by method of treatment and other parameters are shown in Table 8–7. Even though these data are historical and not based on random selection, they can still serve as a basis for decision making, pending a controlled clinical trial.

The conclusions from these data were that epidermoid carcinomas of the anal margin having a size of 2 cm or less, a histologic grade of 0 or 1, and a circumscribed or pushing margin could be treated by wide local excision. All other carcinomas required an abdominoperineal resection, dictated by the frequency of mesenteric lymph node metastases and local recurrence with lesser operations.

The morbidity and mortality from simultaneous abdominoperineal resection and groin dissection were found to be too great to justify the use of both procedures. Staged operation was better when indicated. There is no statistical justification for prophylactic groin dissections for any anal cancer. People developing enlarged groin nodes from metastases do so during a remarkably well-defined period of risk from each site, including the anus. Monthly follow-up and self-palpation are indicated during this period (see Fig. 8–5). All delayed groin metastases from carcinoma of the anus were palpable within 18 months after resection of the primary cancer. As soon as lymph nodes

Table 8–6. **RELATION OF SURFACE AREA OF EPIDERMOID CARCINOMAS OF THE ANUS TO PRESENCE OF MESENTERIC AND ILIOINGUINAL LYMPH NODE METASTASES***

Surface Area of Cancer (cm²)	No. of Cases	No. with Metastases to Mesenteric Nodes	Percentage	No. with Metastases to Inguinal Nodes	Percentage
0– 0.9	0	0	0	0	0
1– 1.9	10	0	0	0	0
2– 3.9	12	0	0	0	0
4– 7.9	13	1	7.7	2	15.4
8– 15.9	5	1	20	4	80
16– 31.9	31	14	45.2	10	32.2
32– 63.9	2	1	50	1	50
64–127.9	6	1	16.7	1	16.7
Total	79	18	22.8	18	22.8
<4 cm^2	22	0	0	0	0
>4 cm^2	57	18	31.6	18	31.6

*From Dillard BM, Spratt JS Jr, Ackerman LV, Butcher HR Jr: Epidermoid cancer of anal margin and canal. Review of 79 cases. Arch Surg 86:772–777, 1963. Copyright 1963, American Medical Association.

Table 8–7. **THE RELATIONSHIP OF CERTAIN PARAMETERS TO SURVIVAL AFTER ABDOMINOPERINEAL RESECTION FOR EPIDERMOID CANCER OF THE ANUS VERSUS LOCAL EXCISION OR IRRADIATION THERAPY***

Clinical Factors	No. of Cases	Abdominoperineal Resection	Local Excision or Irradiation	Chi Square	P Value
Greater Chordal Dimension					
<2 cm	35	12	23	13.54	0.001†
>2 cm	38	38	0		
Total	73	50	23		
Grade Tumor					
≤2	5	0	5	11.7	0.001†
>2	68	50	18		
Total	73	50	23		
Sex					
Male	27	17	10	0.60	0.4‡
Female	46	33	13		
Total	73	50	23		
Race					
Caucasian	64	43	21	0.41	0.50‡
Black	9	7	2		
Total	73	50	23		
Fistula in ano					
Present	23	15	8	0.24	0.50‡
Absent	50	35	15		
Total	73	50	23		
Location					
Anal Margin	23	13	10	2.28	0.10‡
Anal Canal	50	37	13		
Total	73	50	23		

*From Dillard BM, Spratt, JS Jr, Ackerman LV, Butcher HR Jr: Epidermoid cancer of oral margin and canal. Review of 79 cases. Arch Surg 86:772–777, 1963. Copyright 1963, American Medical Association.

†Null hypothesis: Higher grade cancers and cancers larger than 2 cm in diameter were treated by abdominoperineal resection with the same relative frequency as they were treated by local excision or irradiation. (Chi-square = 13.54 and 11.7, respectively, probability of sameness 0.001.) Reject hypothesis. Conclusion: Larger, higher grade cancers were treated more frequently by abdominoperineal resection than they were treated by local excision or irradiation, or both.

‡No significant difference existed between the frequency of abdominoperineal resection and the frequency of local excision and irradiation according to sex, race, presence or absence of associated fistula in ano, or location of the cancer with respect to the anal margin.

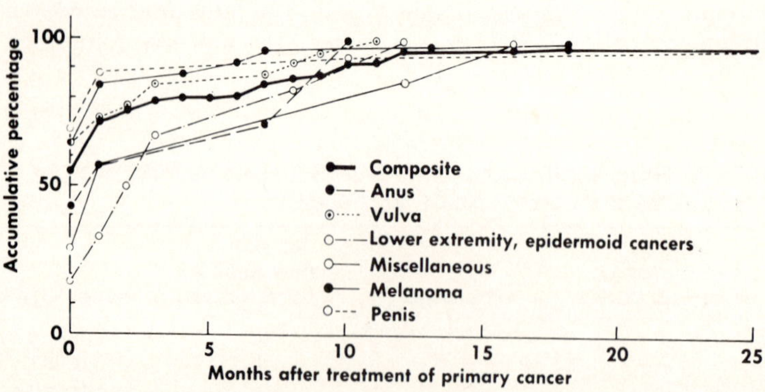

Figure 8–5. This graph shows the accumulative percentage of groin dissections performed for lymph nodes that contained metastatic cancer on pathologic examination as a function of the number of months elapsing after the diagnosis and treatment of primary cancer. Only two operable cases (a penile cancer and a melanoma producing contralateral metastases) presented past the eighteenth posttreatment month. When prophylactic groin dissections are not performed at the time of, or soon after the treatment of, the primary cancer, the patients must be followed very closely by means of monthly palpatory examinations of the groin during this 18-month period of risk. After this 18-month period, they must be educated to examine their groins at least monthly and to report promptly the discovery of newly palpable or enlarging nodes. (From Spratt JS Jr, Shieber W, Dillard BM: Anatomy and Surgical Technique of Groin Dissection. St Louis, CV Mosby Company, 1965.)

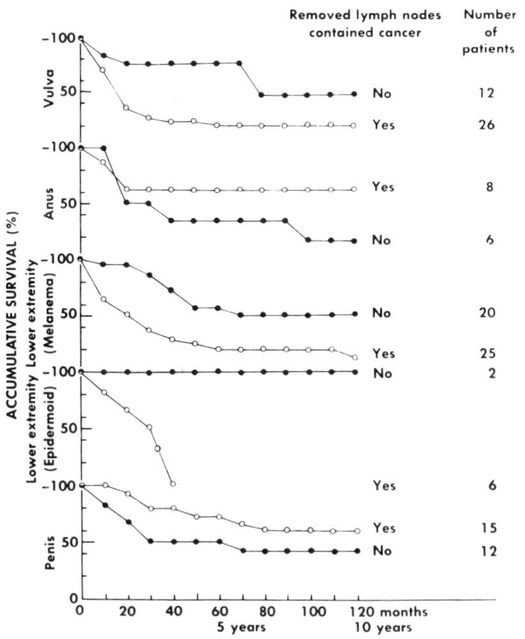

Figure 8–6. Accumulative survival (percentage) after radical groin dissection. (From Spratt JS Jr, Shieber W, Dillard BM: Anatomy and Surgical Technique of Groin Dissection. St Louis, CV Mosby Company, 1965.)

become palpable, an ilioinguinal lymph node dissection is indicated.

The end results after groin dissection for metastases from anal cancer are remarkably good using this approach (Fig. 8–6).

The techniques for performing nearly trouble-free groin dissections are reported in a monograph (Spratt et al., 1965). However, I have made a few modifications in the basic techniques described. For example, graded elastic stockings should be substituted for Ace bandages. The patient is measured for these stockings *preoperatively*. The stockings *must* be available and on the patient *before* postoperative ambulation and preferably in the immediate postoperative period. For unilateral groin dissections, the stockings go to the upper thigh. For bilateral groin dissections, the upper-thigh stockings may be used bilaterally, but the girdle-stocking combination works better. These stockings *must* be worn for at least 3 months postoperatively. Thereafter, both patient and physician must be alert to the development of any trace of infection or edema in the lower extremities. Prompt treatment of infection and the elimination of all traces of edema by elevation, reinstitution of the stockings, or use of a lymphedema pump are essential. Chronic lymphedema with fibrosis develops from untreated acute or trace lymphedema as a result of fibrosis stimulated by the persistence of protein-rich lymph in the tissues. Fibrotic lymphedema or "milk leg" is a permanent anatomic change that is largely preventable.

A second modification is the use of a second incision at the lower end of the quadrilateral block of Anson where the inguinal lymph nodes are known to lie (Daseler et al, 1948). At first, this incision is made just through the skin and most superficial fat (see Figs. 8–7 and 8–8). The skin is then elevated from the underlying block of fatty lymph node-bearing tissue partially through this lower incision. Then, a vertical incision is made through the fat pad suture, ligating the distal fat pad to include major trunks of the valvular lymphatics and the saphenous vein. The incision carries through the deep fascia.

This approach, in conjunction with the inguinal incision and flap elevation described previously, permits an easier identification and transection of the medial and lateral boundaries of the quadrilateral block, allowing mobilization into the inguinal incision for completion of the groin dissection with less retractor-imposed pressure on the flaps.

The final modification came with improved techniques for inserting Hemovac catheters for postoperative wound suction. The large-sized catheters are screwed on to a large trocar, which can be threaded subcutaneously to exit *laterally* through skin on the lower lateral thigh and the lower lateral abdomen, without going through the base of the skin pedicles. With the transfer of the sartorius to cover the femoral vessels and with a light plain catgut stitch over the top of these catheters, they can be kept away from contact with the femoral vessels. After double layer airtight skin closure, the catheters are placed on suction for at least 5 days. No pressure (i.e., as with a pressure dressing) should be placed over these catheters. The skin between the pressure dressing and the catheters is subjected to a tourniquet effect and will necrose. After the fifth day, the catheters are cut several inches from the skin surface and then are advanced daily until out. The remainder of the technique is otherwise unchanged from that previously reported (Spratt et al., 1965). Major steps of that technique are reviewed here owing to the limited availability of the original monograph.

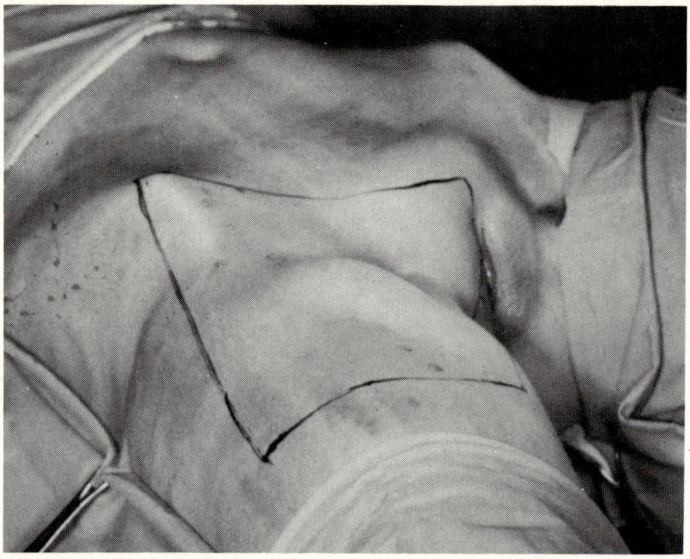

Figure 8–7. The square delineates the quadrilateral block of superficial fascia and fatty areolar tissue containing the superficial inguinal lymph nodes. The four corners of the block are situated at (1) the anterior-superior iliac spine, (2) a point 20 cm distally on the thigh measured from the anterior-superior iliac spine, (3) a point cephalad from the pubic tubercle at the level of the upper margin of the external inguinal ring, and (4) a point distal from the pubic tubercle on the inner thigh at the same level as the point on the outer thigh. The line joining the two points on the thigh crosses the apex of the femoral triangle, where the sartorius muscle overlaps the adductor muscles. The skin flaps have to be elevated to the margins of this block, but care should be taken to ensure that subcutaneous dissection does not extend beyond the margins of the block, unnecessarily interrupting blood supply to the flaps. Before dissection starts, a light mark on the skin outlining the block will simultaneously ensure completeness of the resection and will prevent unnecessary extension of the subcutaneous dissection. Two nearly parallel incisions are made about 2 cm distal to the cephalad border of the block and at the lower border of the block. A bipedicle flap will thus be made.

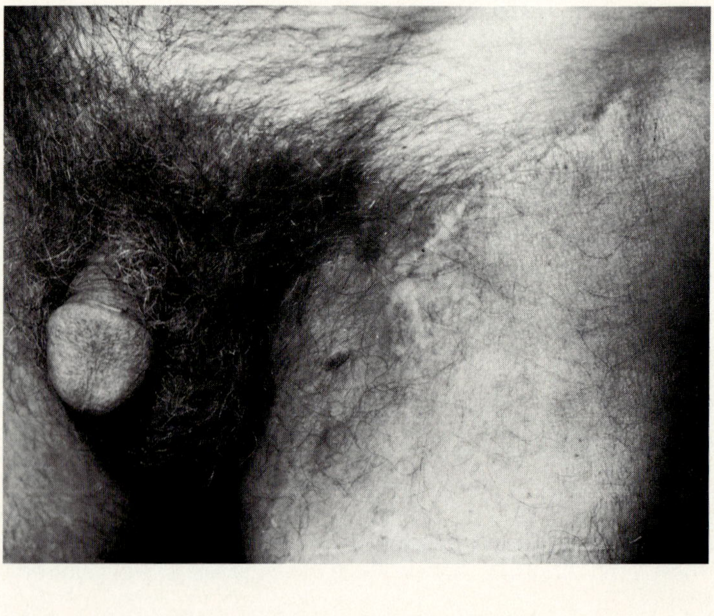

Figure 8–8. The healed results of a groin dissection performed using the two nearly parallel incisions described in the legend of Figure 8–7.

SURGICAL TECHNIQUE OF GROIN DISSECTION

Groin dissection should generally be carried out only if the primary cancer is controllable by the operation planned. In the preoperative evaluation, the presence of metastases beyond the ilioinguinal region should be excluded insofar as possible. In general, results of palpatory examination of the abdomen and the supraclavicular region, a thoracic roentgenogram, and roentgenographic evaluation of any localized skeletal pain should all be within normal limits. If cancerous nodes are palpable in the groin and the diagnosis of distant metastases is uncertain, it is better to proceed with the groin dissection. Doing so will ensure control of the cancer in the groin, even in the absence of cure. Resection of enlarging nodes in the groin provides excellent palliation.

The postoperative management of the bowels can be simplified by preoperative preparation. Patients should have a standard bowel preparation, as for colon surgery (see Chapter Seven). When the planned operation includes a dissection close to the anus, one additional procedure should be carried out. After the patient has been positioned on the table and anesthetized, as a standard part of the antiseptic perineal preparation, a large Pezzer catheter should be inserted through the anus and attached to a drainage tube and bottle. This provides assurance of last-minute mechanical cleansing and decompression of the rectal ampulla during the ensuing operation.

The positioning of the patient on the operating table deserves consideration and planning. Most of the standard positions have been employed by the author. One in particular is considered most adaptable to the performance of groin dissection with or without en bloc organ resections. In this position, the patient is placed on an operating table with orthopedic attachments, making possible abduction of the lower extremities. However, this position does not provide good exposure for the lesions posterior to the anus. When it is anticipated that skin grafts will be needed, a donor site that is easy to manage postoperatively can be selected and prepped.

An exposed or open cancer is a potential source of wound seeding. A sponge thoroughly soaked with either 10 percent formalin or absolute alcohol should be sutured in place over these exposed areas. The solutions will desiccate the tumor surface, ensuring a cleaner surgical field. The instruments used to suture the sponge in place are best discarded, and the surgeon should change gloves before proceeding with the dissection.

The blood vascular supply to the skin flaps that must be elevated to attain access to the lymph node-bearing areas of the groin is peculiarly critical. Much of the bad name of groin dissections is related directly to the frequency of ischemic necrosis in these flaps. In the moist glabrous folds of the groin and the perineum, such necrosis has been complicated by secondary infection and long delay in wound healing. The blood supply of the flaps is derived primarily from the superficial external pudendal, superficial circumflex iliac, and inferior (superficial) epigastric arteries. All three of these vessels are transected and ligated during the course of the dissection, and the flaps must rely on anastomotic branches. These branches lie in Camper's fascia, and they tend to parallel the natural skin creases. In the inguinal region, the skin creases and subcutaneous anastomotic plexus tend to parallel the inguinal ligament. Consequently, the most physiologic skin incision parallels the natural skin folds, transecting as few anastomotic vessels in Camper's fascia as possible. Both Baronofsky (1948) and Woodhall (1953) emphasized the importance of making the skin incision parallel to the inguinal ligament to ensure the maximum likelihood of primary wound healing without flap necrosis.

Delay in wound healing or flap necrosis invariably results in a prolongation of hospital stay. The length of hospital stay has been correlated with the types of incisions employed. There are three basic types of incisions. The oblique incision is a straight line cut made parallel to the inguinal ligament, extending from the anterior-superior iliac spine to the pubic tubercle. The straight vertical and S-shaped incisions both cut across the anastomotic vessels in Camper's fascia and are associated with a high incidence of flap slough and wound separation. The length of hospital stay after groin dissection as a function of wound morbidity is dramatically correlated with the incision type. Seven chief surgeons at the Ellis Fischel State Cancer Hospital employed all three types of incisions over a 24-year period, and the greatest likelihood for primary wound healing occurred with the oblique incision, regardless of the surgeon or the year. Consequently, only the straight oblique incision parallel to the inguinal ligament is recommended.

At the lower edge of the quadrilateral block of Anson a second incision is now made similar to the first (see Figs. 8–7 and 8–8). This incision delineates the distal extent of the dissection on the thigh, and no flap distal to this incision is elevated. Through this incision, the distal end of the quadrilateral block and of the saphenous vein may be transected with ease and with no pressure on the flap.

The inguinal incision permits ready access with good exposure for the iliac dissection and the obturator dissection. The peritoneal cavity can be entered readily through this incision for the purpose of exploration, should this be indicated. Bilateral oblique inguinal incisions can be joined across the midline, and by transection of the rectus muscles suprapubically, an incision is provided that gives superb exposure to the pelvic cavity. This procedure is mentioned because a pelvic surgical procedure in conjunction with a groin dissection is occasionally indicated but is not generally recommended.

The sacrifice of skin and the need for skin grafts should be anticipated in the preoperative planning. Skin must be sacrificed when it is involved, suspected of being involved, or overlying enlarged lymph nodes and elevation of overlying skin would risk exposure of the nodes. The oblique incision is modified simply to circumscribe this skin, and the sacrificed skin is removed en bloc with the node-bearing tissue. Never approximate the skin margins under tension for primary closure. It is better to approximate the margins of the flaps to the deep tissues without tension and to apply split-thickness skin grafts to the defects. Consequently, the need for skin graft should be recognized preoperatively. When preoperative planning anticipates the need for a split-thickness skin graft, a donor site sould be prepared and the graft taken before the groin dissection begins. The graft is then stored in Ringer's lactate solution, to which 1,000,000 units of aqueous penicillin has been added. It is kept on the nurse's sterile table while the rest of the operative procedure is in progress, to be used at the time of closure.

Preliminary delineation of the extent of the superficial portion of the groin dissection with a marking pencil will help prevent the unnecessary elevation of skin flaps beyond the extent of the node-bearing fat. The extent to which flaps need to be elevated is determined by the limits of the quadrilateral block described by Daseler, Anson, and Reimann (1948). These authors, on the basis of 450 anatomic dissections, concluded that inguinal lymph nodes are rarely present outside this quadrilateral block. The four corners of the block are as follows: the anterior-superior iliac spine, a point 20-cm distal from the anterior-superior iliac spine on the thigh, a point about 2-cm cephalad from the pubic tubercle at about the upper margin of the external inguinal ring, and a point on the medial thigh at the intersect of lines drawn transversely from the lower lateral point and vertical from the pubic tubercle. The lower margin of the block crosses the lower extent of the femoral triangle where the sartorius muscle passes over the adductor muscles. This block is outlined with respect to the external landmarks in Figures 8–7 and 8–8. Light marks on the skin made before dissection starts can be referred to as the flaps are elevated, and the subcutaneous dissection is discontinued when these marks are reached. Extensive elevation of flaps beyond these marks adds an unnecessary interruption to the critical blood supply of the skin flaps. A second incision is now made at the lower end of the block to transect the block and the saphenous vein.

The flaps are elevated by sharp dissection to the prescribed lines. The margins of the flaps are retracted gently with skin hooks. A 2-mm thickness of fat is left on the undersurface of the skin. Whenever the skin is so close to enlarged nodes as to preclude the leaving of this margin of fat safely, the skin overlying the nodes should be circumscribed by the incision and removed with the nodes. Exposure under the inferior extent of the lower flap can be secured with a large, blunt-forked rack retractor or a Deaver retractor.

Superficial and Deep Inguinal Dissection

The superficial inguinal nodes accompany the divisions of the saphenous vein and are situated in the fatty areolar tissue lying between the superficial fascia and the fascia lata. The deep inguinal nodes lie in the fibrofatty layer within the femoral sheath adjacent to the femoral vessels and in a plane continuous with the node-bearing areolar tissue about the iliac vessels. These deep inguinal nodes lie between the fascia lata (superficial to the femoral vessels) and the muscular fascia. The objective is to perform a clean dissection in the avascular plane outside of the encompassing fascial layers. After the skin flaps have been elevated, the fatty areolar tissue is incised straight through around the entire circumference of the quadrilateral block.

On the lower abdomen, the incision is carried down to the external oblique aponeurosis at the upper margin of the external inguinal ring (Fig. 8–9). The incision through the fat at this level parallels the inguinal ligament throughout its length. The fat is cleanly reflected from the aponeurosis inferiorly to the inguinal ligament. When operating for cancers arising in the genitalia, the presymphyseal lymphatic plexus containing the prepubic nodes and the areolar tissue of the spermatic cord must be included in the dissection. In the female patient, the spermatic cord analogue does not have to be preserved. The external ring can be opened laterally, and the round ligament can be transected and ligated flush with the internal inguinal ring. The cord is then reflected toward the genitalia for en bloc resection.

The fat is similarly transected at the lateral, medial, and inferior extent of the quadrilateral block (Fig. 8–10). At the deep point of the incision, the fascia lata will be encountered. This is also incised around the periphery of the block down to bare muscle. In dividing the fat of the superficial fascia and the fascia lata, large afferent lymphatics, although not visible, are also being transected. If these are left open, they will weep lymph into the wound for several days and will sometimes become the source of troublesome lymphatic fistulas. As a precaution, this tissue at the margins of the quadrilateral block can be transected between clamps and ligated. The greater saphenous vein is found at the medial inferior extent of the block, and it must be transected and doubly ligated.

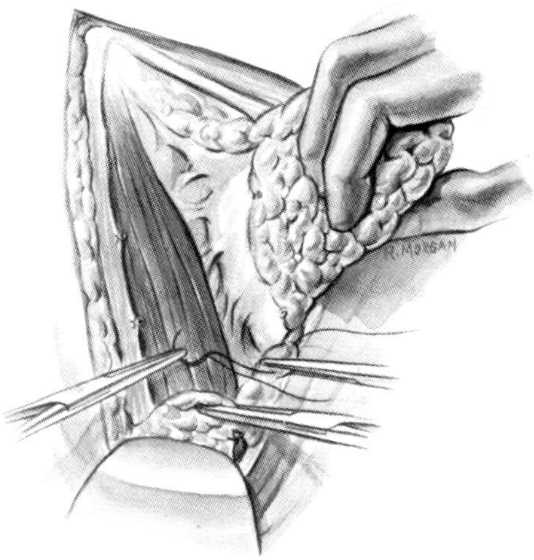

Figure 8–10. The inferior flap is retracted with a Deaver retractor to expose the margins of the quadrilateral block. The lateral margin is exposed first, and the superficial fascia and the fascia lata are incised down to bare muscle. Laterally, the fascia lata is dissected cleanly from the sartorius muscle to the lateral margin of the femoral triangle. Muscular branches of the femoral vessels are clamped individually and ligated as they are encountered. As the margins of the quadrilateral block are incised, particularly along the most distal margin traversed by the larger afferent lymphatics, the areolar tissue may be cross-clamped and suture-ligated to prevent the leakage of lymph into the wound postoperatively. (From Spratt JS Jr, Shieber W, Dillard BM: Anatomy and Surgical Technique of Groin Dissection. St Louis, CV Mosby Company, 1965.)

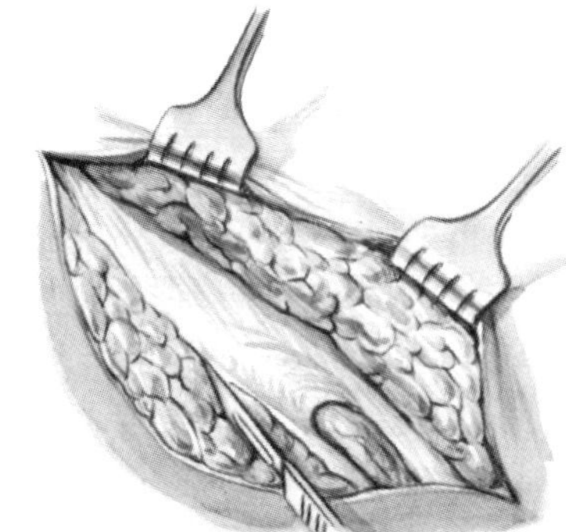

Figure 8–9. After the superior flap has been elevated to the upper margin of the quadrilateral block, the incision is extended vertically through the fatty areolar tissue and superficial fascia down to the external oblique aponeurosis. The incised tissue is then dissected cleanly from the aponeurosis down to the inguinal ligament. In the male patient, the spermatic cord is cleaned of fatty areolar tissue during this dissection. In the female patient, when operating for vulvar or perineal cancer, the round ligament may be taken at this point by dividing the inguinal ring laterally and transecting and ligating the round ligament at the internal inguinal ring. Also, when operating for penile or female genital cancer, the areolar tissue overlying the pubis must be removed cleanly to ensure resection of the presymphyseal lymphatics and nodes. (From Spratt JS Jr, Shieber W, Dillard BM: Anatomy and Surgical Technique of Groin Dissection. St Louis, CV Mosby Company, 1965.)

After the fatty areolar tissue has been completely incised, the fascia over the muscles is lifted up laterally over the sartorius muscle and is dissected off of the underlying muscle (Fig. 8–11). As reflection of the fascia progresses medially, muscular divisions of the femoral nerve will be encountered, and these can be followed upward for a clean dissection of the anterior surface of the main trunk of the nerve. Cutaneous branches passing through the quadrilateral block must be transected. The block of areolar tissue is detached laterally from the inferior edge of the inguinal ligament to the margin of the femoral sheath, exposing the main trunk of the femoral nerve completely as it appears beneath the ligament. Medially, the deep fascia is reflected up from the adductor

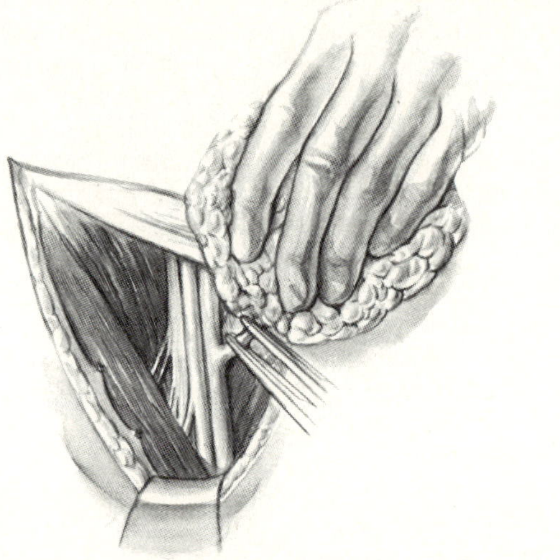

Figure 8–11. Near the medial margin of the sartorius muscle, the lower branches of the femoral nerve will be encountered. These are traced upward to the appearance of the main trunk of the nerve. The fascial attachments to the inguinal ligament are detached laterally. The femoral sheath is entered, and the femoral artery and vein are dissected clean. The saphenous vein will be encountered a second time as it traverses the fossa ovalis to enter the femoral vein. It is divided and tied with a No. 2-0 silk ligature reinforced with a suture ligature. Medially, the quadrilateral block has been incised over the pectineal muscle, and the specimen remains attached only by the lymphatic cord and surrounding fat passing into the femoral space medial to the femoral vein. (From Spratt JS Jr, Shieber W, Dillard BM: Anatomy and Surgical Technique of Groin Dissection. St Louis, CV Mosby Company, 1965.)

muscles to the medial margin of the femoral sheath. During the course of this dissection, muscular divisions of the femoral artery and vein will be encountered, and these must be transected individually.

The deep inguinal nodes lie in the areolar tissue about the femoral vessels beneath the fascia lata and superficial to the muscular fascia. At the inferior extent of the femoral triangle, the dissection must be carried down to the adventitial surface of the femoral artery and vein. These vessels are then cleanly dissected of all adherent areolar tissue. All branches on the anterior, medial, and lateral surfaces are transected individually and are ligated near the main vessel. Included among these will be the upper end of the saphenous vein (see Fig. 8–11). After it traverses the fossa ovalis of the fascia lata, it enters the femoral vein and must be ligated with a simple ligature and a suture ligature a second time flush with the main trunk of the femoral vein. The lymphatics of the femoral region are confluent with the iliac lymphatics through the femoral space. Here, also, lies the major deep inguinal lymph node, Cloquet's node.

At this point, further dissection in the groin is discontinued. When another perineal procedure is to be combined with a groin dissection, the medial division of the superficial and deep fascia overlying the pectineal muscle is delayed until the iliac and obturator dissections have been performed. The iliac lymph cord subsequently will be brought beneath the inguinal ligament and will be reflected medially with perineal ablation by dissecting deep to fascia overlying the pectineal muscle.

Approach for Iliac Dissection

The oblique incision permits easy access with good exposure for dissection of the iliac nodes. First, the external oblique aponeurosis is incised in line with its fibers at the upper margin of the external inguinal ring for the entire length of the incision. The plane beneath the lower flap of external oblique aponeurosis is laid open sharply down to the inguinal ligament. In the male patient, the spermatic cord is retracted superiorly. In the female patient, the round ligament is transected at an earlier point in the operation and is reflected inferiorly with the superficial inguinal dissection.

At the lateral margin of Hesselbach's triangle, overlying the inferior epigastric vessels, is the interfoveolar ligament, a thickened extension of the transverse fascia attaching the fascia to the inguinal ligament. This ligament is incised, and the inferior epigastric artery and vein are individually ligated and transected at the abdominal margin of the ligament (Fig. 8–12). These epigastric vessels will be transected a second time flush with the external iliac vessels. The tissue intervening between the two points of ligation will be included in the dissection. The lateral suprafemoral lymph node lies in the areolar tissue about the origin of the inferior epigastric and deep circumflex iliac arteries (Rouviere, 1938). Aside from the interfoveolar ligament, the attachment of the transvere fascia to the inguinal ligament is loose and easily divided.

The dissection is then continued deeply and laterally, dividing some of the fibers of the lower transverse muscles of the abdomen and the fibers of the internal oblique muscles of the abdomen laterally along the inguinal ligament to the anterior-superior iliac spine (see Fig. 8–12). The peritoneum is exposed

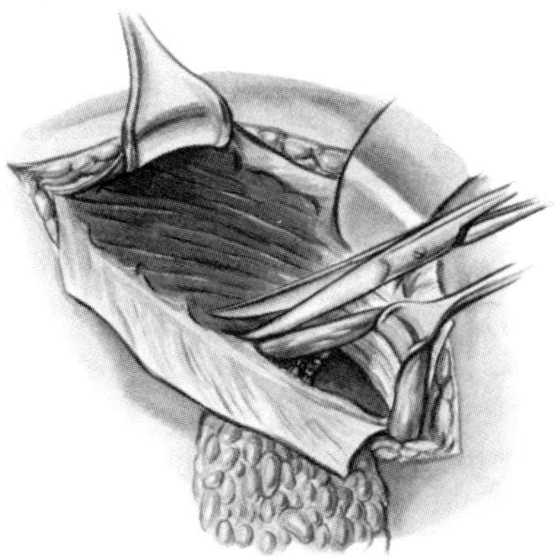

Figure 8–12. The external oblique aponeurosis has been divided at the upper margin of the external inguinal ring for the length of the oblique incision. The fibers of the transversus abdominis and obliquus internus muscle are being separated from the inguinal ligament. In Hesselbach's triangle, the attachments of the transversalis fascia to the inguinal ligament are thin and easily divided, except for the thickened interfoveolar ligament containing the inferior epigastric vessels. This ligament and the vessels must be divided before the retroperitoneal space can be entered. (From Spratt JS Jr, Shieber W, Dillard BM: Anatomy and Surgical Technique of Groin Dissection. St Louis, CV Mosby Company, 1965.)

throughout the depth of the wound. Then the peritoneum is stripped up from the lateral pelvic wall by gentle blunt dissection. The ureter will be seen at the upper extent of the dissection and will remain adherent to the peritoneum. The ureter marks the bifurcation of the common iliac artery, and the upper point of the dissection is just proximal to this bifurcation. Exposure of the iliac region is assured by placing a gauze-covered Deaver or Harrington retractor against the peritoneum to hold it away from the lateral pelvis.

Iliac Dissection

From the surgical standpoint, the major femoral lymph cord of the thigh is continuous with the deep inguinal lymph cord coming through the femoral space. Viewed from above, the femoral space is continuous with the inguinopectineal triangle (Uhlenhuth and Hunter, 1953). This triangle is bounded by the inguinal ligament, the external iliac artery, and the pectineal crest. The apex of the triangle is at the pubic tubercle, and the base is on the artery. The object of the en bloc operation is to dissect the iliac lymph cord from above down, free it from its fibrous attachments to the margin of the inguinopectineal triangle, pass the cord beneath the elevated inguinal ligament, and remove it en bloc with the deep and superficial inguinal dissections (Figs. 8–13 to 8–15). The three chains of iliac lymph nodes lie in a plane of fatty areolar tissue bounded on one margin by the genitofemoral nerve lying on the anterior surface of the psoas muscle and on the other margin by the tendinous arch at the origin of the levator ani muscle. The deep surface of the plane is the parietal layer of the endopelvic fascia. The inner surface is composed of the visceral endopelvic fascia from which the peritoneum was stripped. Between these fascial layers lies the areolar tissue containing the iliac lymphatic cords. The parietal and visceral fasciae are confluent laterally on the psoas muscle. The dissection begins by incising the endopelvic fascia just medial to the genitofemoral nerve, from the inguinal ligament to above the bifurcation of the common iliac artery (see Fig. 8–15). Dissecting on the adjacent psoas muscle, the fascia is reflected medially to the lateral margin of the iliac vessels.

As Rouviere reported in 1938, nodes of the lateral iliac chain tend to nestle in the interstices between the iliac artery and the psoas muscle. Consequently, the external iliac artery should be rolled medially, and the enveloping fascia of the vascular sheath should be incised deep in the interstices and then be reflected up and over the artery. The space between the artery and the muscle must be dissected clean. The dissection then continues by reflecting the vascular sheath away from the external artery and vein down to the deep margin of the vein. The origin of the inferior epigastric artery and vein will be exposed, and these are transected a second time adjacent to the iliac vessels. At this point, the upper end of the lymph cord can be transected overlying the distal iliac artery (see Fig. 8–15). The bundle of areolar tissue and fascia present at the apex of the dissection should be transected and ligated to occlude the lymphatics.

The medial chain of external iliac nodes is a very important one. The most peripheral or inferior node in this chain lies on the iliopectineal line and is a direct extension of the chain of deep inguinal nodes (Rouviere, 1938). The complete removal of the medial chain of iliac lymph nodes requires that a clean and complete dissection of the obturator fossa be performed. To do this, the external iliac vein must be retracted ventrally and laterally. The endopelvic fascia forming the vascular sheath is dissected completely from the undersurface of

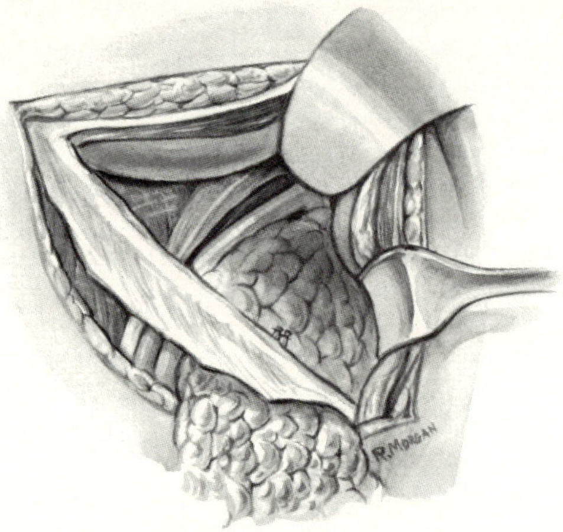

Figure 8–13. After the steps outlined in Figure 8–12, the peritoneum will be exposed, and this is stripped away from the lateral pelvis up to the bifurcation of the iliac vessels. The ureter remains adherent to the peritoneum and should be well visualized at the apex of this dissection. The spermatic cord, ureter, bladder, and peritoneum are retracted medially with one or two deep-bladed retractors. Laterally, the genitofemoral nerve will be seen through the endopelvic fascia overlying the psoas muscle. The fascia is incised just medial to the nerve and is reflected from the underlying muscle, from the angle between the muscle and the external iliac artery, and from the artery to a point just above the iliac bifurcation. (From Spratt JS Jr, Shieber W, Dillard BM: Anatomy and Surgical Technique of Groin Dissection. St Louis, CV Mosby Company, 1965.)

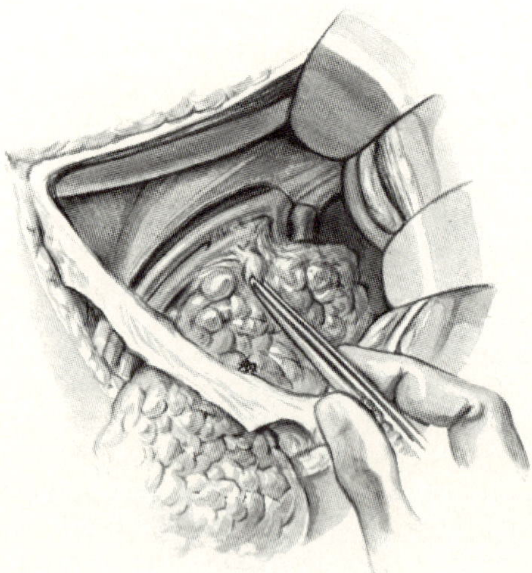

Figure 8–14. The previous dissection of the endopelvic fascia now forming the sheath of the iliac vessels is continued to expose the external iliac vein. The relation of the iliac lymphatic cord to this dissection is described in detail in the text. (From Spratt JS Jr, Shieber W, Dillard BM: Anatomy and Surgical Technique of Groin Dissection. St Louis, CV Mosby Company, 1965.)

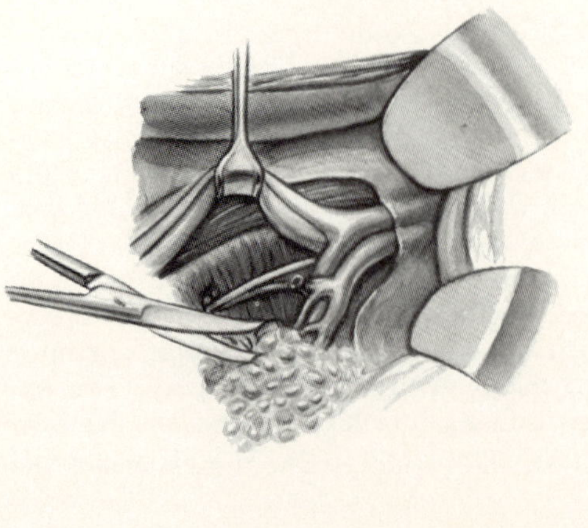

Figure 8–15. The external iliac vein is elevated with a vein retractor to expose the obturator fossa containing the medial chain of the obturator lymph nodes. The obturator fascia is dissected away from the obturator internus muscle, and the obturator nerve is isolated from the fascia. Superiorly, the lymphatic cord has been transected, overlying the common iliac artery. Dorsally, the obturator fascia will be detached from the arcus tendineus to complete the iliac dissection. (From Spratt JS Jr, Shieber W, Dillard BM: Anatomy and Surgical Technique of Groin Dissection. St Louis, CV Mosby Company, 1965.)

the iliac vein from the iliopectineal triangle to the bifurcation of the vein. This dissection must be continued through the endopelvic fascia enveloping the iliac vessels at the deep part of the vascular sheath.

When the deep portion of the vascular sheath has been incised, the bare muscle fibers of the internal obturator muscle will be exposed. A plane then exists between the parietal layer of the endopelvic fascia and the internal obturator muscle that can be opened completely by the gentle spreading of the scissor points. The obturator veins are encountered during this step. These veins go from various points on the iliac veins to the obturator foramen. They are inconsistent in their anatomic location and must be watched for and ligated or hemoclipped as they are encountered. Careless transection of these vessels or avulsion of them from either the obturator foramen or the iliac vein can result in very troublesome hemorrhage. The management of operative hemorrhage from pelvic veins is discussed in the following paragraphs.

The obturator nerve is located near the midpoint in the obturator fossa. Here it passes from beneath the medial border of the psoas muscle near the brim of the pelvis, going toward the upper part of the obturator foramen. It passes beneath the iliac vessels near the bifurcation of the common iliac vein. The shiny fibers of this nerve, which is about 2 to 3 mm in diameter, can be seen through the thin covering layer of fascia. It is dissected from the fascia throughout its length in the obturator fossa and is reflected laterally. Occasionally, enlarged cancerous lymph nodes in the medial chain will involve the obturator nerve. It can be sacrificed unilaterally with negligible morbidity. It the obturator nerves are sacrificed bilaterally, the patient will have a great deal of difficulty walking because of resultant adductor palsy in both lower extremities.

Deep in the obturator fossa and dorsal to the medial chain of the iliac lymph cord, the areolar tissue and fascia become attenuated and can be transected at the tendinous arch formed on the inner surface of the internal obturator muscle by the origin of the levator ani muscle. The tendinous arch extends from the ischial spine to the pubis and marks the junction between the intrapelvic and extrapelvic obturator fascia (Gray, 1959). The iliac lymph cord is now completely mobilized and can be freed from the margin of the inguinopectineal triangle. The inguinal ligament is elevated by a retractor, and the lymph cord is delivered into the femoral triangle for completion of the en bloc dissection (Fig. 8–16). If the iliac lymph cord will not pass easily beneath the inguinal ligament, the ligament may be transected near the pubic tubercle, laying open the roof of the inguinopectineal triangle. A typical specimen is shown in Figure 8–17.

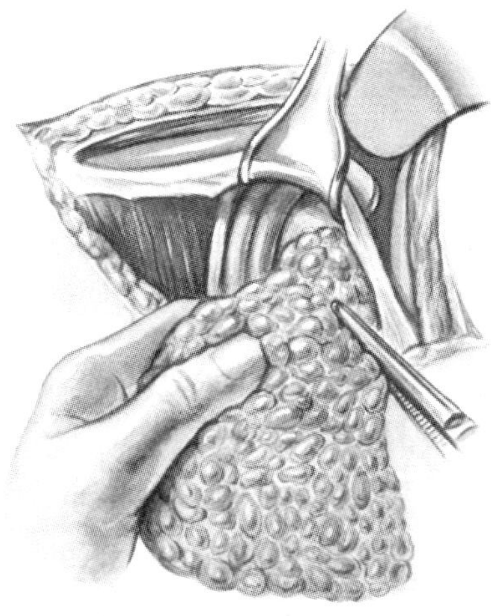

Figure 8–16. The inguinal ligament is then elevated. The iliac lymph cord is passed beneath the inguinal ligament and is detached from the inguinopectineal triangle to complete the en bloc ilioinguinal dissection. (From Spratt JS Jr, Shieber W, Dillard BM: Anatomy and Surgical Technique of Groin Dissection. St Louis, CV Mosby Company, 1965.)

The dissection of the iliac lymph cord can be exceedingly simple in a thin individual with a clean pelvis. The dissection can be very tedious in people who are excessively obese, have received irradiation to the lateral pelvis, have had pelvic inflammation, or have enlarged lymph nodes. In these latter instances, the technical pitfall causing most trouble to the occasional operator is an entry into one of the deep pelvic veins or avulsion of small, unsuspected branches. Blood from the major deep pelvic veins can well up and obscure an operating field in an instant, and a unit of blood can be transferred from the patient to the wall suction bottle in the time it takes a slow scrub nurse to get a suture ready. Blind clamping in a bloody field can do irreparable damage.

The first principle is to avoid these situations by maintaining careful stepwise exposure with anatomically oriented avascular plane dissection. The veins are thin, and in difficult cases, even the careful, experienced surgeon will have an occasional episode of major venous bleeding. Generally, the thin-walled deep pel-

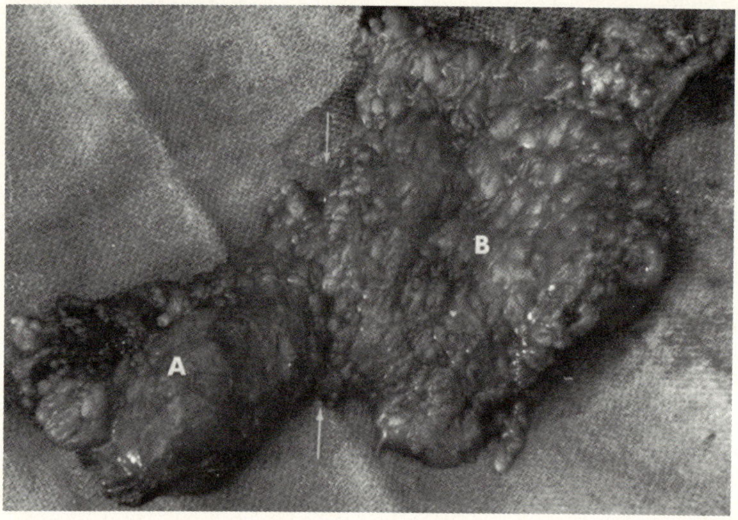

Figure 8–17. Specimen of en bloc ilioinguinal dissection of lymph node–bearing fatty areolar tissue. As many as 39 lymph nodes have been cleared from the specimen of a unilateral dissection, but the mean number of nodes recovered is 16. The arrows mark the crease made by the inguinal ligament and the iliopectineal line. *A* shows the iliac dissection, and *B* shows the superficial and deep inguinal dissections. (From Spratt JS Jr, Shieber W, Dillard BM: Anatomy and Surgical Technique of Groin Dissection. St Louis, CV Mosby Company, 1965.)

vic veins are easily torn by clamps. Preferably, the veins to be ligated should be identified and isolated by careful dissection. Then ligatures can be passed around the veins, and they can be ligated proximal and distal to the point of intended transection—no clamps need to be placed on the veins. Smaller veins can be secured by hemoclips before transection. Small rents in the iliac vein produced by direct trauma or the avulsion of small branches are managed by immediate occlusive pressure from a sponge stick. Sponge sticks are then applied firmly above and below the rent. The covering sponge is removed from the rent, and the rent is closed with continuous 5-0 swaged-on arterial silk sutures while an assistant keeps the field dry.

If a vein is avulsed flush with the lateral pelvic parietes, the end will retract and cannot be clamped. Hemorrhage can be controlled at once by sponge pressure over the aperture. The anatomic aperture into which the vessel retracts can then be sewn closed over the end of the vein by 0-chromic catgut sutures swaged onto a general closure needle (CT-1 Ethicon). The use of sturdy swaged-on sutures is important because larger caliber needles may compound the avulsion, and smaller needles and needles not swaged onto the suture may be lost in the field. A 10-inch needle holder is required.

The management of arterial hemorrhage is generally simpler than the management of venous hemorrhage. The arterial wall is tough enough to tolerate both suture closure of small rents and the cross-clamping of transected ends.

Closure of the Wound

Careful anatomic reconstruction of the lower abdominal wall is pertinent to primary wound healing and the prevention of late herniations. Medially, the iliopectineal triangle is covered with fascia, as for a direct hernia repair. If this is not done, a direct hernia through Hesselbach's triangle can be a late complication of the operation. The free margin of the conjoined tendon, including transverse fascia, is approximated to the pectineal line (pectineal ligament or Cooper's ligament), from the pubic tubercle to the medial margin of the femoral vein, by a row of interrupted heavy silk sutures

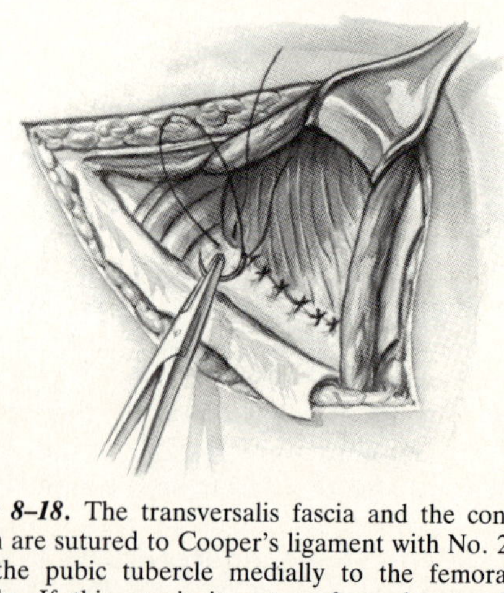

Figure 8–18. The transversalis fascia and the conjoined tendon are sutured to Cooper's ligament with No. 2-0 silk from the pubic tubercle medially to the femoral vein laterally. If this repair is not performed properly, the patient may have a direct inguinal or femoral hernia. (From Spratt JS Jr, Shieber W, Dillard BM: Anatomy and Surgical Technique of Groin Dissection. St Louis, CV Mosby Company, 1965.)

(Fig. 8–18) or by running heavy Prolene sutures. To place these sutures properly through the thickened periosteum of the pectineal line, a Mayo needle (ECT-3 Ethicon) or its equivalent is employed. Laterally, the transected fibers of the transverse muscles of the abdomen and the internal oblique muscles are sutured to the deep portion of the inguinal ligament with interrupted 2-0 sutures. Closure of the external oblique aponeurosis is by simple approximation by interrupted medium sutures.

The sartorius muscle is then transected adjacent to the anterior-superior iliac spine, and the muscle is reflected medially to cover the femoral artery and vein. The end of the muscle is sutured to the inferior margin of the inguinal ligament directly over the upper end of the femoral vessels (Fig. 8–19). Lateral and medial to the vessels, the free margin is sutured to deeper muscles, completing the secure coverage of the femoral vessels.

After completion of the deep closure, the skin flaps are inspected carefully. If a portion of the flap margin has become dusky or no longer blanches with pressure, this portion is best excised. Whenever skin has been sacrificed, as by the removal of a portion of the groin dissection flap or by the performance of a vulvectomy, primary closure is rarely possible except under tension. Aside from producing distraction of the wound margins, tension frequently tents the flaps up across underlying dead space, permitting fluid collection and delayed healing, with the risk of infection. All skin margins should be permitted to fall smoothly onto the contour of the wound in complete approximation to all of the underlying structures. Where skin edges fall together, they may be approximated with interrupted subcutaneous catgut sutures (3-0) and continuous fine silk sutures (4-0) (Fig. 8–20). Where

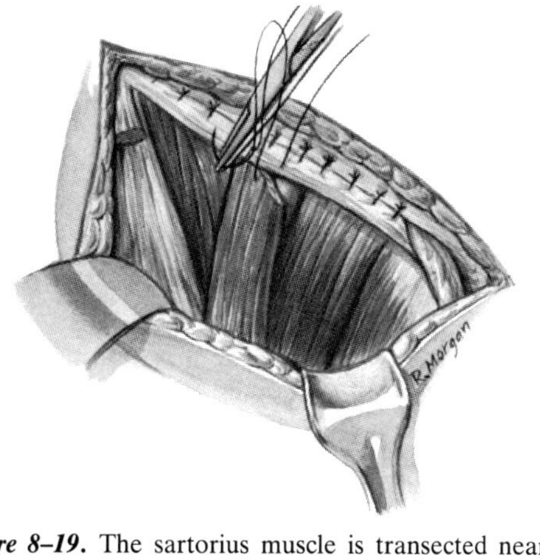

Figure 8–19. The sartorius muscle is transected near its origin, with care being taken to preserve its blood and nerve supplies. The sartorius muscle is then transposed over the femoral vein, artery, and nerve; the proximal edge of the muscle is then sutured to the inguinal ligament with No. 3-0 interrupted silk, and the lateral and medial edges are sutured to the underlying muscle. This maneuver is essential to provide coverage of the femoral vessels when skin overlying enlarged nodes has been sacrificed and to serve as a precaution against exposure of the femoral vessels should a flap infarction occur later. Suction catheters are then inserted through the flaps laterally, after which the skin can be closed. (From Spratt JS Jr, Shieber S, Dillard BM: Anatomy and Surgical Technique of Groin Dissection. St Louis, CV Mosby Company, 1965.)

skin edges do not approximate, the margins of the skin flaps should be sutured to the underlying muscle with interrupted catgut sutures between the subcutaneous layer of the flap and the muscle.

The bare muscle not covered primarily by skin flap is covered by a split-thickness skin graft. The skin graft is sutured to the margin of the flaps by interrupted fine silk sutures, and the suture ends are left on. All air bubbles and fluid are expressed from beneath the sur-

Figure 8–20. Freshly closed oblique incision, with suction catheters in place. (From Spratt JS Jr, Shieber W, Dillard BM: Anatomy and Surgical Technique of Groin Dissection. St Louis, CV Mosby Company, 1965.)

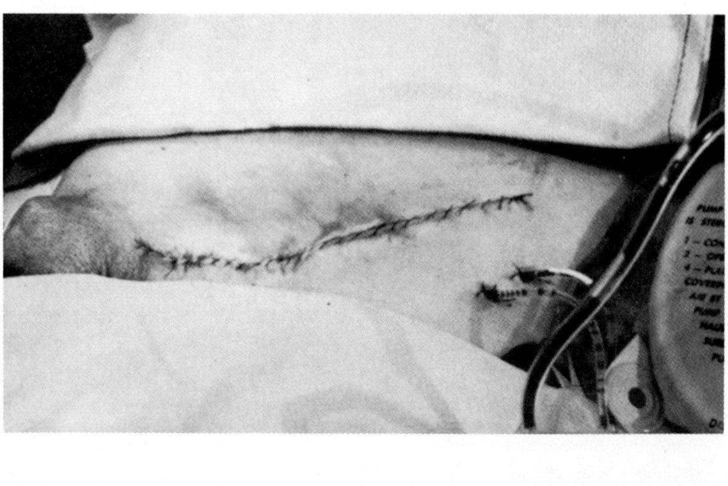

face so that nothing is interposed between the deep surface of the graft and the muscle. The graft is then covered with Telfa and fluffed gauze, and the long ends of the sutures are tied firmly over the fluffed gauze, crisscrossed in all directions to ensure even pressure on the underlying skin graft. The stent remains in place for 5 days and is then removed cautiously to avoid avulsing the graft.

With either complete primary closure or partial closure with skin grafting, it is pertinent that the wound be made as airtight as possible. This is necessary because suction catheters are used routinely for drainage. The application of pressure by heavy dressings on the thin flaps is to be avoided. Two large Hemovac catheters are used. The proximal ends of the catheters are brought out through stab incisions slightly smaller than the catheters, situated, preferably, on the lateral thigh and abdomen. One catheter passes transversely across the wound under the upper flap, and one passes under the lower flap. The proximal ends are attached to a T-tube and then to continuous suction or to a Hemovac system. These catheters should be inserted before the skin flaps are closed or a skin graft is placed over any open areas. The catheters should not lie under either base of the bipedicle flap, where they could exert a tourniquet effect.

POSTOPERATIVE CARE

The proper postoperative management of the patient after a groin dissection is as pertinent to the reduction of morbidity as is a well-executed surgical procedure. The general principles of postoperative care in relation to the care of the cardiopulmonary system, urinary tract, fluid therapy and alimentation, care of the bowels, and general nursing care are not discussed in detail in this chapter. Rather, those procedures peculiar to the care of patients having groin dissections and related organ resections will be enumerated.

The preoperative mechanical cleansing of the bowels simplifies the postoperative management. A bowel movement is not necessary for several days, and the risk of fecal contamination of a fresh wound is avoided. If a bowel movement has not occurred by the fifth postoperative day, the patient should receive a small enema or a Dulcolax suppository, well supervised by the nurse, so that the passage does not contaminate the wound. Additional planned eliminations under nursing supervision to avoid soilage may be required every several days if the patient is restricted to bed.

Urinary Tract

Catheterization with all aseptic and antiseptic precautions should be performed in the operating room after the patient is anesthetized in order to keep the bladder empty during the iliac dissection. The amount of pelvic manipulation involved in a groin dissection, the advanced age of the patient, the delay in ambulation attending this operation, and the need to keep the wounds dry of urine require that the catheter be left in place as long as the patient is confined to bed postoperatively. Sufficient intake of fluid to maintain an adequate urinary output of medium range specific gravity is important. Antibiotics probably will not prevent an invasive urinary tract infection secondary to catheterization, but specific drugs should be used when the presence of invasive urinary tract infections is suspected.

Drainage, Lymph, and Lymphatic Regeneration

Numerous major afferent lymphatics are transected during a groin dissection, and large segments of lymphatics are resected. The open flow of lymph into a groin dissection is simple to demonstrate by lymphography. This flow can be reduced by the operative precaution of cross-clamping and ligating the areolar tissue and fascia at the periphery of the quadrilateral block and at the apex of the iliac lymph cord. In the postoperative period, the following physiologic principles governing the volume and rate of flow of lymph from an extremity should be kept in mind. Essentially no lymph comes from a still and motionless extremity, but the flow increases proportionately to the degree of either active or passive motion in the extremity. Isometric exercise will increase lymph flow but will not provide assistance to lymph egress that is obtained by active muscular contraction. Consequently, isometric exercises should be avoided in favor of active muscular and joint exercises. In the postoperative period, lymph flow from the lower extremity must be kept at a minimum until the inguinal incisions are completely healed and until ample time has elapsed to permit the regeneration of lymphatics or the development of anastomotic lymphatics.

The rate and density of lymphatic regeneration are influenced by the healing of the wound. Butcher and Hoover (1955) demonstrated by sky-blue dye injection of the superficial dermal lymphatics that these lymphatics convey dye across linear incisions in humans at about the fifteenth postoperative day in wounds healing per primam. In 1926, Reichert showed in the dog that superficial lymphatics can become confluent across a cleanly healing, well-approximated wound as early as the fourth postoperative day, but the deeper lymphatics regenerate more slowly than do the superficial ones. Reichert observed that lymphatics are functional enough to keep an extremity free from edema after the eighth postoperative day, with healing per primam. When segmental resection of lymphatics is performed, as in a groin dissection, the establishment of anastomotic channels is an important mechanism for re-establishing lymph flow (Gray, 1940). In wounds healing per secundam, the superficial dermal lymphatics remain sparse in number many years after healing. Regeneration is delayed by infection and excessive scar tissue formation and radiation therapy.

To prevent persistent lymphedema, the extremity must never be permitted to become dependent or active until the inguinal incision has healed completely with no residual fluid beneath the flaps. If an extremity below a groin dissection is permitted to become and remain edematous, the cycle of fibrosis and further lymphatic obstruction begins, secondary to the stagnation of protein-rich lymph. The extremity may develop subcutaneous fibrosis, and the lymphedema may become intractable (Smith and Conway, 1962).

In the case of either unilateral groin dissection or bilateral groin dissection without any associated perineal or genital surgery, the management is relatively simple. The lower extremities are kept in graded elastic stockings measured and obtained preoperatively. The drain catheters are kept on suction until the daily fluid output is negligible and are then removed. Their removal before the fifth postoperative day is rarely advisable. The patient must then remain in bed for several additional days. By about the tenth postoperative day, it should be obvious whether the wound is healing per primam without fluid accumulation beneath the flaps. When this is evident, the patient can be permitted to ambulate, but effective compression of the feet, calf, and lower thigh by the elastic stocking must be maintained for at least 6 additional weeks. The patient should be instructed not to let his feet hang dependently when he sits to rest. A footstool should be available when he sits, and the feet should be elevated at night. This postoperative period should contain a patient education program emphasizing lifelong management of the extremity to avoid delayed infections or trace soft edema that can evolve slowly into chronic fibrotic lymphedema.

Complication of the postoperative course by fluid accumulation beneath the flaps, the development of a lymph fistula, or delay in wound healing necessitates the prompt and complete immobilization of the lower extremity to arrest the flow of lymph. This can be done by applying a molded posterior splint extending from the ends of the toes to the upper one third of the thigh. The splint should remain in place until the groin incision is completely healed without residual drainage.

In spite of all precautions, ischemic infarction of flaps may occur during the postoperative period. The resulting eschar produces a closed-space infection beneath it. If left unattended, this infection cannot drain to the surface and may disseminate beneath the upper and lower flaps, producing a massive wound infection. Patients developing areas of obvious flap infarction should be returned to the operating room as soon as the completeness of the infarction is certain. With complete operating room asepsis, as for the primary operation, a split-thickness skin graft is taken from a remote donor site, and the donor site is dressed. Then, the area of flap infarction is excised completely, and a meshed split-thickness graft or stamp grafts are placed on the wound base. If excision of the infarcted area is delayed until infection beneath the eschar has intervened, skin grafting may have to be delayed. Bacterial cultures should be taken of all infected tissue. Contaminated open wounds clean up most rapidly if managed as infected burns.

Exposure of the Femoral Artery

In earlier years there were several instances of exposure of the femoral artery in an infected wound. At least one instance of major hemorrhage resulted. This complication has never been seen by the author, since the sartorius muscular pedicle to cover the femoral vessels has been used routinely. It is still possible, however, if the sartorius muscular pedicle ever retracts. The exposure of a major artery in an open wound always creates a dangerous and urgent situation because of the risk of rupture. Immediate coverage with the tissues at hand or by prompt split-thickness skin grafting is advised. As soon as there is no danger of covering an infected area with a pedicle, thereby leaving the artery exposed in an abscess cavity, a full-thickness pedicle can be elevated from the lower abdominal wall and slid inferiorly over the exposed artery.

In summary, a groin dissection performed for complete ablation of the node-bearing areolar tissue in the inguinal and iliac regions and with negligible morbidity is a procedure that requires careful attention to the regional anatomy and the pathophysiology of cancer in lymphatics, to preoperative and postoperative care, and to surgical technique, including coordinated utilization of general, plastic, vascular, and orthopedic surgical principles. The operation is an important procedure for the control of cancers when indicated, but it must be performed properly with negligible morbidity by paying attention to the surgical principles involved.

MULTIMODALITY THERAPY

Recent studies from several centers report the responses of anal carcinomas to various combinations of treatment. In chapters Eighteen and Nineteen, the fields of chemotherapy and radiation therapy are covered. The purpose here is to consider several studies in which combinations of treatment have provided responses. Although these studies provide leads for future research, they all have been compromised in experimental design by small numbers of cases and the variegated nature of anal cancers.

In 1980, Green and associates divided 33 patients seen between 1966 and 1979 into six groups: (1) localized favorable disease (21 patients); (2) localized unfavorable disease (3 patients); (3) primary lesion and inguinal metastases (3 patients); (4) inguinal metastases only (3 patients); (5) metastatic disease (2 patients); and (6) a miscellaneous group (6 patients). All patients received external supervoltage radiation therapy and one patient had an iridium interstitial implant. Gallium-67 (^{67}Ga) scanning was carried out in nine patients and was positive in six. The primary tumor only was seen in two cases, metastases only in three cases, and both primary and metastatic sites in one case. The metastases were seen in the inguinal nodes, liver, and brain.

Although this series was larger than average in total numbers, it was divided into many small groups, and over half of the total series was apparently composed of patients with cloacogenic cancer. The overall response rate was good, and only three cases came to abdominoperineal resection requiring colostomy. No patient in this series received adjuvant chemotherapy.

Cummings and associates (1980) reported six cases with previously untreated operable squamous cell carcinomas of the anal canal that were managed by a combination of simultaneously administered radiation therapy and chemotherapy consisting of mitomycin-C (10 mg/m^2) by bolus intravenous injection, and 5-fluorouracil (1000 mg/m^2/24 hours, maximum of 1500 mg/24 hours) by continuous intravenous infusion over 96 hours. Radiation consisted of 5000 rads given in 20 fractions in 4 weeks to the primary site, and 3000 rads in 2.5 weeks to the lymph nodes. Hospitalization for 16 to 38 days was required for all patients. For 6 to 20 months of follow-up the patients had local control and retention of anal continence. These early results are encouraging.

Wanebo and associates (1981a) reported seven patients with locally advanced anal cancer, three with recurrent or persistent disease, and four with advanced primary cancers. Five had groin metastases. The treatment protocol consisted of a continuous 5-day infusion of 5-fluorouracil (750 mg/m^2) and mitomycin-C (15 mg/m^2), by bolus injection, and radiation to 3000 rads. All patients received one or two cycles of chemotherapy preoperatively and four (not previously irradiated) received radiation. Tumor regression of more than 50 percent occurred in five patients, minor regression of 25 to 50 percent occurred in one patient, and no regression occurred in one who received chemotherapy only. All patients then underwent total resection of all gross tumor, and five had groin dissection. Two patients had residual cancer on microscopic examination at the site of the primary cancer, and four of the five patients undergoing groin dissection had microscopic residual cancer. Three of the seven patients were dead within 5 months and a fourth was dead with disease by the 34th post-treatment month. Three patients were disease free for 2 years.

References

Abbas JS, Karakousis CP, Holyoke ED: Anorectal melanoma: clinical features, recurrence and patient survival. Int Surg 65:423–426, 1980.

Baronofsky ID: Technique of inguinal node dissection. Surgery 24:555–567, 1948.

Beahrs OH, Wilson SM: Carcinoma of the anus. Ann Surg 184:422–428, 1976.

Boey J, Choi TK, Wong J, Ong GB: The surgical management of anorectal malignant melanoma. Aust NZ J Surg 51:132–136, 1981.

Bolivar JC, Harris JW, Branch W, Sherman RT: Melanoma of the anorectal region. Surg Gynecol Obstet 154:337–341, 1982.

Boman BM, Moertel, CG, O'Connell MJ, et al: Carcinoma of the anal canal—a clinical and pathologic study of 188 cases. Cancer. Accepted for publication, 1983.

Brennan JT, Stewart CF: Epidermoid carcinoma of the anus. Ann Surg 176:787–790, 1972.

Breslow A: Tumor thickness, level of invasion, and node dissections in Stage I cutaneous melanoma. Ann Surg 182:572–575, 1975.

Butcher HR, Hoover AL: Abnormalities of human superficial cutaneous lymphatics associated with stasis ulcers, lymphedema, scars and cutaneous autografts. Ann Surg 142:633–653, 1955.

Christiansen J, Vitturp M: Squamous cell carcinoma of the anus. Acta Chir Scand 141:554–556, 1975.

Chiu YS, Unni KK, Beart RW Jr: Malignant melanoma of the anorectum. Dis Colon Rectum 23:122–124, 1980.

Clark WH Jr, From L, Bernardino EA, Molin MC: The histogenesis and biologic behavior of primary human malignant melanomas of the skin. Cancer Res 29:705–727, 1969.

Cleveland BR, Green WO Jr: Squamous cell carcinoma arising in a pilonidal sinus. Surgery 55:381–386, 1964.

Cooper HS, Patchefsky AS, Marks G: Cloacogenic carcinoma of the anorectum in homosexual men: an observation of four cases. Dis Colon Rectum 22:557–558, 1979.

Cortese AF: Surgical approach for treatment of epidermoid anal carcinoma. Cancer 36:1869–1875, 1975.

Cullen PK Jr, Pontius EE, Sanders RJ: Cloacogenic anorectal carcinoma. Dis Colon Rectum 9:1–12, 1966.

Cummings BJ, Harwood AR, Keane TJ, et al: Combined treatment of squamous cell carcinoma of the anal canal: radical radiation therapy with 5-fluorouracil and mitomycin-C, a preliminary report. Dis Colon Rectum 23:389–391, 1980.

Daling JR, Weiss NS, Klopfenstein LL, et al: Correlates of homosexual behavior and the incidence of anal cancer. JAMA 247:1988–1990, 1982.

Daseler EH, Anson BJ, Reimann AF: Radical excision of the inguinal and iliac lymph glands. A study based upon 450 anatomical dissections and upon supportive clinical observations. Surg Gynecol Obstet 87:679–694, 1948.

Denning JS, Frederick JF, Gold D, Poth EJ: Pilonidal disease: review of the literature and a method of closure. Am Surg 20:1250–1257, 1954.

Dillard BM, Spratt JS Jr, Ackerman LV, Butcher HR Jr: Epidermoid cancer of anal margin and canal. Review of 79 cases. Arch Surg 86:772–777, 1963.

Golden GT, Horsley, JS: Surgical management of epidermoid carcinoma of the anus. Am J Surg 131:275–280, 1976.

Gray JH: Studies on the regeneration of lymphatic vessels. J Anat 74:309–335, 1940.

Gray H: *In* Goss CM (ed): Gray's Anatomy. Philadelphia, Lea and Febiger, 1959.

Green JP, Schaupp WC, Cantril ST, Schall G: Anal carcinoma: current therapeutic concepts. Am J Surg 140:151–155, 1980.

Grinvalsky HT, Helwig EB: Carcinoma of the anorectal junction. I. Histological considerations. Cancer 9:480–488, 1956.

Grodsky L: Current concepts on cloacogenic transitional cell anorectal cancers. JAMA 207:2057–2061, 1969.

Gupta S, Kumar A, Khanna AK, Khanna S: Pilonidal sinus epidermoid carcinoma: a clinicopathologic study and a collective review. Curr Surg 38:374–381, 1981.

Kheir S, Hickey RC, Martin RG, et al: Cloacogenic carcinoma of the anal canal. Arch Surg 104:407–415, 1972.

Klotz RG Jr, Pamukcoglu T, Souilliard DH: Transitional cloacogenic carcinoma of the anal canal: clinicopathologic study of 373 cases. Cancer 20:1727–1745, 1967.

Knutson CO, Hori JM, Spratt JS Jr: Melanoma. Curr Probl Surg December 1971, pp. 3–5.

Kuehn PG, Eisenberg H, Reed, JF: Epidermoid carcinoma of the perianal skin and anal canal. Cancer 22:932, 1968.

Lone F, Berg JW, Stearns MW Jr: Basaloid tumors of the anus. Cancer 13:907–913, 1960.

McAnally AK, Dockerty MB: Carcinoma developing in chronic draining cutaneous sinuses and fistulas. Surg Gynecol Obstet 88:87–96, 1949.

Nigro ND, Vaitkevicius VK, Considine B Jr: Combined therapy for cancer of the anal canal: a preliminary report. Dis Colon Rectum 17:354–356, 1974.

O'Grady JF, Bacon HE, Koohdary A: Squamous cell carcinoma of the anus. Dis Colon Rectum 16:39–41, 1973.

Pang LS, Morson BC: Basaloid carcinoma of the anal canal. J Clin Pathol 20:128–135, 1967.

Prasad ML, Abcarian H: Malignant potential of perianal condyloma acuminatum. Dis Colon Rectum 23:191–197, 1980.

Probstein JG: Malignant melanoma of the anorectum. Arch Surg 75:253–255, 1957.

Probstein JG: Personal communication, 1983.

Quinn D, Selah C: Malignant melanoma of the anus in a Negro: report of a case and review of the literature. Dis Colon Rectum 20:627–631, 1977.

Reichert FL: The regeneration of lymphatics. Arch Surg 13:871–881, 1926.

Rouviere H: Anatomy of the Human Lymphatic System. Translated by Tobias MJ. Ann Arbor, MI, Edwards Brothers, 1938.

Sawyers JL: Current management of carcinoma of the anus and perianus. Am Surg 43:424–429, 1977.

Sink JD, Kramer SA, Copeland DD, Seigler HF: Cloacogenic carcinoma. Ann Surg 188:53–59, 1978.

Smith JW, Conway H: Selection of appropriate surgical procedures in lymphedema. Plast Reconstr Surg 30:10–31, 1962.

Spratt JS Jr: The lognormal frequency distribution and human cancer. J Surg Res 9:151–157, 1969.

Spratt JS Jr, Shieber W, Dillard BM: Anatomy and Surgical Technique of Groin Dissection. St. Louis, CV Mosby Company, 1965.

Spratt JS Jr, Spratt TL: Rates of growth of pulmonary metastases and host survival. Ann Surg 159:161–171, 1964.

Stearns MW Jr, Quan SH: Epidermoid carcinoma of the anorectum. Surg Gynecol Obstet 131:953–957, 1970.

Strauss RJ, Fazio VW: Bowen's disease of the anal and perianal area, a report and analysis of twelve cases. Am J Surg 137:231–234, 1979.

Svenson EW, Montague ED: Results of treatment in transitional cloacogenic carcinoma. Cancer 46:828–830, 1980.

Uhlenhuth E, Hunter DT: Problems in the Anatomy of the Pelvis; an Atlas. Philadelphia, Lippincott Company, 1953.

Wanebo HJ, Futrell W, Constable W: Multimodality approach to surgical management of locally advanced epidermoid carcinoma of the anorectum. Cancer 47:2817–2826, 1981a.

Wanebo HJ, Woodruff JM, Farr GH, Quan SH: Anorectal melanoma. Cancer 47:1891–1900, 1981.

Welch JP, Malt RA: Appraisal of treatment of carcinoma of the lanus and anal canal. Surg Gynecol Obstet 145:837–841, 1977.

Wolff H: Karzinom auf dem Boden des Dermoids. Arch Klin Chir 62:731, 1900.

Woodhall JP: Radical groin surgery with particular reference to postoperative healing. Surgery 33:886–895, 1953.

NINE

Pathology of Neoplasms

H. J. Spjut, M.D.

An important aspect of the pathologic study of large bowel disease is the interpretation of biopsies. The number of biopsies performed has increased remarkably with the use of colonoscopy. With this technique, disease is seen at an earlier phase and in different settings. The colonoscope provides access to lesions for biopsy that were previously out of reach of the rigid sigmoidoscope, thus enabling pathologists to gain and provide much pertinent information about large bowel diseases and their evolution. The biopsied tissue often comes in small pieces, although polypectomies may be performed using the colonoscope. With the small pieces, particularly of suspected neoplasms, it is important for the pathologist to have information concerning the appearance of the whole lesion and the site of the biopsied tissue, i.e., whether it is from within the lesion, from a site near the lesion, or from the edges of the lesion. These data are important, particularly when the biopsy specimens have been taken from the edge of or near a lesion, in the interpretation of alterations in colonic glands, which may merely reflect injury to the mucosa or regenerative phenomenon. When interpreting biopsy specimens of large tumors, such as villous tumors, it may be difficult to determine whether there is or is not a malignant neoplasm present. When this occurs it is often recommended that additional biopsies be performed in order to diminish the chance of there being a hidden carcinoma in the villous tumor. Well-differentiated adenocarcinomas may be mistaken for adenomatous polyps with various degrees of atypical nuclear changes. Such an error may be avoided if information is available regarding the colonoscopic features of the lesion. In addition to yielding diagnostic information, biopsies may have value in predicting the course of disease; for example, a biopsy may identify certain dysplastic mucosal alterations seen in patients with chronic ulcerative colitis.

Many of the epithelial neoplasms of the large bowel do not have distinctive gross features, thus biopsies are important in the differentiation of these lesions. For example, it may be difficult to distinguish between a small villous tumor and an adenomatous polyp, and a polypoid carcinoma and a large adenomatous polyp. Also, there are many benign lesions that project into the lumen of the bowel that are difficult to define specifically without biopsy. Even with a biopsy it may be a problem to specifically diagnose a lesion, e.g., a carcinoid of the rectum in which there is glandular formation. If one is not considering the possibility of carcinoids, these lesions may be misdiagnosed as adenocarcinomas. Colitis cystica profunda may be mistaken for mucinous carcinoma unless one is aware of this lesion and its histologic features. With a small biopsy specimen, differentiation between an invasive or metastatic adenocarcinoma to the large bowel and a primary adenocarcinoma may be difficult. If the biopsy is representative and the proper configuration of the metastasis is noted, that is, an intact mucosa, then metastatic or invasive adenocarcinoma can be suggested in the diagnosis.

Sarcomas and malignant lymphomas are usually diagnosable by biopsy, but determining whether there is secondary involvement of the large intestine is a major question that cannot be answered by biopsy alone. Inflammatory disease may mimic neoplasms of the large intestine, both clinically and radiographically. These include inflammatory polyps; various ulcerative diseases, such as tuberculosis, amebiasis, and nonspecific ulcers; diverticulitis; and irradiation effect. Thus it is important that biopsies of the diseased tissue be done. Endometriosis may lead to an erroneous diagnosis of a neoplasm, clinically, radiographically, or pathologically.

Much information can be obtained from biopsies in addition to a diagnosis. For example, with a carcinoma one can determine the degree of differentiation and invasiveness and, at times, discover evidence of vascular or nerve involvement. It is often difficult to determine depth of invasion from the small biopsy specimens, since they generally consist almost entirely of tumor without submucosa or muscularis propria. In general, the use of special stains does not aid in answering many of the questions related to neoplasms of the large intestine. At times, mucin stains may be needed in order to differentiate a carcinoma from a sarcoma or undifferentiated malignant neoplasm. Step sections of the small biopsy specimens are important because they show various aspects of the lesion at different depths through the biopsy; in some cases only one or two of the sections will contain the neoplasm. Generally, step sections are routinely done on small biopsy specimens.

With the use of the colonoscope, many polypectomy specimens are now received in the laboratory. It is our routine to block in the entire epithelial polyp, with orientation toward the excisional margin. This allows the proper classification of the polypoid lesion, and if carcinoma is present, the involvement of the stalk and depth of invasion can be determined.

For resected specimens of the large intestine, I prefer to pin the specimen out on a cork board and allow fixation overnight before making the blocks. Better blocks are obtained from fixed rather than from fresh material. In neoplasms and suspected neoplasms, lymph nodes are always searched for in the attached mesentery. After fixation, the tumor is sliced in thin blocks through the entire thickness of the wall so that the deepest point of penetration of the tumor can be used for histologic examination. This has bearing on the Dukes' classification of carcinomas. When pertinent, any other mucosal lesions and the lines of resection are sampled.

Electron microscopic studies are not needed for the classification of most neoplasms of the large intestine. However, they may be helpful in classifying poorly differentiated carcinomas when the possibility of a lymphoma exists or a metastatic undifferentiated carcinoma from some other site. Electron microscopic studies may aid, for example, in the classification of carcinoids and some of the cloacogenic carcinomas of the anus by the identification of neurosecretory granules.

Immunopathologic preparation using immunoperoxidase techniques are helpful in distinguishing invasive or metastatic tumors of the large bowel from primary carcinomas. Specific prostatic proteins are now stainable, allowing identification of prostatic carcinoma as opposed to adenocarcinoma of the rectum. Although it is not specific for colonic carcinoma, carcinoembryonic antigen (CEA) will help the pathologist to determine whether a lesion is epithelial or sarcomatous, since it is specific for epithelial lesions, and few, if any, sarcomas stain with this antigen. Also, it has been shown that a gland-forming carcinoma that is negative for CEA staining is unlikely to be of colonic origin (O'Brien et al., 1981). Detection of CEA and blood group substances may have prognostic implications for carcinoma of the large intestine. Wiley and associates (1981) demonstrated that tumors negative for CEA and blood group substances are more likely to have metastases than those that are positive, especially for the blood group substances.

NON-NEOPLASTIC DISEASES OF THE LARGE INTESTINE THAT MAY MIMIC NEOPLASMS

A wide variety of non-neoplastic lesions of the large intestine mimic benign and malignant neoplasms. Isolated rectal or colonic pseudopolyps (inflammatory polyps) composed of granulation tissue are readily mistaken for true epithelial polyps (Fig. 9–1). Pseudopolyps have an epithelial component; the epithelium closely resembles colonic mucosa. Glands may be dilated. In inflammatory bowel diseases, the pseudopolyps are usually multiple and composed of mucosal elements but may be granulation tissue.

Juvenile polyps (retention polyps) are most frequently seen in children (see Chapter Sixteen). However, despite the name, this disease may occur in adults. Grossly, the lesions are red, polypoid, and often superficially ulcerated. Histologically dilated, inflamed colonic glands are associated with edema and acute and chronic inflammatory cells in the stroma. These lesions have often been considered of inflammatory origin and self-limited. However, as is discussed elsewhere in this book, these lesions, particularly when multiple, may have other implications.

Solitary ulcers are common in the upper

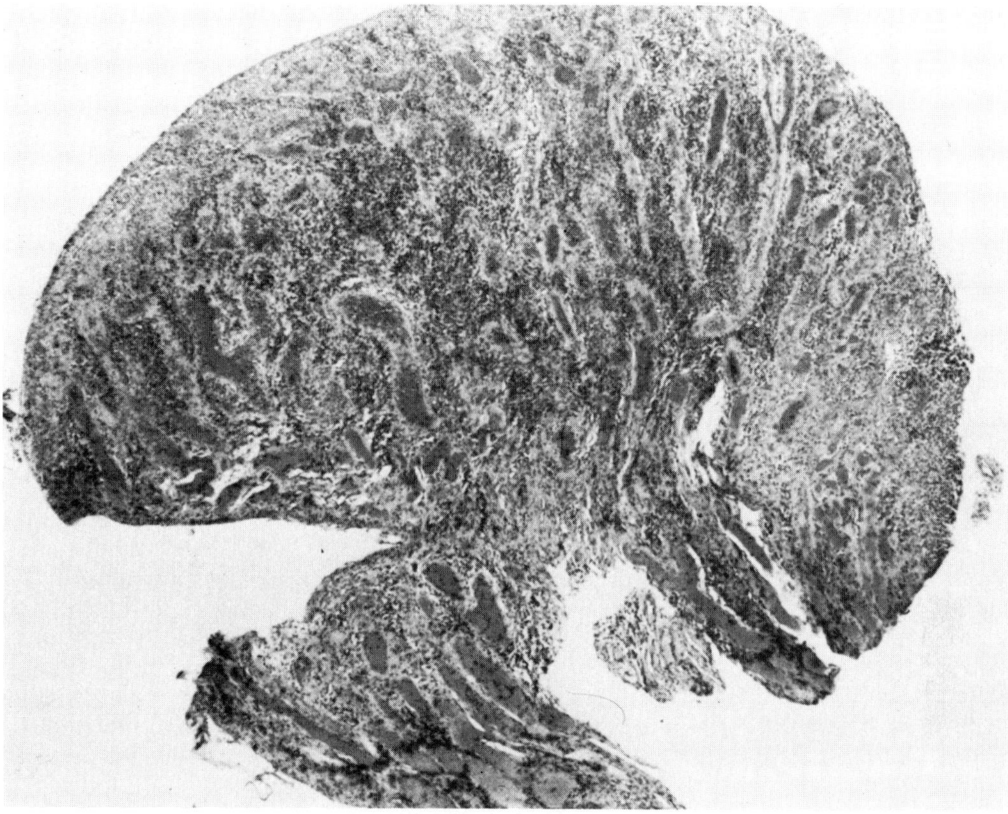

Figure 9–1. A granulation polyp of the rectum mistaken for an adenomatous polyp.

gastrointestinal tract but are less common in the large intestine and therefore less often considered in the differential diagnosis of diseases of the large intestine (Butsch et al., 1969). Recently, it has been demonstrated that solitary ulcers can be mistaken for carcinomas of the large intestine because they often present an annular configuration radiographically (Gardiner and Bird, 1980). A few have been described as polypoid. Because of their radiographic features, ulcers of the large intestine are seldom diagnosed preoperatively. The majority of ulcers of the large intestine are solitary. The most common location is in the cecum, followed by the ascending colon, the transverse colon, and the descending colon and sigmoid, in that order. The etiology of isolated ulcers of the large intestine remains unknown, although many possible causes have been considered, including the intake of medications, solitary diverticulitis, mucosal trauma, and inflammatory and infectious agents. Histologically, the ulcers are nonspecific, showing the loss of the mucosa associated with granulation of the base. There may be scarring at the base and margins, suggesting that some of the ulcers have been present for some period of time. Occasional primary cancers present as mucosal ulcers (see Chapter Ten).

Granulomatous diseases, such as tuberculosis, amebiasis, and histoplasmosis, may cause constricting or polypoid masses of the large intestine that are mistaken radiographically for malignant disease. Even at gross pathologic examination, the ulcerative form of tuberculosis or histoplasmosis may be difficult to differentiate from a neoplasm (Fig. 9–2). Histologic examinations, of course, are conclusive. About 90 percent of tuberculosis of the gastrointestinal tract occurs in the ileocecal area (Bentley and Webster, 1967). Tuberculosis results in ulcerative and stenotic zones, which are interpreted as possible carcinomas by barium enema study. In addition, hypertrophic and hyperplastic changes in tuberculosis in combination with ulcers and stenosis result in thickened segments of the large intestine that mimic carcinoma radiographically. Histologically, gastrointestinal tuberculosis is identical to that seen in other parts of the body, that is, there are granulomas and confluent granulomas with caseous necrosis. The granulomas

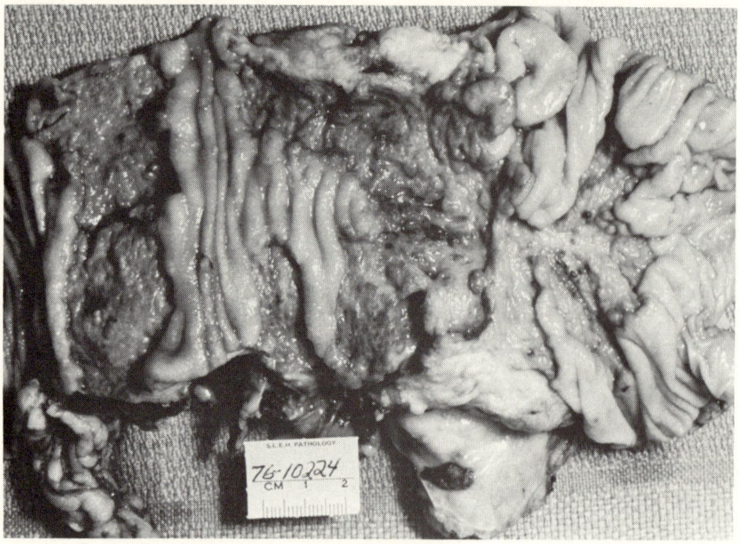

Figure 9–2. Tuberculous ulcers in the ileocecal region. The ulcers are irregular and circumscribe the bowel wall. The patient was a 22-year-old man.

are not specific, and stains for acid-fast organisms must be done; cultures for mycobacteria are important as a means of confirming the diagnosis and classifying the organism.

Histoplasmosis of the gastrointestinal tract is generally associated with a disseminated disease. There are rare examples of involvement of the large intestine with stenosis, which can result in a mistaken radiologic diagnosis of carcinoma (Perez et al., 1966). Histologically the granulomas are similar to those of tuberculosis. The organisms may be identified by special stains and by cultural techniques.

Amebiasis causes stenotic or mass lesions that may be mistaken for neoplastic diseases of the large intestine. Cicatricial stenosis of the colon as well as of the rectum has been described. In either instance, a previous history of amebiasis or signs and symptoms that suggest the disease are helpful in clinically delineating the stenotic or mass lesions of the large intestine. Amebomas may be found in any part of the large intestine but occur most frequently in the cecum, rectosigmoid, and hepatic flexure (Morrey and Wolma, 1972). They may be multiple. Amebomas usually are submucosal nodules that have a granulomatous pattern in which the presence of *Entamoeba histolytica* may be demonstrable. Amebomas may vary in size from a few millimeters up to several centimeters in greatest dimension. Characteristically, an ameboma has an outer zone of fibroblastic tissue associated with fibrosis, an inner zone that consists of granulation tissue with chronic inflammatory cells, and a central zone that is necrotic, resembling caseous necrosis. Usually the organism *Entamoeba histolytica* can be found in the ameboma (Recio, 1965; Levine et al., 1971).

Malacoplakia, although more commonly found in the urinary tract, may present as a mass lesion of the large bowel. In adults the mass may be mistaken clinically for carcinoma. Malacoplakia of the colon has been reported in a child. Histologically, the lesion consists of large macrophages and inflammatory cells with the characteristic Michaelis-Gutmann bodies. Malacoplakia is thought to be of inflammatory origin, as evidenced by detailed studies (Madara et al., 1983; Terner and Lattes, 1965).

Endometriosis may involve any portion of the gastrointestinal tract. The rectum and the sigmoid colon are the most frequent sites in the large intestine. It is in these two sites that the clinical problems related to gastrointestinal endometriosis most often arise and that endometriosis mimics a carcinoma radiographically, surgically, and pathologically (Spjut and Perkins, 1959). Small implants on the serosa of the large bowel are generally not of consequence, but if endometriosis involves the wall of the rectum or sigmoid, an obstructing lesion may form. In these areas, the mucosa is intact, and this allows the radiologist to differentiate an endometrioma from a primary carcinoma. Grossly, endometriosis presents as a firm, constricting mass that resembles carcinoma. The lesion shows a remarkable thickening of the wall of the bowel that histologically correlates with hypertrophy of the muscularis propria (Fig. 9–3). In addition to muscular hypertrophy, there is evidence of fibrosis. If the endometrial component involves the muscularis mucosae, it also undergoes hypertrophy. Mucosal

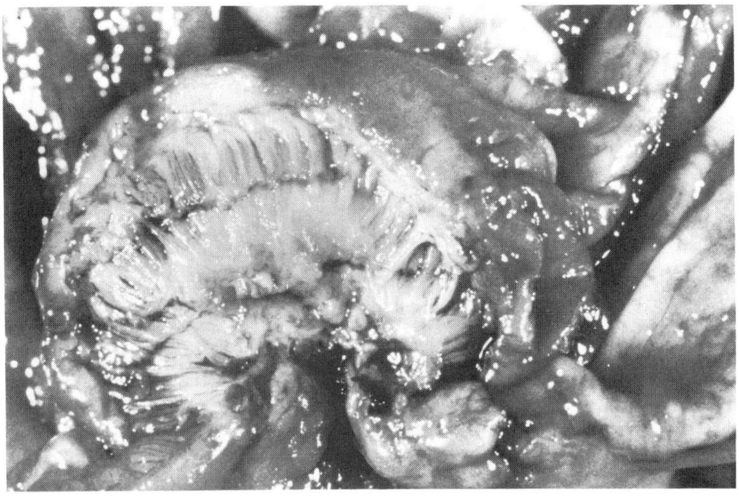

Figure 9–3. Endometriosis of the sigmoid. A mucosa-covered nodule protrudes into the bowel lumen. Most of the thickness of the nodule is due to hypertrophy of muscle. The discolored slits are foci of endometriosis.

involvement is uncommon; therefore bleeding is seen infrequently with endometriosis.

Patients with endometriosis of the large intestine may have a variety of symptoms, including evidence of obstruction, diarrhea, pain, tenderness on palpation, and, occasionally, cyclic rectal pain associated with menses. Examples of endometriosis of the appendix are rarely associated with findings of acute appendicitis, although chronic lower quadrant pain may suggest so-called chronic appendicitis (Uohara and Kobara, 1975).

Besides muscular hypertrophy, endometrial glands accompanied by an identifiable endometrial stroma are present in muscle and serosa, and, rarely, in mucosa (Fig. 9–4). Evidence that these glands participate in the menstrual cycle is the presence of hemosiderin in the glands and the surrounding tissues.

Diverticular disease of the large intestine is important in the discussion of neoplasms not because diverticula are neoplastic but because the sequelae of the diverticular disease may mimic carcinoma. It is estimated that more than a third of patients coming to autopsy have diverticula of the large bowel. In addition, approximately 90 percent of the diverticula involve the sigmoid. Diverticula usually occur along the antimesenteric border of the large intestine (Shindo, 1981). They represent protrusions of the mucosa, submucosa, and the muscularis mucosae through a defect in the muscularis propria caused by penetrating vessels. For all practical purposes, the only time

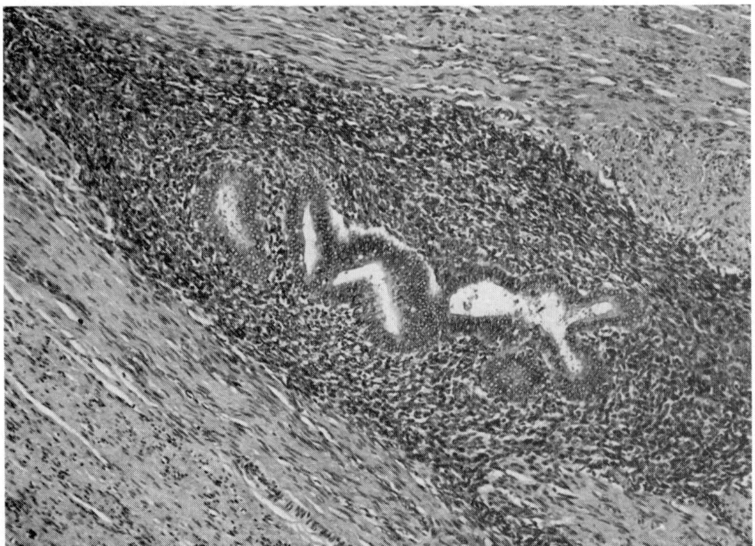

Figure 9–4. Endometrial glands and stroma in the muscularis of the sigmoid colon.

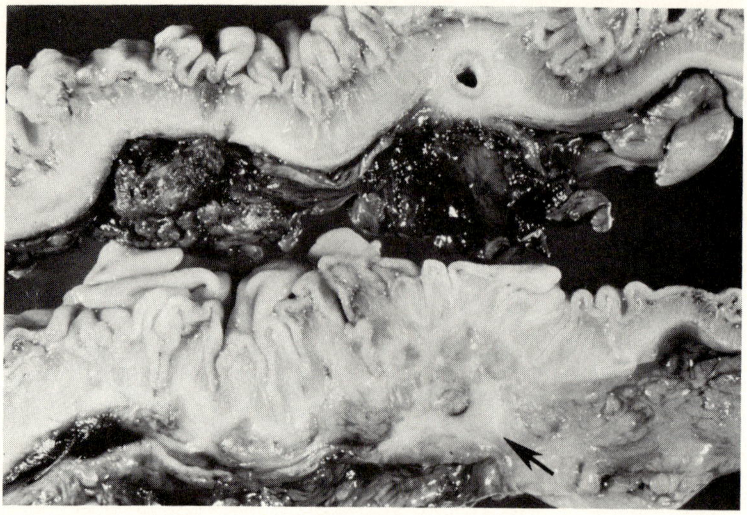

Figure 9–5. Slices of a segment of sigmoid colon removed for diverticular disease. The muscularis is hypertrophied. Diverticula can be seen penetrating the muscularis. A fibrous mass representing diverticulitis is present (arrow).

that diverticular disease is mistaken for carcinoma is when inflammation occurs. Inflammation follows ulceration of the diverticular mucosa and then perforation into pericolic tissue. This results in an inflammatory mass that causes deformity and perhaps constriction of the bowel. It has been observed by Morson (1963) that there is hypertrophy of the muscle in a large number of specimens resected for diverticular disease (Fig. 9–5). Muscular hypertrophy causes remarkable thickening of the wall of the bowel that may present as a constricted zone when seen radiographically or pathologically. Often diverticulosis with muscular thickening is not associated with inflammation. Thus Morson (1963) suggested that, in part, diverticular disease is a dysfunction of the colonic musculature.

Diverticula are not confined to the left side of the colon but may be present in the cecum. Interestingly, in younger patients, diverticula of the right side of the colon are seen more often than those of the left side. Again, these remain asymptomatic unless associated with inflammation or perforation (Shapiro, 1974).

Although carcinoma and diverticula may be seen in the same segment of the large intestine, there seems to be no evidence to suggest that diverticulitis or the presence of diverticula is associated with large-bowel carcinogenesis.

Heterotopic gastric epithelium is rare in the large bowel and rectum. Only a few cases have been reported in patients ranging in age from newborn to middle age. Heterotopic tissues have been associated with a variety of symptoms, including diarrhea and the passing of blood and mucus per rectum. Occasional examples of multiple sites of heterotopic gastric mucosa have been recorded. Because of the symptoms, the occasional ulcer, and the presence of a nodule, these lesions may be mistaken for neoplasms, benign or malignant. Histologically, they should not be confused with neoplasms of the large intestine, as they closely resemble gastric mucosa, usually fundic or pyloric (Wolff, 1971).

A benign lesion that may be mistaken for mucinous carcinoma is colitis cystica profunda. It presents by physical examination or by barium enema study as a polypoid mass of the rectum or sigmoid; at times it is a nondescript mass. The overlying mucosa is intact, and histologically, collections of mucus and proliferating glands in the submucosa form the polypoid mass. These lakes of mucin, shown in small biopsy specimens, have been misinterpreted as evidence of mucinous carcinoma. Colitis cystica profunda may be associated with inflammatory bowel disease. It has been suggested that colitis cystica profunda is a hamartoma, but the consensus is that it is of inflammatory origin. Colitis cystica profunda is most frequently seen in patients in their third, fourth, and fifth decades, although it has been occasionally reported in teenagers (Herman and Nasbeth, 1973; Wayte and Helwig, 1967).

Radiation damage to the large intestine may result in an area of stenosis some months or years after completion of irradiation therapy. The stenotic segments may vary from a few millimeters to 4 to 5 cm in length. The main differential diagnostic problem is related to barium enema studies that show a stenotic segment that mimics carcinoma of the sigmoid or rectum. Often the segments are longer than one would expect for stenosis caused by pri-

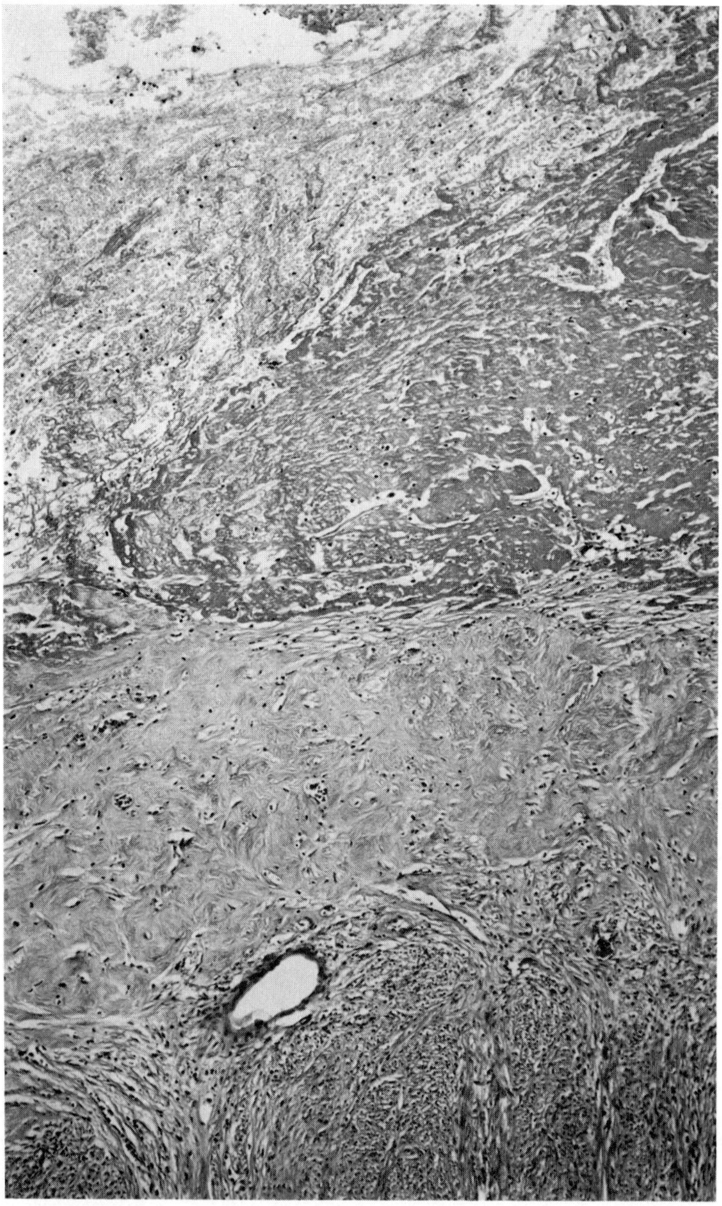

Figure 9–6. Fibrin covers the surface of the sigmoid colon, and there is submucosal fibrosis.

mary carcinoma of the bowel. Radiographically, with radiation damage there is more gradual tapering of the stenosis at the edges than that seen with carcinoma, and there is a lack of sharp demarcation between normal and abnormal bowel segments. These differences help distinguish the two lesions. Grossly, the radiation damage is not likely to be mistaken for carcinoma, as the muscularis propria often remains intact throughout the stenotic and ulcerated zone. In addition, the lesions are flat and do not have the piled-up edges typical of a carcinoma. Histologically, there is ulceration, fibrosis, mucosal atrophy, degenerative changes in the muscularis, inflammation, and varied degrees of vascular damage (Perkins and Spjut, 1962) (Figs. 9–6 and 9–7).

BENIGN NEOPLASTIC DISEASES OF THE LARGE INTESTINE

Epithelial Polyps

One of the most controversial lesions of the large intestine is the "polyp." This has been so especially since Spratt, Ackerman, and Moyer (1958) questioned the relationship be-

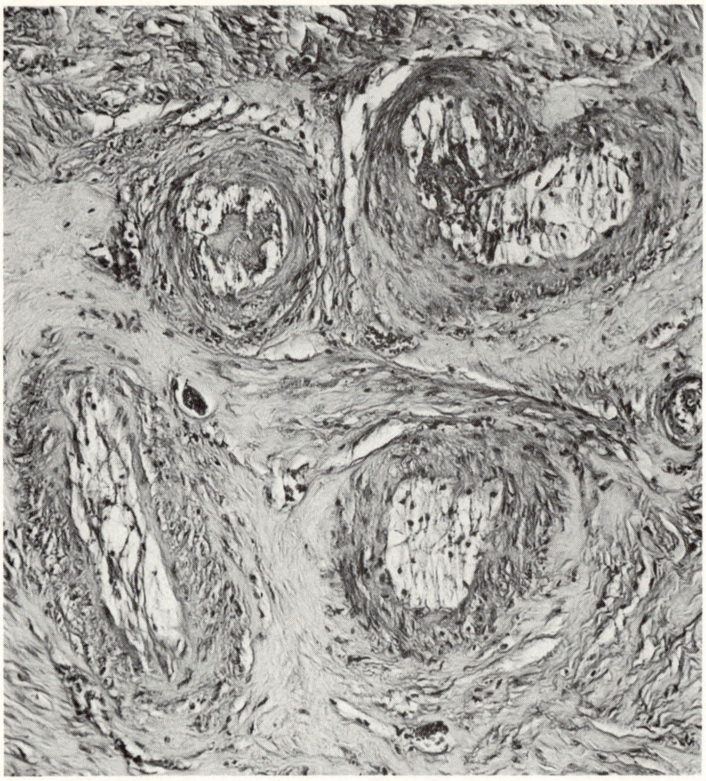

Figure 9–7. Submucosal vessels exhibiting foamy macrophages are often seen as the result of irradiation damage.

tween adenomatous polyps and carcinomas of the large bowel. They doubted there was a relationship, whereas others did not. The controversy is aided and abetted by the poor understanding of just what polyps and, in particular, epithelial polyps, are. A polyp is a mass that protrudes into a lumen. However, in relation to the large bowel, the word polyp is used synonymously with adenomatous polyp. The word is used loosely, and it should be recognized, especially by endoscopists, radiologists and pathologists, that there are many lesions of the large intestine that mimic adenomatous polyps. In order to clarify some of the confusion that surrounds the epithelial polyp, careful definitions by the pathologist of the lesions of the large intestine, especially epithelial polyps, must be adhered to. Among the many lesions that have been designated as polyps of the large intestine, usually endoscopically, are redundant mucosa, granulation tissue, retention polyps, lymphoid nodules, colitis cystica profunda, hemangiomas, lipomas, leiomyomas, carcinoids, and hamartomatous polyps. Many are difficult to identify grossly, and therefore biopsies or excisions are needed. This is also true for epithelial polyps in that polypoid carcinomas, villous tumors, and various types of adenomatous polyps (pure glandular or mixed glandular and villous) are difficult to identify grossly and must be defined histologically. An epithelial polyp that may be diagnosable grossly is the hyperplastic polyp. But even this polyp has variations and therefore cannot always be identified.

Epithelial polyps are distributed widely throughout the large intestine, with the largest concentrations in the rectum and sigmoid (Ekelund, 1974). Villous tumors and hyperplastic polyps have a strong tendency (about 85 percent) to occur in the rectum and sigmoid (Spjut and Estrada, 1977). Epithelial polyps that are purely adenomatous (tubular adenomas) or adenomatous with different degrees of a villous component may be seen throughout the large intestine, but they have a predilection for the sigmoid and rectum (Figs. 9–8 to 9–11).

At times there are gross features that allow one to identify the epithelial polyps, e.g., villous tumors are generally large, often exceeding 3 cm in greatest dimension, broad-based, and frequently multilobulated and possibly villous (Fig. 9–12). However, some villous tumors may be on a stalk and indistinguishable from other types of epithelial polyps.

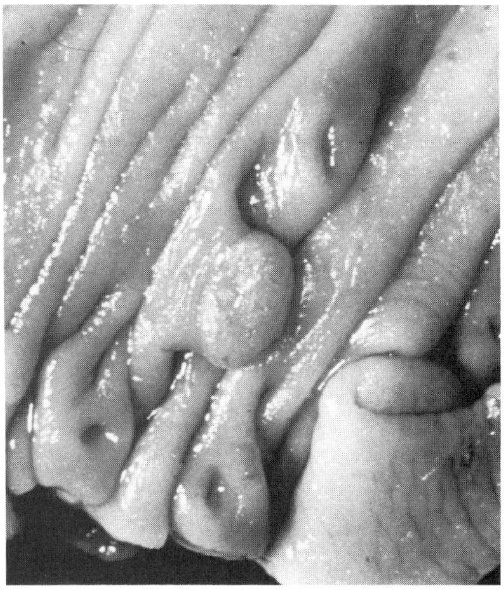

Figure 9–8. A hyperplastic polyp of the sigmoid colon; it measures 7 mm in diameter.

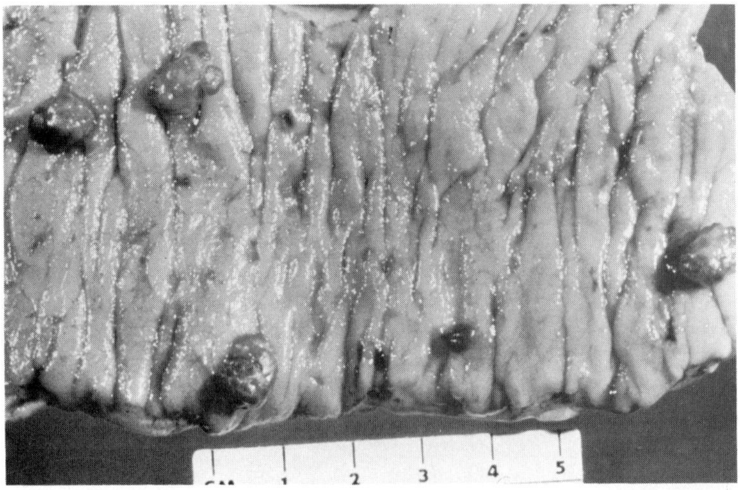

Figure 9–9. Five adenomatous polyps in a segment of large bowel. They vary from 3 to 12 mm in diameter.

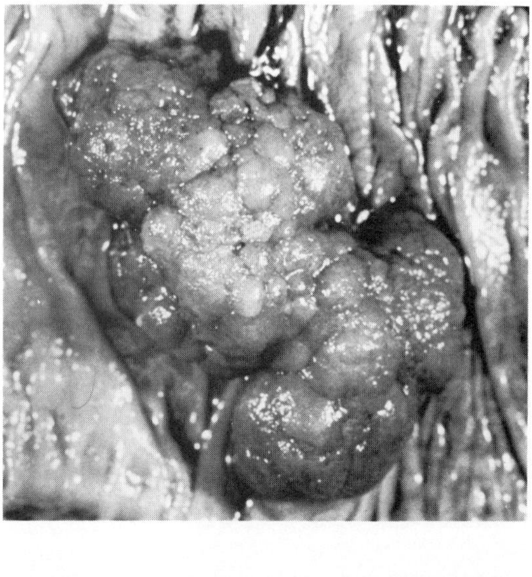

Figure 9–10. A benign villoglandular polyp of the sigmoid colon. It measures 6 cm in greatest dimension and has a broad base.

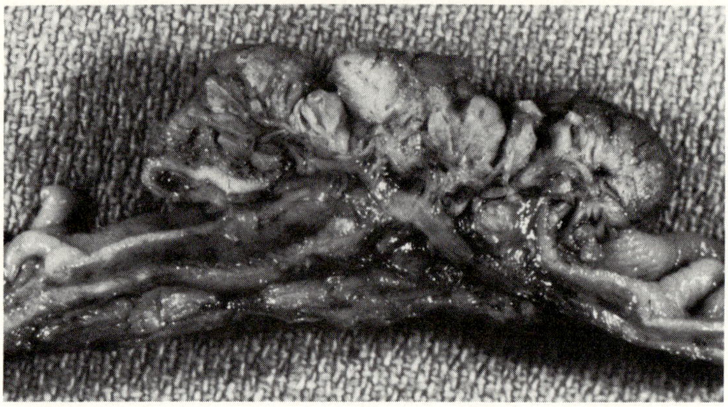

Figure 9–11. A cross-section of the polyp in Figure 9–10 shows a lobate and partly villous pattern.

Generally, hyperplastic polyps are small and broad-based and seldom measure more than 5 mm in their greatest dimension; however, hyperplastic polyps measuring up to 2 cm in greatest dimension and hyperplastic polyps on stalks have been seen (Estrada and Spjut, 1980). A pure adenomatous polyp is indistinguishable from a mixed (villoglandular) polyp grossly. They are both 2 mm to 4.5 cm in size. Because of the overlap in size and gross configuration, epithelial polyps can be distinguished only by biopsy.

Careful histologic definition of epithelial polyps is necessary in order to understand the relationship between carcinomas of the large intestine and epithelial polyps. For example, it is often stated that adenomatous polyps harboring a carcinoma give rise to metastases. However, if one carefully reviews the publications stating this, it becomes apparent from the illustrations that the lesions in question are not adenomatous polyps but villous tumors or adenomatous polyps with a striking villous component (Kraus, 1965; Lane and Kaye, 1967; Shatney, 1974). The pathologist's role in these misinterpretations is well emphasized in a paper written by Castleman and Krickstein (1962) in which a review of carcinomas in situ and carcinomas arising in polyps demonstrated that the majority of these were not carcinomas but adenomatous polyps with different degrees of atypical or dysplastic alterations.

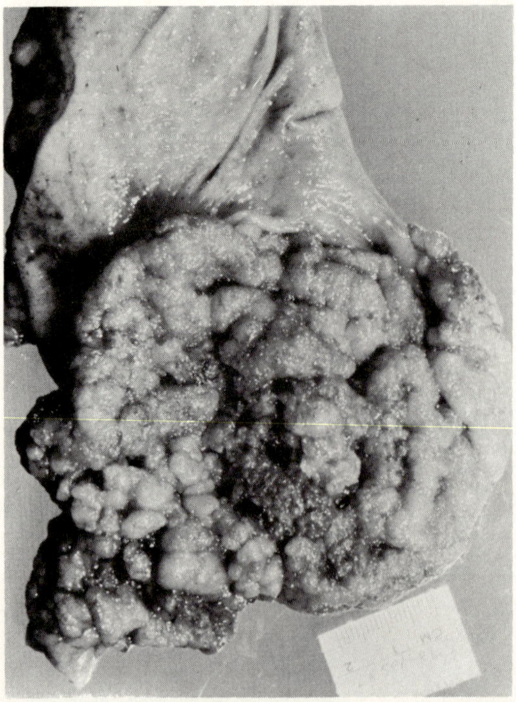

Figure 9–12. A villous tumor of the rectum that measures 11 cm in greatest dimension. Its surface is multilobate.

In order to determine whether a strict definition of epithelial polyps is important, we have reviewed over 800 epithelial polyps removed using the colonoscope or sigmoidoscope or with resected specimens. By defining a pure adenomatous polyp as one composed entirely of glandular elements versus one in which there is a definable villous element, we observed that no carcinomas in situ arose in polyps that were purely glandular. As the estimated villous component increased, so did the risk of finding a carcinoma or a carcinoma in situ in the polyp. The veracity of these findings remains to be proved by repeated studies (Spjut and Estrada, 1977). Others have made similar observations in regard to the villous pattern in epithelial polyps (Kurzon et al., 1974).

Histologically, pure adenomatous polyps consist of glands that are different from the normal colonic epithelial gland in that they have diminished numbers of goblet cells, nuclear stratification, elongation of nuclei (Figs.

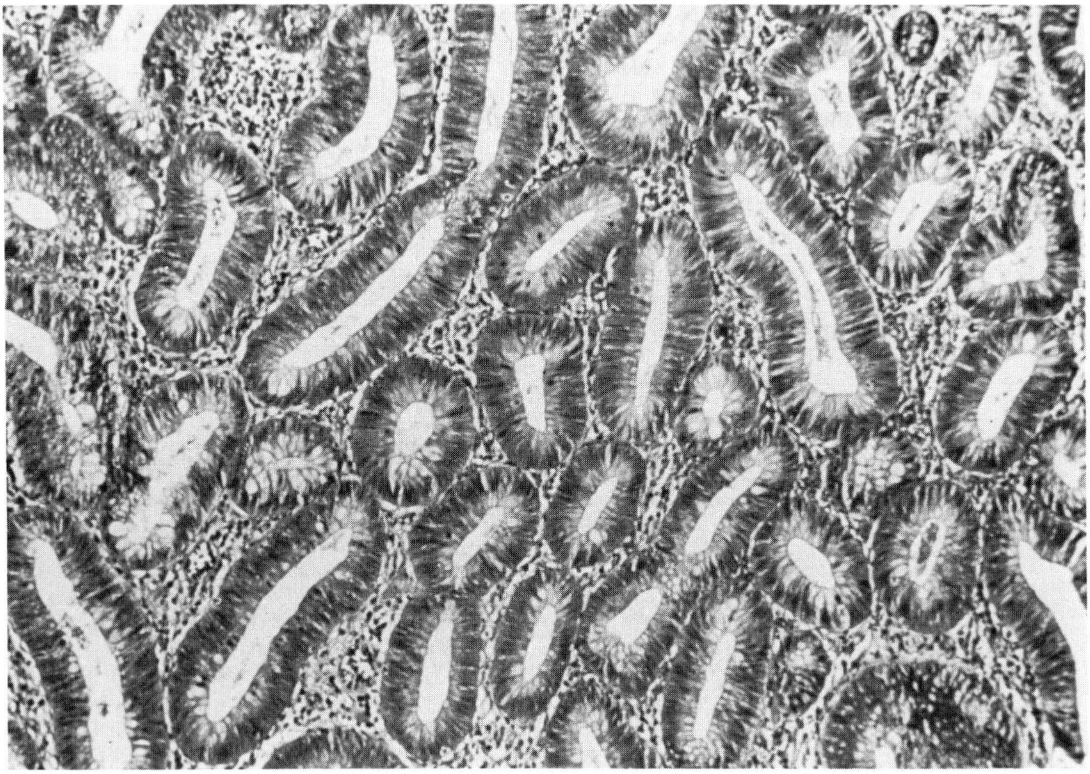

Figure 9–13. A purely glandular (adenomatous) polyp.

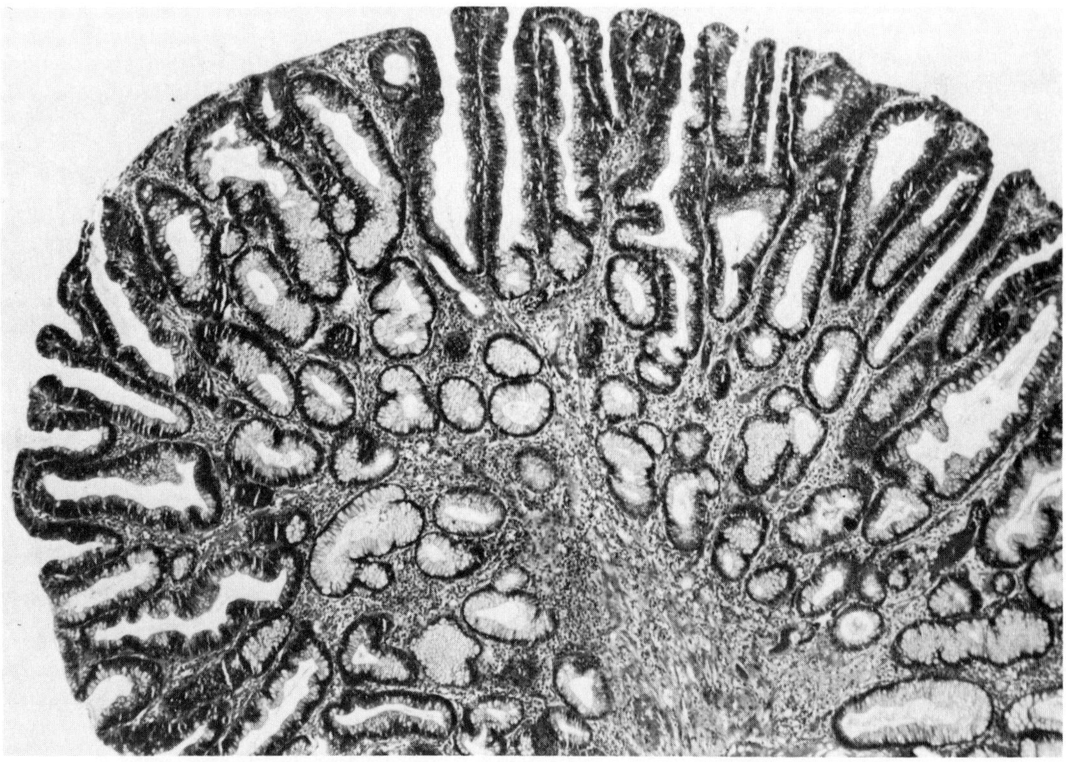

Figure 9–14. An adenomatous polyp with a minor villous component.

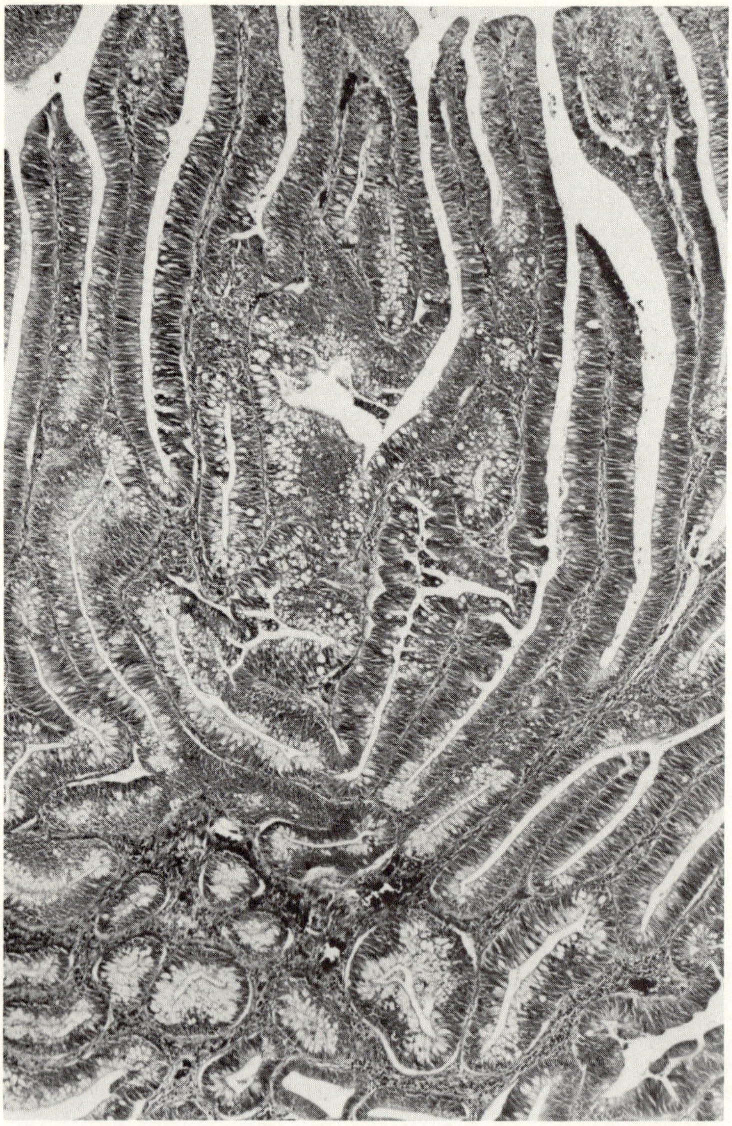

Figure 9–15. An adenomatous polyp with a prominent villous component.

9–13 and 9–14), at times nuclear pleomorphism, and the presence of mitotic figures. The epithelial polyps that contain this glandular component, in addition to villous components, are designated as villoglandular polyps or mixed polyps (Fig. 9–15). The villous component should be truly villous, i.e., having epithelium similar to that of the glands covering a narrow fibrovascular core. The villi should not be merely accentuations of the surface pattern. In general, we have roughly estimated the villous component as a percentage of the surface. If the estimate exceeds 50 percent, these polyps are arbitrarily designated as villous tumors. Degrees of dysplasia (atypia) within the epithelial polyps are recognized, but their significance is not clear. However, Konishi and Morson (1982) state that severe dysplasia in epithelial polyps may be an important marker indicating patients who require careful follow-up. Indications of carcinoma in situ include nuclear pleomorphism, stratification, and mitoses, but more important is the presence of intricate glandular formations with glandular budding and bridging of epithelium (Fig. 9–16). We have not accepted only nuclear alterations as evidence of carcinoma in situ. Invasiveness of the stalk may be difficult to determine. If this is a problem histologically, then step sections through the block must be made to determine whether there is true invasion through the muscularis mucosae or pseudoinvasion (Muto et al., 1973).

There is continuing controversy about the

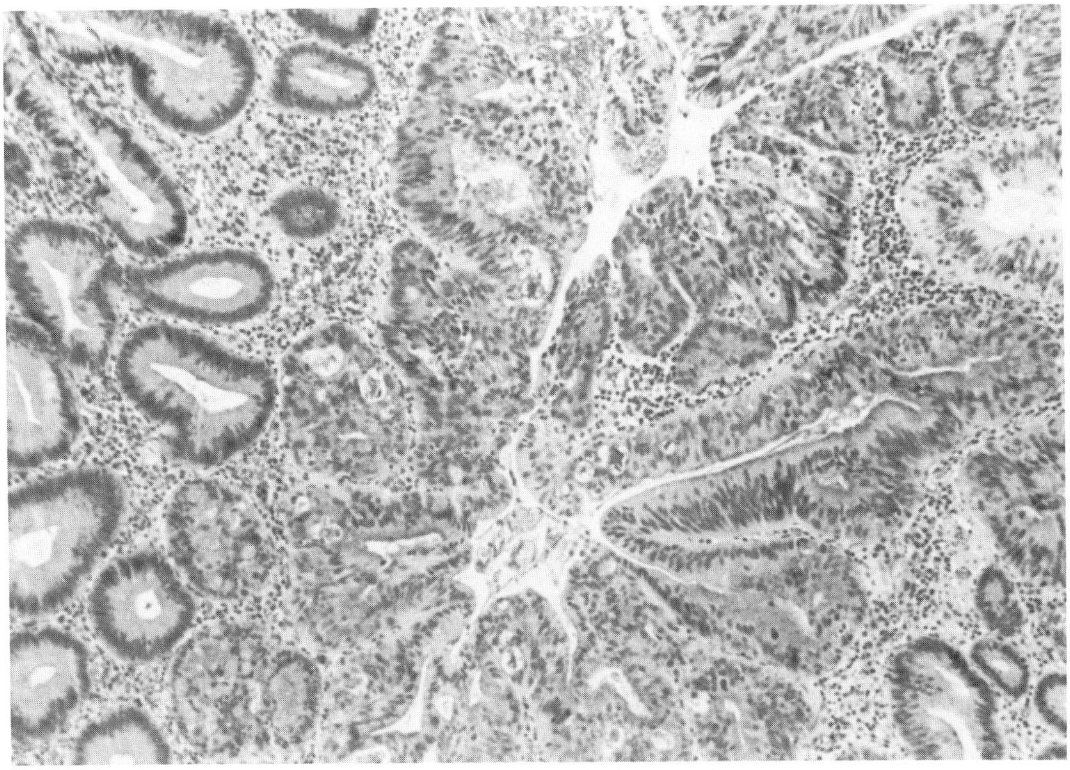

Figure 9–16. Carcinoma in situ arising in a villoglandular (mixed) polyp. Glandular complexity and budding of glands are seen.

role of epithelial polyps in carcinogenesis of the large intestine. The evidence in favor of this relationship includes the polypoid form of some carcinomas, the so-called residual adenomatous polyp seen at the edges of carcinomas, the occurrence of epithelial polyps in the same segment as a carcinoma, the frequent appearance of carcinomas in the most common sites of epithelial polyps, evidence of carcinoma in situ and of carcinomas with metastases residing in recognizable epithelial polyps, and the apparent occurrence of carcinomas in the sites of previously resected epithelial polyps. However, it can be pointed out that there is a more uniform distribution of epithelial polyps in the large bowel than carcinomas. Also, if epithelial polyps are precursors of adenocarcinoma, there should be a widespread distribution of carcinomas of the large bowel in patients with familial polyposis. But, this is not so. Bussey (1975) points out that the location of carcinoma in these patients is essentially identical to that in the general population. For exampe, 53.6 percent of carcinomas occur in the rectum in polyposis patients compared with 57.5 percent in patients who do not have polyposis. As for "residual adenomatous polyps" seen at the edges of large carcinomas, these may be reactive rather than residual. Morson (1966) has stated that 56.6 percent of Dukes' A carcinomas show evidence of preexisting benign tumor. Dukes' A carcinomas are not usually small carcinomas but may measure 5 cm or more in diameter. It seems unreasonable that residual polyps would be found with this frequency and not be seen in small carcinomas, i.e., those 15 mm or less in diameter. A review of small carcinomas measuring less than 15 mm in diameter and many measuring only 5 mm failed to reveal evidence of residual polyps (Spjut et al., 1979). As has been pointed out previously, carcinomas said to arise in "adenomatous polyps" and associated with nodal metastases are not pure adenomatous polyps but either are villous tumors or have a major villous component. Histologic definitions need to be carefully applied, since all epithelial polyps do not seem to have the same potential, i.e., patients with epithelial polyps with villous components seem to be at greater risk for carcinoma in situ or carcinomas than those with pure adenomatous polyps. There are many arguments for and against the polyp-carcinoma sequence, yet the major ques-

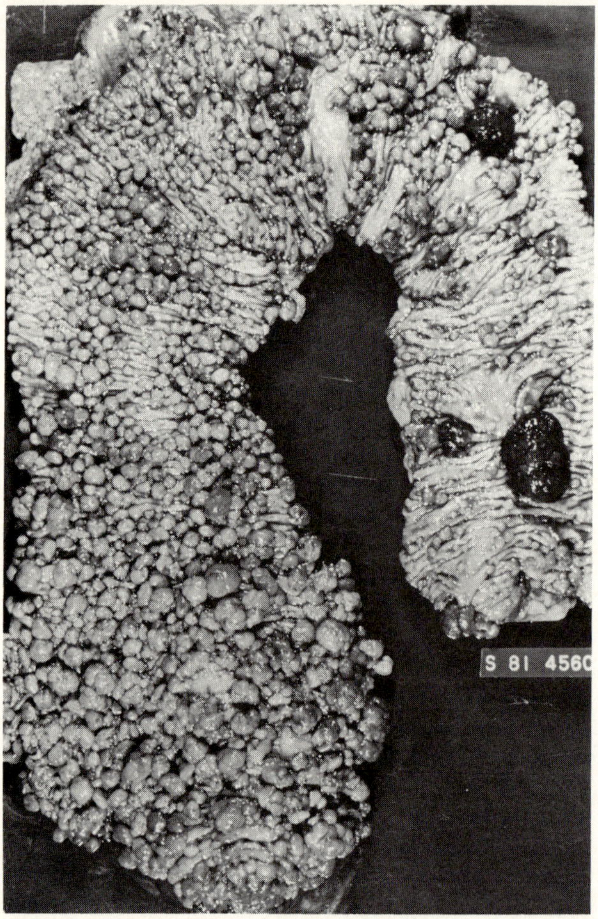

Figure 9–17. The myriad polyps of the large intestine of a 28-year-old man with Gardner's syndrome. Two adenocarcinomas were present (Dukes' B) in the large polyps. Fibromatosis of the mesocolon was diagnosed.

tion is, What is the risk for any given patient who has epithelial polyps of the large intestine of developing a carcinoma? The fact that epithelial polyps and carcinomas occur in the same segment does not mean that the epithelial polyps gave rise to the carcinoma. It may signify that the same etiologic factors that provoked the epithelium to form the carcinoma may have provoked formation of the epithelial polyps. Therefore, epithelial polyps may signify that the patient is at risk for having or developing a carcinoma not that the epithelial polyps will become carcinoma inevitably. Furthermore, there is evidence from studies of small carcinomas of the large bowel that carcinomas do arise de novo from the mucosa (Spjut et al., 1979; Spratt and Ackerman, 1962).

The fact that a myriad of epithelial polyps occur in familial polyposis and other related syndromes with a high risk for carcinoma does not necessarily signify that carcinomas in patients who do not have these genetic diseases arise from epithelial polyps. In a study of many epithelial polyps from patients with familial polyposis and Gardner's syndrome (Fig. 9–17), it was found that there are the same variety of histologic patterns in these disorders as are found in patients with sporadic occurrence of epithelial polyps or multiple epithelial polyps. Further discussion of the polyposis syndromes is found in Chapter Three.

The hyperplastic polyp is often stated to be the most common of the epithelial polypoid lesions of the large intestine. This may be true; however, if one considers polyp size, that is, adenomatous polyps or hyperplastic polyps measuring less than 3 mm in greatest dimension, then the number of hyperplastic and adenomatous polyps is about equal in biopsy material (Estrada and Spjut, 1980). Nevertheless, hyperplastic polyps are usually small, that is, less than 5 mm in diameter, and are nearly always sessile. In our studies, we have found that approximately 3 percent of hyperplastic polyps have a distinct stalk. In addition, they may measure as much as 2 cm in their greatest dimension. About 13 percent of hyperplastic polyps have an adenomatous component. The significance is not evident. In general, it is accepted that hyperplastic polyps bear no relationship to the genesis of carcinoma of the large intestine (Estrada and Spjut, 1980). Hyperplastic polyps are apparently the result of overgrowth of mature columnar and goblet cells secondary to slow cell migration from the crypts to the surface epithelium. Typically, the glands have a serrate luminal configuration, with the cytoplasm being acidophilic. The nuclei remain at the base of the cells (Fig. 9–18).

Nine to 15 percent of epithelial polyps of the large bowel are villous tumors (papillary adenoma), with 75 percent or more occurring in the left side. Villous tumors are often the largest of the epithelial polyps, but because of overlap of measurements, diagnosis cannot always be made on this basis alone. In Shinya and Wolff's (1979) study of 519 villous tumors, 230 measured 2 cm or more in greatest dimension. Spjut and Estrada (1977) noted a size range of 0.6 cm to 8.5 cm among 123 villous tumors.

Grossly, villous tumors are multilobate, tan-pink, broad-based, and often soft. Only occasionally are they pedunculated. They do not generally appear villous (Fig. 9–19); this is a microscopic feature. In the examination of the specimen or, for that matter, of the lesion in situ, firm areas, ulceration (not from biopsy), and fixation of the tumor to the muscularis propria are features that suggest an accompanying carcinoma. Grossly, one would not expect to see carcinoma in situ.

Microscopically, villous tumors have an abundance of fingerlike projections (villi) associated with a few glands (Fig. 9–20). At least 50 percent of an epithelial polyp should be villous before it is designated as a villous tumor. Villi should be slender and epithelium covered and have a fibrovascular core. The nuclei are elongated, with stratification; goblet cells are scarce. Various degrees of atypia may be present, indicated by nuclear pleomorphism, mitotic figures, nuclear enlargement, and prominent nucleoli. If the tumors also have epithelial bridging and glandular budding confined to the mucosal component of the tumor, the lesion can be designated as a villous tumor with carcinoma in situ. However, the line dividing severe dysplasia from carcinoma in situ is vague, if existing at all.

The histologic differentiation of villous tu-

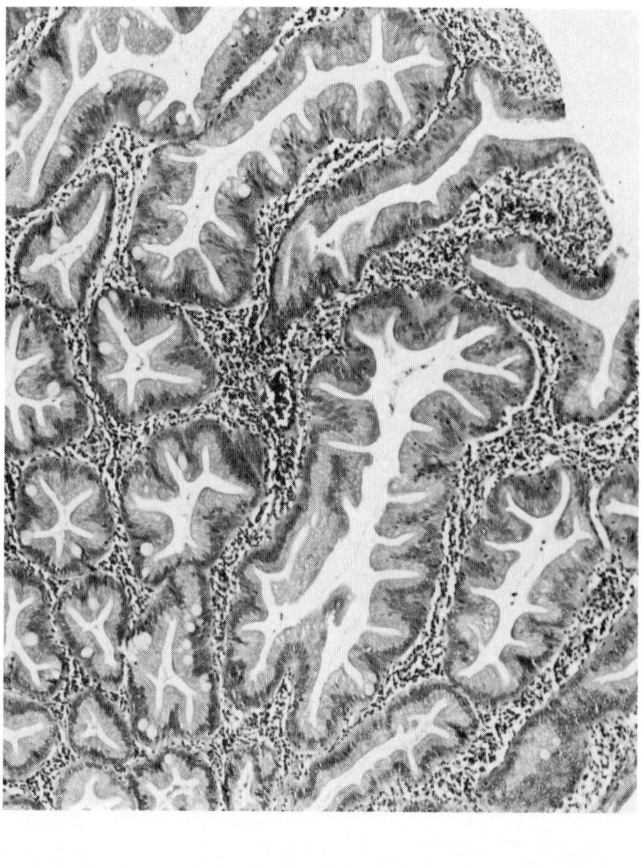

Figure 9–18. A characteristic hyperplastic polyp showing few goblet cells, fairly dense cytoplasm, and serrate luminal configuration.

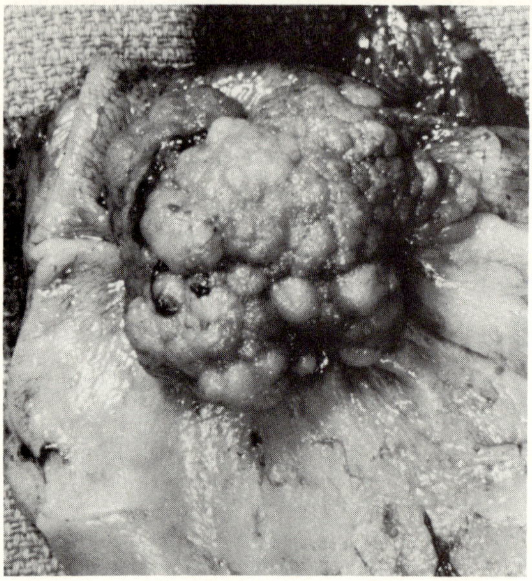

Figure 9–19. A villous tumor measuring 4.5 cm in greatest dimension. Histologically it contained an invasive carcinoma, but this was not apparent from the outer surface.

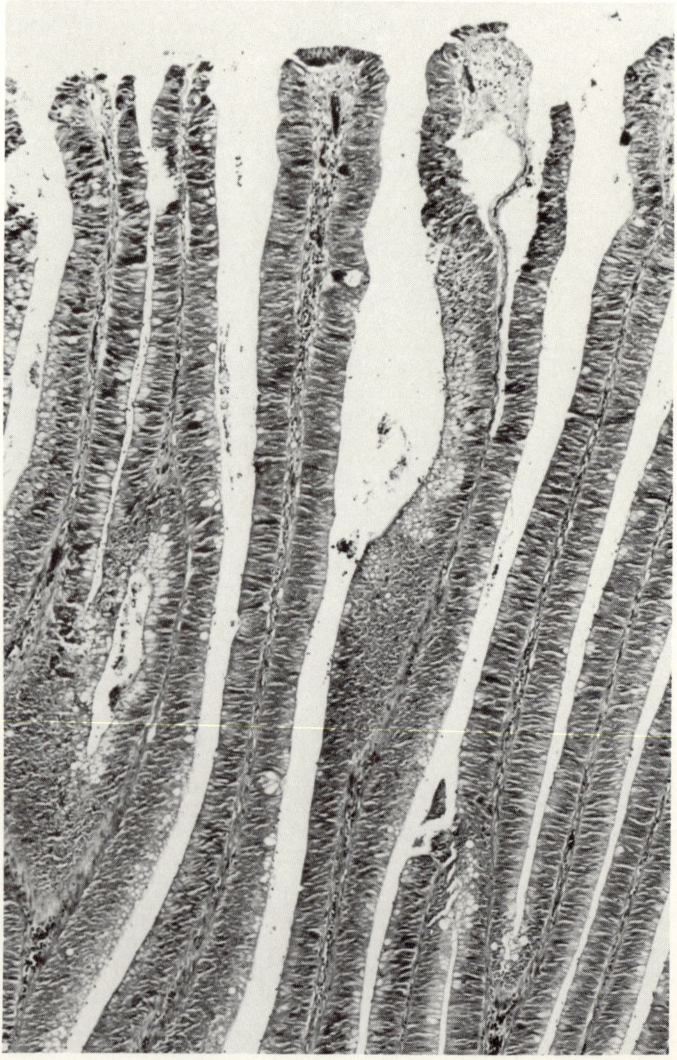

Figure 9–20. Villous tumor showing slender villi, with the epithelium exhibiting nuclear stratification and only sparse goblet cells.

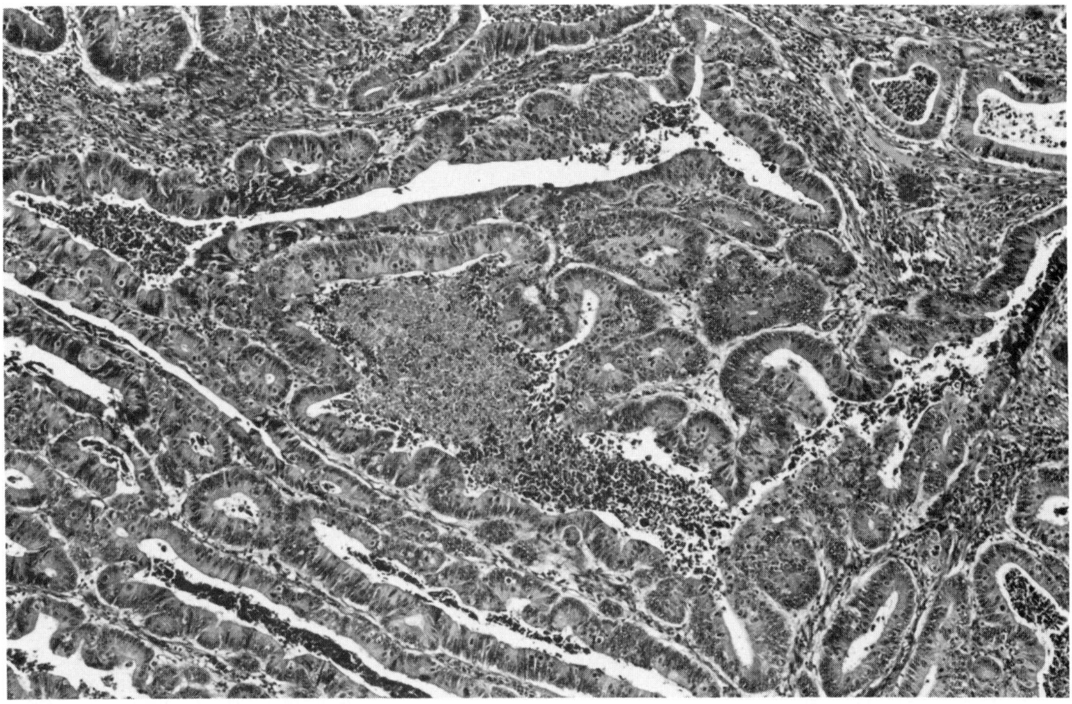

Figure 9–21. A well-differentiated adenocarcinoma in a villous tumor. Necrosis of the tumor is seen in the center.

mors from other epithelial polyps has a practical purpose because of the known risk of malignancy. In a study of 519 villous tumors, Shinya and Wolff (1979) observed that 15 percent were carcinomas in situ and 10 percent were invasive carcinomas. In our own study of 123 villous tumors, 6 percent were carcinomas in situ and 8 percent were invasive carcinomas (Spjut and Estrada, 1977) (Fig. 9–21).

Other Benign Tumors

Hamartomatous polyps may be found in the large intestine and are frequently associated with Peutz-Jeghers syndrome. Occasionally they seem to arise sporadically without clinical or physical evidence of Peutz-Jeghers syndrome. The polyps may be large, measuring up to 4 to 5 cm in their greatest dimension. Histologically, they are similar to the hamartomatous polyps found in the upper gastrointestinal tract. There is a proliferation of the colonic mucosa, which is often demarcated by slender "fingers" of smooth muscle. The mucosal glands may be somewhat distorted and abundant.

Hemangiomas of the large bowel are concentrated in the sigmoid and rectum. Only rarely are they found in other portions. They may be diffuse, forming what seems to be a thickened wall, but with an intact mucosa (Fig. 9–22). Hemangiomas may be polypoid also. Grossly, the lesions may present as bright red or blue-red spots or elevations. As would be expected, when a hemangioma is biopsied, bleeding might be profuse. Histologically, hemangiomas usually have large, thin-walled veins with areas of smaller vessels (Allred and Spencer, 1974; Bell et al., 1972).

Lymphangiomas of the large bowel occur less frequently than hemangiomas, with only some 20 examples reported. They present as smooth polypoid lesions. Patients may have diarrhea and bleeding. Histologically, lymphangiomas are composed of thin-walled lymphatic channels that are free of blood (Camilleri et al., 1982).

Lipomas are considered to be among the most common of the nonepithelial benign tumors of the large bowel. The majority occur in the region of the cecum or ileocecal valve, with only a scattered few appearing beyond the ascending colon (Fig. 9–23). Their importance lies in the fact that radiographically and clinically they can be mistaken for carcinomas or epithelial polyps, which can at times result in a major surgical procedure. In addition, lipomas may be the source of bleeding and may serve as a point for intussusception.

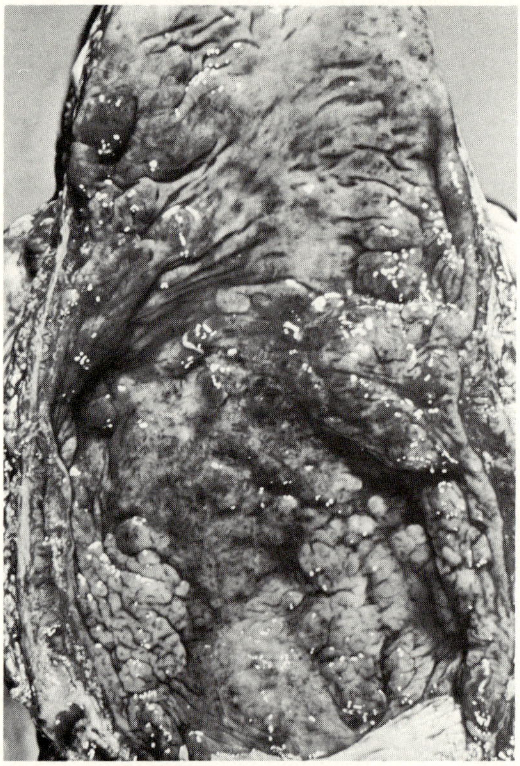

Figure 9–22. A rectal hemangioma that presents a thickened raised but visibly intact mucosa. The dark areas of the mucosa define the extent of the lesion. This occurred in a 45-year-old man who had rectal bleeding for years.

Grossly, a lipoma may be polypoid or merely an elevation of the mucosa and may measure up to 6 cm in its greatest dimension. The overlying mucosa is frequently intact but may be ulcerated. Histologically, lipomas consist of mature adult fat that is mainly submucosal and may extend into the muscularis propria. The mucosa is often thinned (Ginzburg et al., 1958; Haller and Roberts, 1964).

Leiomyomas are frequently encountered in the large intestine, but in contrast to lipomas, most are located in the rectum and sigmoid. In one group of 28 leiomyomas of the large intestine, 19 were found in the rectum (Quan and Berg, 1962). They may present as a smooth nodular mass or a polypoid mass in the rectum. They may be ulcerated (Fig. 9–24). Leiomyomas may be a cause of rectal bleeding and constipation. Grossly, leiomyomas are submucosal, often with an intact mucosal covering. Leiomyomas are well circumscribed and may vary from 10 mm to 5 cm in size. Histologically, they contain intertwining bundles of smooth muscle cells, without nuclear atypia or mitotic figures. Ordinarily, it is possible to trace the transition between the smooth muscle of the muscularis mucosae or muscularis propria and the leiomyoma. Only rarely do leiomyomas recur after adequate excision.

Occasional solitary neurilemmomas, neurofibromas, and ganglioneuromas have been reported in the large intestine. The tumors are usually submucosal and may result in intestinal obstruction. Histologically, neurilemmomas and neurofibromas have the same pattern as those located in the skin, that is, the spindle cells with tight fascicles of nuclei often associated with areas of degeneration. Ganglioneu-

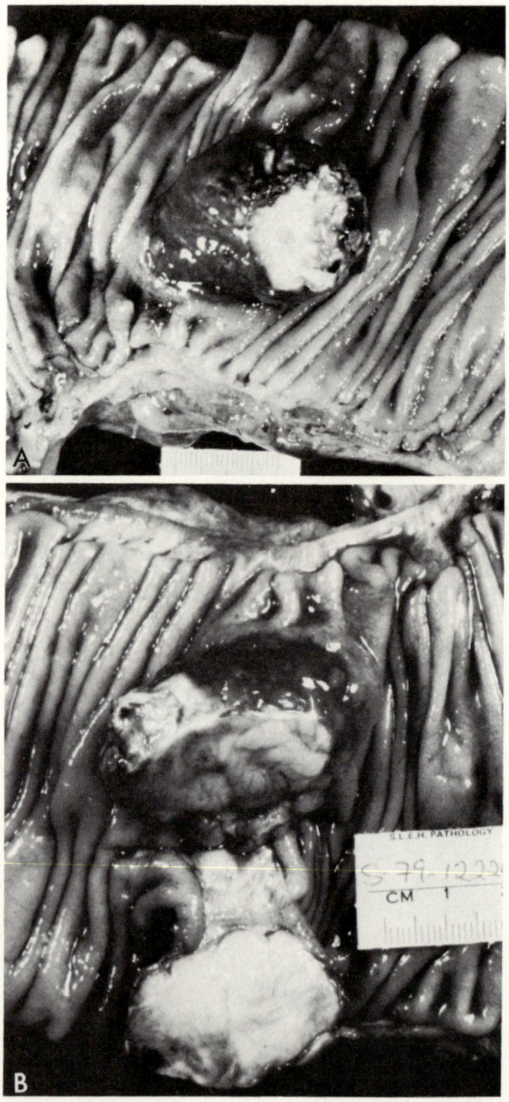

Figure 9–23. *A* and *B*, A lipoma of the ascending colon, with surface ulceration (white area). Cut surface shows lobular fat.

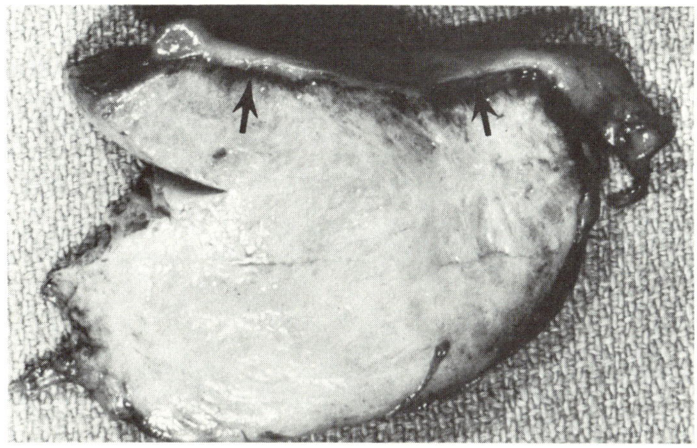

Figure 9–24. Leiomyoma of the rectum. The mucosa is intact (arrow). The tumor measures 10 cm in greatest dimension, has a gray-white cut surface, and is well circumscribed. The patient was a 19-year-old woman.

romas have a similar histologic pattern, but ganglion cells are a prominent characteristic. Any of these neurogenic tumors may involve the muscularis propria and extend to and through the serosa (Bibro et al., 1980; Doyle et al., 1968; Raszkowski and Hufner, 1971). Multiple ganglioneuromas and plexiform neurofibromas are often associated with neurofibromatosis.

The most common site of granular cell tumors (myoblastomas) in the gastrointestinal tract is the esophagus. However, they do occur in the large intestine. Johnston and Helwig (1981) reported 32, with 11 in the rectum, 12 in the cecum, and the others scattered in the large bowel. The tumors are submucosal nodules that are histologically similar to granular cell tumors of the skin.

Lymphoid nodules (hyperplasia) are most commonly found in the rectum; only rarely are they found in other portions of the large intestine. For the most part they are solitary, raised nodules and vary in size from 3 mm to 1.5 cm. Occasionally they may be multiple. In one series, some 22 percent of the patients had two or more polypoid lymphoid lesions. Most of the lesions are sessile but approximately 20 percent may be pedunculated. Occasionally they are ulcerated, giving rise to rectal bleeding. A variety of diagnoses are suggested from the clinical appearance of the lymphoid hyperplasia: hemorrhoid, polyp, lymphoma, carcinoma, inflammation. Polyp seems to be the commonest clinical diagnosis. A few examples of multiple diffuse nodular lymphoid hyperplasia of the large intestine have been described. Most occur in children. Frequently, radiographic studies indicate that these patients have multiple familial polyposis or some other syndrome associated with polyposis (Edelman and Sternberg, 1977; Franken, 1970).

Grossly, the lesions are smooth, rounded, brown to gray-brown, and, for the most part, mucosal. However, they can also be submucosal and occasionally involve the muscularis propria. The cut surfaces are homogeneous and moist and suggest lymphoid tissue. Histologically, the lesions consist of lymphoid tissue in which the germinal centers are readily identified. The major histologic differential diagnosis is that of malignant lymphoma. If germinal centers are identified, the lesion is lymphoid hyperplasia rather than a malignant lymphoma (Fig. 9–25). One must take care to differentiate lymphoid hyperplasia from nodular lymphoma; this may be difficult with small biopsy specimens. The etiology of lymphoid hyperplasia remains unknown; however, most observers believe that it represents an inflammatory response. There does not appear to be an association between lymphoid hyperplasia and the development of a malignant lymphoma.

Various degrees of dysplasia (atypical hyperplasia) and carcinoma in situ may occur in the large intestine. Generally these lesions are associated with epithelial polyps. Isolated dysplastic glands are occasionally found in normal or granular-appearing colonic mucosa from specimens resected for carcinoma (Lewin et al., 1978). Dysplastic alterations in normal-appearing colonic mucosa are common in familial polyposis (Bussey, 1975). In addition, it is well known that dysplastic alterations occur in the large bowel of patients having inflammatory bowel disease.

The significance of these dysplastic changes and carcinoma in situ in epithelial polyps is

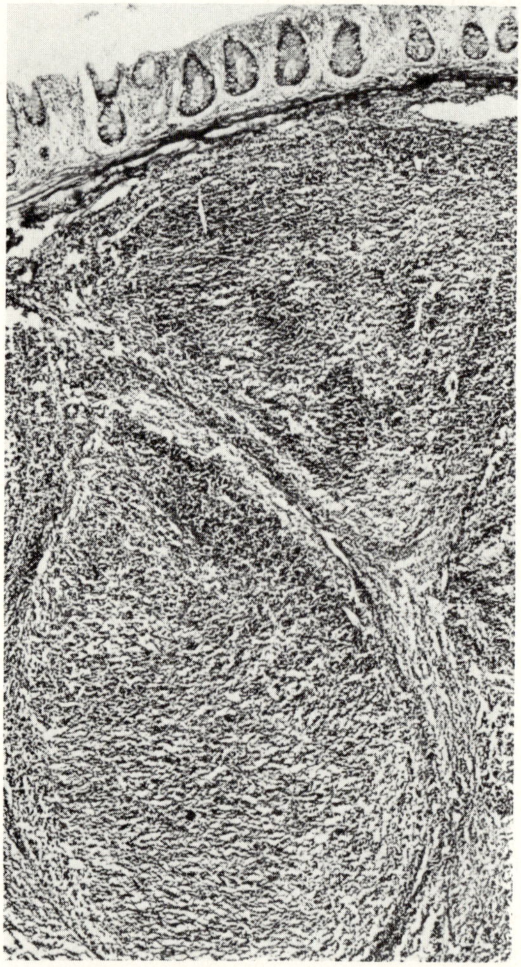

Figure 9–25. A lymphoid nodule of the rectum shows a large germinal center.

not entirely clear. It seems reasonable, however, to assume that in the genesis of adenocarcinoma of the large intestine a series of dysplastic alterations of different degrees of severity and carcinoma in situ precede invasive carcinoma. Both of these could take place in the normal-appearing mucosa or in epithelial polyps. This sequence of events is difficult to prove, although dysplastic changes and carcinoma in situ have been seen in epithelial polyps and colonic mucosa of rats that have received carcinogens, e.g., dimethylhydrazine. Transition from the lesions to carcinoma has not been demonstrated and some believe that carcinomas may arise de novo but Madara and associates (1983) have demonstrated that at least some carcinomas in rats apparently arise from pre-existing adenomas. The fact that the stepwise genesis of adenocarcinoma of the large bowel has not been observed does not contradict this theory; however, it will be difficult to prove pathologically.

Although the relationship of carcinoma in situ in an epithelial polyp to adenocarcinoma remains unclear, if carcinoma in situ is clearly demonstrated histologically, there are certain treatment implications. With carcinoma in situ, there will probably not be any metastases to lymph nodes or evidence of vascular dissemination. Thus, in a polypectomy specimen in which carcinoma in situ has been diagnosed, removal of the polyp is sufficient treatment for that form of carcinoma. However, if carcinoma is present at the line of resection, the chance of residual carcinoma in the resection specimen is increased. Otherwise, resection of a portion of colon is not indicated (Lipper et al., 1983). It has been suggested that individuals with carcinoma in situ are at risk for associated invasive carcinoma or for the development of an invasive carcinoma in the future; this has implications for patient follow-up (Kalus, 1972).

MALIGNANT NEOPLASTIC DISEASES OF THE LARGE INTESTINE

Carcinomas

Carcinomas of the large intestine occur in different sizes and shapes; they vary in size from a few millimeters to several centimeters. If one was to classify adenocarcinomas on the basis of their gross characteristics, they could be characterized as polypoid, ulcerative, bulky, or circumscribing. The most common form of carcinoma of the large intestine is the ulcerative lesion with raised, somewhat lobate margins. Frequently carcinoma occupies a major portion of the circumference of the segment involved. If one excludes villous tumors, polypoid carcinomas are uncommon. Bulky lesions have the reputation for occurring in the right side of the colon, but they are not exclusive to that site. The same could be said for circumscribing lesions, which reputedly occur most frequently in the left side of the colon. However, as more and more carcinomas are observed, it is apparent that there are probably no characteristic features of carcinomas occurring in either the right half or the left half of the large intestine (Gellhoed and Crossland, 1981). Circumscribing lesions are seen in the cecum and ascending colon, although perhaps a little more commonly in the left side of the colon. However, bulky lesions are seen in the

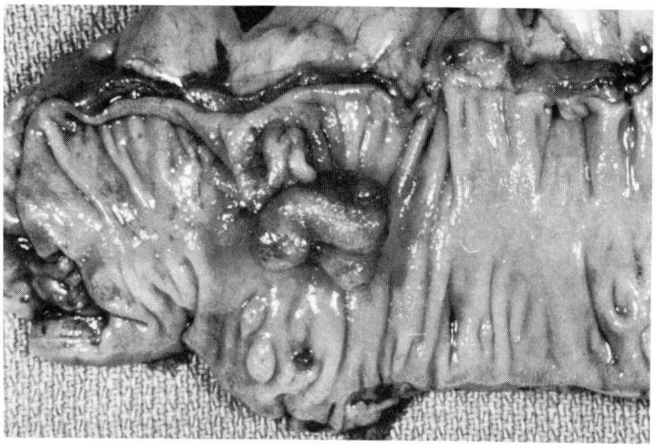

Figure 9–26. A polypoid carcinoma of the sigmoid. It measured 22 mm in greatest dimension. There was no invasion into the muscularis, and the nodes were negative for metastases.

rectum or sigmoid but are perhaps found a little more frequently in the cecum and ascending colon. In other words, no general conclusions can be made about carcinomas of the large intestine in regard to their segmental location (Figs. 9–26 to 9–30).

Because of the varied gross morphologic features of carcinomas, it is easy to understand why the diagnosis of large intestinal carcinoma is difficult radiographically. As is indicated previously in this chapter, there are many lesions that mimic the patterns of large intestinal carcinoma, leading to difficulties in diagnosis. On the other hand, carcinomas may simulate other neoplastic and non-neoplastic diseases of the large bowel. Consequently, biopsy is an important definitive diagnostic procedure in patients suspected of having large intestinal carcinomas.

It is well known that most large intestinal carcinomas occur in the rectum and the rectosigmoidal and sigmoidal areas. In fact, the incidence of large intestinal carcinomas has been reported as high as 80 percent, with an average generally above 65 percent, in these sites (Spratt et al., 1958; Welch and Burke, 1962). In recent years it has been noted that an increasing number of carcinomas are occurring in the right half of the colon, although the majority still arise in the left half of the large intestine (Abrams and Reines, 1979; Snyder et al., 1977). We have made similar observations in regard to epithelial polyps of the large intestine, that is, in follow-up of patients who have had previous removal of polyps, the additional polyps found in follow-up of the patient were more likely to occur beyond the splenic flexure than in the original location of the polyps (Spjut and Appel, 1979). Explanations for the change in location of large intestinal carcinomas in polyps are not apparent. However, with the introduction of the colonoscope, tumors not diagnosed by barium enema study are being found in the right colon. Whether this "shift to the right" is real or simply a perception based on selection bias is yet to be determined.

Synchronous carcinomas of the large intestine occur relatively frequently. They were found in 1.5 to over 6 percent of resected specimens (Snyder et al., 1977). Often the second or third carcinoma is not detected until the specimen is examined (Fig. 9–31). They have the same gross and histologic characteristics as the primarily detected carcinoma. As a result of such procedures as colonoscopy, the diagnosis of synchronous carcinomas has increased, and carcinomas are being found in new locations in the large intestine. Thus it would seem reasonable that all patients who have carcinoma of the large intestine for which resection is proposed should have a colonoscopic examination in order to detect other lesions, particularly second carcinomas.

More than 95 percent of carcinomas of the large intestine are adenocarcinomas. A few adenosquamous carcinomas and squamous carcinomas have been described. About 80 percent of adenocarcinomas are differentiated to the point that easily recognizable tubular formations are identified. Undifferentiated carcinomas are those in which there is no discernible gland formation; about 11 percent of carcinomas are undifferentiated. The remainder are mucinous, adenosquamous, or squamous. Histologically, there are no features specifically diagnostic of adenocarcinoma of the large bowel. The glands may be ovoid to rounded. Papillary structures may be present. Small islands of mucin production are often seen, but unless these make up about 60 percent of the tumor, the carcinoma is not classi-

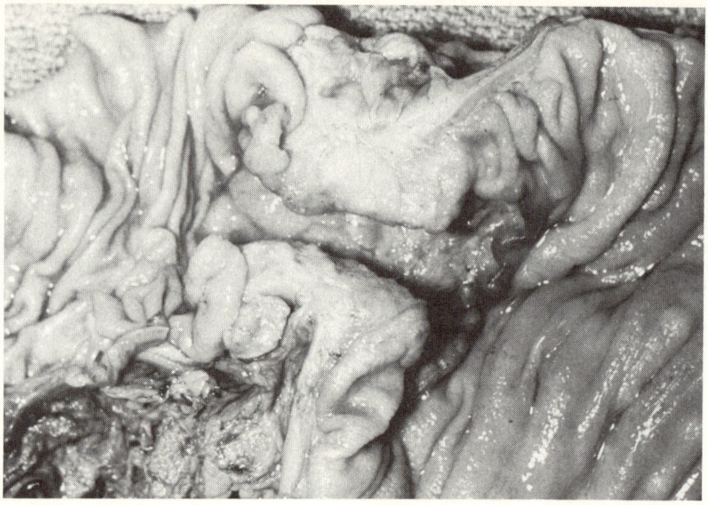

Figure 9–27. Adenocarcinoma of the descending colon. The carcinoma constricts the bowel wall, appears ulcerated, and has raised margins. The cut surfaces show invasion through the muscularis propria, with kinking of the bowel wall.

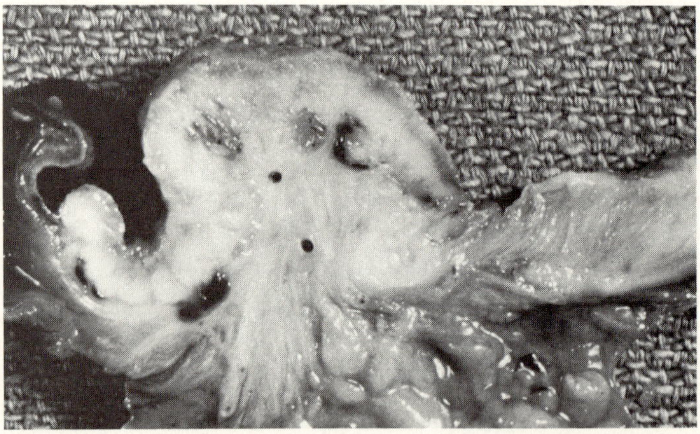

Figure 9–28. A raised adenocarcinoma of the cecum, with obliteration of the muscularis propria. Pericecal fat is drawn into the tumor. The regional lymph nodes were free of metastases.

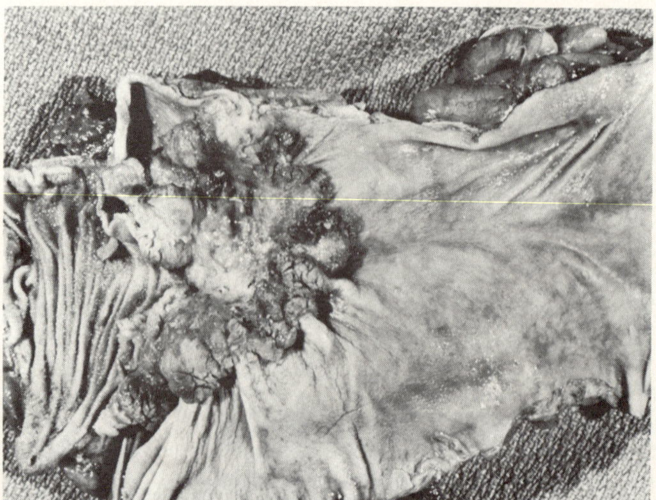

Figure 9–29. Adenocarcinoma of the ascending colon. The tumor is raised but not especially bulky.

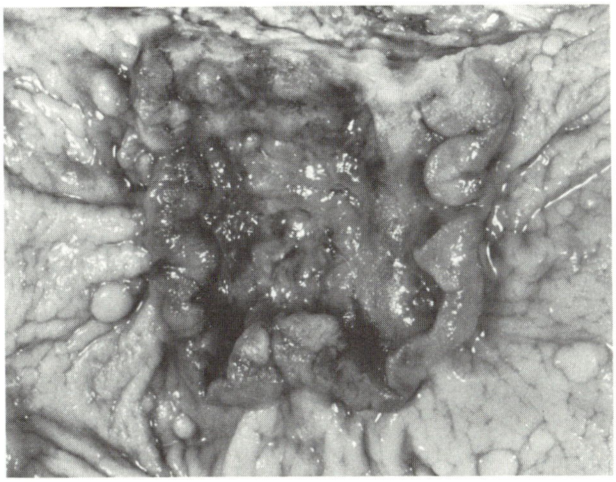

Figure 9–30. Rectal adenocarcinoma 2 cm above the dentate line. The margins are raised, and the carcinoma is ulcerated.

fied as mucinous. Special stains for mucins will show intracytoplasmic mucin and intraglandular mucin. Malignant cells are positive for CEA. Undifferentiated carcinoma does not form glandular structures, is richly cellular, and often exhibits considerable necrosis. Rarely lakes of mucin are found in undifferentiated carcinoma, which in reality indicates an attempt at differentiation. Occasionally, undifferentiated carcinoma is found in a villous tumor. Using the electron microscope, Hickey and Seiler (1981) reported characteristics of adenocarcinoma of the large bowel that are quite distinctive. These include microvilli with dense cores of microfilaments, electron-dense bodies in the apex of the cells, and numerous glycocalyceal bodies.

The prognosis of carcinoma of the large bowel relates to many factors. A time-tested guide to prognosis is the Dukes classification, which is based upon histologic findings. Dukes' classification was originally limited to rectal carcinomas, but it was eventually applied to large bowel carcinomas and other gastrointestinal carcinomas. The classification is based upon pathologic examination of resected specimens (Dukes, 1932):

Dukes' A. Carcinoma is confined to the bowel wall and has not penetrated the muscularis propria.

B. Carcinoma extends through the entire bowel wall and serosa if present.

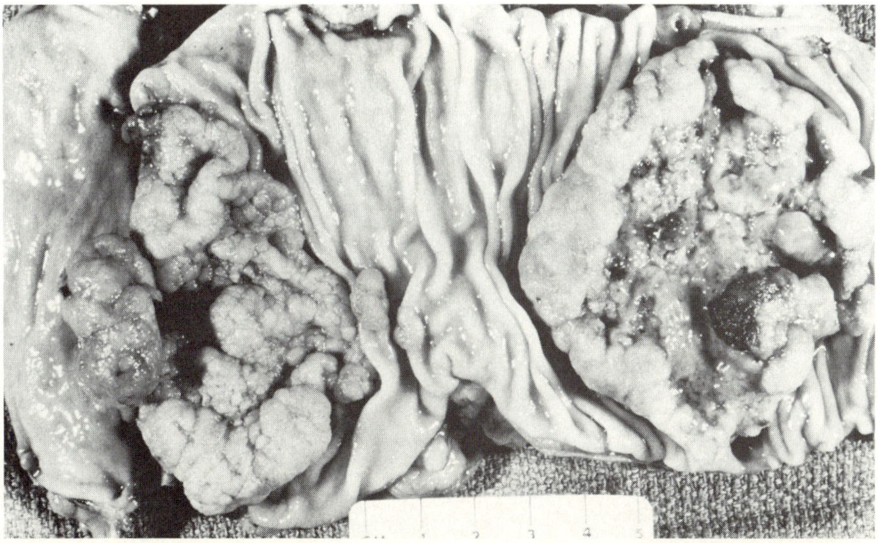

Figure 9–31. Synchronous carcinomas of the sigmoid colon of a 44-year-old woman. Metastases to regional lymph nodes were found.

C. A or B with metastases to lymph nodes.

The classification has been modified to make it more accurate in terms of prognosis (Astler and Coller, 1954):

A. Carcinoma confined to the mucosa; nodes are negative.
B1. Carcinoma into the bowel wall but not through it; nodes are negative.
B2. Carcinoma extends through the bowel wall; nodes are negative.
B3. Carcinoma invades or is adherent to surrounding structures or organs; nodes are negative.
C1. Carcinoma limited to the bowel wall; nodes are positive.
C2. Carcinoma extends through the bowel wall; nodes are positive.
C3. Carcinoma is adherent to or invasive of adjacent structures or organs; nodes are positive.

Many other characteristics of cancer relate to prognosis; pushing or infiltrative margins (Fig. 9–32), differentiation of the carcinoma to some extent, presence or absence of inflammation around the edges of the carcinoma, vascular invasion, and perineural invasion (Spratt and Spjut, 1967). Margins, poor differentiation, minimal or no inflammation around the advancing margin of the tumor, and presence of perineural and vascular invasion all contribute to a poor prognosis. In regard to vascular invasion, Talbot and associates (1981) have noted that with extramural vein invasion, a 33 percent 5-year survival rate can be expected, but with intramural vein invasion a 60 percent 5-year survival rate is attained. Similarly there is a greater chance of hepatic metastases with extramural than with intramural venous invasion.

There are other lesions that mimic adenocarcinoma of the large intestine, particularly on biopsy. These include carcinoids of the rectum; invasive adenocarcinomas from the prostate, ovary, or uterus; and metastases from other adenocarcinomas within the abdomen, e.g., the stomach. Electron microscopy is useful to differentiate metastatic or invasive lesions from primary carcinomas of the large intestine; special stains for silver-positive granules may be used in the case of carcinoids; and immunopathologic stains may aid in the differentiation of adenocarcinoma of the prostate from adenocarcinoma of the large intestine.

Metastases from carcinomas of the colon and the rectum have a fairly similar distribution. There are some variations. For example, approximately 48 percent of carcinomas from

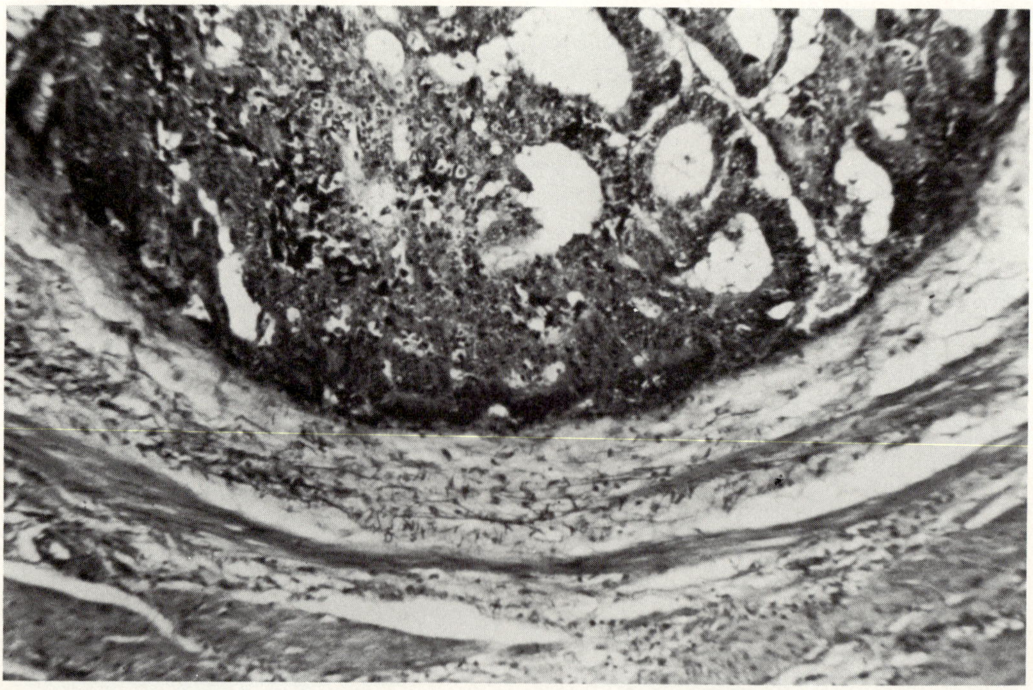

Figure 9–32. Pushing margin of an adenocarcinoma of the sigmoid. The advancing edge of the tumor is rounded; the smooth muscle fibers conform to this contour.

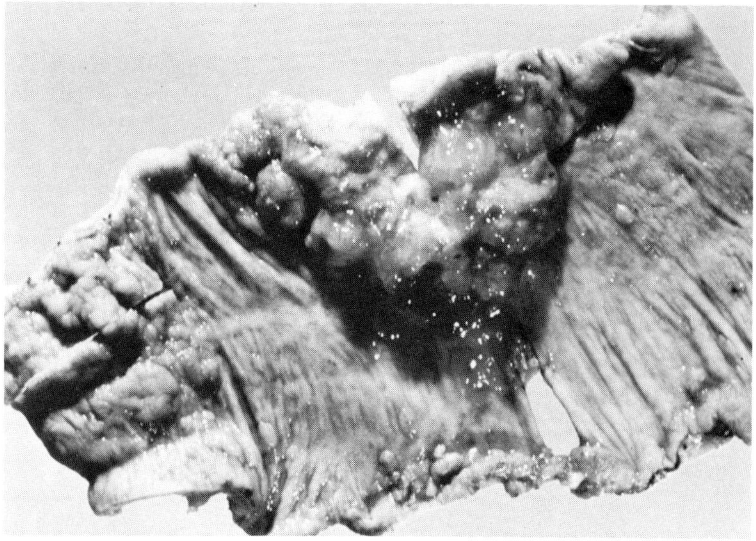

Figure 9–33. A mucinous carcinoma in a patient with a quiescent chronic ulcerative colitis. The patient was a 28-year-old woman who had suffered chronic ulcerative colitis for more than 10 years. There were no nodal metastases.

the colon have metastases to the lung, whereas 64 percent of rectal carcinomas have pulmonary metastases. Likewise, skeletal metastases are more common from rectal carcinomas than from colonic carcinomas. However, metastases to the liver occur in approximately 76 percent of patients with colonic carcinomas and 62 percent of patients with rectal carcinomas. Peritoneal metastases occur in 49 percent of patients with colonic carcinomas and 25 percent of patients with rectal carcinomas. As would be expected, nodal metastases are similar in both locations. In the autopsy series from which the preceding figures were taken, 77 percent of patients with colonic carcinoma had nodal metastases and 78 percent of patients with rectal carcinomas had nodal metastases. There is widespread distribution of metastases to various organs and structures of the body. The sites of metastases described previously are the most common (Berge et al., 1973).

It has long been recognized that carcinoma may be a complication of inflammatory bowel disease, particularly chronic ulcerative colitis. In general, carcinoma of the large intestine occurs earlier in patients who have inflammatory bowel disease than in patients who do not. Patients with carcinoma and inflammatory bowel disease have not fared well. Consequently, a means of predicting or detecting carcinomas in these patients has been sought. Random biopsies of the colon have revealed histologic lesions designated as "precancer" dysplasia or atypical hyperplasia. It was observed that dysplastic changes present in the mucosal glands of the biopsies were predictive of a higher risk for cancer than if the changes were absent. Histologically, these changes consist of nuclear pleomorphism, mitotic activity, and irregularity of glandular shape and size (Myrvold et al., 1974). Minor changes are not predictive, but those that are severe or border on glandular carcinoma in situ are of significance (Dobbins, 1977). Recently, Blackstone and associates (1981) reported that the occurrence of dysplasia with an associated mass, such as a plaquelike lesion or a polypoid mass, was most significant; seven of 12 patients with this condition had carcinomas, whereas only one of 27 patients with dysplasia in a flat mucosa had carcinoma. Dysplastic lesions occur also in Crohn's disease of the colon, but it is not clear whether their significance is the same as that of lesions in chronic ulcerative colitis (Craft et al., 1981).

Carcinoma occurs in patients with chronic ulcerative colitis more frequently than in patients at large. The frequency varies from less than 1 percent to 14 percent (Budd and Fink, 1981). Butt and Morson (1981) reported a 2 percent frequency and were uncertain whether Crohn's disease of the large bowel increases the risk for carcinoma. The carcinomas vary from vague plaques to tumors with characteristics of adenocarcinoma of the conventional type (Fig. 9–33). They may be multiple; eight of 37 patients in one study had two or more carcinomas (Farmer et al., 1971). There seems to be a tendency for a more random distribution of these carcinomas than occurs in the conventional form of adenocarcinoma. Even in those series with carcinomas clustered in the rectosigmoidal area, there are a large number of carcinomas in the right half of the colon (Farmer et al., 1971; Hulten et al., 1979; Thorlakson, 1956).

Histologically, the carcinomas of patients with ulcerative colitis are similar to those in the noncolitic patient. In one study of patients 40 years of age or less there was a predominance of mucinous carcinomas (Hultén et al., 1979). Rarely, other malignancies are associated with inflammatory bowel disease, e.g., Kaposi's sarcoma and adenosquamous carcinoma (Aldersberg, 1970; Patterson, 1973).

Of the variants of adenocarcinoma, mucinous carcinomas occur most frequently, representing 4.5 percent to 50 percent of adenocarcinomas. Generally, the number of mucinous carcinomas falls into the range of 4.5 to 12 percent. The discrepancy undoubtedly is related to the definition of mucinous carcinoma. Our definition is similar to that of Symonds and Vickery (1976), who defined it as a carcinoma that is 60 percent mucinous. Two varieties of mucinous carcinoma are identifiable. The most common type consists of large lakes of mucin, with clusters and strands of neoplastic epithelial cells floating in the

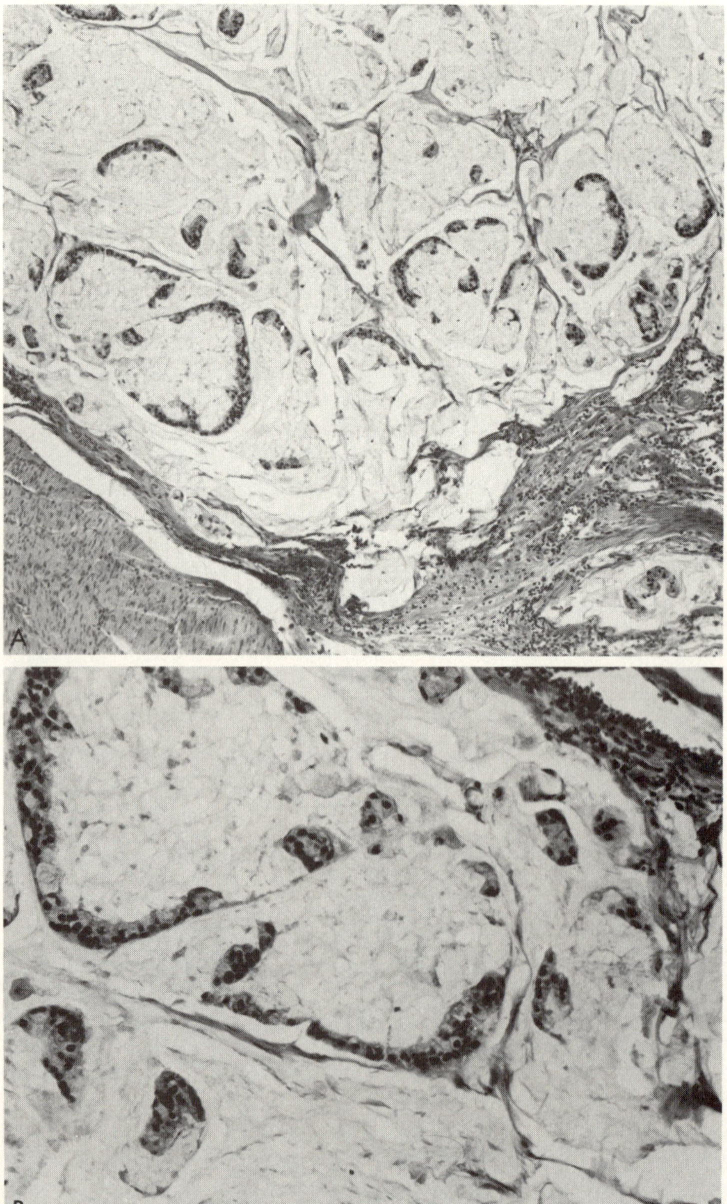

Figure 9–34. *A* and *B*, Mucinous carcinoma in which malignant epithelium lies in pools of mucin.

mucin or at the edges of the mucinous components (Fig. 9–34). The second form is signet ring cell carcinoma, which is poorly differentiated and often diffusely infiltrative.

Patients having mucinous carcinomas of the large intestine suffer the same symptoms as do patients with conventional carcinomas; bleeding is the commonest symptom. Constipation, loose bowel movements, or alternating diarrhea and constipation may plague these patients. Occasionally, a slimy discharge on the stools is noted. This has been recorded in 36 percent of patients in one series (Symonds and Vickery, 1976).

The location of mucinous carcinomas is similar to that of conventional adenocarcinomas of the large intestine. Approximately 60 percent of mucinous carcinomas are found in the rectum and sigmoid. However, mucinous carcinomas make up a large percentage of carcinomas of the cecum and ascending colon. Symonds and Vickery (1976) noted that 22 percent of cecal adenocarcinomas and 23 percent of ascending colonic carcinomas were mucinous. Grossly, mucinous carcinoma may be indistinguishable from the conventional adenocarcinoma. It may cause stenosis of the bowel or present as a bulky mass. Often the cut surface has a shiny, gray, gelatinous mucinous appearance, particularly when the carcinoma is extensive.

Linitis plastica of the rectum may result from diffuse infiltration by signet ring cells (Mathews, 1982). Linitis plastica of the colon is more likely to occur at a younger age and is less likely to metastasize to the liver than conventional adenocarcinoma. It also has a poorer prognosis than conventional adenocarcinoma (Amorn and Knight, 1978). Histologically, mucinous carcinomas are frequently associated with a villous component (Fig. 9–35), and this type of carcinoma is commonly associated with villous tumors. Sundblad and Paz (1982) observed a rather frequent association between villous adenomas, mixed villous adenomas, and tubular adenomas, and mucinous carcinomas. Not only did they find more epithelial polyps in other segments of the large bowel when compared with conventional carcinomas, but mucinous carcinomas apparently arose in villous and mixed adenomas in 11 of 44 cases.

An interesting feature of mucinous carcinoma is that there is usually little reaction by the invaded tissue, there being some fibrosis and little or no inflammation. This is in contrast to adenocarcinoma, in which there is frequently an inflammatory infiltrate associated with the advancing tumor margins. In mucinous carcinoma, the extracellular mucin stains positively with different stains for mucin, whereas the epithelial component often stains poorly. This is in contrast to signet ring cell carcinoma, in which the cytoplasm stains strongly for mucin. As with other carcinomas of the large intestine, the majority of mucinous carcinomas are Dukes' B or C.

The significance of mucinous carcinomas is that, in general, patients with this condition have a poorer prognosis than those with conventional adenocarcinomas. In a large series reviewed by Symonds and Vickery (1976), the 5-year survival rate for patients with mucinous carcinomas was 34 percent compared with 53 percent for patients with nonmucinous adenocarcinomas. Those with carcinomas located in the rectum have a poorer prognosis than those with carcinomas in other sites. Patients having signet ring cell carcinomas of the large intestine have a particularly poor prognosis, with the expected 5-year survival rate being very near zero. Fortunately, these carcinomas make up a small percentage of carcinomas of the large intestine.

Mucinous carcinomas have been described in one cancer family (Budd and Fink, 1981). Mucoid colonic carcinoma is considered an autosomal-dominant inherited syndrome. Of 14 family members with mucoid carcinoma, five have survived.

An interesting aspect of mucinous carcinomas is that they occur more frequently in the younger age group, accounting for a large proportion of carcinomas of the large intestine in patients in the first four decades of life. The number decreases in frequency in the third to fourth decades. In one group of 16 patients, 12 had mucinous carcinomas, with the majority having the signet ring cell variety. The distribution of metastases with mucinous carcinomas is similar to that of conventional adenocarcinomas; regional lymph nodes are the most frequent site of metastases. Dissemination may occur with peritoneal seeding, and distant metastases have been recorded.

Adenoacanthoma and squamous cell carcinoma are rare carcinomas of the lage bowel. Perhaps a better name for adenoacanthoma is adenosquamous carcinoma (Fig. 9–36). Some 50 cases of adenosquamous carcinoma have been reported; the location in the large bowel is similar to adenocarcinomas, with the majority localized in the sigmoid. Grossly, the lesions are not distinctive, with most being ul-

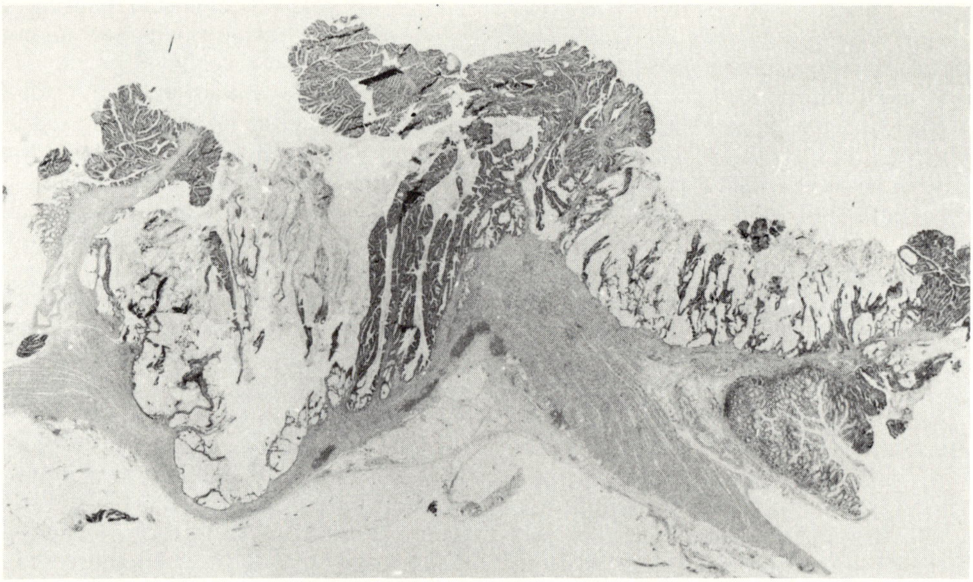

Figure 9–35. A whole-mount section of a mucinous carcinoma of the large intestine. It is associated with a well-differentiated adenocarcinoma. Note that there is no inflammatory response to the invasive margins of the tumor.

cerated and occasional ones polypoid. Squamous cell carcinomas of the large intestine, of which there are 17 reported cases, are most commonly found in the cecum; grossly, they are usually ulcerative and infiltrative (Pittella and Torres, 1982). Those occurring in the rectum must be distinguished from squamous cell carcinomas of the anus. Adenosquamous carcinoma has been known to complicate chronic ulcerative colitis.

Histologically, squamous cell carcinoma of the large intestine is similar to a squamous cell carcinoma seen elsewhere. Adenosquamous carcinoma, as the name suggests, is a combination of identifiable adenocarcinoma and a squamous component that is histologically malignant. Occasionally tumors are seen in which the squamous component appears to be benign. These lesions are probably better designated as adenocarcinoma with squamous metaplasia, although the term adenoacanthoma is often applied. The biologic behavior of adenosquamous and squamous cell carcinomas is difficult to determine simply because there are so few cases. However, a collected series from the Mayo Clinic indicates that the 5-year survival rate is considerably less for these carcinomas than for conventional adenocarcinoma (Comer et al., 1971). A reason for this can be related to a study made by Berg and Goodwin (1974) in which nearly 40 percent of the patients with adenosquamous and squamous cell carcinomas had distant spread compared with 22 percent of patients with conventional adenocarcinoma at the time of treatment. The frequency of metastases to regional lymph nodes was similar. Rare examples of basaloid carcinomas of the sigmoid colon have been reported. Histologically, they are similar to those of the anus. (Craggs and Toker, 1982).

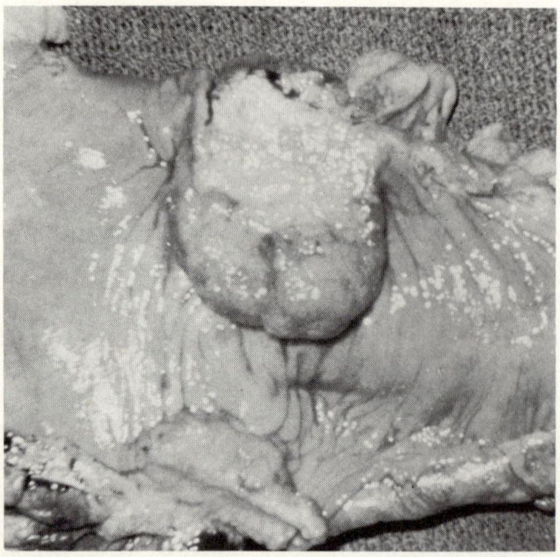

Figure 9–36. An adenoacanthoma of the large bowel. The tumor is polypoid, and the mucosa appears intact.

Lymphomas

When compared with primary carcinomas, malignant lymphomas of the gastrointestinal tract are uncommon, and in the gastrointestinal tract, one of the least common sites for primary lymphoma is the large intestine. Approximately 10 percent of gastrointestinal lymphomas occur in the large intestine. In children, most of the intestinal lymphomas that occur are found in the ileocecal region. Most lymphomas occur in the cecum and right side of the colon. The remainder are scattered in other parts of the bowel. However, in one collected series, 44 lymphomas of the rectum were reported. Grossly, malignant lymphomas present varied patterns; some are polypoid some stenotic, and others ulcerated. Occasionally, they may be multiple, and examples of multiple polypoid lymphomas throughout the large intestine have been recorded (Fig. 9–37). Histologically, the mucosa, submucosa, and often the muscularis propria are replaced by the lymphoma. Even though these lesions are often ulcerated, the mucosa in portions of the lesion that are not ulcerated remains intact, although at times attenuated. Histologically, the majority are histiocytic lymphomas of the diffuse type. Diffuse lymphocytic lymphomas of different degrees of differentiation are the next most common type of lymphoma. Nodular lymphomas may occur but are less common than diffuse forms. Hodgkin's disease is distinctly rare. Symptoms associated with lymphomas of the large intestine include abdominal pain, diarrhea, nausea, vomiting, weight

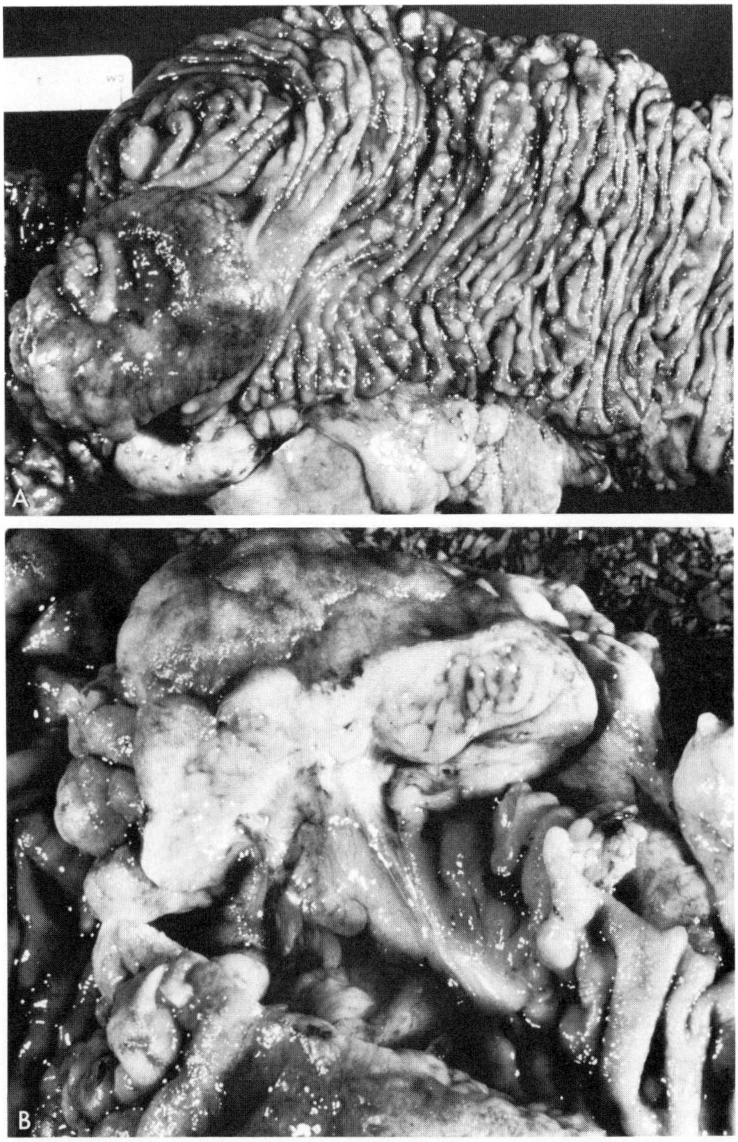

Figure 9–37. *A* and *B*, A polypoid malignant lymphoma (mixed histiocytic), with numerous lymphoid nodules. The cut surfaces show a somewhat lobular homogeneous surface. The patient was a 57-year-old man.

loss, and bleeding. Bleeding is the most common symptom. Thus, in general, the symptoms do not differ from those associated with adenocarcinomas of the large bowel, but constipation generally is not a feature. Occasionally, malignant lymphomas of the large bowel will be associated with chronic ulcerative colitis.

It has been demonstrated that there is no relationship between the histologic pattern of lymphoma of the large bowel and the expected survival rate. In general, the survival rates are fairly similar for lymphoma in all areas of the gastrointestinal tract; for example, the 2-year survival rate for lymphoma in the stomach is 55 percent and that for lymphoma in the large intestine is 38 percent (Culp and Hill, 1962; Jenkin et al., 1969; Lewin et al., 1978; Wychulis et al., 1966).

Sarcomas

Sarcomas of the large intestine are rare, with leiomyosarcomas occurring most frequently. Even so, there are only some 40 known leiomyosarcomas of the large bowel, and interestingly, they are more common than leiomyomas. Rare fibrosarcomas have occurred in the rectum, presenting as submucosal or polypoid masses (Russell and Hughes, 1964). Pararectal rhabdomyosarcomas presenting in adults and children have been described (Sasajiima et al., 1980). Patients having sarcomas of the large intestine present with symptoms similar to those of adenocarcinoma. The distribution of sarcomas is random throughout the large intestine. From the gross appearance, these lesions are often bulky and may be ulcerated (Fig. 9–38). A few may be polypoid or diffusely infiltrative. Histologically, the sarcomas are similar to soft tissue sarcomas. The histologic pattern of leiomyosarcomas in regard to pleomorphism is not necessarily correlated with the behavior of the lesions (Fig. 9–39). As with leiomyosarcomas located in other parts of the body, the mitotic figures give some indication as to the expected behavior of the lesions (Lev and Grover, 1981).

Hemangiopericytomas rarely arise in the large intestine. They may present as red, sessile, polypoid masses. They have the same histologic and electron microscopic characteristics as those that occur in the soft tissue (Genter et al., 1982).

Kaposi's sarcoma involves the intestinal tract as well as the large intestine. Ordinarily Kaposi's sarcoma is considered a systemic disease, frequently involving the skin. Occasionally, the first manifestations of this tumor suggest gastrointestinal disease. It has been reported that patients with Kaposi's sarcoma have been considered to have colitis. Grossly, the lesions may be nodular and appear to be mucosa-covered, although they may be ulcerated. Histologically, Kaposi's sarcoma is frequently confined to the mucosa and submucosa. The familiar spindle cell pattern, with slits containing red blood cells, is present. The lesion may

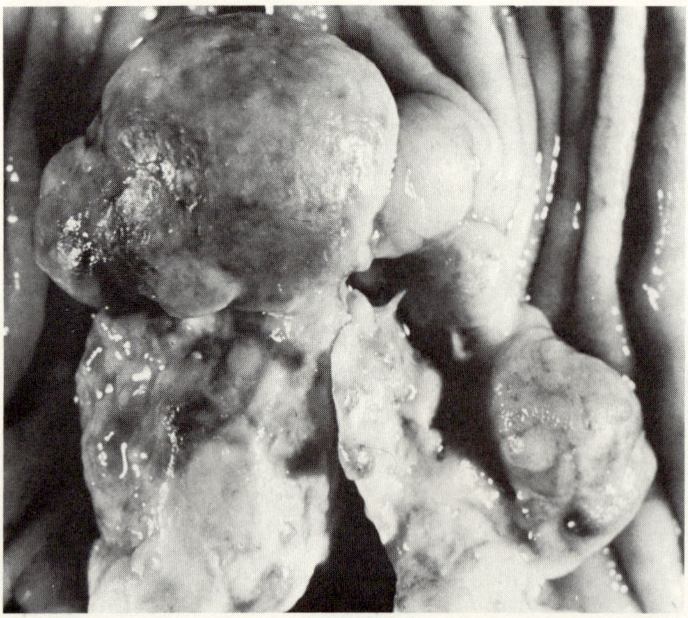

Figure 9–38. A polypoid leiomyosarcoma of the large bowel.

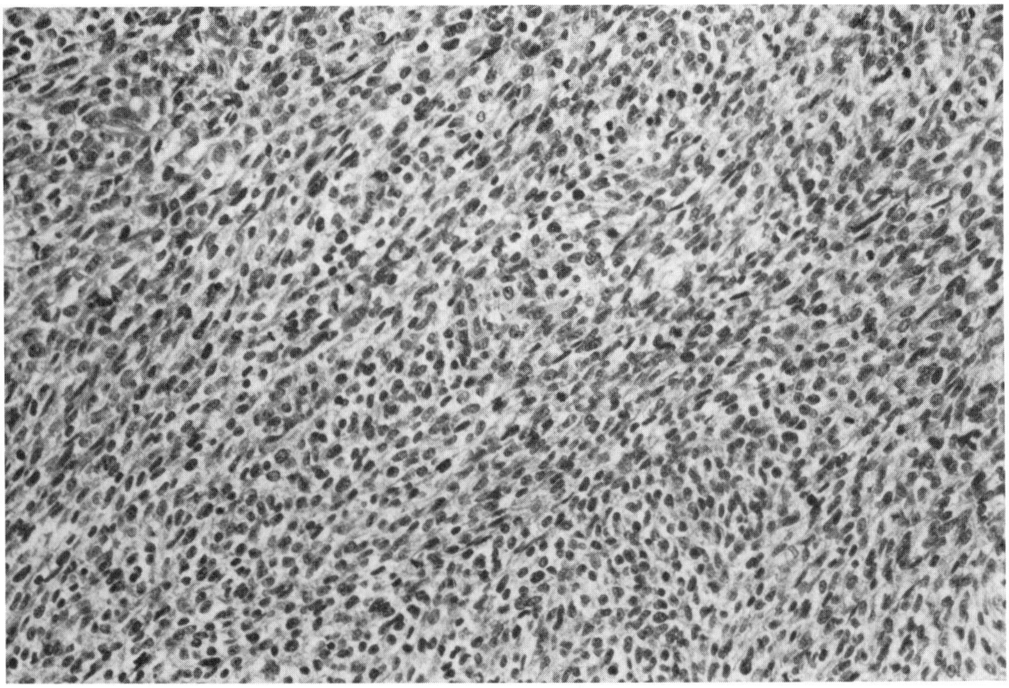

Figure 9–39. A well-differentiated leiomyosarcoma. The cells are spindled; a few mitoses were found.

also contain larger vessels. In one autopsy series, five of 19 patients dying from Kaposi's sarcoma had involvement of the large intestine (Roth et al., 1978).

Carcinoids

Approximately 20 percent of carcinoids occur in the large intestine. The largest concentration of carcinoids is, of course, in the appendix. In a review of 2837 carcinoids, 569 or 20 percent occurred in the large intestine. Of these, 400 or 70 percent of the 569 occurred in the rectum. There were fewer scattered throughout the remainder of the large intestine, with the cecum having the next largest concentration, with 79 carcinoids (Goodwin, 1975). The distribution of carcinoids throughout the length of the rectum is random, with

Figure 9–40. A carcinoid of the descending colon of an 86-year-old woman. It is raised, with a rolled margin and an ulcerated surface. It measured 5 cm in diameter and had metastases to one node.

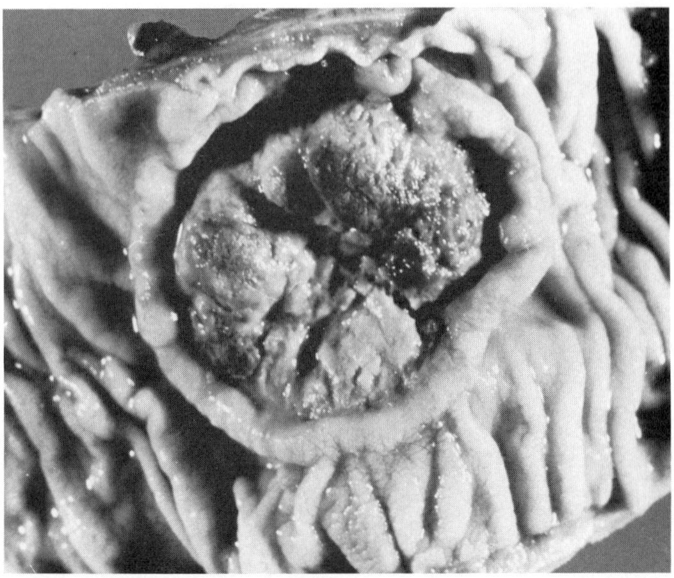

no particular localization. Carcinoids vary in size from a few millimeters to more than 3 cm in greatest dimension (Fig. 9–40). Occasional carcinoids in the right side of the colon have been described as large as 10 cm. Most of the lesions are sessile or raised plateaus, and only rarely are carcinoids pedunculated. At times there may be multiple carcinoids. Grossly, rectal carcinoids may be diagnosed by the endoscopist because they may shine through the mucosa as a yellowish or yellowish-tan lesion. In addition, carcinoids are firm, if not hard, lesions because of the associated fibrous proliferation. Thus, if palpation is possible, a diagnosis may be suggested by the firmness of the nodule. Histologically, carcinoids of the large intestine have the same pattern as those seen in other portions of the body. Frequently

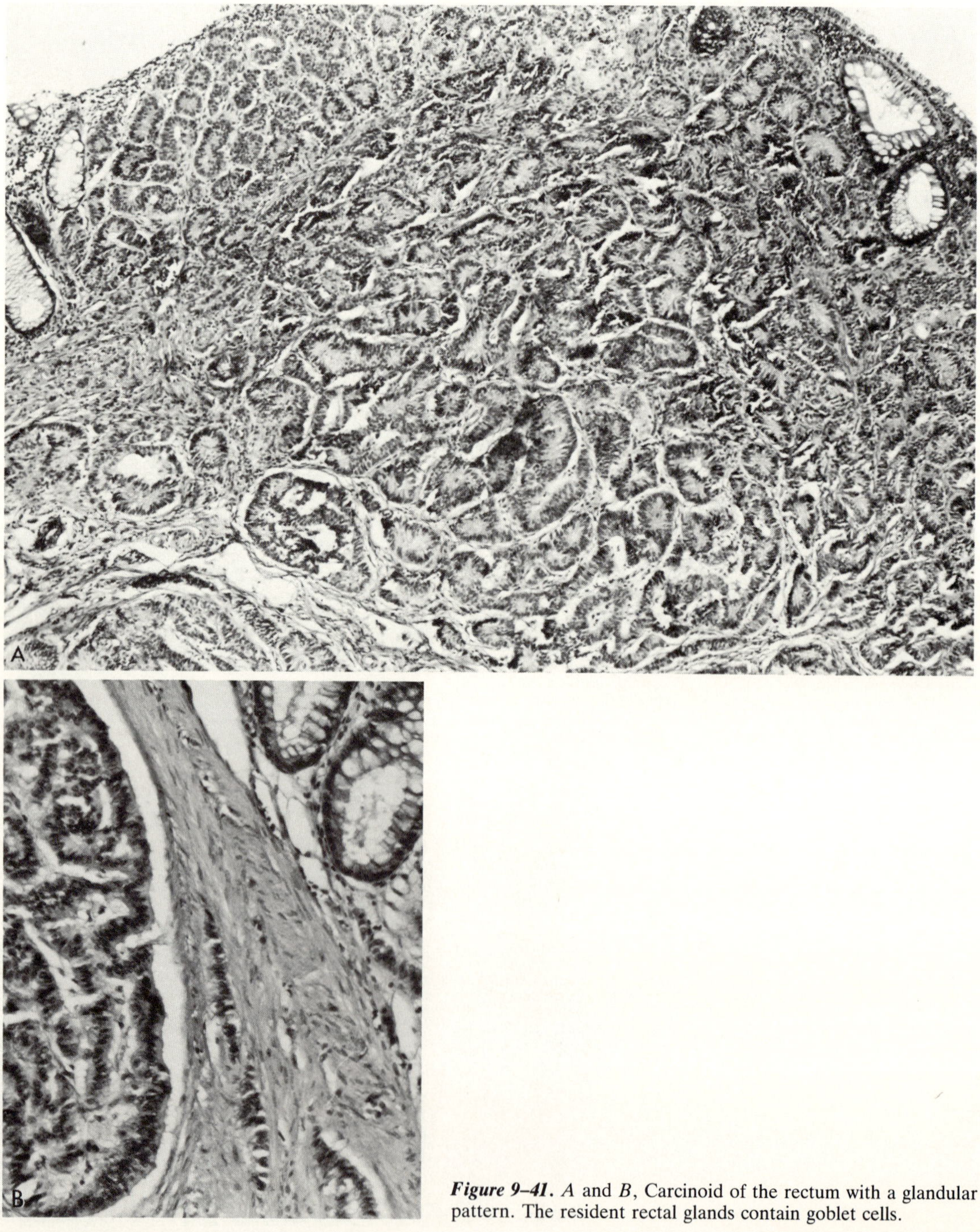

Figure 9–41. *A* and *B*, Carcinoid of the rectum with a glandular pattern. The resident rectal glands contain goblet cells.

in colonic and particularly in rectal carcinoids, a glandular pattern is present (Ponka and Walke, 1971). The glandular pattern may lead to the incorrect diagnosis of adenocarcinoma on the basis of biopsies or small excisional specimens (Fig. 9–41). It is at times difficult to differentiate a glandular carcinoid from adenocarcinoma because rectal carcinoids, as carcinoids in other parts of the body, may at times produce considerable mucin. Therefore, a mucin stain is not a differentiating feature in all instances (Hernandez and Fernandez, 1974). Ordinarily the mucosa is uninvolved unless small clusters of cells or the small glands of the carcinoid involve it. This characteristic may be used to differentiate carcinoids from adenocarcinomas. Special stains for argyrophilic or argentaffin granules are helpful also because most, but not all, rectal carcinoids will stain positively. Immunoperoxidase stains for serotonin may prove useful in the differentiation of carcinoids from other gland-forming tumors (Taxy et al., 1980). In addition, electron microscopic studies are helpful in diagnosis in that membrane-bound secretory granules will be present in carcinoids but not in adenocarcinomas.

In general, the size of the lesion is related to the chance of metastases. Those lesions measuring less than a centimeter rarely metastasize, but on occasion metastases have been identified in lesions that are less than 5 mm in diameter (Sabback and O'Brien, 1979).

Carcinoids may present as well-defined nests of uniform cells with poorly defined cytoplasmic boundaries. These nests are often surrounded by fibrous tissue, setting them off clearly from their neighbors. Other carcinoids may be purely glandular in structure, with a ramifying glandular pattern, and again, groups of glands are set off by a fibrous stroma. In some carcinoids there is a combination of these two histologic patterns. In addition, carcinoids of the rectum on occasion may be mucin producing (Hernandez and Fernandez, 1974). Carcinoids metastasize to the regional lymph nodes, the liver, the skeleton, and the lungs. Other sites are less frequent. Johnson and associates (1983) have defined five histologic patterns of carcinoids: insular, trabecular, glandular, undifferentiated, and mixed. The relationship between these patterns and patient survival is important. The insular pattern is associated with the best median survival time, and the undifferentiated pattern is associated with the worst.

Apparently, the carcinoid syndrome is rarely associated with carcinoids of the large intestine and rectum. However, there appears to be an increased incidence of malignancies in other sites associated with carcinoids, e.g., in the gastrointestinal tract and uterus (Sabback and O'Brien, 1979).

Metastatic Neoplasms

Metastatic neoplasms to the large intestine may present in various forms; most are polypoid and ulcerated (Fig. 9–42). They may be the site of an intussusception. The transverse colon may be the target of invasive gastric or pancreatic carcinomas. Gastric carcinomas often involve the superior border of the transverse colon, and carcinoma of the pancreas the inferior border. Neoplasms that metastasize to the large intestine are most frequently from malignant melanomas, carcinomas of the

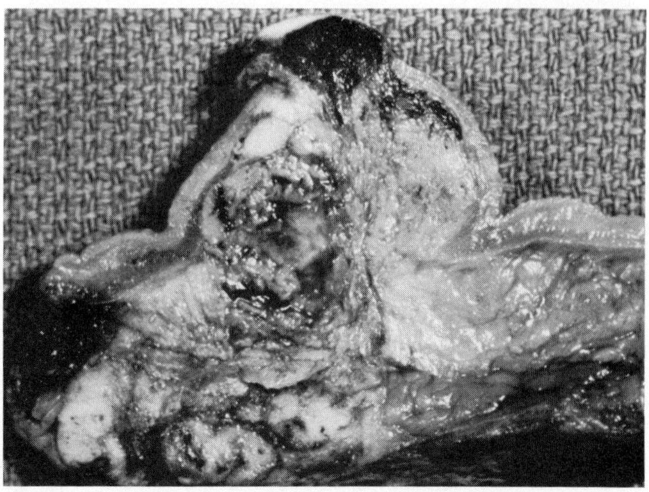

Figure 9–42. Ovarian carcinoma metastatic to the sigmoid colon. It forms a polypoid mass that involves the full thickness of the wall. The dark area at the apex of the mass represents an area from which bleeding occurred.

breast, or carcinomas of the lung; they have a predilection for antimesenteric localizations. Rarely, metastases may be so widespread in the large intestine as to simulate inflammatory bowel disease.

Most metastases may be distinguished from primary adenocarcinomas because they tend to localize submucosally, preserving the overlying mucosa. Histologically, malignant melanomas are readily identified, but some adenocarcinomas, for example, those from the stomach or biliary tract, may be difficult to specifically identify as being metastatic. Invasive carcinomas from the stomach and pancreas may be difficult to differentiate from a primary carcinoma of the transverse colon, but ordinarily the mucosa again will be preserved or, if ulcerated, will not have the mucosal alterations frequently associated with primary carcinomas.

BENIGN DISEASES AND NEOPLASMS OF THE ANUS

Non-neoplastic diseases of the anus and perianal skin are common. They include such lesions as hemorrhoids, fibrous polyps, fissures, fistulas, and various infectious processes (Fig. 9–43). They are important in terms of neoplasms in that they may produce lesions that are mistaken for neoplastic diseases, particularly carcinomas. It is important to examine many of these lesions histologically because approximately 1 to 2 percent of hemorrhoidectomy, fistulectomy, and fissurectomy specimens will be characterized by carcinoma or dysplastic epithelium. This has been demonstrated in two rather large series (Fenger and Nielsen, 1981; Grodsky, 1967). In the series reported by Fenger and Nielsen (1981) only dysplastic lesions were found; in the follow-up there was no progression to a more serious disease. In one report, approximately 150 mucinous carcinomas developed from anal fistulas (Getz et al., 1981). For a carcinoma to qualify as arising from a fistula, these researchers stipulated that the fistula must be of long standing and that there should be no evidence of a rectal neoplasm. Squamous cell carcinoma may also originate in anal fistulas (Kline et al., 1964).

Grossly, tuberculosis of the anus has been mistaken for carcinoma, usually because of ulceration. At times, tuberculosis may produce verrucoid masses that resemble carcinoma papillomas or condylomas (Walsh and Mulholland, 1981).

Another disease that may simulate carcinoma is lichen sclerosus et atrophicus. It most often involves the vulva but may spread to the perianal skin. Lichen sclerosus presents as a gray-white, somewhat firm area on the skin. It was stated in one review that approximately 5 percent of patients having this lesion will develop a carcinoma (Sloan and Goepel, 1981). Malacoplakia rarely involves the anus but may be mistaken both grossly and histologically for a malignancy. It is described earlier in this chapter.

Aside from anal skin tags, which are often designated clinically as polyps, inflammatory cloacogenic polyps occur in the anus. They vary from 1 to 3 cm in their greatest dimension and apparently arise from the transitional zone of the anus. Histologically, they are composed of glandular and stromal elements, with a major portion of the polyps often covered by

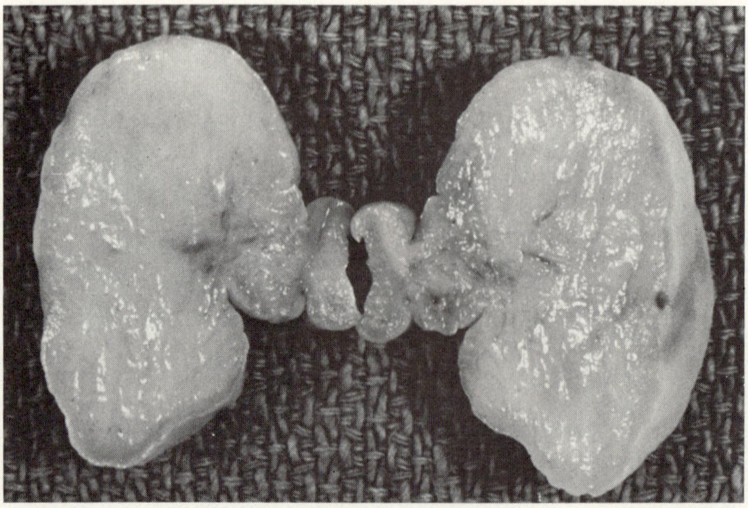

Figure 9–43. Fibrous anal polyp that measured 3 cm in greatest dimension. It was covered by stratified squamous epithelium.

stratified squamous epithelium. Histologically, an inflammatory cloacogenic polyp can be mistakenly diagnosed on biopsy as an infiltrating, well-differentiated adenocarcinoma from the rectum. As far as can be determined, there is no evidence of transformation from cloacogenic polyp to carcinoma (Lobert and Appelman, 1981).

Apocrine fibroadenomas arise from sweat glands of the anus and perianal area. They are composed of sweat glands and a fibrous stroma, with a pattern that is similar to a fibroadenoma of the breast (Assor and Davis, 1978).

Condylomas are rather common in the anal and perianal areas (Moore et al., 1978). Condylomas may be flat or papillomatous. Histologically, they are composed of well-differentiated stratified squamous epithelium, and they are frequently associated with chronic inflammation. There may be hyperkeratosis on their surfaces. A diagnostic feature is the presence of cells within the epidermis that have a clear, sometimes colorless, cytoplasm and a dark, somewhat irregular nucleus. These may be common or rather infrequent, but they serve to separate condylomas from other hyperplastic lesions of the squamous epithelium. Lee et al. (1981) reported on nine patients with malignant transformation of condylomas to carcinomas in situ or invasive squamous carcinomas. In most instances the follow-up of these patients was relatively short; thus, the biologic behavior of this malignancy is difficult to determine. In the nine cases, there were four local recurrences.

A few granular cell tumors have been described as occurring in the anal canal or anal verge. They often present as a painless mass or nodule. Histologically, anal tumors have the same appearance as tumors that occur elsewhere in the skin, that is, there are aggregates of large acidophilic, somewhat granular cells. In the anus, pseudoepitheliomatous hyperplasia of the overlying stratified squamous epithelium may occur and lead to a mistaken diagnosis of squamous cell carcinoma. Anal granular cell tumors have also been mistaken for giant cell tumors, malignant melanomas, and ganglioneuromas (Johnston and Helwig, 1981).

MALIGNANT TUMORS OF THE ANUS

Malignant epithelial tumors of the anus are often divided into squamous cell carcinomas and cloacogenic carcinomas. They are also classified as keratinizing and nonkeratinizing carcinomas, with the keratinizing carcinomas being squamous cell carcinomas and the nonkeratinizing tumors consisting of basal cell, basaloid, basosquamous, and the transitional carcinomas. On the basis of biologic behavior, all these various carcinomas are considered by some to be variants of squamous cell carcinoma. However, it is customary to divide the carcinomas of the anus into the various named categories mentioned previously (Pang and Morson, 1967; Stearns et al., 1980).

The etiology of carcinoma of the anus is unknown. However, there are a number of associated lesions such as fistulas, anal abscesses, lymphogranulomas, and condylomas that are related to an increased risk of carcinoma (Stearns et al., 1980). Rarely, carcinoma in situ complicates Crohn's disease of the anus. Recently, it has been observed that there is apparently an increased incidence of carcinoma of the anus associated with homosexual behavior (Daling et al., 1982).

Carcinomas of the anus and anal verge account for approximately 1 to 2 percent of carcinomas of the large intestine. The majority are squamous cell carcinomas or variants, which are often designated as cloacogenic carcinomas. Adenocarcinomas of the anus make up a small proportion, less than 10 percent, of all carcinomas of that region. Anatomically, squamous cell carcinomas are located throughout the length of the anus and the anal verge. The largest number occur at the mucocutaneous line or pectinate line. A fewer number occur in the anal canal and at the anal verge. Tumors designated as cloacogenic originate in the transitional zone, with some apparently arising below or above the pectinate line. Electron microscopic studies have verified a relation between cloacogenic tumors and the transitional epithelium. There seems to be nearly equal distribution between anterior and posterior locations in the circumference of the anus. A smaller number are located laterally, and approximately 10 to 11 percent of carcinomas will circumscribe the anus. The majority of anal carcinomas present as intraluminal ulcerated masses. They may have fungating raised margins, and their centers may be rather deeply excavated. Only occasionally will a carcinoma of the anus present as a smooth polypoid mass (Figs. 9–44 to 9–46). (Gillespie and MacKay, 1978; Klotz et al., 1967; Kuehn et al., 1968).

Histologically, squamous cell carcinoma of the anus has the same patterns as squamous cell carcinoma occurring in other parts of the

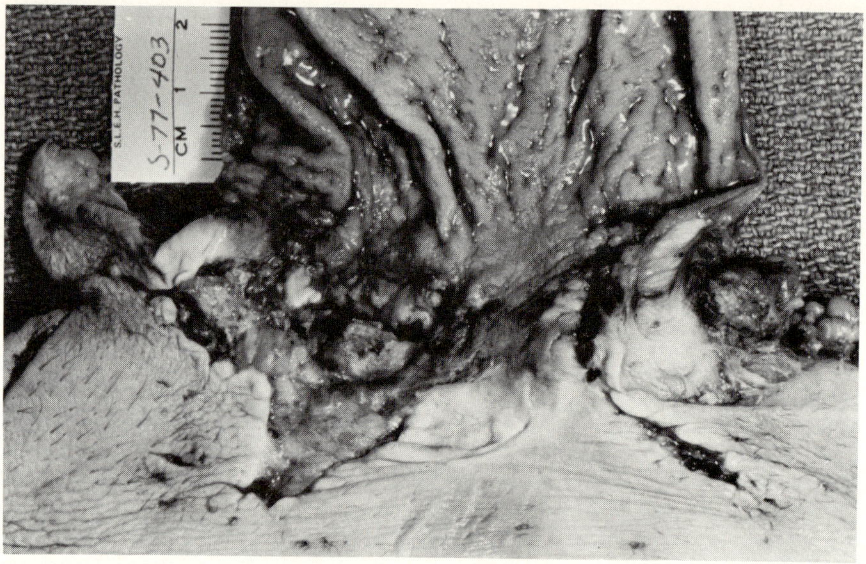

Figure 9–44. An ulcerative squamous cell carcinoma of the anal canal that has extended to involve perianal skin. The patient was a 43-year-old woman.

the body (Fig. 9–47). There may or may not be evidence of keratinization. The carcinomas vary from well to poorly differentiated. The anal soft tissues and muscles are often infiltrated. Cloacogenic carcinomas have the variety of patterns described previously. The transitional variant resembles squamous cell carcinoma, but the cells and the nuclei are smaller and there is some resemblance to urothelium. Electron microscopic studies have noted the differences between this carcinoma and squamous and urothelial carcinomas. Other tumors in this group have a basaloid pattern, that is, they often have discrete cluster cells with peripheral palisading of nuclei, resembling basal cell carcinomas to some degree. The degrees of differentiation vary; some carcinomas have been designated as small cell carcinomas of the anus because they are similar to small cell carcinomas of the lung (Pang and Morson, 1967). A combination of transitional cell carcinoma and glandlike structures is also

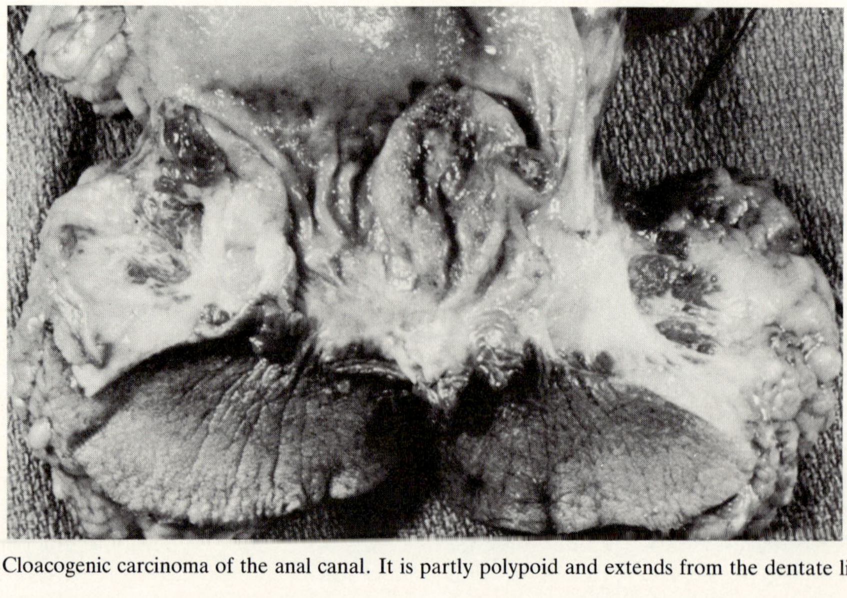

Figure 9–45. Cloacogenic carcinoma of the anal canal. It is partly polypoid and extends from the dentate line to the anal verge.

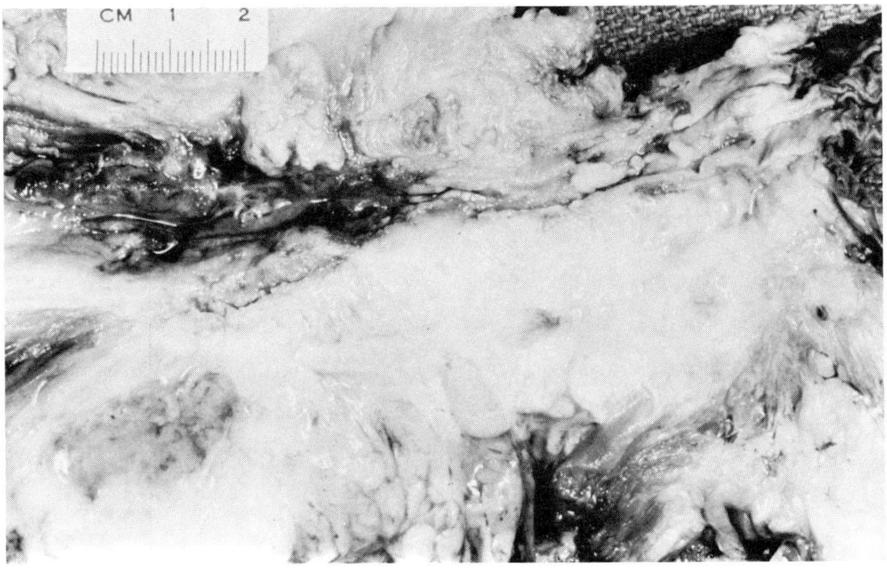

Figure 9–46. A sagittal section through a cloacogenic carcinoma showing extensive perianal invasion by tumor that practically circumscribes the anal canal.

seen. This has often been designated as a mucoepidermoid carcinoma because mucus is produced by the glandular component (Stearns et al., 1980).

Another form of squamous cell carcinoma that occurs in the anus and perianal area is verrucous carcinoma. This has also been designated as giant condyloma. This form of carcinoma is invasive and apparently rarely if ever metastasizes. It is unclear from the literature how many verrucous carcinomas of this region have been reported (Gingrass et al., 1978).

Adenocarcinomas make up less than 10 percent of malignant neoplasms of the anus and perianal tissues (Fig. 9–48). Many adenocarcinomas developing in this area occur in the presence of chronic fistulas or fissures. Histologically, it is necessary to determine that an

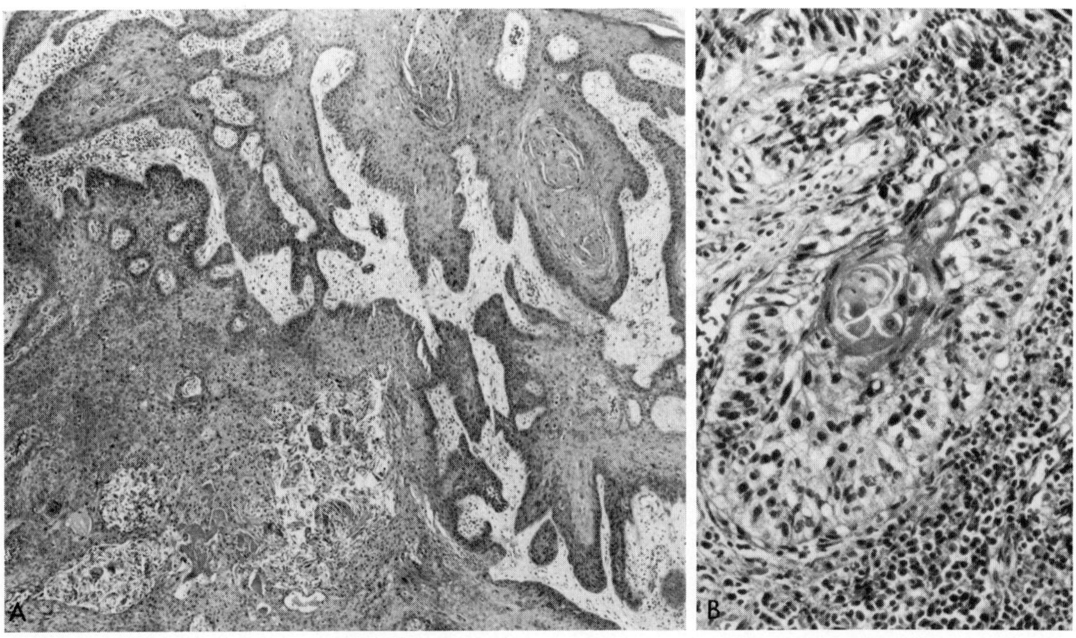

Figure 9–47. *A* and *B*, Well-differentiated squamous cell carcinoma with keratinization occurring in a 57-year-old woman.

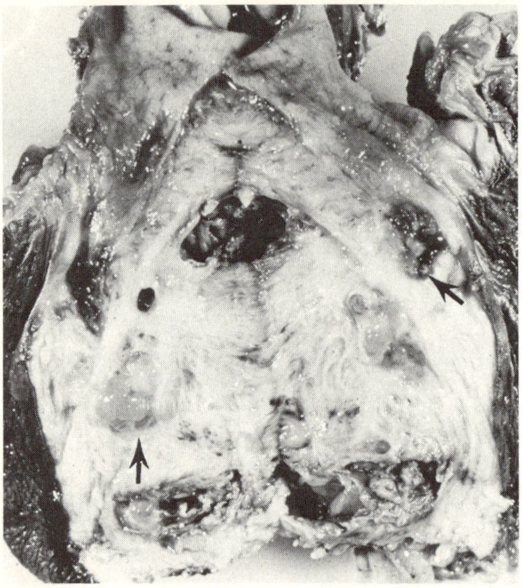

Figure 9–48. Adenocarcinoma of the anal canal that has diffusely infiltrated surrounding tissues. Loculi of mucus are evident (arrows).

adenocarcinoma in this area is not an extension downward from the rectum. This obviously is an important prerequisite to the diagnosis of adenocarcinoma of the anus. Histologically, the lesions have features similar to those of adenocarcinomas of the large intestine (Cabrera et al., 1966; Getz et al., 1981).

Basal cell carcinomas, similar to those that might occur on the face, occasionally are seen in the perianal region, usually at the anal margin or perianal skin. Occasionally they may extend into the anal canal. Clinically, these lesions have been mistaken for hemorrhoids, fissures, and eczema. In a group of 34 cases reported by Nielsen and Jensen (1981), one patient had metastases to the inguinal lymph nodes. There was a local recurrence rate of 29 percent associated with local excision.

In the perianal skin there may be erythematous, pruritic areas that on biopsy show a thickened epithelium with enlarged single cells and clusters of cells. The cytoplasm of these cells is pale compared with that of the adjacent squamous cells. The enlarged cells usually stain for mucin. This lesion, known as extramammary Paget's disease, is often but not always associated with an underlying carcinoma, usually an adenocarcinoma. It may be mistaken for a malignant melanoma, Bowen's disease, or another form of carcinoma, such as transitional carcinoma of the anus, but the mucin-positive cells are helpful in distinguishing Paget's disease from other types of tumors (Helwig and Graham, 1963).

Lymph nodes are the most frequent site of spread of carcinomas of the anus. Approximately 50 percent of patients will have evidence of inguinal lymph node involvement, depending somewhat on the extent of the lesion, its location, and the depth of invasion. Pelvic lymph nodes will be involved in as many as 50 percent of patients; again, the involvement is related to the size, extent, and location of the lesion. In one study, nodal metastases were more common with basaloid carcinoma than with squamous carcinoma, 18 percent and 32 percent, respectively (Beahrs, 1979). Interestingly, metastases that travel by way of the bloodstream are rather uncommon with anal carcinomas. Less than 10 percent of patients will have pulmonary or hepatic metastases; fewer will have skeletal metastases (Stearns et al., 1980). Local recurrence is dependent on the stage of the carcinoma. For example, when the sphincter muscles are invaded, the rate of recurrence approaches 60 percent. Recurrence rates are similar for squamous and cloacogenic carcinomas (Wolff, 1971).

Shindo (1981) recently reviewed and compared squamous cell carcinomas with adenocarcinomas of the anus. He observed that the 5-year survival rates are similar for both, but there is slight difference in the incidence of metastases to the inguinal node, with nodal metastases from squamous cell carcinomas being more frequent than from adenocarcinomas. However, the overall incidence of nodal metastases is the same for both lesions. Shindo also observed that adenocarcinomas are usually more deeply invasive than the squamous cell carcinomas.

Melanomas of the anus often present as ulcerative lesions, polypoid lesions, or lesions that are mistaken for hemorrhoids. There apparently is nothing distinctive about the gross presentation. The lesions are located most often in the anal canal, with fewer located in the anorectal area; a few arise in the lower rectum, and others at the anal verge or perianal skin (Stearns et al., 1980). Histologically, junctional activity is often associated with the melanomas. Melanomas of the anus have the same histologic patterns as those of the skin, although many cells of the former have a spindled pattern (Fig. 9–49). In contrast to melanomas of the skin, it is difficult to apply a Clark's level system because of the difference in thickness of the overlying epithelium when

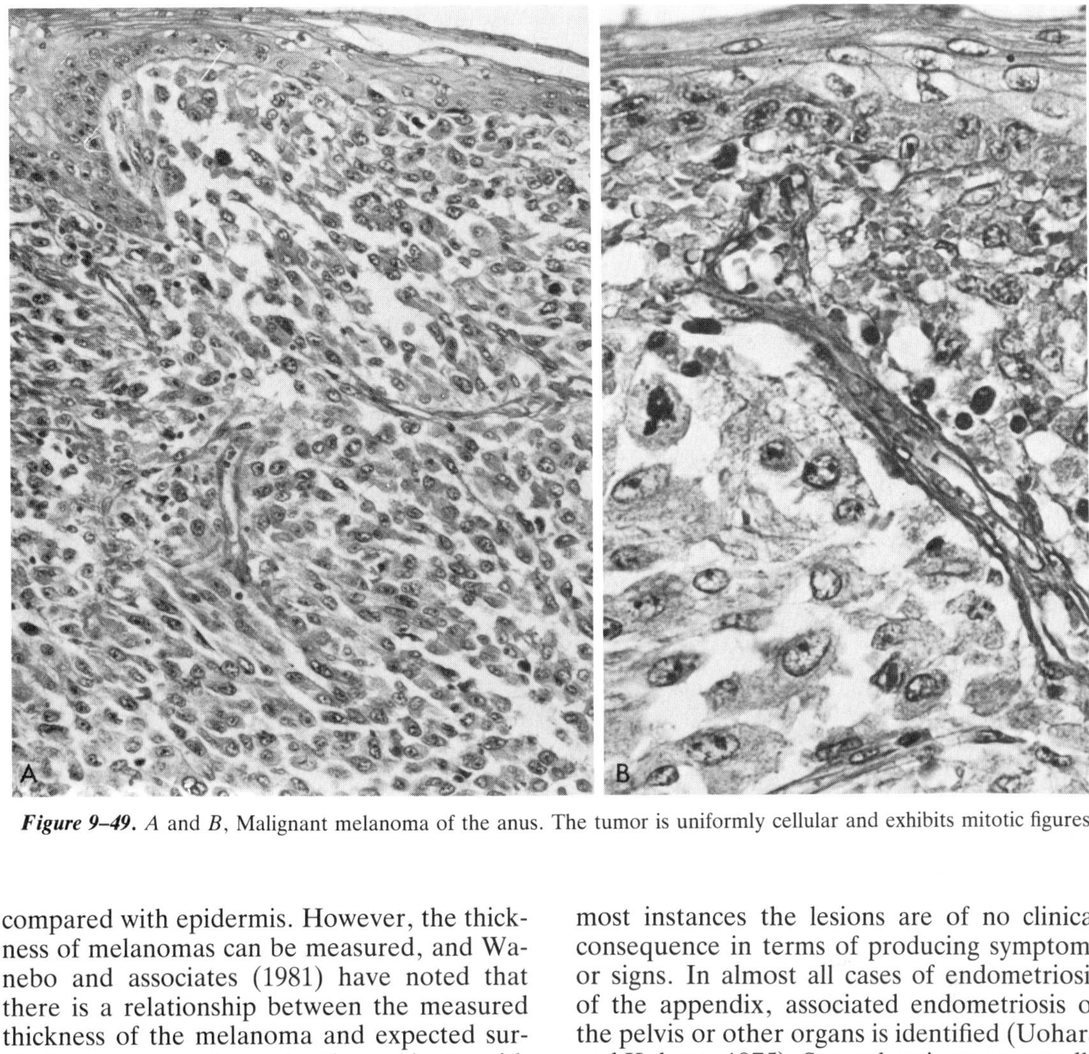

Figure 9–49. *A* and *B*, Malignant melanoma of the anus. The tumor is uniformly cellular and exhibits mitotic figures.

compared with epidermis. However, the thickness of melanomas can be measured, and Wanebo and associates (1981) have noted that there is a relationship between the measured thickness of the melanoma and expected survival. For example, only the patients with melanomas less than 2 mm thick survived (13 years or more), whereas those with melanomas greater than 2 mm in thickness died of their disease (no survivors at 5 years).

The anus may be invaded by adjacent carcinomas, particularly from the rectum. But, metastases from distant sites are distinctly rare. An example of carcinoma of the lung metastatic to the anus has been reported (Ger and Reuben, 1968).

THE APPENDIX

The appendix may be affected by various non-neoplastic diseases. Among them are endometriosis, malacoplakia, heterotopic gastric mucosa, and intussusception (Aubrey, 1970; Blackshear, 1970; Howard et al., 1970). In most instances the lesions are of no clinical consequence in terms of producing symptoms or signs. In almost all cases of endometriosis of the appendix, associated endometriosis of the pelvis or other organs is identified (Uohara and Kobara, 1975). Several patients reportedly had symptoms related to appendiceal endometriosis, but as with endometriosis in other areas, this is questionable. Endometriosis can cause a mass or an enlargement of the appendix that may be mistaken for an appendiceal tumor (Fig. 9–50). Histologically, endometriosis in the appendix is similar to endometriosis in other areas of the gastrointestinal tract.

Occasionally, intussusception of the appendix has been described, and on barium enema study, it has been mistaken for a carcinoma of the cecum.

As in other portions of the gastrointestinal tract, epithelium of the appendix may form neoplasms that vary from mucosal hyperplasia (MacGillivray, 1972) to adenocarcinoma. Hyperplasias have characteristics similar to those of hyperplastic polyps of the large intestine, such as acidophilic cytoplasm and the typical

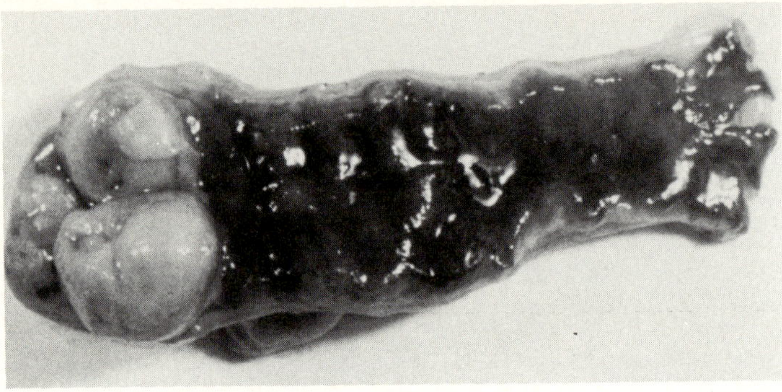

Figure 9–50. Endometrioma at the tip of the appendix. The lesion is a nodular submucosal lesion.

saw-tooth arrangement of the cells in the glandular lumens. Areas may be papillary. Mucosal hyperplasia in which considerable mucus is produced is seen also. In addition to the hyperplastic lesions, benign epithelial neoplasms, such as villous adenomas and adenomatous polyps, originate in the appendix. Histologically, these two lesions are identical to those found in the large intestine. To be sure they are rare, and of 42 benign epithelial neoplasms described by Wolff and Ahmed (1976), 36 were cystadenomas, four were papillary adenomas, one was a pedunculated adenomatous polyp, and one was a sessile adenomatous polyp. An interesting observation made by Wolff and Ahmed was that about 25 percent of patients having these epithelial neoplasms of the appendix also had associated synchronous or metachronous neoplasms in other portions of the large intestine. Several patients also had carcinoma of the breast, kidney, or ovary.

An important finding with epithelial neoplasms is mucocele. Approximately 50 percent of epithelial lesions will be associated with a mucocele. This leads to the question of what is the relationship between a mucocele and pseudomyxoma peritonei. A mucocele per se does not give rise to pseudomyxoma peritonei, since the former is an enlarged cystic appendix that contains mucus and may or may not have identifiable lining epithelium. It has been suggested that a mucocele be designated as a retention cyst of the appendix so that it cannot be associated with pseudomyxoma peritonei. The latter lesion is associated, however, with neoplasms, such as cystadenomas or cystadenocarcinomas. Cystadenomas are histologically identifiable as proliferative, often papillary, lesions of the appendiceal mucosa. Histologically, nuclear alterations, particularly nuclear stratification and some pleomorphism, resemble those seen in the epithelium of adenomatous polyps (Gibbs, 1973).

Should a mucocele rupture, the resultant spillage of mucus is self-limited, whereas if a cystadenoma ruptures, the free mucus can result in pseudomyxoma peritonei because viable mucus-producing epithelium may be implanted in the region of the appendix or elsewhere in the peritoneum. Ordinarily, if the cystadenoma is benign and the appendix is removed, the disease is self-limited. Only with cystadenocarcinoma does pseudomyxoma peritonei represent a malignant disease. Histologically, cystadenocarcinoma and cystadenoma may be difficult to distinguish. Both lesions may be well differentiated. Usually only the observation of invasiveness allows the diagnosis of cystadenocarcinoma. In some instances, the epithelial changes will be cytologically malignant, thus also allowing a diagnosis of cystadenocarcinoma.

There are two types of adenocarcinomas of the appendix: the colonic type of adenocarcinoma and the microglandular or signet ring cell type of carcinoma. Only some 200 examples of adenocarcinoma of the appendix have been reported (Lee and Song, 1982). The prognosis is related to the extent of the neoplasm and correlates well with the Dukes classification of carcinoma. The well-differentiated colonic type of carcinoma has a better prognosis than the mucinous carcinoma. Wolff and Ahmed (1976) have observed that a third of their patients having adenocarcinoma of the appendix also had juxtaposed polyps, suggesting that the adenomatous polyp is a precursor of adenocarcinoma of the appendix. Metastases from adenocarcinoma of the appendix have a distribution similar to those from carcinoma of the cecum; thus treatment ordinarily requires a right hemicolectomy.

Carcinoids are the most common of the malignant neoplasms of the appendix. Frequently they are discovered incidentally by the surgeon or pathologist when examining an appendix. Occasionally patients with a carcinoid tumor of the appendix present with signs and symptoms suggesting appendicitis. As least three fourths of carcinoids are located in the distal one third of the appendix, with the remainder located in the mid and proximal thirds. Grossly, carcinoids are firm masses that may enlarge the appendix, and their cut surfaces are often yellow, allowing for gross diagnosis (Fig. 9–51). As with carcinoids located in other portions of the gastrointestinal tract, the size of the lesion is important and thus should be measured by the pathologist. It has been demonstrated that those that exceed 2 cm are at high risk to metastasize, whereas those that are smaller than 2 cm are at a considerably lower risk to metastasize (Glasser and Bhagavan, 1980). Histologically, carcinoids of the appendix have the same pattern as carcinoids elsewhere. This pattern has been described previously in this chapter. It is uncommon to find a carcinoid of the appendix that does not invade the submucosa and the muscularis. Often they invade through the full thickness of the wall of the appendix. The depth of invasion is not necessarily related to metastases; the size seems to be more important. For example, Hajdu and associates (1974) have classified carcinoids of the gastrointestinal tract as "deeply invasive" on the basis of invasion halfway through the wall of the organ or when the lesion was larger than 2.5 cm. They noted, for example, that all of the so-called deeply invasive carcinomas ranged in size from 2.5 to 11 cm in greatest dimension. Syracuse and associates (1979) suggested that invasion of the mesoappendix may indicate nodal metastases, and when invasion is present, they recommend hemicolectomy. The rate of metastases from carcinoids of the appendix is extremely low. Of 60 cases reported by Hajdu and associates (1974), none showed evidence of nodal metastases.

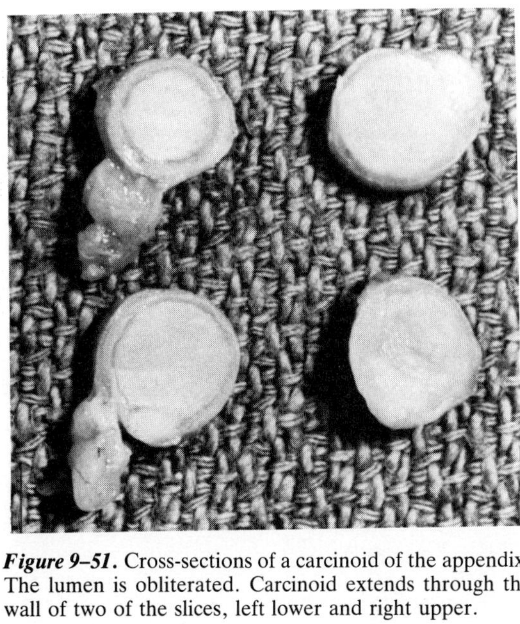

Figure 9–51. Cross-sections of a carcinoid of the appendix. The lumen is obliterated. Carcinoid extends through the wall of two of the slices, left lower and right upper.

A histologic variant of a carcinoid tumor has been designated a goblet cell carcinoid or a mucinous carcinoid. In this lesion the pattern of infiltration is similar to that of other carcinoids, except that in many instances signet ring cells that stain readily for mucin are part of the tumor. In addition, glands that have a colonic pattern are seen frequently and stain for mucin. These carcinoids apparently have no greater capability for metastases than the more conventional form. However, there are examples in which metastases have occurred to lymph nodes and the peritoneum (Klein, 1974; Subbuswamy et al., 1974). We have seen one patient in whom there was extensive dissemination of the tumor throughout the abdomen.

Other benign and malignant tumors of the appendix are rare, and these include leiomyoma, lipoma, neurofibroma, hemangioma, liposarcoma, malignant schwannoma, and malignant lymphoma (Collins, 1963).

Metastases to the vermiform appendix are rare. At times, the metastases cause signs and symptoms that suggest appendicitis. Carcinoma of the breast is the most frequent contributor to metastases to the appendix (Burney et al., 1974).

CARCINOGENESIS

Over the years there has been considerable interest in the experimental production of colonic tumors in animals because of the prevalence of the disease in humans. In addition, certain factors, such as the role of adenomatous polyps in the genesis of carcinoma, are of special interest. Numerous carcinogenic agents have been used to produce colonic tumors, such as the cholanthrenes, aromatic amines, hydrazine derivatives, alkylnitrosamides, and aflatoxins. Of this group, the most productive has been the hydrazine derivative 1,2-dimethylhydrazine (DMH). In addition to these chemical compounds, many substances occurring in our daily diet have been observed to be related to the carcinogenesis. These include food additives, plant foods, and spices and beverages. These may act as mutagens, carcinogens, or promoters of neoplasia (LaMont and O'Gorman, 1978).

In addition to the interest in extraneous carcinogens, there has been considerable interest in the role of bile acids in the production of carcinomas of the intestinal tract, particularly of the large bowel. It has generally been considered that bile acids may act as cocarcinogens; it has also been postulated that clostridia in the bowel may produce a carcinogen from a bile acid cell nucleus. Intestinal flora may have an influence on carcinogenic compounds (Hill, 1975). The study of the intestinal flora is complex, as pointed out by Gustafsson (1982). It has not been clearly demonstrated that bile acids are related to the carcinogenesis in the large intestine. In a recent study, Gelb and associates (1982) determined the bile acid content of normal tissue, adenomatous polyps, and carcinomas of the large intestine. They could find no relationship between the histologic findings and the bile acid content. This would not necessarily negate the association between bile acids and the genesis of neoplasia. Rodents, particularly rats and mice, have been the favorite subjects of carcinogenic studies of the large intestine. An advantage of using these animals, aside from their size, is that spontaneous colonic carcinomas are particularly rare in rodents. Thus the evaluation of the induced neoplasms is not obscured by spontaneous tumors (Burn et al., 1966).

The most effective way to administer carcinogens is subcutaneously. Rats subjected to a carcinogen in a dose related to body weight will develop neoplasms within 3 to 6 months. The lesions are often multiple and present gross features similar to their counterparts found in humans. With the use of DMH, at least 90 percent of the animals develop neoplasms of the intestinal tract. The distribution of the tumors is similar to that expected for large intestinal carcinomas of humans, with a dominance on the left side and a concentration near the major flexure (Rosengren, 1977). Experiments using 3:2′-dimethyl-4-aminobiphenyl show that the distribution of neoplasms in rats is quite similar to that expected in humans (Fig. 9–52). Because of the interest in the relationship of adenomatous polyps to carcinomas of the large bowel in humans, this has been the focal point of animal experiments. Histologically, it has been difficult if not impossible to demonstrate a relationship between experimentally induced adenomatous polyps and adenocarcinomas. Most observers believe that the carcinomas arise de novo from the colonic epithelium (Maskens and Dujardin-Loits, 1981; Spjut and Spratt, 1965). Histologically, the neoplastic lesions are similar to those seen in humans, including a focus of carcinoma in situ. Pohzarisski (1975) believes that carcinoma develops through various stages of proliferation to carcinoma in situ and then to an invasive carcinoma. Madara and associates (1983) take the opposite view. In their experiments using DMH, they noted histologic evidence of adenomatous epithelium. Electron microscopic studies comparing the experimentally induced neoplasms with similar human neoplasms show a remarkable similarity between the two (Spjut and Smith, 1967).

The experimentally produced carcinomas seldom metastasize, but in one large group of neoplasms induced by DMH there were extensive distant metastases from signet ring cell carcinomas (Pohzarisski, 1975). Another interesting observation in this experiment was that the majority of mucinous and signet ring cell carcinomas were in the right side of the colon. This latter observation compares with a human study in which 23 percent of the carcinomas arising in the ascending colon were mucinous (Symonds and Vickery, 1976).

In mice injected with DMH, squamous cell carcinomas of the anal region have been in-

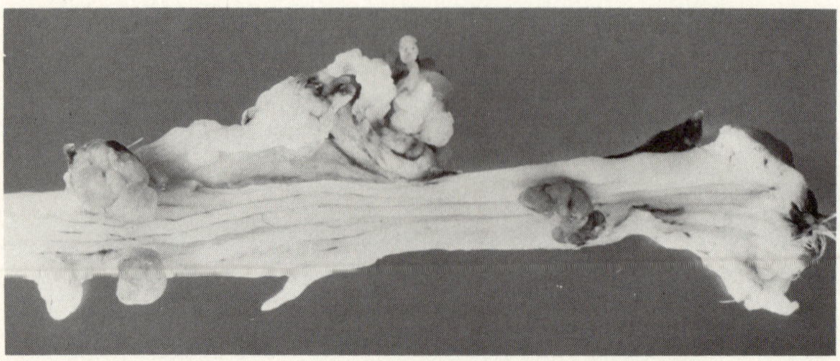

Figure 9–52. Epithelial polyps in a male rat that received 3:2′-dimethyl-4-aminobiphenyl subcutaneously.

duced in addition to intestinal neoplasms. The large bowel neoplasms are similiar to those seen in rats, with a distribution dominantly on the left side. Injection of alkylnitrosoguanidines into rats produces numerous gastric tumors and occasionally sarcomas and carcinosarcomas of the large intestine. Thus a range of neoplasms of the large intestine and anus are produced by the different agents (Schoental and Bensted, 1969).

The role of feces has often been considered in relation to carcinogenesis in the large bowel. In order to determine the effects of the presence of and the passage of feces in relation to carcinogenesis, various diversions of fecal flow have been made. In one experiment, a distal colostomy was performed and then the animals were given subcutaneous injections of a carcinogen. As a result, there were no polypoid or epithelial lesions distal to the colostomy, which was the excluded portion of the large intestine (Navarrete and Spjut, 1967). In other experiments using DMH, transection of the proximal colon with anastomosis to the rectum resulted in fewer adenomatous polyps and carcinomas in the excluded segment than expected with the use of this carcinogen (Lewin et al., 1981). Thus, there is some evidence to support the fact that the fecal flow or elements in the feces act as cocarcinogens in experimental situations.

Experiments to demonstrate the effects of injury of the colonic mucosa and the genesis of neoplasia have been done. Rats received enemas of 5 percent and 10 percent acetic acid; DMH was given subcutaneously. There is evidence that this type of injury to the large intestine caused increased numbers of large bowel epithelial neoplasms as compared with control groups. Results such as these at least raise the possibility that injury, as seen in the inflammatory bowel disease, may be a factor in the genesis of carcinomas in those diseases (Hagihara, 1982).

References

Abrams JS, Reines HD: Increasing incidence of right-sided lesions in colorectal cancer. Am J Surg 137:522, 1979.

Aldersberg R: Kaposi's sarcoma complicating ulcerative colitis. Am J Clin Pathol 54:143, 1970.

Allred HW Jr, Spencer RJ: Hemangiomas of the colon, rectum, and anus. Mayo Clin Proc 49:739, 1974.

Amorn Y, Knight WA Jr: Primary linitis plastica of the colon. Cancer 41:2420, 1978.

Assor D, Davis JB: Multiple apocrine fibroadenomas of the anal skin. Am J Clin Pathol 68:397, 1978.

Astler VB, Coller FA: The prognostic significance of direct extension of carcinoma of the colon and rectum. Ann Surg 139:846, 1954.

Aubrey DA: Gastric heterotopia in the vermiform appendix. Arch Surg 101:628, 1970.

Beahrs OH: Management of cancer of the anus. AJR 133:790, 1979.

Bell GA, McKenzie AD, Emmons H: Diffuse cavernous hemangioma of the rectum: Report of a case and review of the literature. Dis Colon Rectum 15:377, 1972.

Bentley G, Webster JHH: Gastrointestinal tuberculosis. Br J Surg 54:90, 1967.

Berg JW, Goodwin JD III: The epidemiologic pathology of carcinoma of the large bowel. J Surg Oncol 6:381, 1974.

Berge T, Ekelund G, Mellner C, et al: Carcinoma of the colon and rectum in a defined population. Acta Chir Scand (Suppl) 1:86, 1973.

Bibro MC, Houlihan RK, Sheahan DG: Colonic ganglioneuroma. Arch Surg 115:75, 1980.

Blackshear WM: Malakoplakia of the appendix: A case report. Am J Clin Pathol 53:284, 1970.

Blackstone MO, Riddell RH, Rogers BHG, Levin B: Dysplasia-associated lesion or mass (DALM) detected by colonoscopy in long-standing ulcerative colitis: an indication for colectomy. Gastroenterology 80:366, 1981.

Budd DC, Fink DL: Mucoid colonic carcinoma as an autosomal-dominant inherited syndrome. Arch Surg 116:901, 1981.

Burn JJ, Sellwood RA, Bishop M: Spontaneous carcinoma of the colon of the rat. J Pathol Bacteriol 91:253, 1966.

Burney RE, Koss N, Goldenberg IS: Acute appendicitis secondary to metastatic carcinoma of the breast. Arch Surg 108:872, 1974.

Bussey HJR: Familial Polyposis Coli. Baltimore, Johns Hopkins University Press, 1975.

Butsch JL, Dockerty MB, McGill DB, Judd ES: "Solitary" nonspecific ulcers of the colon. Arch Surg 98:171, 1969.

Butt JH, Morson B: Dysplasia and cancer in inflammatory bowel disease. Gastroenterology 80:865, 1981.

Cabrera A, Tsukado Y, Pickren JW: Adenocarcinomas of the anal canal and perianal tissues. Ann Surg 164:152, 1966.

Camilleri M, Satti MB, Wood CB: Cystic lymphangioma of the colon. Dis Colon Rect 25:813, 1982.

Castleman B, Krickstein HI: Do adenomatous polyps of the colon become malignant? New Engl J Med 267:469, 1962.

Collins DC: 71,000 human appendix specimens. A final report, summarizing forty years' study. Am J Proctol 14:365, 1963.

Comer TP, Beahrs OH, Dockerty MB: Primary squamous cell carcinoma and adenoacanthoma of the colon. Cancer 28:1111, 1971.

Cornes JS, Wallace MH, Morson BC: Benign lymphomas of the rectum and anal canal: A study of 100 cases. J Pathol Bacteriol 82:371, 1961.

Craft CF, Mendelsohn G, Cooper HS, Yardley JH: Colonic "precancer" in Crohn's disease. Gastroenterology 80:578, 1981.

Craggs MH, Toker C: Basaloid tumor of the sigmoid colon. Hum Pathol 13:497, 1982.

Culp CE, Hill JR: Malignant lymphomas involving the rectum. Dis Colon Rectum 5:426, 1962.

Culver GJ, Pereira RM, Seibel R: Radiographic features of rectosigmoid endometriosis. Am J Obstet Gynecol 76:1176, 1958.

Daling JR, Weiss NS, Klopfenstein LL, et al: Correlates of homosexual behavior and the incidence of anal cancer. JAMA 247:1988, 1982.

Daly JJ, Madrazo A: Anal Crohn's disease with carcinoma in situ. Dig Dis Sci 25:464, 1980.

Dobbins WO III: Current status of the precancer lesion in ulcerative colitis. Gastroenterology 73:1431, 1977.

Doyle JL, Bryant FJ Jr, Voltz PW: Neurilemoma of the cecum. Tex Med 64:42, 1968.

Dukes CE: The classification of cancer in the rectum. J Pathol Bacteriol 35:323, 1932.

Edelman MJ, Sternberg SS: Nodular lymphoid hyperplasia of the colon in an adult. Clin Bull 7:146, 1977.

Ekelund G: On colorectal polyps and carcinoma with special reference to their interrelationship. Ph.D. thesis. University of Lund, Malmö, Sweden, 1974.

Estrada RG, Spjut HJ: Hyperplastic polyps of the large bowel. Am J Surg Pathol 4:127, 1980.

Farmer RG, Hawk WA, Turnbull RB Jr: Carcinoma associated with mucosal ulcerative colitis and with transmural colitis, and enteritis (Crohn's disease). Cancer 28:289, 1971.

Fenger C, Nielsen VT: Dysplastic changes in the anal canal epithelium in minor surgical specimens. Acta Pathol Microbiol Scand (A) 89:463, 1981.

Franken EA Jr: Lymphoid hyperplasia of the colon. Radiology 94:329, 1970.

Gardiner GA, Bird CR: Nonspecific ulcers of the colon resembling annular carcinoma. Radiology 137:331, 1980.

Gelb AM, McSherry CK, Sadowsky JR, Mosbach EH: Tissue bile acids in patients with colon cancer and colonic polyps. Am J Gastroenterol 77:314, 1982.

Gellhoed GW, Crossland SG: Carcinoma of the right colon. A change in characteristic configuration? South Med J 74:1436, 1981.

Genter B, Mir R, Strauss R, et al: Hemangiopericytoma of the colon: Report of a case and review of literature. Dis Colon Rectum 25:149, 1982.

Ger R, Reuben J: Squamous-cell carcinoma of the anal canal: A metastatic lesion. Dis Colon Rectum 11:213, 1968.

Getz SB, Ough YD, Patterson RB, Kovalcik PJ: Mucinous adenocarcinoma developing in chronic anal fistula: Report of two cases and review of the literature. Dis Colon Rectum 24:562, 1981.

Gibbs NM: Mucinous cystadenoma and cystadenocarcinoma of the vermiform appendix with particular reference to mucocele and pseudomyxoma peritonei. J Clin Pathol 26:413, 1973.

Gillespie JJ, MacKay B: Histogenesis of cloacogenic carcinoma. Hum Pathol 9:579, 1978.

Gingrass PJ, Bubrick MP, Hitchcock CR, Stroma RL: Anorectal verrucose squamous carcinoma: Report of two cases. Dis Colon Rectum 21:120, 1978.

Ginzburg L, Weingarten M, Fischer MG: Submucous lipoma of the colon. Ann Surg 148:767, 1958.

Glasser CM, Bhagavan BS: Carcinoid tumors of the appendix. Arch Pathol Lab Med 104:272, 1980.

Goldgraber MB, Humphreys EM, Kirsner JB, Palmer WL: Carcinoma and ulcerative colitis; a clinical-pathologic study. Gastroenterology 34:809, 1958.

Goodwin JD II: Carcinoid tumors. An analysis of 2837 cases. Cancer 36:560, 1975.

Grodsky L: Unsuspected carcinoma found histologically after minor anorectal operations. Calif Med 106:44, 1967.

Gustafsson BE: Intestinal microflora and carcinogenesis. In Accomplishments in Cancer Research, 1981. Fortner JG, Rhoads JE (eds): Philadelphia, JB Lippincott Co, 1982.

Hagihara PF: Experimental colitis as a promoter in a large-bowel tumorigenesis. Arch Surg 117:1304, 1982.

Hajdu SI, Winawer SJ, Meyers WPL: Carcinoid tumors. Am J Clin Pathol 61:521, 1974.

Haller JD, Roberts TW: Lipomas of the colon: A clinicopathologic study of 20 cases. Surgery 55:773, 1964.

Heald RJ, Bussey HJR: Clinical experience at St. Mark's Hospital with multiple synchronous cancers of the colon and rectum. Dis Colon Rectum 18:6, 1975.

Helwig EB, Graham JH: Anogenital (extramammary) Paget's disease. Cancer 16:387, 1963.

Herman AH, Nasbeth DC: Colitis cystica profunda: Localized segmental and diffuse. Arch Surg 106:337, 1973.

Hernandez FJ, Fernandez BB: Mucus-secreting colonic carcinoid tumors: light and electron microscopic study of three cases. Dis Colon Rectum 17:387, 1974.

Hickey WF, Seiler MW: Ultrastructural markers of colonic adenocarcinoma. Cancer 47:140, 1981.

Hill MJ: The role of colon anaerobes in the metabolism of bile acids and steroids and its relation to colon cancer. Cancer 36:2387, 1975.

Hishida Y, Ishida M: Smooth-muscle tumors of the rectum in Japanese. Dis Colon Rectum 17:226, 1974.

Howard RJ, Ellis CMC, Delaney JP: Intussusception of the appendix simulating carcinoma of the cecum. Arch Surg 101:520, 1970.

Hultén L, Kewenter J, Aorén C, Ojerskog B: Clinical and morphological characteristics of colitis carcinoma and colorectal carcinoma in young people. Scand J Gastroenterol 14:673, 1979.

Jaworski RC: Benign mesenchymal tumours of the colon and rectum: A retrospective study. Aust NZ J Surg 50:586, 1980.

Jenkin RDT, Sonley MJ, Stephens CA, et al: Primary gastrointestinal tract lymphomas in childhood. Radiology 92:763, 1969.

Johnson LA, Lavin P, Moertel CG, et al: Carcinoids: The association of histologic growth pattern and survival. Cancer 51:882, 1983.

Johnston J, Helwig EB: Granular cell tumors of the gastrointestinal tract and perianal region. Dig Dis Sci 26:807, 1981.

Kalus M: Carcinoma and adenomatous polyps of the colon and rectum in biopsy and organ tissue culture. Cancer 30:972, 1972.

Kasulke RJ, Anderson WJ, Gupta SV, Gleidman ML: Primary tuberculous enterocolitis. Arch Surg 116:110, 1981.

Klein HZ: Mucinous carcinoid tumor of the vermiform appendix. Cancer 33:770, 1974.

Kline RJ, Spencer RJ, Harrison EG Jr: Carcinoma associated with fistula-in-ano. Arch Surg 89:989, 1964.

Klotz RG, Pamukcoglu T, Souilliard DH: Transitional cloacogenic carcinoma of the anal canal. Cancer 20:1727, 1967.

Konishi F, Morson BC: Pathology of colorectal adenomas: a colonoscopic survey. J Clin Pathol 35:830, 1982.

Kraus FT: Pedunculated adenomatous polyp with carcinoma on the tip and metastasis to lymph nodes. Dis Colon Rectum 8:283, 1965.

Kuehn PG, Eisenberg H, Reed JF: Epidermoid carcinoma of the perianal skin and anal canal. Cancer 22:932, 1968.

Kurzon RM, Ortega R, Rywlin AM: The significance of papillary features in polyps of the large intestine. Am J Clin Pathol 62:447, 1974.

Lammer J, Dirschmid K, Hügel H: Carcinomatous metastases to the colon simulating Crohn's disease. Gastrointest Radiol 6:89, 1981.

LaMont JT, O'Gorman TA: Experimental colon cancer. Gastroenterology 75:1157, 1978.

Lane N, Kaye GI: Pedunculated adenomatous polyp of the colon with carcinoma lymph node metastasis and suture-line recurrence. Am J Clin Pathol 48:170, 1967.

Lee SH, McGregor DH, Kuziez MN: Malignant transformation of perianal condyloma acuminatum. Dis Colon Rectum 24:462, 1981.
Lee SS, Song KT: Primary adenocarcinoma of the appendix: A report of two cases. J Surg Oncol 21:162, 1982.
LeMole G, Goldman LI, Rosemond GP: Leiomyosarcoma of the colon—a revised prognosis: Report of a case. Dis Colon Rectum 11:306, 1968.
Lev R, Grover R: Precursors of human carcinoma: A serial section study of colectomy specimens. Cancer 47:2007, 1981.
Levine SM, Stover JF, Warren JG, et al: Ameboma, the forgotten granuloma. JAMA 215:1461, 1971.
Lewin KJ, Ranchod M, Dorfman RF: Lymphomas of the gastrointestinal tract. Cancer 42:693, 1978.
Lewin MR, Ferulano GP, Cruse JP, Clark CG: Experimental colon carcinogenesis is facilitated by endogenous factors in the intestinal contents. Carcinogenesis 2:1363, 1981.
Lipper S, Kahn LB, Ackerman LV: The significance of microscopic invasive cancer in endoscopically removed polyps of the large bowel: A clinicopathologic study in 51 cases. Lab Invest 48:51A, 1983 (Abstract).
Lobert PR, Appelman HD: Inflammatory cloacogenic polyp. Am J Surg Pathol 5:761, 1981.
Lou TY, Teplitz C: Malakoplakia: pathogenesis and ultrastructural morphogenesis. Hum Pathol 5:191, 1974.
MacGillivray JB: Mucosal metaplasia in the appendix. J Clin Pathol 25:809, 1972.
Madara JL, Harte P, Deasy J, et al: Evidence for an adenoma-carcinoma sequence in dimethylhydrazine-induced neoplasms of rat intestinal epithelium. Am J Pathol 110:230, 1983.
Maskens AP, Dujardin-Loits RM: Experimental adenomas and carcinomas of the large intestine behave as distinct entities: Most carcinomas arise de novo in flat mucosa. Cancer 47:81, 1981.
Mathews JL, Coyle D Jr, Little WD: Primary linitis plastica of the rectum. Dis Colon Rectum 25:448, 1982.
Meyers MA, McSweeney J: Secondary neoplasms of the bowel. Radiology 105:1, 1972.
Moore GE, Norton LW, Meiselbaugh DM: Condyloma. A new epidemic. Arch Surg 113:630, 1978.
Morrey B, Wolma FJ: Cicatricial stricture in intestinal amebiasis: A review of 121 cases of intestinal amebiasis. South Med J 65:678, 1972.
Morson BC: The muscle abnormality in diverticular disease of the sigmoid colon. Br J Radiol 36:385, 1963.
Morson BC: Factors influencing the prognosis of early cancer of the rectum. Proc Roy Soc Med 59:607, 1966.
Muto T, Bussey HJR, Morson BC: Pseudo-carcinomatous invasion in adenomatous polyps of the colon and rectum. J Clin Pathol 20:25, 1973.
Myrvold HE, Kock NG, Ahrén C: Rectal biopsy and precancer in ulcerative colitis. Gut 15:301, 1974.
Navarrete A, Spjut HJ: Effect of colostomy on experimentally induced neoplasms of the colon of the rat. Cancer 20:1466, 1967.
Nielsen OV, Jensen SL: Basal cell carcinoma of the anus—a clinical study of 34 cases. Br J Surg 68:856, 1981.
O'Brien MJ, Zamcheck RN, Burke B, et al: Immunocytochemical localization of carcinoembryonic antigen in benign and malignant colorectal tissues. Am J Clin Pathol 75:283, 1981.
Pang LSC, Morson BC: Basaloid carcinoma of the anal canal. J Clin Pathol 20:128, 1967.
Patterson FK: Adenoacanthoma and ulcerative colitis: Case report and review of the literature. South Med J 66:681, 1973.
Perez CA, Sturim HS, Kauchoukos NT, Kamberg S: Some clinical and radiographic features of gastrointestinal histoplasma. Radiology 86:482, 1966.
Perkins DE, Spjut HJ: Intestinal stenosis following radiation therapy. AJR 88:953, 1962.
Pittella JEH, Torres AV: Primary squamous cell carcinoma of the cecum and ascending colon. Dis Colon Rectum 25:483, 1982.
Pohzarisski KM: Morphology and morphogenesis of experimental epithelial tumors of the intestine. JNCI 54:1115, 1975.
Ponka JL, Walke L: Carcinoid tumors of the rectum. Dis Colon Rectum 14:46, 1971.
Quan SHQ, Berg JW: Leiomyoma and leiomyosarcoma of the rectum. Dis Colon Rectum 5:415, 1962.
Raszkowski HJ, Hufner RF: Neurofibromatosis of the colon. A unique manifestation of von Recklinghausen's disease. Cancer 27:134, 1971.
Recio PM: Ameboma of the colon. Philipp J Surg 20:61, 1965.
Rosengren JE: Radiographic investigations of experimentally induced colonic tumors in the rat. Ph.D. Thesis. University of Lund, Malmö, Sweden, 1977.
Roth JA, Schell S, Panzarino S, Coronato A: Visceral Kaposi's sarcoma presenting as colitis. Am J Surg Pathol 2:209, 1978.
Russell IS, Hughes ESR: Fibrosarcoma of the rectum. Aust NZ J Surg 34:27, 1964.
Sabback MS, O'Brien PH: Clinical study of 81 gastrointestinal carcinoid tumors. South Med J 72:386, 1979.
Sasajiima K, Okawa K, Sasamoto Y, et al: Pararectal rhabdomyosarcoma: Report of a case. Dis Colon Rectum 23:576, 1980.
Schoental R, Bensted JPM: Gastro-intestinal tumours in rats and mice following various routes of administration of N-methyl-N-nitro-N′-nitroguanidine and N-ethyl-N-nitroso-N′-nitroguanidine. Br J Cancer 23:757, 1969.
Shapiro JL: Diverticular disease of the colon. South Med J 67:710, 1974.
Shatney CH: The treatment of penduncculated adenomatous colorectal polyp with focal cancer. Surg Gynecol Obstet 139:845, 1974.
Shindo K: Epidermoid carcinoma compared with adenocarcinoma of the anal canal. Aust NZ J Surg 51:426, 1981.
Shinya H, Wolff WI: Morphology, anatomic distribution and cancer potential of colonic polyps. Ann Surg 190:679, 1979.
Singh R, Nime F, Mittelman A: Malignant epithelial tumors of the anal canal. Cancer 48:411, 1981.
Sloan PJ, Goepel J: Lichen sclerosus et atrophicus and perianal carcinoma: A case report. Clin Exper Dermatol 6:399, 1981.
Snyder DN, Heston JF, Meigs JW, Flannery JT: Changes in site distribution of colorectal carcinoma in Connecticut, 1940–1973. Am J Dig Dis 22:791, 1977.
Spjut HJ, Appel MF: Epithelial polyps of the large bowel: A pathological and colonoscopic study. Curr Probl Cancer 4:23, 1979.
Spjut HJ, Estrada RG: The significance of epithelial polyps of the large bowel. Pathol Annu 12:147, 1977.
Spjut HJ, Frankel NB, Appel MF: The small carcinoma the large bowel. Am J Surg Pathol 3:39, 1979.
Spjut HJ, Perkins DE: Endometriosis of the sigmoid colon and rectum. AJR 82:1070, 1959.
Spjut HJ, Smith MN: A comparative electron microscopic study of human and rat colonic polyps and carcinomas. Exper Mol Pathol 6:11, 1967.
Spjut HJ, Spratt JS Jr: Endemic and morphologic similarities existing between spontaneous colonic neoplasms in man and 3:2′-dimethyl-4-aminobiphenyl induced colonic neoplasms in rats. Ann Surg 161:309, 1965.

Spratt JS Jr, Ackerman LV: Small primary adenocarcinomas of the colon and rectum. JAMA 179:337, 1962.

Spratt JS Jr, Ackerman LV, Moyer CA: Relationship of polyps of the colon to colonic cancer. Ann Surg 148:682, 1958.

Spratt JS Jr, Spjut HJ: Prevalence and prognosis of individual clinical and pathologic variables associated with colorectal carcinoma. Cancer 20:1976, 1967.

Stavorovsky M, Morag B, Stavorovsky H, Papo J: Smooth muscle tumors of the alimentary tract. J Surg Oncol 22:109, 1983.

Stearns MW Jr, Urmacher C, Sternberg SS, et al: Cancer of the anal canal. Curr Probl Cancer 4:1, 1980.

Subbuswamy SG, Gibbs NM, Ross CF, Morson BC: Goblet cell carcinoid of the appendix. Cancer 34:338, 1974.

Sundblad AS, Paz RA: Mucinous carcinomas of the colon and rectum and their relationship to polyps. Cancer 50:2504, 1982.

Symonds DA, Vickery AL Jr: Mucinous carcinoma of the colon and rectum. Cancer 37:1891, 1976.

Syracuse DC, Perzin KH, Price JB, et al: Carcinoid tumors of the appendix. Mesoappendiceal extension and nodal metastases. Ann Surg 190:58, 1979.

Talbot IC, Ritchie S, Leighton MH, et al: Spread of rectal cancer within veins. Am J Surg 141:15, 1981.

Taxy JB, Mendelsohn G, Gupta PK: Carcinoid tumors of the rectum. Silver reactions, fluorescence and serotonin content of the cytoplasmic granules. Am J Clin Pathol 74:791, 1980.

Terner JY, Lattes R: Malakoplakia of colon and retroperitoneum. Am J Clin Pathol 44:20, 1965.

Thorlakson RH: Carcinoma of the colon and rectum associated with chronic ulcerative colitis. Surg Gynecol Obstet 103:41, 1956.

Uohara JK, Kobara TY: Endometriosis of the appendix. Am J Obstet Gynecol 121:423, 1975.

Walsh TJ, Mulholland JH: Laryngeal and perianal tuberculosis simulating laryngeal and perianal carcinoma. John Hopkins Med J 149:135, 1981.

Wanebo HJ, Woodruff JM, Farr GH, Quan SH: Anorectal melanoma. Cancer 47:1891, 1981.

Watson LC, Mueller EO, Thompson JC: Leiomyosarcoma of the colon. South Med J 71:726, 1978.

Wayte DM, Helwig EB: Colitis cystica profunda. Am J Clin Pathol 48:159, 1967.

Welch CE, Burke JF: Carcinoma of the colon and rectum. New Engl J Med 266:211, 1962.

Wiley EL, Mendelsohn G, Eggleston JC: Distribution of carcinoembryonic antigens and blood group substances in adenocarcinoma of the colon. Lab Invest 44:507, 1981.

Wolff M: Heterotopic gastric epithelium in the rectum: A report of three new cases with a review of 87 cases of gastric heterotopia in the alimentary canal. Am J Clin Pathol 55:604, 1971.

Wolff M, Ahmed N: Epithelial neoplasms of the vermiform appendix (exclusive of carcinoid). I. Adenocarcinoma of the appendix. Cancer 37:2493, 1976.

Wolff M, Ahmed N: Epithelial neoplasms of the vermiform appendix (exclusive of carcinoid). II. Cystadenomas, papillary adenomas, and adenomatous polyps of the appendix. Cancer 37:2511, 1976.

Wychulis AR, Beahrs OH, Woolner LB: Malignant lymphoma of the colon. Arch Surg 93:215, 1966.

TEN

Adenocarcinomas of the Colon and Rectum
Primary Anatomic Extent, Histopatholgy, and Management Factors Correlating with Prognosis

J. S. Spratt, M.D.

The prognosis for cancer of the colon and rectum depends on many variables describing the clinical state of the patient, including biologic factors in the cancer-host relationship, the anatomic extent of the cancer, and the treatment being used. This relationship is not easy to study because of the numerous variables involved; the changing technology of treatment over time; the length of follow-up necessary to measure end results accurately; the number of cases needed to obtain statistically significant end points; and the difficulties in designing controlled studies, such as costs and the problems of human acceptance and compliance. With the aim of organizing the mass of available data, this chapter attempts to correlate end results with the past and present technologies of management and the anatomic extent, clinical presentation, and histopathology of the cancers. The chapter cannot be all-encompassing, since too many urgent, infrequent, and often immediately life-threatening circumstances exist that clutter the path toward simplification.

EVOLVING TECHNOLOGY AND END RESULTS

The impact of all therapeutic systems on cancer is in a constant state of flux. The unplanned introduction of new technologies and temporal variations in the incidence of disease are major reasons for this. Mortality and survival rates with colorectal cancers are classic examples of this phenomenon. I participated in reviews covering almost the entire spectrum of colorectal cancer management in a single university hospital (Barnes Hospital, St. Louis) in a period of rapid technologic change (1914 to 1951) (Polk et al., 1964). During this period, a sustained improvement in the 5-year survival rate occurred, and the reviews clearly confirmed that the improvement was due to reduced operative mortality and increased operability and resectability rates (Fig. 10–1). Both anastomotic dehiscence and fatal peritonitis declined steadily during this period (Fig. 10–2).

The introduction of blood banking is most responsible for the great changes in surgical mortality and enhanced resectability rates between 1935 and 1939 and 1940 and 1944. Antibiotics were not generally used at Barnes until after 1947.

These early studies and others at Barnes Hospital and, subsequently, at the Ellis Fischel State Cancer Hospital (EFSCH) stimulated a continuing interest in these complex cancers. As stated previously, the intent of this chapter is to review the associations between prognosis and various factors. The general convention for defining these subsets is the clinical and anatomic staging systems. However, as the early Barnes' studies confirmed, changing prognosis is continually affected by uncontrolled application of evolving technology.

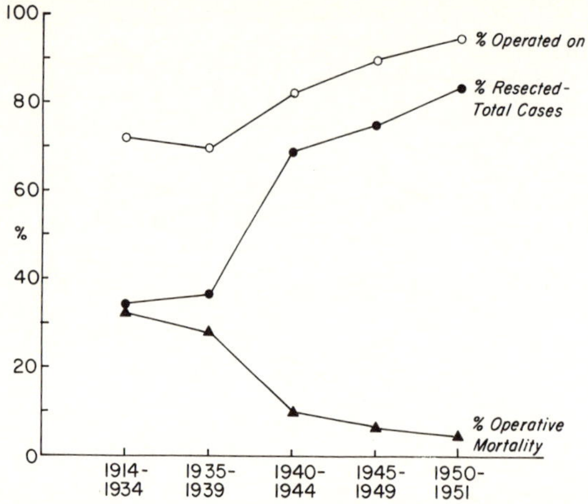

Figure 10–1. Operability, resectability, and operative mortality rates for carcinomas of the colon and rectum presenting at Barnes Hospital from 1914 to 1951. (From Polk HC Jr, Spratt JS Jr, Bennett D, et al: Surgical mortality and survival from colonic carcinoma. Arch Surg 89:16–23, 1964. Copyright 1964; American Medical Association.)

ANATOMIC AND CLINICAL STAGING SYSTEMS

Staging systems currently in use tend to group large numbers of variables under the various stages with incomplete consideration of whether the variables are independent of or dependent on one another (Dukes, 1932; Gabriel et al., 1935; Dukes, 1940; Dukes et al., 1948; Astler and Coller, 1954; Polk et al., 1964; Shepherd and Jones, 1971; Goligher, 1976; Beart et al., 1978; American Joint Committee on Cancer, 1983). Also, histologic variables, independent of the factors determining clinical staging, have often proved to have highly significant associations with prognosis. Grouping variables for classification can obscure the significance of individual factors and interdependent sets of factors.

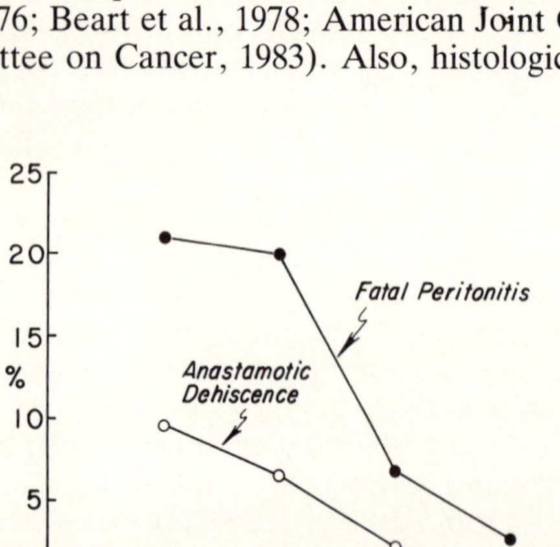

Figure 10–2. Frequency of fatal peritonitis or anastomotic dehiscence as a complication of operations for carcinoma of the colon and rectum at Barnes Hospital from 1914 to 1951. (From Polk HC Jr, Spratt JS Jr, Bennett D, et al: Surgical mortality and survival from colonic carcinoma. Arch Surg 89:16–23, 1964. Copyright 1964, American Medical Association.)

In the precomputer days, these groupings were necessary to reduce the categories into convenient numbers, usually four stages and grades, and to determine the efficacy of therapy on the different groups. The state of the art use of electronic data processing (EDP) has made these gross empirical groups anachronistic. EDP can perform the mathematical work needed for more precise identification of the prognosis associated with individual variables. Computer-stored information can permit the rapid comparison of individual variables and groups of variables, and important information is not lost by arbitrary grouping. Powerful statistical methods can then be used to manipulate data through various analyses essential for improved understanding of these data and, ultimately, the specificity of treatment.

A major concern is that staging systems based largely on a limited number of anatomic or pathologic characteristics might conceal information about various subsets of cases, particularly those that may have either an exceptionally good or an exceptionally bad prognosis. This information is essential to ascertain with the greatest possible accuracy the specificity of primary treatment and the need for additional clinical research when current treatment does not lead to control of the cancer. Inadequate classification systems can put subsets in jeopardy of both overtreatment and undertreatment.

The major conventional staging systems in wide use include Dukes' classification with several subsequent modifications, and the TNM system, adopted by the American Joint Commission on Staging and End Results (AJC). This latter system is superior to earlier ones because it considers more variables. However, much information is still lost and time is wasted by the TNM system as a result of the horizontal transfer of information, which groups measured characteristics together into categories (T, N, M) at considerable cost and often with a reduction in specificity. These categories are then further reduced in specificity by an additional horizontal transfer of information into stages. The groupings have often been defined with incomplete consideration of the independence or dependence of

Table 10–1. STAGING SYSTEMS FOR CARCINOMA OF THE COLORECTUM*

AJCC 1982	UICC 1978 (3rd ed)	Dukes (1932, 1935)†	Astler-Coller‡
Stage 0	*Stage 0*		*Stage 0*
Carcinoma in situ			
Tis NO MO	Tis, NO, MO		0
Stage I	*Stage I*	*A*	*Stage I*
IA Tumor confined to mucosa or submucosa	1A		
T1, NO, MO			
IB Tumor involves muscularis propria but not beyond	T1, NO, MO	A	A
	1B		
T2, NO, MO	T2, NO, MO	A	B1
Stage II	*Stage II*	*B*	*Stage II*
Involvement of all layers of bowel wall with or without invasion of immediately adjacent structures T3, NO, MO	T3, T4, NO, MO (T3a with fistula) (T3b without fistula)		B2
Stage III	*Stage III*	*C (1932)*	*Stage III*
Any degree of bowel wall with regional node metastasis	Any T, N1, MO	C1 (1935) C2 (1935)	C1 C2
Any T, N1–N3, MO			
Extends beyond contiguous tissue or immediately adjacent organs with no regional lymph node metastasis			
T4, NO, MO			
Stage IV	*Stage IV*	*Type 4*	*Stage IV*
Any invasion of bowel wall with or without regional lymph node metastasis but with evidence of distant metastasis	Any T, any N, M1	(so-called D)	D
Any T, any N, M1			

*American Joint Committee on Cancer. *In* Beahrs OH, Myers MH: Manual for Staging of Cancer. 2nd ed. Philadelphia, JB Lippincott Company, 1983.

†Dukes: A = Limited to bowel wall; B = Spread to extramural tissue; C = Involvement of regional nodes (C1: Near primary lesion; C2; Proximal node involved at point of ligation); Type 4 (so-called D) = Distant metastasis.

‡Astler-Coller: A = Limited to mucosa; B1 = Same as AJCC Stage IB (T2a); B2 = Same as AJCC Stage IB (T2b); C1 = Limited to wall with involved nodes; C2 = Through all layers of wall with involved nodes.

the variables. Each variable measured and any stage defined has to be viewed as a "snapshot" of a continual spectrum of events. A cancer is a seething mass of intracellular and extracellular biochemical actions in a constant state of flux progressing over time at highly variable rates, which are associated with a complex interaction of many variables relating both to treatment decisions and prognosis.

As a matter of documentation, the major staging systems are provided in Table 10–1. Suggested staging forms for new cases are provided in Figure 10–3.

The TNM Classification

The AJC staging of colorectal cancers uses a method of evaluation based on the following rules:

Clinical-Diagnostic Staging. Clinical assessment includes medical history, physical examination, routine and special roentgenograms (including barium enema and fluoroscopy), sigmoidoscopy, colonoscopy biopsy, cytologic examination of colon washings, laboratory examinations, e.g., occult blood determination in the stool, carcinoembryonic antigen (CEA) assay, and special examinations used to demonstrate the presence of extracolonic metastasis, such as chest and bone films, computed axial tomography (CAT) scans, blood counts, tests of CEA levels, isotopic scans of liver and bone, and liver chemistries.

Surgical-Evaluative Staging. This should include all the data obtained for clinical classification, as well as the information obtained at the time of exploratory laparotomy, including biopsy, but not including information obtained by complete histopathologic examination of a therapeutically resected specimen.

Postsurgical Treatment–Pathologic Staging. This classification describes the known extent of the colorectal carcinoma after complete examination of the resected specimen. Important determinants of survival in this classification are the depth of tumor penetration, involvement of regional lymph nodes, and presence of distant metastasis. Other histopathologic factors associated with survival are

Data Form for Cancer Staging

Patient identification
Name ______
Address ______
Hospital or clinic number ______
Age ____ Sex ____ Race ______

Institutional identification
Hospital or clinic ______
Address ______

Oncology Record

Anatomic site of cancer ______
Chronology of classification* [ ] Clinical-diagnostic (cTNM) [ ] Surgical-evaluative (sTNM)
Date of classification ______

Histologic type† ______ Grade (G) ______
[ ] Postsurgical resection–pathologic (pTNM)
[ ] Retreatment (rTNM) [ ] Autopsy (aTNM)

Definitions: TNM Classification

Primary Tumor (T)

[ ] TX Minimum requirements to assess the primary tumor cannot be met.
[ ] T0 No evidence of primary tumor
[ ] Tis Carcinoma *in situ*
[ ] T1 Tumor confined to mucosa or submucosa
[ ] T2 Tumor limited to bowel wall but not beyond
  [ ] T2a Partial invasion of muscularis propria
  [ ] T2b Complete invasion of muscularis propria
[ ] T3 Tumor invasion of all layers of bowel wall with or without invasion of adjacent or contiguous tissues; fistula may or may not be present.
[ ] T4 Tumor spread by direct extension beyond contiguous tissue or the immediately adjacent organs
[ ] T Multiple primary carcinoma; classify most extensive tumors. (Indicate number in brackets.)

Nodal Involvement (N)

[ ] NX Minimum requirements to assess the regional nodes cannot be met.
[ ] N0 Nodes not involved
[ ] N1 One to three involved regional nodes adjacent to primary lesion [ ]
[ ] N2 Regional nodes involved extending to line of resection or ligature of blood vessels [ ]
[ ] N3 Nodes contain metastasis, location not identified. Specific number examined [ ]; number involved [ ]

Distant Metastasis (M)

[ ] MX Minimum requirements to assess the presence of distant metastasis cannot be met.
[ ] M0 No (known) distant metastasis
[ ] M1 Evidence of distant metastasis
Specify ______

Stage Grouping

[ ] Stage 0		Tis, N0, M0
[ ] Stage I		
	IA	T1, N0, M0
	IB	T2, N0, M0
[ ] Stage II		T3, N0, M0
[ ] Stage III		Any T, N1–N3, M0
		T4, N0, M0
[ ] Stage IV		Any T, any N, M1

*Use a separate form each time a case is staged.
†See reverse side for additional information.

Site-Specific Information

History
  Symptoms ______
  Duration ______
Physical examination
  Rectal ______
  Abdominal palpation ______
Proctosigmoidoscopy ______
  Fiberoptic colonoscopy ______
  Laparoscopy ______
    Liver edge palpable Yes ____ No ____
Roentgenographic Studies
  Type ______
  Findings ______
  Site or level ______
Laboratory studies
  Hb ______
  CEA (serum) ______ ng
  Other markers (Specify) ______
  Fecal occult blood smear [ ] Positive [ ] Negative [ ] Not done
  Cytology [ ] Positive [ ] Negative [ ] Not done
Pathologic findings
Primary tumor Biopsy [ ] Resected tumor [ ]
  Site (note diagrams):
    Indicate by numeral ______
    Size greatest diameter ______
  Gross characteristics ______
  Depth of penetration of bowel wall ______
  Blood vessel invasion: Venous ______
    Arterial ______
    Not stated ______
  Additional tissues involved: Adjacent ______
    Distant ______
  Complications: Fistula ______ Other ______
  Other neoplasms: Number [ ] Location ______
    Type ______
Nodal involvement
  Cannot assess ______
  None ______
  Regional ____ (Specify ______)
  Distant ____ (Number ______ Proved ______)
Metastasis
  None ____ Yes ____ Specify ______
  Proved ______ Histologically confirmed Yes ____ No ____

Examination by ______ M.D.
Date ______

A

Figure 10–3. *A* and *B*, Staging forms for cancer of the colon (ICD-O 152) and rectum (ICD-O 154). (From Beahrs OH, Myers MH: Manual for Staging of Cancer. 2nd ed. American Joint Committee on Cancer, Philadelphia, JB Lippincott Company, 1983.)

Illustration continued on opposite page

Histologic Type of Cancer

The predominant cancer is adenocarcinoma (98%).

Histologic Grade

[ ] G1 Well differentiated
[ ] G2 Moderately well differentiated
[ ] G3–G4 Poorly to very poorly differentiated

Postsurgical Resection–Pathologic Residual Tumor (R)

[ ] R0 No residual tumor
[ ] R1 Microscopic residual tumor
[ ] R2 Macroscopic residual tumor
Specify ______________________

Performance Status of Host (H)

Several systems for recording a patient's activity and symptoms are in use and are more or less equivalent as follows:

AJCC	*Performance*	*ECOG Scale*	*Karnofsky Scale (%)*
[ ] H0	Normal activity	0	90–100
[ ] H1	Symptomatic but ambulatory; cares for self	1	70–80
[ ] H2	Ambulatory more than 50% of time; occasionally needs assistance	2	50–60
[ ] H3	Ambulatory 50% or less of time; nursing care needed	3	30–40
[ ] H4	Bedridden; may need hospitalization	4	10–20

Anatomic Areas of Colon and Rectum

1. Cecum
2. Ascending colon
3. Hepatic flexure
4. Transverse colon
5. Splenic flexure
6. Descending colon
7. Sigmoid
7.5. Rectosigmoid
8. Rectum
9. Anal canal

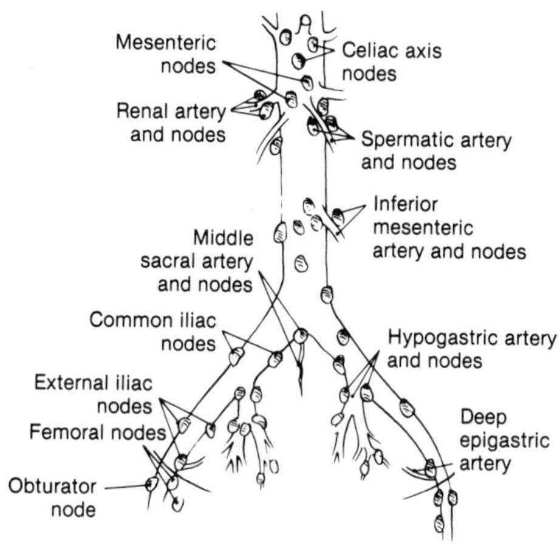

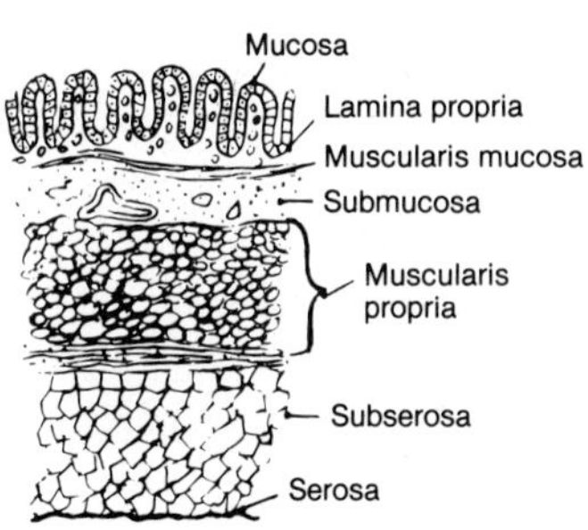

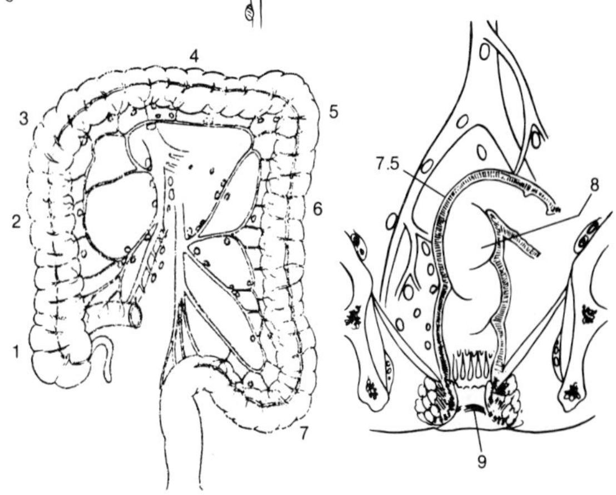

For anatomic areas corresponding to numbers, see list above.

B

Figure 10–3 *Continued.*

local intravasal invasion (venous or lymphatic), grade, and, eventually, the thymidine labeling index when available (see Chapter Two).

Definitions of TNM Categories

The definitions of TNM categories for carcinoma of the colon and rectum follow. Each case must be assigned the highest category of T, N, and M that describes the full extent of disease in that case.

Primary Tumor (T)

TX: Depth of penetration not specified.
TO: No clinically demonstrable tumor.
Tis: Carcinoma in situ (no invasion of lamina propria).
T1: Lesion confined to the mucosa or submucosa (e.g., carcinoma de novo, and/or carcinomatous adenoma, either polypoid or papillary/villous).
T2: Tumor limited to wall of colon or rectum but not beyond—viz., invading into muscularis propria or subserosa (colon and proximal rectum) and into muscularis propria but not beyond (distal rectum).
T2a: Tumor extending into muscularis propria but not penetrating through it.
T2b: Tumor extends through the wall with complete penetration of the muscularis propria.
T3: Tumor invades all layers of bowel wall including serosa (colorectal), with or without extension to adjacent or contiguous tissues. Fistula may or may not be present.
T4: Tumor has spread by direct extension beyond contiguous tissue or the immediately adjacent organs.
( )T: Multiple primary carcinoma. The greatest extent of the tumor is indicated as usual by a suffix as described previously, and the number of multiple tumors is indicated by a parenthetical numerical prefix.

Regional Nodal Involvement (N)

NX: Minimum requirements to assess the regional nodes cannot be met.
NO: Nodes not believed to be involved.
N1: One to three involved regional nodes adjacent to primary lesion.
N2: Regional nodes involved extending to line of resection or ligature of blood vessels.
N3: Nodes contain metastasis; location not identified. Specify number examined ( ); number involved ( ). (Cases cannot be properly staged.)

Distant Metastasis (M)

MX: Minimum requirements to assess the presence of distant metastasis cannot be met.
MO: No (known) distant metastasis.
M1: Distant metastasis present, including extra-abdominal nodes; intra-abdominal nodes proximal to mesocolon and inferior mesenteric artery (juxtaregional); peritoneal implants; liver; lungs; and bones. Specify __________.

Specify sites according to the following notations:

Pulmonary	PUL	Bone Marrow	MAR
Osseous	OSS	Pleura	PLE
Hepatic	HEP	Skin	SKI
Brain	BRA	Eye	EYE
Lymph Nodes	LYM	Other	OTH

Add "+" to the abbreviated notation to indicate that the pathologic condition (p) is proved.

Postsurgical Treatment Residual Tumor (R)

RO: No residual tumor.
R1: Microscopic residual tumor.
R2: Macroscopic residual tumor.
Specify __________.

Stage Grouping

Stage O

Tis NO MO; carcinoma in situ.

Stage I

Stage 1A: T1, NO, MO; tumor confined to mucosa or submucosa.
Stage 1B: T2, NO, MO; tumor involves muscularis propria but not beyond.

Stage II

T3, NO, MO; tumor involvement of all layers of bowel wall with or without invasion of immediately adjacent structures.

Stage III

Any T, N1–3, MO; any degree of bowel wall invasion with regional node metastasis. T4 NO MO; tumor extends beyond the contiguous tissue or immediately adjacent organs with no regional node metastasis (see Astler and Coller, 1959; Spratt et al., 1970).

Stage IV

Any T, any N, M1; any degree of invasion of bowel wall with or without metastasis to regional lymph nodes but with evidence of distant metastasis.

Histopathologic Classification

The predominant cancer is adenocarcinoma, but a pathologic diagnosis is required to utilize this classification. Tumor grading is required (Sobin et al., 1978; Morson et al., 1976; Wood, 1967). Reference to World Health Organization (WHO) nomenclature is advised.

The basic tumor grades (G) are as follows:

GX: Grade or differentiation not determined, not stated, or not applicable.
G1: Well differentiated.
G2: Moderately differentiated.
G3: Poorly differentiated.
G4: Undifferentiated.

Other characteristics of importance that merit further evaluation in prospective studies are tumor margin circumscription, histopathologic differentiation (e.g., nuclear grade, growth pattern, and mucin production), and host-cellular reaction (lymphocyte and plasma cell infiltration in and about the tumor as well as in contiguous tissues). In each case the specific histologic type and the presence or absence of intravasal permeation (lymphatic, venous, or both) must be recorded routinely.

Definition of the Anatomic Segments of the Colon and Rectum

Accurate definition of the anatomic segments of the colon and rectum is also essential in staging. Exclusive of the designation of the anatomic segment, it is useful for the pathologist to record the centimeter distance between the border of a cancer and an anatomic landmark, such as the ileocecal valve or pectinate line, when available. The length, breadth, and thickness should also be measured and recorded by the pathologist.

Primary Site. The large intestine (or colon) extends from the terminal ileum to the anal canal, although for simplicity it may be divided into three subdivisions exclusive of the rectum: right, middle, and left. Still more simply, the large intestine may be divided into the intraperitoneal colon and the rectum (distal 10 cm). All intraperitoneal colonic lesions are categorized similarly. The rectal lesions are classified differently. The subdivisions will be reiterated, since they may be of relevance in prospective studies.

Ileocecal Valve. The junction of the ileum and cecum is marked by the ileocecal valve, which is an anteroposterior slit formed by the partial invagination of the distal end of the ileum into the cecum.

Cecum. The cecum is a large pouch that constitutes the proximal segment of the large intestine. It measures about 6 by 9 cm and is invested completely by the peritoneum. The vermiform appendix arises from the medial and posterior aspects of the cecum below the ileocecal junction. The appendix may lie in any axis of a circle whose center is the cecal attachment. The ascending colon is 15 to 20 cm long and is ordinarily retroperitoneal.

Hepatic Flexure. Lying at the undersurface of the right lobe of the liver and close to the duodenum and the right kidney is the hepatic flexure. Cancers in this segment frequently invade contiguous organs and mimic other disorders, which may sometimes complicate the differential diagnosis.

Transverse Colon. The transverse colon lies in a more anterior position than do other portions of the colon. Cancers here are often palpable. The transverse mesocolon is attached to the pancreas. Anteriorly, its serosa is contiguous with the gastrocolic ligament attached to the stomach forming the ventral boundaries of the lesser sac.

Splenic Flexure. The splenic flexure lies at a more cephalad level than the transverse colon and is more fixed than the hepatic flexure. It is related intimately to the spleen, the tail of the pancreas, and the left kidney. The descending colon, 10 to 15 cm long, is only partially invested by peritoneum, the posterior portion being in a retroperitoneal position.

Sigmoid Loop. The sigmoid loop extends from the medial border of the left psoas major muscle to the beginning of the rectum. It is suspended by a variable length of mesocolon (the sigmoid mesocolon). When the mesocolon is excessively long, the resulting "redundant" sigmoid may come to lie in the right lower quadrant of the abdomen. This same redundancy also increases the risk of volvulus.

Rectum. The rectum, about 10 to 12 cm long, extends from a point opposite the third sacral vertebra down to the apex of the prostate in the male and to the apex of the perineal body in the female, to a point about 4 cm anterior to the tip of the coccyx. It is defined for convenience as the distal 10 cm of the large intestine, as measured by preoperative sigmoidoscopy from the anal verge. The rectosigmoid area is considered as extending from 10 to 15 cm from the anal mucocutaneous junction. The rectum has no omental appendages, no haustrations, and no taeniae. It is covered by peritoneum in front and on both sides in its upper third and on the anterior wall only in its upper and middle thirds. There is no peritoneal covering on the lower third. In the lower rectum, the mucosa is thrown into longitudinal folds known as the rectal columns or the columns of Morgagni. Between them, just above the white line of Hilton, are the anal pits or sinuses.

Anal Canal. The anal canal extends 4 cm in from the apex of the prostate or the perineal body. The anocutaneous line, or white line of Hilton, at the base of the rectal columns marks the site of the original anal membrane that separated the entodermal gut from the ectodermal proctodeum.

Assessment of Lymph Nodes

Whenever possible, at surgical exploration and in the surgical pathologic evaluation, the status of the principal lymph nodes at the base of the mesocolon should be observed and recorded. Nodes to be assessed are those proximal to the origins of the ileocolic, right colic, middle colic, and inferior mesenteric arteries. In staging for N, involvement of the principal (periaortic) lymph nodes, in contrast to involvement of intervening nodes, constitutes distant metastasis. Intervening, or regional, nodes are (1) intermediate (along the course of the major vessels supplying the colon), (2) paracolic (following the vascular arcades of the marginal artery), and (3) omental (in close proximity to the colon, being found along the mesocolic border of the colon and often in the epiploic appendages).

Although the flow of lymph usually traverses each group of nodes in sequence, it can flow directly to the intermediate or even to the principal nodes, bypassing intervening nodes. Use of the "no-touch" isolation technique in resecting colonic lesions has been considered a contraindication to the intraoperative assessment of lymph node involvement. Certainly, extreme gentleness is in order with any palpation intended to assess the extent of cancer.

Table 10–2 lists the regional lymph nodes for each colorectal segment. Lymph nodes between and about origins of the inferior and superior mesenteric arteries are more difficult to dissect, and this dissection is not always done as a routine. Although these nodes are regional in the anatomic sense, they are designated "distant" for purposes of clinical stage classification. Colonic resections are distal to the superior mesenteric artery and its contiguous nodes. Similarly, lymph flow from the lower rectum may be to regional lymph nodes, i.e., internal iliac (hypogastric), which are not routinely resected at the time of an abdominoperineal resection. They may be resected as a separate procedure (Spratt et al., 1965; Spratt et al., 1973) (see Chapter Eight).

Table 10–2. **LOCATION OF REGIONAL LYMPH NODES FOR EACH COLORECTAL SEGMENT**

Segment	Regional Lymph Nodes
Cecum	Anterior cecal; posterior cecal; ileocolic
Ascending colon	Ileocolic; right colic; middle colic
Hepatic flexure	Right colic; middle colic
Transverse colon	Middle colic
Splenic flexure	Middle colic; left colic
Descending colon	Left colic; inferior mesenteric
Sigmoid colon	Inferior mesenteric; sigmoid mesenteric
Rectosigmoid	Perirectal; left colic; sigmoid mesenteric; inferior mesenteric
Rectum	Perirectal; left colic; sigmoid mesenteric; inferior mesenteric; internal iliac (hypogastric); lateral sacral; common iliac; sacral promontory (Gerota)
Anus	Same as rectum plus femoral

In summary, regional lymph nodes have to be distinguished from juxtaregional lymph nodes in these sites.

Colon. Regional lymph nodes are the pericolic nodes and the nodes located along the ileocolic, right colic, middle colic, and inferior mesenteric arteries. The juxtaregional lymph nodes are the periaortic and other subdiaphragmatic intra-abdominal nodes.

Rectum. Regional nodes are the perirectal nodes and the nodes distal to the origin of the inferior mesenteric artery. The juxtaregional nodes are the periaortic and other subdiaphragmatic intra-abdominal nodes.

Turnbull's Staging System

Turnbull and associates (1967) reported an important compilation of end result data using a different clinical pathologic staging system:

Stage A: Tumor confined to the colon and its coats.

Stage B: Tumor extension into pericolic fat.

Stage C: Tumor metastasis to regional mesenteric lymph nodes, but no evidence of distant spread.

Stage D: Tumor metastasis to liver, lung, bone; seeding of tumor; tumor irremovable because of parietal invasion; adjacent organ invasion.

Comment on the Relationship of End Result Data to Staging Systems

As reported in Chapter One, the end results by the AJC TNM staging system obtained in the treatment of cancers of the colon and rectum in various hospitals in the United States are remarkably uniform. There are many explanations for this outcome, such as standards and quality of practice are uniform in reporting institutions and the biologic behavior of the cancer and not the anatomic extent or treatment are the overriding predeterminants of outcome. Also the variance of end results using the common staging systems may not permit the identification of small differences.

Many special studies looking for these small differences have been reported that review the evolution of end results, the impact of special situations unique but not systematically included in staging schema (obstruction, perforation, ovarian metastases), and the impact that special techniques exhibit on outcome (early ligation of lymph vascular bundle, intraluminal irrigants, iodized suture, etc.).

Few reports on various management approaches have been subjected to the scrutiny of controlled clinical trials to evaluate impact on end results. The variegated nature and urgency of many clinical situations produced by these neoplasms have often required life-saving surgical action. However, there is often more than one life-saving approach. Infrequency and dissimilarities in cases have made rigid experimental design difficult. In discussing end results in these special situations, the results can rarely be separated from the management approach and the condition of the patient. As was shown in the introduction to this chapter, technology changing over time has affected end results without there being rigid verification that observed associations are causally related. Special characteristics of and problems created by colorectal neoplasms and the methods of surgical management in uncontrolled studies have often been associated with highly different end results, as will be reviewed next.

RELATIONSHIP OF THE SIZE OF COLONIC TUMORS TO THEIR CELLULAR COMPOSITION AND BIOLOGIC BEHAVIOR

An early study (Spratt and Ackerman, 1960b) investigated the relationship between the sizes of tumors of the colon and their cellular composition and biologic behavior (lymph nodal metastases and lethality). The sample consisted of 243 consecutive single adenocarcinomas and 132 noncarcinomatous polypoid tumors removed surgically from the colon and rectum between 1952 and 1955 and 34 untreated colonic cancers found among 4210 consecutive necropsies performed between 1950 and 1957. The entire sample was from the Barnes Hospital population and was not random. It consisted predominantly of people seeking medical care because of symptoms related to the colonic tumors.

The greatest linear dimension of that portion of the tumor lying within the lumen of the colon had been recorded for 258 of the 275 cancers and 126 of the 132 polyps. This measure was called the "diameter." The pedicles of pedunculated tumors were excluded from measurement. The seriations of the diameters of the tumors (Fig. 10–4) were based on the changes in diameter that would occur with a quadrupling of the volume of a spherical tumor. Although the relationship between the greatest intraluminal linear dimension of an irregularly shaped tumor and the diameter of a true sphere is crude, it is a satisfactory basis for seriation of the sizes of tumors so as to permit the direct correlation of tumor size with its duration. Ackerman reclassified two of the 132 polyps as cancers. A complete follow-up of 4 to 7 years was obtained for 53 persons with cancer of the colon.

The relationship between tumor size and histologic nature was considered. Figure 10–4 demonstrates that only 12 percent of the tumors having a diameter of 1.24 to 1.97 cm were cancers and that the proportion of tumors that were cancers rapidly increased as the size of the tumors increased. All colonic tumors greater than 3 cm in diameter were cancers. In the population of tumors smaller than 1.26 cm in diameter, only 1 of 91 tumors was a cancer.

These observations had three clinical implications. First, all tumors of the colon located beyond the range of a sigmoidoscope measuring over 12 mm in diameter on a roentgenogram could be regarded as cancers and resected as such without the need for prior biopsy. Second, in order that an iatrogenic mortality rate not be substituted for a neoplastic one, persons of poor operative risk and extreme age rarely needed to be operated on for a colonic tumor beyond the range of the sigmoidoscope that measured 12 mm or less in

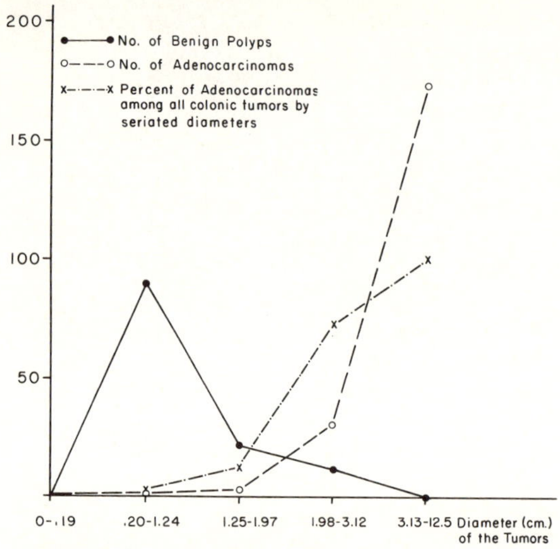

Figure 10–4. The distribution of 228 adenocarcinomas and 124 benign polyps of the colon and rectum according to the seriated diameters of the tumors. (From Spratt JS Jr, Ackerman LV: Relationship of the size of colonic tumors to their cellular composition and biological behavior. Surg Forum 10:56–61, 1960).

diameter on the roentgenogram. The percentages in Figure 10–4 define the upper limits of acceptable operative mortality for the removal of very small colonic tumors. Otherwise, an iatrogenic mortality rate would be substituted for a neoplastic one even if benign polyps might once in a while progress to cancer (Spratt et al., 1958). Third, all rectal and lower colonic tumors visible through a sigmoidoscope should be removed in whole or in part for histologic examination regardless of the size of the tumor because the mortality risk attending these procedures is less than 0.02 of 1 percent, a figure lower than the actual frequency of cancer within the sigmoid and rectum (Dorn and Cutler, 1959). The impact of the colonoscope on these conclusions is still incompletely defined but is discussed in Chapter Six.

The Small Primary Cancer

The need to define further the properties of small cancers was addressed by Spratt and Ackerman (1962). They reported the biologic characteristics of 20 small primary adenocarcinomas of the colon and rectum, all measuring 2 cm or less in diameter, collected from the experience of Ackerman between 1950 and 1959. None of the cancers was associated with a previous or simultaneous carcinoma in another part of the colon or rectum nor with a benign adenomatous polyp.

These cancers were of three gross morphologic types: the pedunculated type (Fig. 10–5), the sessile type (Fig. 10–6), and the ulcerated

Table 10–3. **CHI-SQUARE TESTING OF THE HOMOGENEITY OF THE PRESENCE OR ABSENCE OF LYMPH NODAL METASTASES FROM RESECTED COLONIC AND RECTAL CANCERS OF SERIATED DIAMETERS***

Number of Doubling Times Equivalent to Diameter of the Cancer	Seriated Diameters of the Cancers (cm)	No. of Cancers with Lymph Nodal Metastases (a′)	No. of Cancers without Lymph Nodal Metastases (a)	P $\left(\frac{a}{a + a'}\right)$	a P
0–33	0 – 1.97	0	2	No Test	No Test
33–35	1.98 – 3.12	16	15	.48	7.2
35–37	3.13 – 4.97	30	28	.48	13.4
37–39	4.98 – 7.89	54	52	.49	25.5
39–41	7.90 –12.50	16	13	.45	5.9
Total		116	108		52.0
		N′	N		Σ(aP)

$$\overline{P} = \frac{N}{N + N'} = .48 \qquad X^2 = \frac{1}{.48 \cdot .52}[52.0 - (108 \cdot .48)]$$

$$\overline{Q} = 1 - \overline{P} = 1 - .48 = .52 \qquad X^2 = .80 \text{ , } N = 3$$

$$X^2 = \frac{1}{\overline{P} \cdot \overline{Q}}[\Sigma(aP) - N \cdot \overline{P}] \qquad P = >.8 \text{ , } <.9$$

Acceptable hypothesis: Among resected colonic cancers the ratio of lymph nodal metastasizing to nonlymph nodal metastasizing cancers (52:48) is the same for all cancers of seriated diameters over 1.97 cm

*From Spratt JS Jr, Ackerman LV: Relationship of the size of colonic tumors to their cellular composition and biologic behavior. Surg Forum 10:56–61, 1960.

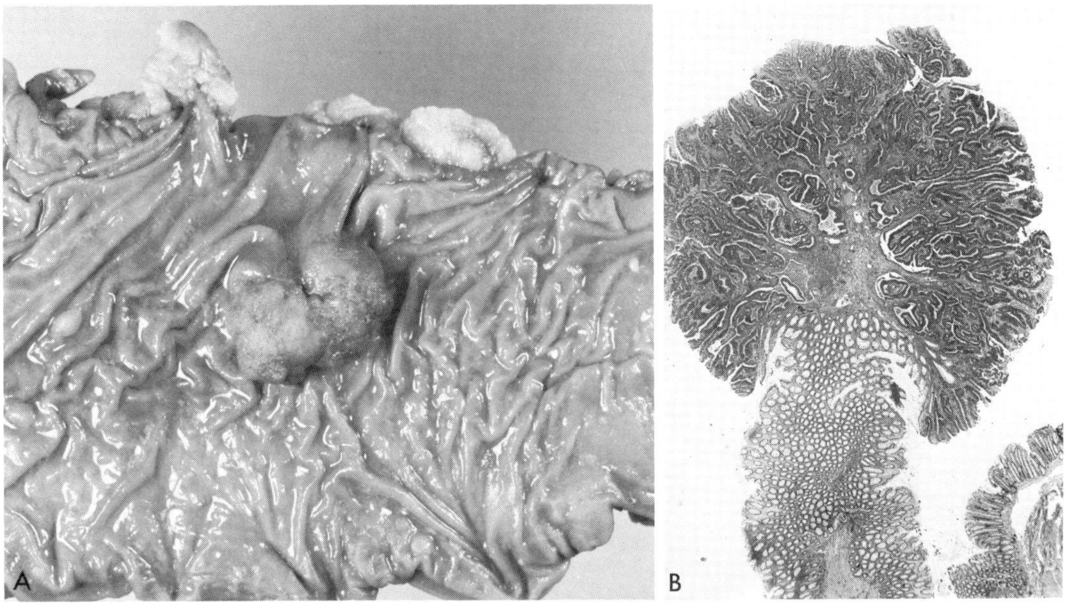

Figure 10–5. *A* and *B*, A polypoid cancer of the colon with a well-formed pedicle of normal mucosa. No metastases were associated with this cancer. No transition zone of benign adenoma separates cancer from normal mucosa. (From Spratt JS Jr, Ackerman LV: Small primary adenocarcinomas of the colon and rectum. JAMA 179:337–346, 1962. Copyright 1962, American Medical Association.)

type (Fig. 10–7). None of the pedunculated polypoid cancers had demonstrable metastases at the time of their removal, and none developed recurrent cancer. One of the eight patients with sessile carcinomas had lymph node metastases at the time of resection. This patient subsequently died from metastases from this cancer. Four of the six patients with ulcerated cancer had lymph node metastases, and a fifth had cancer in the lymphatics but not in the nodes at the time of resection. One of these patients had died of cancer at the time of the report.

The smallest cancer among the 20 cases was only 2 mm in diameter. All cancers were sectioned subserially for microscopic study, and no remnant of adenomatous polyp was found within them or upon their peripheries.

Of pertinence to the discovery of small cancers, Mottram (1934, 1935) showed that even skin tumors did not become visible to the unaided eye until they attained a diameter of 1 to 3 mm. Consequently, a visceral cancer 2 mm in diameter was considered at the lower extent of visual distinction on a routine proctoscopic examination. This cancer was removed by proctoscopic biopsy (Fig. 10–8).

Only four of these 20 small cancers produced symptoms. All were discovered by digital rectal examination, proctoscopic examination, or barium enema study. The four that were symptomatic had caused minor hemorrhage manifested as blood-streaked feces.

There were fundamentally two types of small cancer: cancer that was circumscribed by a fibrous stroma, into which the cancer did not infiltrate (none of this type had metastasized to lymph nodes), and cancer that infiltrated the tissues of the host. The small ulcerated cancers were the most infiltrative (Fig. 10–9). Of the six polypoid cancers, none was infiltrative, although two patients did have carcinoma in the lymphatics of the submucosa of the pedicle.

Unequivocal blood vascular invasion was discovered in only two cases; in neither case was there recurrence of the cancer after resection of the bowel.

Three of the polypoid cancers were treated by local excision alone, and none of these recurred. The remaining cancers were removed by resections that are standard for the treatment of cancer. Only 2 of the 20 persons bearing these cancers developed persistent cancer, but in 1 of these 2 patients a terminal carcinomatosis occurred that was probably of mammary gland origin.

Before the preceding observations were reported, Gilchrist (1938) stated that "the size of tumor (rectal adenocarcinoma) is of little

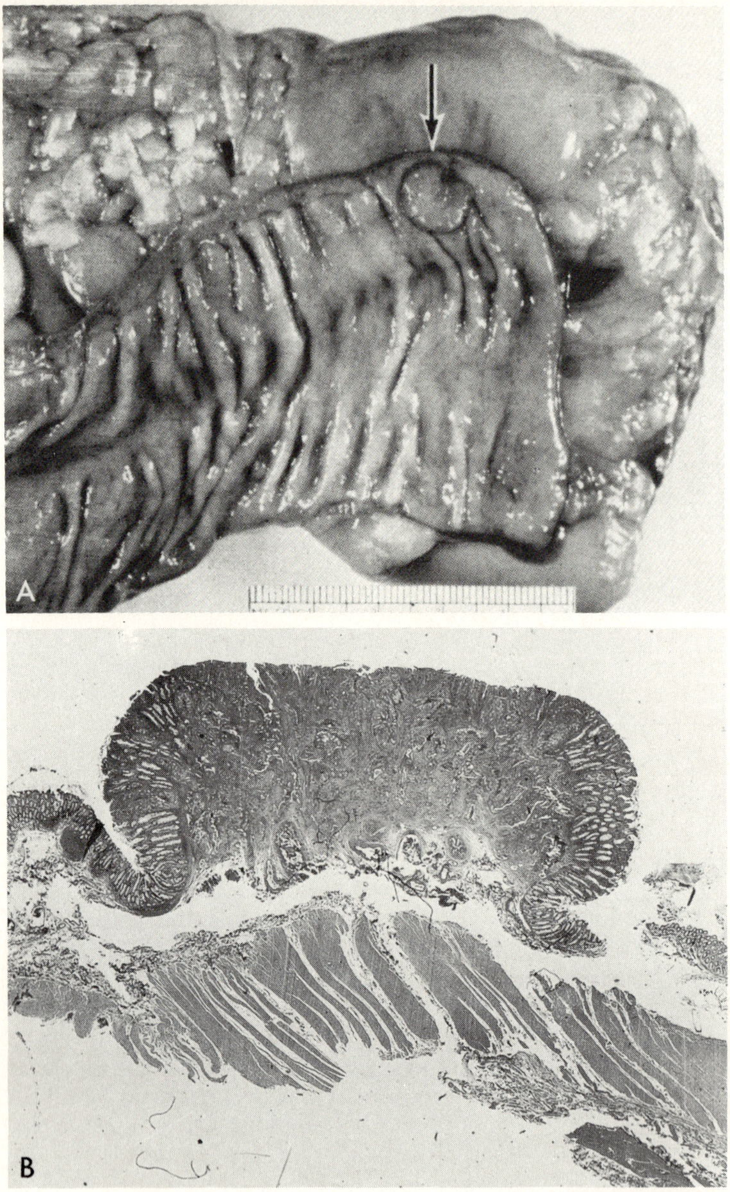

Figure 10–6. *A* and *B*, Small sessile adenocarcinomas of the colon evolve into the classic "medallion cancer," with no polyp formation.No benign adenomatous tissue was associated with this cancer. (From Spratt JS Jr, Ackerman LV: Small primary adenocarcinoma of the colon and rectum. JAMA 179:337–346, 1962. Copyright 1962, American Medical Association.)

value in determining the presence or absence of lymph node metastases." In 1956, Stearns and Deddish observed that the size of a rectal cancer had no relationship to its penetration of the bowel, its frequency of lymph node metastases, or its curability. The lack of correlation between the size of colonic and rectal cancers and the frequency of lymph node metastases was reaffirmed by Spratt and Ackerman (1960b). The general agreement of these separate bodies of data concerning this point implies that some colonic and rectal adenocarcinomas frequently metastasize while they are still very small and others never metastasize at all. Consequently, study of the biologic characteristics of colonic cancers smaller than 2 cm remains especially pertinent, since the smallest size at which a metastasizing colorectal adenocarcinoma disseminates is a critical datum for the design and analysis of screening programs (see Chapter Four).

An estimate of this datum was made by assuming that the primary cancer and the largest lymph node metastasis from it grew at approximately the same rate. Assuming this, the calculation of the approximate volume of the primary tumor at the time it metastasizes was made from measurements of the volume

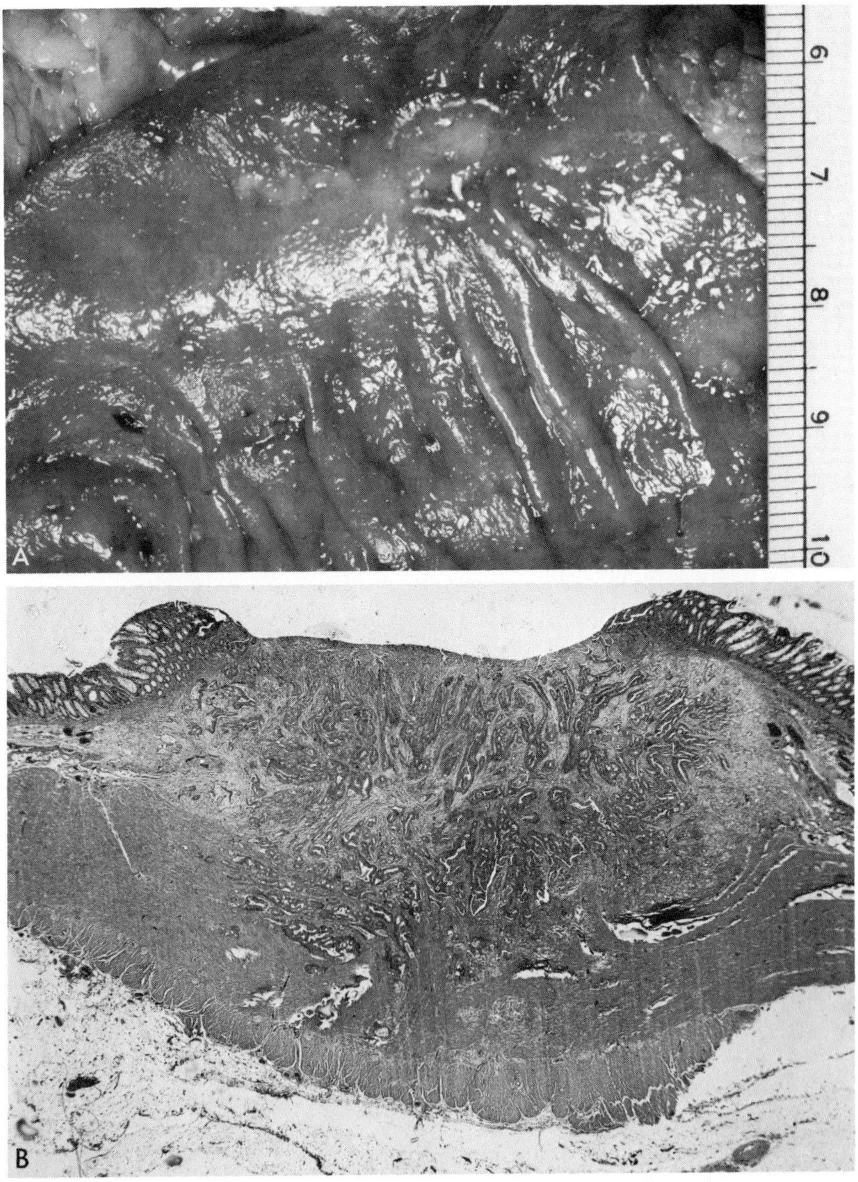

Figure 10–7. *A* and *B*, The most virulent adenocarcinomas of the colon and rectum begin as ulcerations, with very infiltrative growth of cancer permeating all layers of the colonic wall. (From Spratt JS Jr, Ackerman LV: Small primary adenocarcinomas of the colon and rectum. JAMA 179:337–346, 1962. Copyright 1962, American Medical Association.)

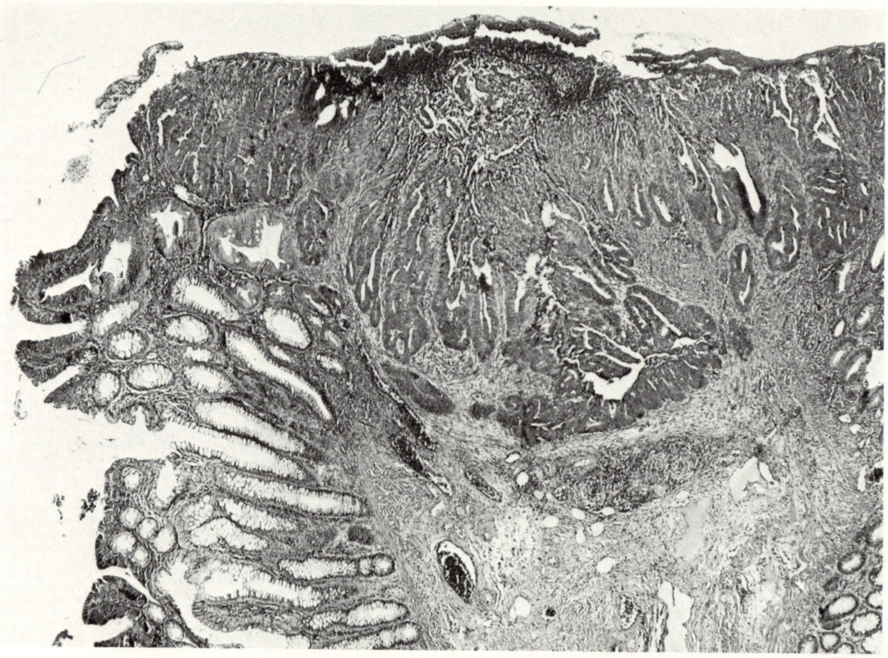

Figure 10–8. Photomicrograph of a primary sessile adenocarcinoma of the rectum, 2 mm in diameter (×33). (From Spratt JS Jr, Ackerman LV: Small primary adenocarcinomas of the colon and rectum. JAMA 179:337–346, 1962. Copyright 1962, American Medical Association.)

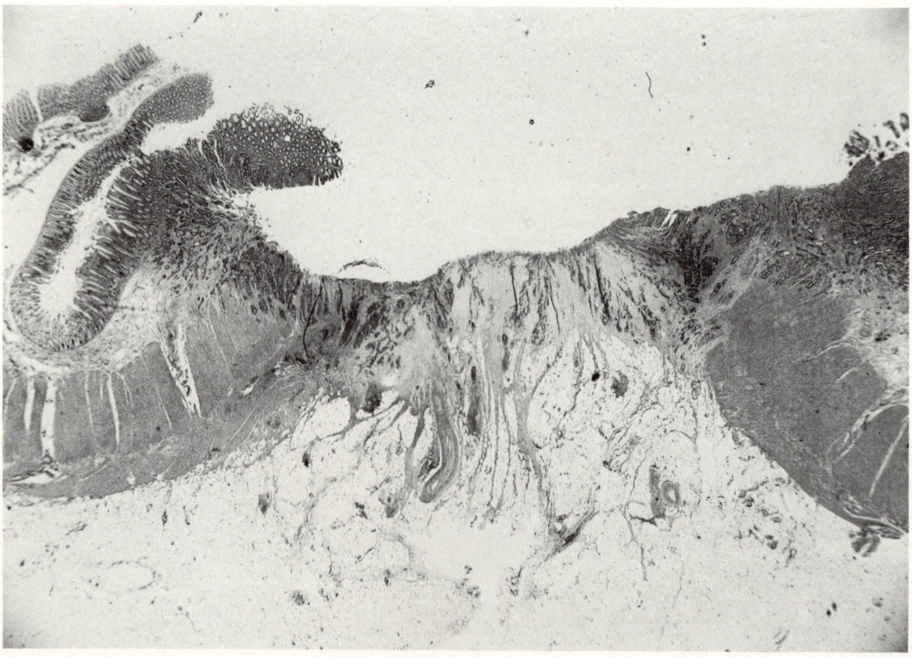

Figure 10–9. This photomicrograph of an ulcerating cancer demonstrates an extreme degree of virulent infiltrative growth well into the mesentery.

of the primary tumor and of the largest metastasis in the lymph nodes. Not even an estimate is available regarding the size at which metastasizing cancers disseminate systemically beyond the locoregional lymph nodes. On an average, cancers in closed spaces may double their volume much faster than cancers growing on a surface where desquamation is occurring (see Chapter Two). If this was generally true, the size of a cancer at first metastasis would be even smaller than the old estimates concluded. Estimates were all of sizes below the range of gross visual distinction.

RELATIONSHIP OF BIOLOGIC PROPERTIES, SIZE, AND METHOD OF RESECTION TO PROGNOSIS

The effect of the performance of local excision of small primary cancers without the performance of colonic or rectal resection on end results is an important issue. The results of Wittoesch and Jackman (1958) following the treatment of even moderately large rectal adenocarcinomas by various methods of local therapy confirmed early that local treatment might be successful in selected patients. In fact, the 46 percent cumulative 5-year survival rate attained by Butcher in treating very large rectal cancers by pelvic exenterations represented primarily the end result of wide local excision of nonmetastasizing cancers, since only a few of the survivors had metastatic cancer in the pelvic and perirectal lymph nodes (Butcher and Spjut, 1959). All these giant cancers had a phase when local excision should have been curative. Only three of the 20 small cancers reviewed were excised locally. None of these recurred. Among the remaining 17 cancers treated by a colonic or rectal resection, eight were not characterized by either lymph node metastases or cancer in the lymphatics. If an infallible method could be devised for selecting the small cancers that do not metastasize, local excision or fulguration could be used more often.

Single cancers of the colon were found by Spratt and Ackerman (1960b) to be associated with the same frequency of metastasis to the regional lymph nodes whether they measured 2 to 3 cm in diameter or 7 to 12 cm in diameter. Colonic cancers of 5 to 8 cm in diameter examined at necropsy were associated with lymph node metastases with the same frequency as larger tumors ($p > .8, < .9$). However, they observed that this finding did not confirm that the frequency of lymph nodal metastasis is not directly related to the sizes of tumors smaller than 2 to 4 cm in diameter. Spratt and Ackerman (1960b) reported that survival was independent of the size of resected cancers larger than 1.5 cm in diameter.

These observations have two significant connotations: (1) Even the very large colonic cancers are curable, with a frequency comparable to that of small tumors, provided that a circumscribing resection including contiguously involved organs together with the perirectal and mesocolic lymph nodes can be performed. (2) The limited resection of many small cancers is unwarranted because 50 percent of the cancers of 3.1 cm in diameter or less had lymph node metastases. Those small cancers with ulceration or excessive mucin production seemed at greatest risk to metastasize, but other characteristics must be considered.

The "early diagnosis" of colonic cancers based on patient response to symptoms is probably a myth. By the time colonic cancers became sufficiently large to bring patients to physicians, all but one of the cancers in this series were larger than 1.2 cm in diameter, and 84 percent of them were larger than 3.1 cm. The implications of growth rates and other factors on the problem of finding the silent cancer in a timely manner are discussed in Chapters Two and Four. Also, see the section entitled Does delay after onset of symptoms affect prognosis? (p. 247).

This led to a question concerning the biologic characteristics of colonic cancer, which is particularly pertinent in an examination of these small cancers: "What is the frequency of origin of colonic cancers from adenomatous polyps?" On statistical grounds the conclusion had already been reached that the probability that benign adenomatous polyps become invasive cancers had to be exceedingly low (Spratt et al., 1958). If these small cancers arose in adenomatous polyps, some microscopic evidence of this origin should have been evident, especially in those that were not ulcerated. After an exhaustive examination of the margins of 14 nonulcerated and six ulcerated small cancers, no sign of an adenomatous polyp was found in any of them. Furthermore, the sizes of these cancers went to the limit of gross visual distinction (2 mm). There was no evidence that these small carcinomas arose in adenomatous polyps. Actually, the frequency with which cancers of the colon arise in the general population can be accounted for without assuming that any of them arose in adenomatous polyps (Spratt et al., 1958). Consequently, stepwise transfiguration of adenomatous polyps to invasive cancers was not confirmed. If adenomatous polyps become invasive cancers, they must do so infrequently. There is no proof that such entities as "focal atypia" and "carcinoma in situ" do not represent some dynamic process other than stepwise metamorphosis from an adenomatous polyp to an invasive metastasizing colonic cancer. If such progression occurs, nothing is known about the time required for this staged metamorphosis (see Chapters One and Nine).

In the 1934 and 1935 reports, Mottram's observations on the dynamics of a system of epitheliomatous growths seemed to have many analogies in the human colon. Mottram observed that neoplasms formed a continuous spectrum ranging from the extremely benign to the highly malignant and that no clear-cut zones of differentiation really existed. He observed that the logarithmic growth rates of the tumors formed a spectrum of rates from the very slow to the very rapid. He established a rough correlation between the rates of growth and the degree of malignancy, i.e., the more rapidly growing tumors were more malignant and more infiltrating, and the more slowly growing tumors frequently disappeared spontaneously. Although he discovered mixed aggregates of cells conforming to different degrees of differentiation in an individual tumor and observed that adjacent benign and malignant tumors became confluent, he noted that it was "uncommon" for an individual tumor to undergo a change in logarithmic growth rate. Rather, the logarithmic growth rate for a particular tumor tended to remain remarkably constant even projected back to the probable moment of cellular origin. He also showed that the host reaction to any neoplasm, i.e., the formation of capillaries, fibroblasts, and monocytic infiltration, was always the same but that the ability of the stroma formed by the host to contain the expanding neoplasm was largely dependent on the growth rate of the neoplasm. Thus, "differentiation" to Mottram was a spectrum of morphologic appearances determined by the growth rates of the tumors with respect to the ability of the stroma formed about the neoplasm and the host tissues to contain the expanding tumor. The mathematical behavior correlated with the morphologic findings. At least two possibly independent variables entered into the equation: (1) the growth rate of the neoplasm and (2) the mechanical resistance of the host tissue to infiltration by the geometrically expanding neoplasm. To these variables might well be added reduced cohesiveness of cells, particularly during cell division, and angiogenic factors needed to maintain nourishment. The rate of growth of colorectal cancers and benign tumors of the colon are related to the histopathologic findings, as discussed in Chapter Two.

Mottram also stated that even the gross morphologic appearance of individual tumors in this system of epithelial neoplasms was related to the growth rate, in that the slowly growing benign tumors tended to pedunculate, whereas the more rapidly growing malignant tumors grew as sessile cancers or as infiltrating cancerous ulcers. In the case of colonic adenocarcinomas and adenomatous polyps, every element or phase of the dynamic system of epithelial neoplasms described by Mottram has been identified. If we are to appreciate the behavior of the system of colonic epithelial tumors in a human population, we must pay increasing attention to the kinetics of the system and determine the extent of correlation existing between the growth parameters of the tumors in the system and their corresponding gross and microscopic appearances, biochemical characteristics, and survivorship.

Among the 20 small cancers reported in the study of Spratt and Ackerman (1962), there were examples of every type of small cancer observed by Mottram, i.e., pedunculated, sessile, and ulcerated. Of these three forms, pedunculated cancers were associated least with metastases, and the ulcerated cancers were most frequently associated with infiltrating metastasizing cancer. With colonic cancers, as with other epithelial cancers, the most lethal form was the infiltrating cancerous ulcer with little intraluminal or exophytic growth. Therefore, it should not be surprising that the frequency and lethality of colonic and rectal cancers have been reduced little by the protracted preoccupation with intraluminal polypoid growths, most of which, when small, are benign (Spratt and Ackerman, 1960a, 1960b). The fundamental problem in improving results of therapy for rectal and colonic adenocarcinomas continues to be the detection of small ulcerated cancers at a stage amenable to curative surgical resection. Preoccupation with the discovery of intraluminal benign or lower-grade malignant polypoid tumors may camouflage the presence of malignant colonic cancers. The alert endoscopist has the peculiar advantage of being able to see small malignant ulcers of the rectum and sigmoid flexure when some of them might still be amenable to cure by surgical resection. However, the endoscopist cannot hope to find an incidence of these ulcers among asymptomatic people that exceeds the age-specific incidence of cancer. Consequently, in order to use the barium enema and proctoscope more efficiently for the periodic examinations of large numbers of people, we must refine and expand our knowledge of the epidemiology of small cancers of the colon and rectum. The problem of finding cancers too small to be seen or felt but large enough to give off lethal metastases has not been solved. The time that elapses between the attainment of a size large enough to detect and the size at which dissemination occurs has been designated the "cancer control window." This is the segment of time in the life history of a cancer when earlier detection is beneficial (see Chapters Two and Six).

END RESULTS ASSOCIATED WITH INDIVIDUAL VARIABLES

The author's (J.S.S.) major study on prognosis is derived from the clinical records and pathologic material on 1141 consecutive patients treated at the Ellis Fischel State Cancer Hospital between 1939 and 1961 (Spjut and Spratt, 1965). Histologic verification of the diagnosis of colorectal cancer was a prerequisite for inclusion in the study. Four cases were unsatisfactory for review, reducing the effective series size to 1137 patients. All patients were followed to death or through December 31, 1963. Over 600 clinical, therapeutic, and pathologic variables and survival data were coded for transfer to Hollerith cards. The histopathologic slides on each case were reviewed and classified for the coded variables by Spjut.

Computer programs tabulated the frequency with which each variable occurred and calculated the survival rates through 10 years by the life-table method for all cases exhibiting a particular variable. Many of the variables considered were so infrequent and so unrelated to the prognosis of colonic cancer that they were not reported. Selected results for the more important and frequent variables are provided in Tables 10–4 to 10–22, along with frequency of observation and the 5- and 10-year accumulative survival rates with standard deviations.

Gross categories of variables that were unrelated to prognosis included occupation; weight of the host (70 to 259 lb, with a median weight of 135 lb); family history of cancer; ABO blood group; Rh type; admission laboratory data for prothrombin time, serum globulin, and serologic test for syphilis; simultaneously discovered colorectal cancer in the same or other segments of the colorectum; presence or absence of adenomatous polyps in the colorectum; method employed in the preoperative preparation of the colon; presenting symptom of the cancer; type of anastomosis or colostomy; nonfatal postoperative complications; and type of postoperative complication. Diseases of other organs did not affect prognosis unless the diseases themselves were potentially lethal, such as mammary cancer or cardiac disease severe enough to require digitalis.

Admission hemoglobin level was not associated with an altered prognosis unless it exceeded 17.0 gm per dl. When the admission blood urea nitrogen exceeded 40 mg per dl, the accumulative 5-year survival rate fell to 10.5 percent, with a standard deviation of 7 percent. Patients whose admission blood urea nitrogen (BUN) level exceeded 50 mg per dl did not survive 5 years.

Whenever the admission serum albumin level was less than 3.4 gm percent, survivorship was lower at both the fifth and tenth year when compared with cases with admission serum

Table 10–4. SURVIVAL RATES OF PATIENTS WITH COLORECTAL CANCER ACCORDING TO RACE AND SEX*

Race	Sex	No. of Patients	Accumulative Survival ± 1 S.D.	
			5-yr	*10-yr*
Caucasian	M	579	0.196 ± 0.018	0.134 ± 0.017
Caucasian	F	494	0.329 ± 0.022	0.226 ± 0.022
Black	M	34	0.270 ± 0.082	0.154 ± 0.078
Black	F	30	0.310 ± 0.088	0.106 ± 0.076

*Adapted from Spratt JS Jr, Spjut HJ: Prevalence and prognosis of individual clinical and pathologic variables associated with colorectal carcinoma. Cancer 20:1976–1985, 1967

Table 10–5. Age at Diagnosis and Survival Rates of Patients with Colorectal Cancer*

Age	No. of Patients	Accumulative Survival ± 1 S.D.		Accumulative 5-yr Survival Corrected for Natural Mortality
		5-yr	*10-yr*	
0–29	9	0.222 ± 0.139	0.222 ± 0.139	.224
30–39	37	0.226 ± 0.070	0.198 ± 0.067	.229
40–49	86	0.299 ± 0.052	0.282 ± 0.051	.309
50–59	200	0.282 ± 0.033	0.204 ± 0.032	.307
60–69	364	0.277 ± 0.025	0.153 ± 0.024	.334
70–79	353	0.256 ± 0.025	0.153 ± 0.024	.404
80–89	87	0.099 ± 0.036		.217
90–99	3	0.333 ± 0.272		.938

*Adapted from Spratt JS Jr, Spjut HJ: Prevalence and prognosis of individual clinical and pathologic variables associated with colorectal carcinoma. Cancer 20:1976–1985, 1967.

albumin values of 3.5 gm percent or greater (Table 10–6).

Variables seemingly associated with variations in prognosis are shown in Tables 10–4 to 10–22. These data were used as a basis for placing variables in groups based on similar end results. For all patients, the cumulative 5-year survival was 25.9 percent, with a 95 percent confidence range from 23.1 percent to 28.7 percent (± 2 S.D.), and the 10-year survival was 17.4 percent, with a 95 percent confidence range from 14.8 percent to 20.0 percent (± 2 S.D.).

A characteristic whose mean survival ± 2 S.D. did not overlap the 95 percent confidence limits for the total experience was considered significantly more lethal or significantly more favorable than the general experience. If some overlap of the confidence limits occurred, then other statistical tests would have been required to determine whether there was a significant difference. These tests were not done, since the interpretation would be in doubt because sample sizes were different and the variances were rarely equal, and the retrospective nature of the study imposed limitations on the value of such statistical refinements.

Host Characteristics and Prognosis

According to the host characteristics in the tables, Caucasian and Black women obviously had a more favorable prognosis than men of the same ethnicity. Only when the host population exceeded 80 years was the observed survival significantly decreased by the age of the host. When a correction for age-specific natural mortality was introduced with data, there was no difference in the mortality from cancer alone between octogenarians and those aged 20 (Spratt and Hoag, 1966).

Laboratory Test Results, Nutritional Assessment, and Prognosis

The only results of routine laboratory tests associated with an altered prognosis were elevated BUN and polycythemia levels and low serum albumin levels (see Table 10–6). The importance of the preoperative serum albumin levels in cancer patients as a measure of nutritional status has been amplified by Copeland (1983). A preoperative serum albumin level of less than 3.4 gm per dl, a recent weight loss of

Table 10–6. SERUM ALBUMIN LEVELS ON FIRST ADMISSION AND SURVIVAL

Albumin (gm/dl)	No. of Patients	Accumulative Survival ± 1 S.D.	
		5-yr	*10-yr*
No test	564	0.247 ± 0.021	0.164 ± 0.019
0–2.4	38	0.129 ± 0.055	0.129 ± 0.055
2.5–3.4	131	0.213 ± 0.037	0.146 ± 0.038
3.5–4.4	262	0.304 ± 0.030	0.204 ± 0.035
4.5–5.4	123	0.304 ± 0.044	0.188 ± 0.041
5.5–6.4	19	0.345 ± 0.114	0.276 ± 0.110

*Adapted from Spratt JS Jr, Spjut HJ: Prevalence and prognosis of individual clinical and pathologic variables associated with colorectal carcinoma. Cancer 20:1976–1985, 1967.

Table 10–7. SURVIVAL RATES OF PATIENTS WITH COLORECTAL CANCER ACCORDING TO ANATOMIC SEGMENT CONTAINING THE PRIMARY TUMOR*

Segment	No. of Patients	Accumulative Survival ± 1 S.D.	
		5-yr	10-yr
Rectum	669	0.222 ± 0.017	0.154 ± 0.016
Rectosigmoid	22	0.141 ± 0.087	0.071 ± 0.066
Sigmoid	208	0.330 ± 0.034	0.196 ± 0.033
Descending	23	0.313 ± 0.102	—
Splenic flexure	15	0.467 ± 0.129	0.311 ± 0.153
Transverse	42	0.410 ± 0.082	0.358 ± 0.086
Hepatic flexure	18	0.286 ± 0.120	0.286 ± 0.120
Ascending	33	0.416 ± 0.087	0.360 ± 0.091
Cecum	98	0.232 ± 0.045	0.175 ± 0.050
Multiple segments	5	0.200 ± 0.179	0.200 ± 0.179
Indeterminable	4	0	—

*Adapted from Spratt JS Jr, Spjut HJ: Prevalence and prognosis of individual clinical and pathologic variables associated with colorectal carcinoma. Cancer 20:1976–1985, 1967.

10 percent or more, and a negative reaction to a battery of standard recall skin test antigens indicated malnutrition, according to the general definition. Smale and associates (1981) have shown that malnourished cancer patients having surgical operations while still malnourished have a much higher morbidity and mortality rate if nutritional repletion is not obtained preoperatively. Preoperative nutritional repletion can be obtained within 10 to 21 days. Solid tumor growth has not been preferentially stimulated when this is done. Nutritional repletion has not been shown to enhance response to anticancer agents, but it may well be of value preoperatively to malnourished patients with resectable cancers who can tolerate a delay of several weeks before operation. The preoperative albumin value may serve to identify patients who should be considered for further nutritional evaluation and possible repletion. The adverse prognostic implications of low serum albumin levels in the EFSCH series may well be attributable to the lack of effective methodology for preoperative nutritional repletion between 1940 and 1961. However, the data were not assessed to see how many patients with low serum albumin levels also had hepatic metastases. Further study is needed in this area.

The anatomic segment containing the primary cancer had an influence on prognosis, as has been previously reported (Table 10–7).

RESECTABILITY AND OPERABILITY

In Tables 10–8 and 10–18, factors affecting resectability of cancers are shown. The resectability rate at EFSCH from 1939 to 1961 was only 74.6 percent (Spjut and Spratt, 1967). This is based on the inclusion of all cases for which histologic confirmation of the diagnosis of colorectal carcinoma was obtained. Even with an aggressive surgical attitude, staff competence in resection of contiguously involved organs, the ability to perform pelvic exenterations for large rectal cancers, if indicated, and in a later period (1961 through 1965), the availability of good blood banking and other necessary ancillary facilities, the resectability rate remained a static 75.3 percent. The operability rate was 86.2 percent for 340 additional cases of colorectal carcinoma managed during this latter period.

Considerations at the Time of Resection

Carcinoma of the colorectum may spread by direct extension, by dissemination through the lymphatics or bloodstream, possibly by transluminal seeding, and by implantation at operation. Efficacy in controlling cancer by particular surgical resection is associated with many of these factors involved in tumor spread. When there is intramural spread, any curative resection has to be performed with sufficient margin on each side of the cancer to provide a tumor-free margin. The freshly resected bowel should be opened for inspection immediately on removal of the cancer. If there is doubt as to the margin, a frozen section can be performed.

First metastases seem to occur in pericolic nodes. The spread extends up the chain of

Table 10–8. **SURVIVAL RATES OF PATIENTS WITH COLORECTAL CANCER ACCORDING TO RESECTABILITY***

Therapeutic Determinants	No. of Patients	Accumulative Survival ± 1 S.D. 5-yr	10-yr
Not resected; patient refusal	24	0.083 ± 0.056	0.042 ± 0.041
Not resected; other illnesses	11	0	—
Not resected; proven metastasis	144	0.021 ± 0.012	—
Not resected; suspected metastasis	18	0	—
Not resected; considered inoperable	87	0.011 ± 0.011	0.011 ± 0.011
Not resected; death from cancer before resection	2	0	—
Not resected; death from other causes before resection	3	0	—
Resected; proven distant metastasis	101	0.097 ± 0.030	0.042 ± 0.033
Resected; distant metastasis suspected	286	0.264 ± 0.028	0.163 ± 0.026
Resected; thought locally incurable	69	0.009 ± 0.012	0.009 ± 0.012
Resected; no proven or suspected distant metastasis	388	0.531 ± 0.027	0.381 ± 0.030
Observed longer than 1 mo before resection	4	0.500 ± 0.250	0.500 ± 0.250

*Adapted from Spratt JS Jr, Spjut HJ: Prevalence and prognosis of individual clinical and pathologic variables associated with colorectal carcinoma. Cancer 20:1976–1985, 1967.

nodes that closely parallel the veins from the affected segment of colon, with probable bypass of some nodes. Perinodal and intranodal blood vascular invasion probably occurs in some cases, leading to transnodal hematogenous spread. Adequate resection must include wide removal of the proximal lymphatic channels. Any lymph node involvement reduced the 5-year survival rate by approximately 50 percent.

Hematogenous metastases may occur when tumor cells invade venous channels or transgress lymph nodes and enter the venous sytem. The usual route is by way of the portal venous system to the liver. After the liver, the lung and bone are most frequently involved by metastasis, with cells reaching them either by passage through the liver into the inferior vena cava or by extension of tumor into tissues drained by systemic veins. Many experimental and clinical studies have shown that after operations for colorectal carcinoma, implantation in the anastomosis can occur. Experimental data show that there are relatively few techniques that are effective in preventing this form of spread (see Chapter Twenty-Two). In addition, tumors of the colorectum may break through the serosa and invade any contiguous organ. Transperitoneal spread is more prevalent with serosal penetration. A review of some surgical techniques used to reduce the risk of local recurrence is to be found in Chapter Twenty-One.

Nonresection and incomplete resection were major prognostic determinants in 459 (40.9 percent) of the cases in the EFSCH series. The use of palliative resections to obtain additional periods of symptom-free survival is to be considered in selected cases, even in the presence of a poor prognosis.

The surgical pathologists at EFSCH customarily recorded certain gross and microscopic characteristics. The permanent tissue slides on file for each case were reviewed by Spjut. The microscopic variables (see Tables 10–9 to 10–13) were his interpretations based on a review of several slides on file for each case and the original report on the gross characteristics. All variables could not be quantified for each cancer. This was particularly a factor for advanced cases that were not resected. Most of these cases have on file only a histologic section from biopsy. Therefore, resectability could have biased the prognosis of many of these variables.

In 11 patients, cancer of signet ring cell or poorly differentiated cancer in ulcerative colitis was uniformly lethal. The accumulative 5-year survival for 115 cases with undifferentiated cancer (grade 3) was only 7.4 percent, with a 95 percent range from 2 percent to 12.8 percent. This is well below the 95 percent confidence interval for the entire group. The cancers in grades 1 and 2 (786 cases) form the buffering central group not differing from the whole in survival. The mean survival rates of the smaller groups all had wide overlapping-variances. Some categories seemed largely hy-

Table 10–9. **SURVIVAL RATES OF PATIENTS WITH COLORECTAL CANCER ACCORDING TO HISTOLOGIC TYPE OF PRIMARY TUMOR***

Type	No. of Patients	Accumulative Survival ± 1 S.D. 5-yr	10-yr
Well-differentiated cancer (grade 1)	121	0.317 ± 0.044	0.154 ± 0.037
Well-differentiated cancer in adenomatous polyp	3	1.000	0.667 ± 0.272
Well-differentiated cancer in villous adenoma	15	0.363 ± 0.136	0.363 ± 0.136
Well-differentiated cancer with adenomatous polyps in same segment	24	0.528 ± 0.104	0.352 ± 0.110
Well-differentiated cancer with generalized polyposis	2	0.500 ± 0.354	0.500 ± 0.354
Well-differentiated cancer with mucinous elements	12	0.571 ± 0.146	0.571 ± 0.146
Poorly differentiated cancer (grade 2)	615	0.260 ± 0.018	0.177 ± 0.018
Poorly differentiated cancer in adenomatous polyp	3	0.333 ± 0.385	0.333 ± 0.385
Poorly differentiated cancer in villous adenoma	8	0.125 ± 0.117	—
Poorly differentiated cancer with adenomatous polyps in same segment	71	0.290 ± 0.062	0.199 ± 0.062
Poorly differentiated cancer with generalized polyposis	5	0.400 ± 0.219	0.400 ± 0.219
Poorly differentiated cancer with ulcerative colitis	1	0	—
Signet ring adenocarcinoma	10	0	—
Poorly differentiated cancer with mucinous adenocarcinoma	34	0.611 ± 0.090	0.611 ± 0.090
Undifferentiated cancer (grade 3)	115	0.074 ± 0.027	0.059 ± 0.025
Undifferentiated cancer with neoplastic polyps in same segment	11	0.091 ± 0.087	0.091 ± 0.087
Malignant tumor, unclassified	13	0.051 ± 0.068	0.051 ± 0.068
Undifferentiated cancer with mucinous elements	4	0.250 ± 0.217	0.250 ± 0.217
Mucinous cancer	64	0.133 ± 0.046	0.111 ± 0.043
Mucinous cancer in villous adenoma	1	1.000	1.000
Mucinous cancer with adenomatous polyps in same segment	3	0.333 ± 0.272	—

*Adapted from Spratt JS Jr, Spjut HJ: Prevalence and prognosis of individual clinical and pathologic variables associated with colorectal carcinoma. Cancer 20:1976–1985, 1967.

pothetical, with no cases in the groups. These categories have been eliminated from the tables published in this chapter.

The correlation between histologic grade and other factors affecting prognosis brings out the overriding importance of the biology of the cancer. Chung and associates (1982) analyzed 246 patients with cancer of the colorectum treated by "curative" surgery alone. They observed that patients with poorly differentiated cancers (grade 3) had an increased likelihood of having deep invasion through the bowel wall and lymph node metastases. When compared with well-differentiated (grade 1) and moderately differentiated (grade 2) cancers, those cancers characterized by poor differentiation, penetration of the bowel wall, and lymph node metastases were associated with a very poor prognosis, independent of the patient's age and sex, large bowel site, or size of the primary cancer. This adverse combination was more frequently associated with both local recurrence and distant metastases.

The depth of penetration (Table 10–10) was determined by microscopic examination of resected cancers. Embolic lymph node metastases were found to occur from cancers whose deep margin was through the muscularis mucosae. Thus, some Dukes' C cancers were found among the more superficial neoplasms. In keeping with the pattern of this study, only a single variable, the direct and contiguous deep extension of the primary cancer through the layers of the intestinal wall, was considered. When the cancer was resectable, depth of penetration had much less effect on prognosis than might be expected unless the excision was incomplete.

Table 10–10. **SURVIVAL RATES OF PATIENTS WITH COLORECTAL CANCER ACCORDING TO DEPTH OF PENETRATION**

Depth	No. of Patients	Accumulative Survival ± 1 S.D.	
		5-yr	*10-yr*
Not through muscularis mucosae	2	0.500 ± 0.354	0.500 ± 0.354
Through muscularis mucosae but not to muscle	20	0.479 ± 0.115	0.423 ± 0.114
To inner muscle	9	0.444 ± 0.166	0.222 ± 0.139
Into but not through muscle	153	0.464 ± 0.044	0.361 ± 0.049
Through muscle but not through serosa or fat	77	0.296 ± 0.053	0.099 ± 0.038
Through serosa	32	0.214 ± 0.076	0.064 ± 0.048
Through muscle and into mesenteric fat	421	0.352 ± 0.025	0.269 ± 0.025
Direct extension into adjacent organs	88	0.167 ± 0.041	0.098 ± 0.039
Depth not determinable	31	0.129 ± 0.060	0.097 ± 0.053
Incompletely excised to margins	2	0	—
Total	835		

*Adapted from Spratt JS Jr, Spjut HJ: Prevalence and prognosis of individual clinical and pathologic variables associated with colorectal carcinoma. Cancer 20:1976–1985, 1967.

The character of the margin could be well evaluated on resected cancers only . When the entire margin of the cancer appeared to be infiltrating into normal tissue, the prognosis was significantly worse than when a well-circumscribed or "pushing" margin or a mixed margin (Table 10–11) was present.

The lack of any inflammatory response, as judged by the intensity of the inflammatory cell infiltration about the periphery of the cancer, had a more ominous prognostic significance than the presence of moderate to intense inflammatory reaction (Table 10–12).

Cases in which there was permeation of lymphatic or blood vascular vessels or of perineural sheaths had significantly worse prognoses than cases with cancers not demonstrating these characteristics. Permeation of all three routes of spread was particularly ominous (Table 10–13).

The pathologist could only measure the size of resected cancers (Table 10–14). Prognosis was remarkably independent of size if the cancer was resectable. However, nonmeasurement for 289 of the 525 unmeasured cancers is attributable to nonresection, and these cases might skew the prognosis downward for the larger cancers if the sizes were known. Greater size was a probable cause for nonresection in an unknown number of patients.

Similarly, the percentage of resected cancers without metastasis in the mesenteric lymph nodes remained constant at 54 percent to 66.7 percent for cases grouped by 1-cm size ranges from 1 through 23 cm respectively. Among the 17 resected cancers whose greatest dimension was 12 cm or more, 11 (65 percent) had no metastasis in the mesenteric lymph nodes (Table 10–15). Other factors possibly related to survivorship include the total length of lower intestine resected (Table 10–16), the total number of mesenteric lymph nodes counted in the resected specimen (Table 10–17), the reason for resecting part or all of a noncolorectal

Table 10–11. **SURVIVAL RATES OF PATIENTS WITH COLORECTAL CANCER ACCORDING TO MARGIN CHARACTERISTIC***

Margin	No. of Patients	Accumulative Survival ± 1 S.D.	
		5-yr	*10-yr*
Pushing	103	0.456 ± 0.054	0.373 ± 0.058
Infiltrating	519	0.283 ± 0.021	0.178 ± 0.020
Mixed	155	0.538 ± 0.042	0.404 ± 0.048
Not determinable	36	0.122 ± 0.059	0.122 ± 0.059

*Adapted from Spratt JS Jr, Spjut HF: Prevalence and prognosis of individual clinical and pathologic variables associated with colorectal carcinoma. Cancer 20:1976–1985, 1967.

Table 10–12. **SURVIVAL RATES OF PATIENTS WITH COLORECTAL CANCER ACCORDING TO DEGREE OF INFLAMMATORY REACTION AROUND CANCER ASSAYED MICROSCOPICALLY***

Degree of Inflammatory Reaction	No. of Patients	Accumulative Survival ± 1 S.D. 5-yr	10-yr
None	127	0.199 ± 0.038	0.166 ± 0.036
Moderate with no abscesses	439	0.359 ± 0.024	0.246 ± 0.025
Intense with abscess formation	223	0.407 ± 0.035	0.270 ± 0.036
Not classifiable	13	0.231 ± 0.117	0.115 ± 0.100

*Adapted from Spratt JS Jr, Spjut HJ: Prevalence and prognosis of individual clinical and pathologic variables associated with colorectal carcinoma. Cancer 20:1976–1985, 1967.

Table 10–13. **SURVIVAL RATES OF PATIENTS WITH COLORECTAL CANCER ACCORDING TO INVASION OF PERINEURAL, LYMPHATIC, OR BLOOD VASCULAR STRUCTURES NEAR PRIMARY CANCER***

Type of Invasion Seen	No. of Patients	Accumulative Survival ± 1 S.D. 5-yr	10-yr
None	417	0.468 ± 0.026	0.337 ± 0.028
Lymphatics only	163	0.199 ± 0.034	0.072 ± 0.032
Blood vascular only	72	0.274 ± 0.055	0.208 ± 0.054
Perineural only	38	0.197 ± 0.069	0.131 ± 0.059
Lymphatic and blood vascular	38	0.166 ± 0.061	0.100 ± 0.052
Lymphatic and perineural	30	0.214 ± 0.087	0.153 ± 0.081
Blood vascular and perineural	20	0.143 ± 0.080	0.143 ± 0.080
Perineural, blood vascular, and lymphatic	36	0.083 ± 0.046	0.056 ± 0.038

*Adapted from Spratt JS Jr, Spjut HJ: Prevalence and prognosis of individual clinical and pathologic variables associated with colorectal carcinoma. Cancer 20:1976–1985, 1967.

Table 10–14. **SURVIVAL RATES OF PATIENTS WITH COLORECTAL CANCER ACCORDING TO GREATEST LONGITUDINAL DIMENSION OF CANCER***

Length (cm)	No. of Patients	Accumulative Survival ± 1 S.D. 5-yr	10-yr
No measurement	525	0.143 ± 0.016	0.248 ± 0.014
0 – 0.9	2	0.500 ± 0.354	—
1 – 1.9	6	0	—
2 – 2.9	17	0.248 ± 0.112	0.248 ± 0.112
3 – 3.9	46	0.243 ± 0.067	0.157 ± 0.059
4 – 4.9	86	0.417 ± 0.057	0.293 ± 0.062
5 – 5.9	121	0.468 ± 0.048	0.340 ± 0.053
6 – 6.9	106†	0.327 ± 0.050	0.264 ± 0.052
7 – 7.9	72	0.420 ± 0.059	0.249 ± 0.057
8 – 8.9	62	0.322 ± 0.065	0.322 ± 0.065
9 – 9.9	36	0.311 ± 0.080	0.198 ± 0.083
10 –10.9	30	0.241 ± 0.081	0.070 ± 0.062
11 –11.9	11	0.455 ± 0.150	0.114 ± 0.105
12 –12.9	8	0.469 ± 0.187	0.469 ± 0.187
13 –16.9	6	0	—
17 –17.9	2	0.500 ± 0.354	0.500 ± 0.354
20	1	1.000	1.000
Total	1137		

*Adapted from Spratt JS Jr, Spjut HJ: Prevalence and prognosis of individual clinical and pathologic variables associated with colorectal carcinoma. Cancer 20:1976–1985, 1967.

†Median.

Table 10–15. **PREVALENCE OF LYMPH NODE METASTASES ACCORDING TO LENGTH OF PRIMARY CANCER***

No. of Lymph Nodes Containing Cancer	No Measurement	Length of Primary Cancer (cm) 1–1.9	2–2.9	3–3.9	4–4.9	5–5.9	6–6.9	7–7.9	8–8.9	9–9.9	10–10.9	11–11.9	12–12.9	13–22.9	Total
None with cancer	100 (51.5)†	4 (66.7)	7 (53.8)	23 (56)	46 (58.2)	64 (57.1)	55 (54.5)	37 (55.2)	33 (54.1)	19 (54.3)	15 (55.6)	6 (54.5)	5 (62.5)	6 (66.7)	420
1–5	71	2	2	15	27	34	28	22	20	12	6	3	2	3	247
6–10	15	0	2	1	4	9	12	4	7	2	3	2	0	0	61
11–15	2	0	2	1	0	1	1	2	0	1	2	0	1	0	13
16–20	1	0	0	0	1	1	1	0	1	1	0	0	0	0	6
21–41	5	0	0	1	1	4	4	2	0	0	1	0	0	0	17
Total Resected	194	6	13	41	79	113	101	67	61	35	27	11	8	9	764
No nodes removed	331	2	4	5	7	9	5	5	1	1	3	0	0	0	373
Total	525	8	17	46	86	122	106	72	62	36	30	11	8	9	1137

*Adapted from Spratt JS Jr, Spjut HJ: Prevalence and prognosis of individual clinical and pathologic variables associated with colorectal carcinoma. Cancer 20: 1976–1985, 1967.

†Figures in parentheses are percentages of cancers having no metastases in the mesenteric lymph nodes removed by surgical resection.

Table 10–16. SURVIVAL RATES OF PATIENTS WITH COLORECTAL CANCER ACCORDING TO LENGTH OF LARGE INTESTINE RESECTED*

Length (cm)	No. of Patients	Accumulative Survival ± 1 S.D.	
		5-Yr	*10-Yr*
1–10	11	0.242 ± 0.138	0.121 ± 0.110
11–20	105	0.328 ± 0.047	0.226 ± 0.045
21–30	197	0.396 ± 0.036	0.251 ± 0.038
31–40	226	0.343 ± 0.034	0.245 ± 0.033
41–50	119	0.357 ± 0.047	0.279 ± 0.048
51–75	46	0.341 ± 0.088	0.213 ± 0.091
75–100	5	0.400 ± 0.219	—
126–150	1	1.000	—
Total colectomy	3	0.333 ± 0.272	—
Colon not resected	295	0.024 ± 0.009	0.010 ± 0.006
Colon resected but not measured	116	0.266 ± 0.043	0.171 ± 0.042

*Adapted from Spratt JS Jr, Spjut HJ: Prevalence and prognosis of individual clinical and pathologic variables associated with colorectal carcinoma. Cancer 20:1976–1985, 1967.

Table 10–17. SURVIVAL RATES OF PATIENTS WITH COLORECTAL CANCER ACCORDING TO NUMBER OF MESENTERIC LYMPH NODES CONTAINED IN SURGICAL SPECIMEN*

No. of Nodes in Specimen	No. of Patients	Accumulative Survival ± 1 S.D.	
		5-Yr	*10-Yr*
None	233	0.075 ± 0.018	0.047 ± 0.016†
1–5	153	0.217 ± 0.035	0.118 ± 0.033
6–10	187	0.377 ± 0.037	0.249 ± 0.041
11–15	138	0.453 ± 0.045	0.328 ± 0.051
16–20	96	0.470 ± 0.054	0.323 ± 0.058
21–25	53	0.453 ± 0.073	0.370 ± 0.073
26–30	26	0.222 ± 0.083	0.133 ± 0.069
31–35	33	0.318 ± 0.087	0.232 ± 0.082
36–40	19	0.189 ± 0.097	0.126 ± 0.083
41	58	0.293 ± 0.061	0.201 ± 0.054

*Adapted from Spratt JS Jr, Spjut HJ: Prevalence and prognosis of individual clinical and pathologic variables associated with colorectal carcinoma. Cancer 20:1976–1985, 1967.

†Includes both unresected cases and cases with sleeve resections with no nodes in the removed mesentery.

Table 10–18. SURVIVAL RATES OF PATIENTS WITH COLORECTAL CANCER ACCORDING TO REASON FOR REMOVING SECOND ORGAN*

Reason	No. of Patients	Accumulative Survival ± 1 S.D.	
		5-Yr	*10-Yr*
Incidental	71	0.520 ± 0.064	0.433 ± 0.071
Other pathologic condition	75	0.352 ± 0.060	0.352 ± 0.060
Involved inflammatory mass	37	0.170 ± 0.063	0.041 ± 0.037
Thought to be involved by direct extension of cancer, but no cancer in other organ on microscopic examination	10	0	—
Involved by direct extension of cancer (proved on microscopic examination)	76	0.201 ± 0.047	0.128 ± 0.045

*Adapted from Spratt JS Jr, Spjut HJ: Prevalence and prognosis of individual clinical and pathologic variables associated with colorectal carcinoma. Cancer 20:1976–1985, 1967.

Table 10–19. SURVIVAL RATES OF PATIENTS WITH COLORECTAL CANCER ACCORDING TO ASSOCIATED RESECTION OF ORGANS OTHER THAN COLORECTUM*

Associated Resection	No. of Patients	Accumulative Survival ± 1 S.D.	
		5-Yr	*10-Yr*
None	837	0.242 ± 0.016	0.157 ± 0.015
Uterus or adnexa	45	0.318 ± 0.073	0.241 ± 0.073
Vagina	16	0.296 ± 0.118	0.099 ± 0.090
Prostate	10	0	—
Bladder	3	0	—
Abdominal wall	3	1.000	—
Omentum	4	0	—
Small intestine†	113	0.405 ± 0.050	0.324 ± 0.054
Kidney	1	1.000	—
Stomach	2	0.500 ± 0.354	0.500 ± 0.354
More than 1	60	0.223 ± 0.056	0.173 ± 0.054
Other	19	0.292 ± 0.108	0.195 ± 0.107

*Adapted from Spratt JS Jr, Spjut HJ: Prevalence and prognosis of individual clinical and pathologic variables associated with colorectal carcinoma. Cancer 20:1976–1985, 1967.

†Includes terminal ileum with right colectomies.

organ simultaneously with the colorectal resection (Table 10–18) and the additional organs resected (Table 10–19). Resection of great lengths of intestine and very large numbers of mesenteric lymph nodes obviously had an upper limit of impact on survivorship. Resection of organs contiguously involved by the primary cancer exerted a definite impact on survivorship in some cases.

CARCINOMA OF THE RECTUM

Carcinomas of the rectum merit further discussion. The earliest symptoms of rectal cancer may be a change in bowel habit and bleeding, but these are not the signs and symptoms of "early" cancer. Most commonly the change in bowel habit is an increase in stool frequency, although the stool may remain formed. Particularly characteristic is an urgent desire to defecate on arising, the so-called morning diarrhea. Less commonly, the patient may complain of obstipation, and a large number of patients with rectal cancer notice both obstipation and diarrhea, sometimes alternating, with this tendency aggravated by laxative use. Other bowel changes include tenesmus, a sense of incomplete evacuation, and a change in stool caliber. Bleeding may be bright or dark, and blood may be mixed with feces or spread on the surface of the feces. Frequently, blood is seen mixed with mucus after ineffectual straining to pass stool. It is seldom seen only on the tissue, as in hemorrhoidal bleeding, and bleeding is seldom exsanguinating. Pain is not an early symptom of rectal cancer, and when present, it usually indicates far advanced disease. As the tumor invades the pararectal tissues, the patient may first complain of a vague rectal fullness. Later the complaint may be of a dull ache confined to the rectum or sacral region. When pain becomes severe with nocturnal awakening and radiation to groin, labia, scrotum, penis, or legs, the neoplasm has almost always reached a very advanced stage. Patients with carcinoma of the large bowel may present with a variety of physical findings, resulting from secondary effects of their disease, such as bowel obstruction, pallor, a mass, cachexia, ascites, hepatomegaly, peripheral lymphadenopathy, weight loss, prostate enlargement, and urinary tract infections.

The digital rectal examination is of prime importance in the diagnosis and staging of carcinoma of the rectum. One third of all rectal cancers are readily palpable on digital examination. The level of the tumor above the anal verge can be assessed at the time of digital examination. During assessment of the level of the tumor, the examiner must be certain that he is feeling the tumor itself and not indirectly feeling it through a fold in the rectal wall. This would incorrectly locate the tumor at a level lower than its actual site. Also the shape of the lesion whether ulcerating, polypoid, or sessile may be determined at the time of the rectal examination. The consistency of the tumor is also important. Soft, velvetlike tumors may have large areas of benign villous adenoma mixed with the cancer; thus, the actual cancer may be smaller than the grossly palpable tumor. The degree of cancer spread along the bowel wall and beyond the rectal wall into adjacent structures should be evaluated. Such spread may occur laterally along the lateral ligaments of the rectum into the walls of the pelvis or posteriorly to the sacrum and anteriorly to involve the vagina, prostate, urethra, or bladder. The degree of fixation of the tumor to these other structures should be assessed. Whenever invasion of the prostate, bladder, or urethra is suspected, urethrocystoscopic examination with biopsy of suspicious areas is indicated as part of the preoperative assessment. The size of the lesion may be estimated at the time of the rectal examination and from roentgenogram measurements. Large tumors may still be resected with a chance for cure, but large growths often have had an opportunity to spread beyond the rectum. Large rectal cancers with uncertain degrees of invasion constitute an indication for the placement of ureteral catheters immediately before exploration that may lead to an abdominoperineal resection, possibly complicated by different patterns of anterior invasion.

The position of the tumor on the bowel wall must be determined. Anterior tumors in women may spread into and through the rectovaginal septum and may require removal of the posterior vaginal wall and uterus as part of the surgical extirpation of the tumor. Pelvic lymph nodes are often palpable in the presence of inflammatory and neoplastic diseases of the anorectal region. The presacral lymph nodes can sometimes be felt through the posterior rectal wall and occasionally along the lateral ligaments and lateral pelvic walls. Nodes may be felt in the presacral region in many patients with cancer of the rectum. These nodes are the first order nodes lying in the rectal mesentery. An assessment of the size and degree of firmness of these nodes may give a useful preoperative clue as to the likelihood of involvement of the nodes by tumor. As the examining finger is removed from the rectum, it should be inspected for the presence of blood or mucus and, when not present on gross inspection, the stool on the examining finger should still be tested for occult blood. The role of the CAT scan and other newer imaging methods in determining the extent of pelvic cancer is still being defined, but will unquestionably be of increasing value for delineating the size and extent of larger rectal cancers.

Proctosigmoidoscopic examination permits direct visualization of the tumor and supplies information additional to that already obtained from the digital rectal examination. High rectal tumors are often not readily palpable, and much of the assessment of the lesion must be made through the use of the proctosigmoidoscope. The size, shape, consistency, location on the bowel wall, level from the anal verge, and even degree of infiltration and fixation of the tumor may be evaluated with this instrument. Tumors involving long segments of the rectum may still permit passage of the proctosigmoidoscope into the tumor, thus permitting assessment of the involvement. However, the length of involvement is often better assessed by barium enema study. Also, the proctosigmoidoscope allows the tumor to be biopsied. A histopathologic diagnosis of biopsy material should be obtained for all accessible neoplasms before surgical treatment. Too many benign conditions can mimic cancer in the rectal area, and they are often best managed by means other than resection. Several samples should be removed from various portions of any lesion for examination. A good marginal biopsy at the junction between the cancer and normal colon often can be used to identify characteristics helpful in assessing the cancer growth patterns at this interface. In the case of villous adenomas, biopsies should be taken from any firm or ulcerated area.

The barium enema study is useful in the assessment of high rectal lesions that cannot be examined adequately by digital and proctosigmoidoscopic means. The major purpose of the barium enema is to evaluate the colon rather than the rectum. Synchronous cancers involving the colon occur in 3 to 5 percent of patients with cancer of the rectum. Such an incidence makes the use of the barium study to investigate these patients valuable. Care must be taken, however, not to use the barium enema in patients in whom the tumor is near obstructing size. The radiologist can often determine how far to proceed during early instillation of barium under fluoroscopic examination. These lesions are more likely to cause obstruction, and once barium has been introduced into the colon above such a lesion it may be difficult to retrieve. Barium may complete a partial obstruction in such a way that a planned anastomotic procedure could become unsafe. The patient may have to have a colostomy that could have been avoided. In the absence of an urgent need for surgical intervention, time should always be taken preoperatively to clear the colon of barium proximal to the cancer.

Other components of the routine physical examination are simple to do and are often very helpful in assessing the extent and behavior of these cancers: Careful palpation of all lymph node clusters, but particularly those in the groin and supraclavicular area, palpation of the abdomen for liver size and consistency, and palpation of the abdomen for masses and fluid. Suspicious lymph nodes merit excisional biopsy preoperatively. This should be done in such a way as to permit a later regional lymph node dissection if indicated.

There are advocates of preoperative percutaneous needle biopsy of suspicious livers. However, when laparotomy is to be performed anyway, this may be a superfluous step generating data without affecting actions or outcome. Biopsy is justified when it is used for a specific research protocol or when its results will lead to an altered treatment plan.

Prognostic Assessment of Stage, Location, and Method of Treatment for Rectal Cancers

Proper function of the anus and control of bowel action require an anorectal stump at least 4 cm in length. Tumors that are palpable by digital rectal examination that lie within 8 or 9 cm of the anal verge generally require total removal of the rectum and anus. The operation used is the abdominoperineal resection of the rectum. The aims of cancer surgery are an encompassing local excision, an adequate distal margin of clearance (5 cm), and an en bloc resection of all regional lymphatics. In the case of a cancer in the upper third of the rectum, taking out the entire rectum may add nothing to the value of the cancer operation. For a growth in the upper rectum, an adequate cancer operation, including a 5-cm margin distal to the tumor, often can be performed with preservation of the rectum and restoration of continuity. The most satisfactory operation is anterior resection. It has the smoothest postoperative course and provides the best rectal function subsequently. The choice is between abdominoperineal resection and a sphincter-saving operation. If the lower margin of the tumor lies 10 cm or more from the anal verge, a sphincter-saving operation can usually be performed. At the 7- to 10-cm level it is less certain that this operation should be performed, and the final decision usually has to be made with the abdomen open after the rectum has been mobilized. Once the rectum has been fully mobilized and straightened out, a point on the rectal wall 7.5 cm from the anal verge may rise to a level of 11 to 12 cm, especially if it lies on the posterior wall. If the lesion lies in the lowest 5 cm of the rectum, then abdominoperineal resection is required because removal of the tumor with a 5-cm distal margin leaves little or no remaining rectum, and a much wider resection of the distal rectum can be performed from the perineal aspect. If 4 cm of rectal ampulla does not remain for anastomosis, the patient may end up with a perineal colostomy. An abdominal wall colostomy is often more manageable. In Chapter Twelve, the technologic improvements in the ability to do low anastomoses with stapling devices is discussed.

Slanetz and associates (1972) presented a comparison of 277 consecutive abdominoperineal resections and 247 consecutive anterior resections, all "curative" in nature, performed at the Columbia-Presbyterian Medical Center between 1944 and 1963. These operations were for tumors situated at the level of 8 to 18 cm from the anal verge. They found that for rectal tumors above the level of 8 cm, anterior resection was the equal of abdominoperineal resection. Anterior resection was accompanied by significantly lower morbidity and mortality rates than was abdominoperineal resection. Between 8 and 18 cm, the level of the tumor could not be related to survival or recurrence rates, and should not influence the surgeon's choice of procedure as long as an adequate distal margin of resection can be provided. In addition they found local recurrence rates after abdominoperineal resection and anterior resection were roughly equal and were determinants more of the pathologic nature of the disease than of the procedure employed. Local extension of the primary tumor to adjacent structures, regardless of lymph node involvement, and inadvertent perforation of the bowel during surgical dissection both significantly prejudiced survival and increased local recurrence rates. Lastly, they found that lymphatic metastases from carcinoma of the rectum were seen more frequently in women than in men, but survival rates after resection for Dukes' C lesions were appreciably higher in women.

Even though abdominoperineal resection is at present the standard surgical treatment for most invasive cancer of the lower rectum, there are several controversial local treatment alternatives, namely, local excision, electrocoagulation, and primary radiation therapy. In no instance has a concurrently controlled test, using well-defined criteria for patient selection, of any local treatment against abdominoperineal resection been reported that placed alternate modalities in proper therapeutic perspective. A policy of local excision or total biopsy for early cancer of the colorectum has been described in several recent studies. In 1977, Morson and associates reported their experiences with local excision of colorectal cancer during 1948 to 1972 based on thorough histologic examination of the excised specimen with special reference to the completeness of the surgical excision, the depth of spread of the cancer into the bowel wall, and the histologic grade of the malignancy. Out of the 119 patients studied, there were ten recurrences of cancer, but only five patients were regarded as policy failures. The authors suggest that because of the good results, this policy of local excision should be regarded as an alternative to resective surgical treatment. In addition, the authors emphasized that there was a high degree of patient selectivity, that more than 80 percent of the cancers treated by local excision were less than 3 cm in diameter, and that about 50 percent of the patients treated were older than 70 years of age.

Another therapeutic local procedure is electrocoagulation, which, by definition, is "coagulation by means of a biterminal high frequency electric current." The results and techniques of electrocoagulation were reported in two large series, one by Crile and Turnbull in 1972 and the other by Madden and Kandalaft in 1973. These compared quite favorably in terms of both surgical salvage and operative mortality and morbidity rates with those reported for abdominoperineal resection. I believe that the cancers managed most successfully by these local means of treatment are the nonmetastasizing cancers described in detail starting on page 238 of this chapter.

There are also several studies that have described the use of radiation therapy alone in treating low-lying rectal cancer successfully (see Chapter Nineteen).

Many complications may be encountered after abdominoperineal resection. Some of these are peritonitis, wound infection and abscess, obstruction as a result of adhesions, wound disruption, stricture or retraction of the colostomy, urinary retention due to benign prostatic hypertrophy, bladder dysfunction, urinary fistulas and impotence in males secondary to injury to the autonomic nerve supply to the genitalia, as well as the cardiovascular or pulmonary problems involved. Breakdown of the anastomosis is the principal source of sepsis after anterior resection and was found in 40 percent of patients after high anterior resection and 69 percent after low anterior resection by Goligher and associates (1977) in a series studying 73 patients using radiologic confirmation. The most current data concerning stapled anastomoses is provided in Chapter Twelve.

The operative mortality rate of abdominoperineal resection varies in large reported series from 4 to 20 percent, with a mean of about 8 percent. The mortality rate of anterior resection is somewhat less, ranging from 2.4 to 20 percent, with a mean of 5 percent. The morbidity rate of abdominoperineal resection is from 27 to 68 percent. The morbidity rate is 15 to 56 percent for anterior resection.

As shown by Polk and Spratt (1971), weight loss and weakness are nonspecific symptoms and are commonly found in elderly patients after surgery. After an abdominoperineal resection perineal pain is an ominous development and perineal recurrence is usually associated with pelvic recurrence. Once recurrence of tumor is discovered, surgical resection clearly results in the best outcomes in a select group of patients with localized disease (see Chapter Twenty-One).

THERAPY ADJUVANT TO SURGERY

Numerous reports have confirmed the fact that the salvage of patients with colorectal cancer treated by surgical resection has reached a plateau in the past two decades and these reports have emphasized the need for additional modalities of therapy. Properly timed resection or more extensive use of adjuvant techniques may result in increased survival of these patients. More detailed studies of patterns of recurrence of the disease are needed as well as prospective trials of adjuvant methods of treatment. As is documented throughout this book and particularly in this chapter, factors associated with the prognosis of patients having colorectal cancers are very numerous. This greatly complicates the stratification of similar cases in sufficient numbers needed for controlled clinical trials, to test the value of adjuvant therapies. This fact accounts for the paucity of controlled clinical trials for colorectal cancers. Chapters Eighteen and Nineteen provide comprehensive reviews of chemotherapy, radiation therapy, and immunotherapy.

The compilation of convincing data to prove the benefit from any adjuvant therapy requires carefully controlled randomized clinical trials. Conclusions are difficult to make about the effects of low-dose preoperative radiation because two major clinical trials have shown differing results. One trial of the Veterans Administration Surgical Adjuvant Group (Higgins, 1975), carried out from 1964 to 1969, employed 2000 to 2500 rad in ten fractions over an elapsed period of 12 days on operable patients with rectal cancers. A subset of patients in the study did show a survival benefit and a lower incidence of lymph node metastasis than the control group. These findings were offset by the results of a randomized trial of low-dose preoperative radiation therapy carried out at Memorial-Sloan Kettering between 1960 and 1967. The results of this trial showed no difference in the incidence of lymph node metastasis between the treated patients and the control group receiving no treatment. Chapter Nineteen expands on the potential role of radiotherapy.

I reported a randomized series of rectal cancers treated by preoperative radiation at EFSCH (Spratt et al., 1968). Although only 3000 rad were given preoperatively over 3 weeks, followed immediately by resection, the treatment was not well tolerated by the elderly patients with advanced cancer. As a result, the cases with preoperative radiation had a greater morbidity rate. The survivorship of the two groups was not significantly different. The existence of the numerous variables affecting prognosis would have required a very large series to rule out biases in case mix among control and treated groups with this study (Spratt et al., 1968).

DETERMINANTS OF PATIENT SURVIVAL

The evidence is clearly available that nonresection and palliative resections for colorectal carcinoma are associated with a very high lethality rate by the fifth post-treatment year (see Table 10–8). Table 10–20 unquestionably showed an inverse correlation between the number of lymph nodes containing metastatic cancer and the prognosis. The presence of any lymph node metastasis makes the prognosis significantly worse, and when patients had 16 or more mesenteric lymph nodes containing cancer, they died.

With this observation it was natural to inquire whether the number of lymph nodes containing metastatic cancer increased as the sizes of the primary cancers increased. A tendency toward this pattern did seem to exist in resected tumors up to about 7 cm. Beyond this, the number of positive lymph nodes decreased with increasing size. Probably, the presence of extensive metastases was responsible for the classification of these larger cancers as nonresectable (see the 144 cases not resected because of proven metastasis in Table 10–8).

If metastasis in 16 or more mesenteric lymph nodes was a universally lethal characteristic, then it appears from Table 10–15 that the cancers prone to develop extensive lymph node metasis would have to be resected before the primary cancer exceeded 3 cm in diameter. This observation makes the following apparent:

1. Certain biologic types of colonic cancers can metastasize extensively while very small.

Table 10–20. SURVIVAL RATES OF PATIENTS WITH COLORECTAL CANCER ACCORDING TO NUMBER OF MESENTERIC LYMPH NODES CONTAINING CANCER*

Lymph Nodes Removed	No. of Patients	Accumulative Survival ± 1 S.D.	
		5-yr	*10-yr*
None removed	373	0.065 ± 0.013	0.033 ± 0.011
Removed but contained no cancer	420	0.488 ± 0.026	0.350 ± 0.028
Contained cancer			
1–5	247	0.241 ± 0.029	0.143 ± 0.027
6–10	61	0.086 ± 0.040	0.086 ± 0.040
11–15	13	0.093 ± 0.087	—
16 or more	23	0	—
Total	1137		

*Adapted from Spratt JS Jr, Spjut HJ: Prevalence and prognosis of individual clinical and pathologic variables associated with colorectal carcinoma. Cancer 20:1976–1985, 1967.

Table 10–21. **CORRELATION OF HOST SURVIVAL TO PATHOLOGIC CHARACTERISTICS***

Proportion Surviving 5 yr	Pathologic Characteristic	No. of Cases
.01 (all dead within 5 yr)	Signet ring adenocarcinoma	10
	Cancer with ulcerative colitis	1
	Metastatic cancer in more than 16 mesenteric lymph nodes	23
	Incompletely excised to margin	2
	†Undifferentiated cancer (grade 3)	115
	Undifferentiated cancer (grade 3) with adenomatous polyps in the same segment	11
	†Malignant tumor, unclassified	13
	†Perineural, blood vascular, and lymphatic permeation	36
	†Metastatic cancer in 6 to 16 mesenteric lymph nodes	74
	No mesenteric lymph nodes removed	373
.101–.2	†Poorly differentiated cancer (grade 2) in villous adenoma	8
	†Mucinous adenocarcinoma	64
	†Direct extension of cancer into adjacent organs	88
	†No inflammatory reaction about cancer	127
	†Lymphatic or perineural permeation only	201
	†Blood vascular and perineural or lymphatic permeation	58
.201–.3	Poorly differentiated cancer (grade 2)	615
	†Poorly differentiated cancer (grade 2) with adenomatous polyps in same segment	71
	†Undifferentiated cancer with mucinous elements	4
	†Deep margin through muscle and serosa	32
	†Infiltrating margin	519
	†Lymphatic and perineural permeation	30
	†Blood vascular permeation without lymphatic or perineural permeation	72
	Metastatic cancer in 1 to 5 mesenteric lymph nodes	247
.301–.4	†Well-differentiated cancer (grade 1)	121
	Well-differentiated cancer (grade 1) in adenomatous polyp	3
	Well-differentiated cancer (grade 1) in villous adenoma	15
	†Poorly differentiated cancer (grade 2) in an adenomatous polyp	3
	†Poorly differentiated cancer (grade 2) with generalized polyposis	5
	†Mucinous cancer with adenomatous polyps in same segment	3
	Through muscle and into but not through mesenteric fat	421
	Moderate inflammatory reaction (no abscesses)	439
.401–.5	†Well-differentiated cancer (grade 1) with generalized polyposis	2
	Deep margin through muscularis mucosae but not through inner muscle	182
	†Pushing or circumscribed margin	103
	Intense inflammatory reaction with gross or microscopic abscess formation	223
	No lymphatic, perineural, or blood vascular permeation	417
	No metastases in mesenteric lymph nodes	420
.501–	†Well-differentiated cancer with adenomatous polyps in same segment	24
	†Well-differentiated cancer with mucinous elements	12
	†Poorly differentiated cancer with mucinous elements	34
	Mucinous cancer in a villous adenoma	1
	†Mixed infiltrating and pushing margins	155

*Adapted from Spratt JS Jr, Spjut HJ: Prevalence and prognosis of individual clinical and pathologic variables associated with colorectal carcinoma. Cancer 20:1976–1985, 1967.

†±2 S.D. (95 percent confidence) would place characteristic in higher and/or lower range.

Table 10–22. **SURVIVAL RATES OF PATIENTS WITH COLORECTAL CANCER ACCORDING TO TYPE OF OPERATIVE THERAPY AND PRIMARY CARE***

Operative Therapy	No. of Patients	Accumulative Survival ± 1 S.D. 5-Yr	10-Yr
Abdominoperineal resection with high ligation (inferior mesenteric)	35	0.369 ± 0.101	0.369 ± 0.101
Abdominoperineal resection with low ligation (superior hemorrhoidal)	418	0.316 ± 0.024	0.210 ± 0.022
Low anterior resection with anastomosis	47	0.335 ± 0.081	0.335 ± 0.081
Posterior proctotomy and local excision	1	0	—
Posterior proctotomy and segmental resection	1	0	—
Local excision per anus without dividing sphincter	1	0	—
Local excision per anus with division of sphincter	2	1.000	0.500 ± 0.354
Pelvic exenteration	15	0.200 ± 0.103	0.200 ± 0.103
Hartmann's procedure	23	0.109 ± 0.071	0.109 ± 0.071
Sigmoid resection with high ligation of inferior mesenteric vessels	15	0.636 ± 0.131	0.538 ± 0.143
Sigmoid resection with low ligation of vessels (superior hemorrhoid)	48	0.401 ± 0.072	0.209 ± 0.075
Sigmoid resection, level of vessel division not determinable	31	0.202 ± 0.074	0.110 ± 0.064
Left colectomy	48	0.446 ± 0.076	0.142 ± 0.073
Transverse colectomy	25	0.520 ± 0.107	0.416 ± 0.126
Right colectomy with ligation of middle colic artery at origin	56	0.364 ± 0.068	0.364 ± 0.068
Right colectomy without ligation of middle colic artery	49	0.477 ± 0.075	0.390 ± 0.083
Laparotomy, biopsy only without opening bowel	16	0	—
Laparotomy, colotomy and excision	5	0.267 ± 0.226	—
Laparotomy, local excision of tumor and bowel wall	1	0	—
Laparotomy, local resection of segmental resection	2	0	—
Laparotomy, closure because inoperable	54	0.037 ± 0.026	—
Laparotomy, colostomy only	112	0	—
Total colectomy with excision of rectum	1	1.000	—
Subtotal colectomy (resection of multiple segments of colon but part of colon other than rectum left in)	6	0.286 ± 0.195	0.286 ± 0.195
Two-stage colectomy with excision of rectum	2	0.500 ± 0.354	0.500 ± 0.354
Roentgenotherapy with colostomy	4	0	—
Roentgenotherapy without colostomy	2	0	—
Roentgenotherapy with resection	1	0	—
Biopsy only of recurrent cancer	11	0.116 ± 0.106	—
Excision only of recurrent cancer	1	1.000	—

*Adapted from Spratt JS Jr, Spjut HJ: Prevalence and prognosis of individual clinical and pathologic variables associated with colorectal carcinoma. Cancer 20:1976–1985, 1967.

2. Extensive mesenteric lymph node dissections should be performed for small but high-grade infiltrating cancers.

3. There is no cancer related justification for delaying the surgical resection of small colonic cancers proven by biopsy or for delay in exploration of the nature of roentgen intracolonic shadows whose diameters exceed 1 cm (Spratt and Ackerman, 1960b; Spratt and Spjut, 1967).

The type of surgical therapy and a ranking of various factors associated with surgical management were correlated with survival (Tables 10–21 and 10–22). Allowing for selection and variance in the smaller samples, one operation is not significantly better or worse than another. All 131 persons having laparotomies without some standard cancer resection died within 5 years; most were determined to have unresectable cancers at the time of the laparotomy. Emphasizing the point that certain colorectal carcinomas can grow very large yet never metastasize is the 20 percent 5-year survival rate for the 76 cases having resections for colorectal cancers that had invaded adjacent organs by direct extension. Many surgical factors had surprisingly little effect on prognosis. However, many surgical decisions and some surgical techniques do affect the prognosis of resectable cancers, as discussed later in this chapter.

The fundamental adverse determinants of host survival with colorectal carcinomas were the patterns of cellular appearance or grade, including cancers of signet ring cell, undifferentiated carcinoma (grade 3), cancer in ulcerative colitis, and unclassified malignant cancers. These accounted for 150 of the 1137 cancers (13.2 percent), and less than 10 percent of the persons having cancers with these characteristics survived 5 years (see rankings in Table 10–21).

When more than six mesenteric lymph nodes contained metastatic cancer, less than 10 percent of the patients survived 5 years. When 16 or more lymph nodes contained cancer, all patients were dead within 5 years. Metastases in six lymph nodes was not observed in cancers less than 2 cm in greatest dimension. Metastases in 16 or more lymph nodes was not observed in cancers less than 3 cm in diameter. The only chance for the surgical cure of high-grade colorectal cancers having a tendency to develop extensive lymph node metastases would require wide resection of the mesenteric lymph nodes while the primary cancer is less than 3 cm and preferably less than 2 cm in diameter.

The EFSCH series had too few patients with carcinomas arising in colons with ulcerative colitis to study. A much larger base of experience with carcinomas arising in colons with ulcerative colitis confirms that this is not a hopeless problem as the earlier data indicated (Lavery et al., 1982). The authors compared the survival statistics of patients with cancer arising in ulcerative colitis with those colon cancer patients with no colitis, using the extended Dukes' classification. They found no significant difference in survivorship, stage for stage. However, there were more colitic patients with incurable disease at the time of diagnosis. They speculated that with close surveillance for premalignant changes the need for prophylactic colectomy in the interest of cancer prevention might be reduced.

Nonresection of colorectal carcinomas for any cause resulted in the death of 92 to 100 percent of the patients within 5 years (see Table 10–8). Local extension or extensive metastases, both functions of tumor size and grade, were the principal causes of nonresection. Even with the ability to perform pelvic exenterations and multiple organ resections when required, the resectability rate at the EFSCH was only 74.6 percent, and in the final 5 years of the study this increased to 75.3 percent.

The effect on prognosis of modifications in surgical technique, such as ligation of the vasculature before mobilization of the tumor, irrigation of the colonic lumen with cytotoxic agents, and technical precautions against implantation metastases, remains incompletely evaluated. These technical changes certainly would not have helped the 25 percent of patients who had cancers that were unresectable for the various reasons outlined. For the resectable cancers, the changes in surgical technique to avoid dissemination and implantation of cancer by surgical manipulation may improve the prognosis, as will be discussed later in this chapter (see Chapter Twenty-One).

RELATION OF SURVIVAL TIME TO CLINICAL, THERAPEUTIC, AND PATHOLOGIC VARIABLES USING THE ANALYSIS OF VARIANCE AND COVARIANCE

EFSCH data on individual variables were studied further using the analysis of variance and covariance (Watson, 1964; Watson et al., 1976). The more stringent manner for the analysis of variance and covariance gives further specificity to prognostic indicators. The EFSCH series was extended over additional years to include 1174 consecutive patients with histologically confirmed adenocarcinomas of the colon and rectum. Follow-up on all cases to the terminus of life or through December 31, 1973 was complete. A minimum of 10 years of follow-up (100Δ) was available on all cases.

The computer program used, called Generalized Regression and Statistical Problem Inquirer (GRASPI), was written in FORTRAN IV. Its use required IBM 360 or 370 with 150K storage or IBM 7040 with 32 K storage or equivalent.

GRASPI was designed to solve generalized linear regression problems and, for easy access by users, featured well-labeled output. In its most general form, linear regression is called analysis of covariance (ANOCOVA). This program was suitable for problems in multiple regression, analysis of variance, and analysis of covariance (orthogonal or nonorthogonal designs, fixed effects model).

No variable could exceed a nine-column field size. There was no limit to the number of cases (subjects) allowed, but there were general limits of 30 analyses of variance type variables. The sum of the levels within the analysis of variance type variables plus continuous variables could not exceed 49. Interaction terms were not solved. Only subjects with complete data for the specified variables were used; other subjects were rejected, probably introducing an additional source of bias.

The solution was computed from the appropriate parts of the data matrix and included means, correlations, regression weights (or effects), and standard errors. The program also computed F tests and contrasted (critical ratios) pairs of levels within each analysis of variance type variable. Chi-square analysis between pairs of analysis of variance type variables was also obtainable.

Although the belief is generally held that the survival time of individual patients is a function of numerous variables concerning him or his cancer, or both, many of these variables have been ignored in existing staging systems. Attempting to use all these variables in a staging system would have led to a very large number of staging categories, each defined in a complex manner. Except for extremely large studies, the number of patients in each group might be too small to provide statistical significance. The permutations and combinations of staging possibilities become almost infinite, supporting the need for a less cumbersome system that is still able to consider as many prognostically significant variables as possible.

When these conditions exist in other areas of knowledge, other statistical techniques are often employed. One such method is generalized regression analysis (Harvey, 1960; Rao, 1952; Scheffe, 1959). Surprisingly, this method had not been employed previously in the analysis of survival times for a group of cancer patients. The major reason for this may be that the distribution of survival times for a group of patients was generally censored on the high side. The fact that the censoring characteristics could not be completely specified made certain estimations and interpretations of regression technique difficult.

To avoid this problem, the investigator could wait to do end-result analyses until all patients in a given group had died. If the last patient survived 40 years, the results of such analysis would be rather late to be of practical use. Consequently, most investigators have turned to methods of analyzing survival curves in which censoring factors are more readily handled, as with cumulative survival rates.

Yet correlation coefficients and variance estimates are not the totality of generalized regression methods. Of equal importance in many studies is the estimate of the regression coefficients. Generally, these estimates are not biased by censoring as are variance estimates. For example, if we wish to estimate the influence of numerous factors upon an individual's survival time, we may set up a generalized regression equation for a group of individuals (Watson, 1964; Watson et al., 1976).

The application of the methods to the clinical setting is based on the fact that each patient has one and only one survival time. However, in the mathematical sense, each patient is composed of many different variables acting simultaneously to determine this uniqueness. These variables act upon each other in highly complex ways often not initially determinable.

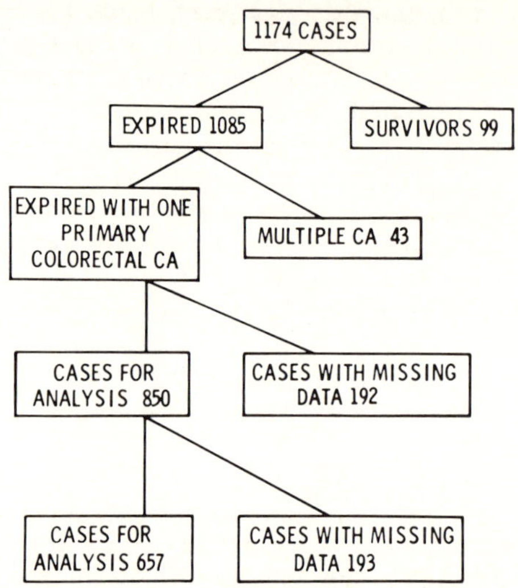

Figure 10–10. Steps in the stratification of 1174 consecutive cases of cancer of the colon and rectum for the analysis of variance and convariance to determine the prognostic score of individual variables. (From Watson FR, Spratt JS Jr, LeDuc RJ: Analysis of variance and covariance for colorectal adenocarcinomas in man as a logical prelude to staging. J Surg Oncol 8:155–163, 1976.)

By the computer program used, it was possible to score up to 49 different variables of potential prognostic significance and then to apply this scoring system to predict the survival of an individual patient with a high degree of accuracy. The analysis to determine the effect of survival time associated with the ten clinical, therapeutic, and pathologic variables was applied as shown in Figure 10–10. The results of the analysis are provided in Table 10–23.

The conclusion was that it is feasible to determine the prognostic score or weight of many prognostically important variables in cancer patients. The combined effect of these weights provides scores of clusters of variables relevant to assaying the outcome of current management and to planning and evaluating clinical trials. This approach provides a higher degree of accuracy, versatility, and scope than do most contemporary staging systems and is reported here as a method useful in studying the prognostic significance of cancer-related variables (see Table 10–24).

NONMETASTASIZING CANCERS

After recognizing that a behavioral variant of adenocarcinoma of the colon and rectum

Table 10–23. **EFFECT ON SURVIVAL TIME IN MONTHS OF TEN CLINICAL, THERAPEUTIC, AND PATHOLOGIC VARIABLES***

Constant	Analysis 1 11.98	Analysis 2 8.81
I. Race and sex		
White male	0.84	0.76
White female	1.13	1.01
Black male	0.87	1.71
Black female	1.22	1.11
II. Intestinal obstruction		
No Yes—subsided with conservative Rx	1.61	1.71
Yes—required colostomy	1.37	1.35
Yes—obstructive resection with anastomosis Yes—obstructive resection with colostomy	0.89	0.84
Yes—produced perforation of proximal colon	0.51	0.51
III. Therapeutic determinants		
Not resected; patient refusal	1.49	None
Not resected; other illnesses Not resected; proven metastases Not resected; suspected metastases Not resected; considered inoperative	0.52	0.45
Resected; proven distant metastases Resected; distant metastases suspected	1.04	1.40
Resected; thought locally incurable	0.57	0.75
Resected; no proven or suspected distant metastases Observed over 1 mo before resection	2.17	2.11
IV. Anatomic segment containing primary tumor		
Rectum Rectosigmoid	0.71	0.70
Sigmoid Descending Splenic flexure Transverse	1.02	1.03
Hepatic flexure Ascending	0.83	0.91
Cecum	0.75	0.97
Multiple segments	2.21	1.57
V. Length of colon resected		
1–30	1.13	1.07
31–100 cm	1.21	1.23
Total colectomy	1.17	1.08
Colon not resected	0.55	0.70
Colon resected but not measured	1.13	1.01
VI. Type of primary tumor		
Well-differentiated carcinoma (grade 1)	0.87	0.73
Poorly differentiated carcinoma (grade 2)	0.94	0.97
Signet ring carcinoma	0.97	1.08
Poorly differentiated carcinoma with mucinous adenocarcinoma	1.70	1.68
Undifferentiated cancer (grade 3) Malignant tumor, unclassified Undifferentiated cancer with mucinous elements Mucinous cancer	0.74	0.78
VII. Margin		
Not through muscularis mucosae Through muscularis mucosae but not to muscle To inner muscle Into but not through muscle	Not Estimated	1.19
Through muscle but not through serosa or fat Through serosa Through muscle and into mesenteric fat	Not Estimated	1.15

Table continued on following page

Table 10–23. **EFFECT ON SURVIVAL TIME OF TEN CLINICAL, THERAPEUTIC, AND PATHOLOGIC VARIABLES*** (*Continued*)

Constant	Analysis 1 11.98	Analysis 2 8.81
Direct extension into adjacent organs Depth not determinable Incompletely excised to margins	Not Estimated	0.73
VIII. Invasiveness		
None seen	Not Estimated	1.50
Lymphatics	Not Estimated	0.95
Blood vascular invasion	Not Estimated	1.18
Neural sheath Lymphatic and blood vascular Lymphatic and neural Blood vascular and neural	Not Estimated	0.97
Lymphatic, blood vascular and neural sheath	Not Estimated	0.61
IX. Number of lymph nodes removed		
None	1.03	1.06
1–10 nodes	0.78	0.75
11–25 nodes	1.26	1.21
>25 nodes	0.98	1.04
X. Admission hemoglobin		
<14	1.03	0.97
14 or more gm/dl	1.14	1.10

*Adapted from Watson FR, Spratt JS Jr, LeDuc RJ: Analysis of variance and covariance for colorectal adenocarcinomas in man as a logical prelude to staging. J Surg Oncol 8:155–163, 1976.

existed that exhibited only contiguous local growth with no metastases, additional studies were carried out to see what characteristics might differentiate the metastasizing from the nonmetastasizing cancers. The EFSCH series, contained on Hollerith cards, were sorted as shown in Figure 10–11. The accumulative percentage of metastasizing and nonmetastasizing cancers had been plotted previously against the logarithm of the greatest chordal dimension of the cancers, producing two almost parallel lines (Fig. 10–12). There was no statistically significant difference between these two distributions (Spratt, 1969) (Fig. 10–13).

Table 10–24. **BASE DATA FROM COLUMN 2 OF TABLE 10–23***

	Prognostic Score from Table 10–23
Constant†	8.81
Caucasian male	0.76
Intestinal obstruction (no)	1.71
Resected, no proven or suspected distant metastases	2.11
Rectum	0.70
Over 30 cm of bowel resected	1.23
Well-differentiated cancer	0.73
Invasion of blood, lymph vessels, or nerve sheaths not seen	1.50
Number of lymph nodes resected was 10 or less	0.75
Admission hemoglobin over 14 gm/dl	1.10
Expected survival time equals constant multiplied by each prognostic score	= 12.26 months

*Adapted from Watson FR, Spratt JS Jr, LeDuc RJ: Analysis of variance and covariance for colorectal adenocarcinomas in man as a logical prelude to staging. J Surg Oncol 8:155–163, 1976.

†Mean survival rate of 657 cases followed until death was 8.81 months.

All distributions that were not similar, with probabilities greater than 0.95 or better, were regarded as significantly dissimilar. The variables that were significantly more likely to denote the presence or absence of metastases in resected lymph nodes are provided in Table 10–25.

Unfortunately, no characteristic that would allow the surgeon to be absolutely correct about the presence or absence of metastases in the regional lymph nodes was identified in this study. There were, however, some interesting correlations. The presence, past or present, of cancers of the skin and of a highly infiltrative cancer margin with little associated inflammatory reaction of this marginal zone significantly increased the chance of metastases in the regional lymph nodes. The presence of cancer cells in lymphatic or blood vessels also

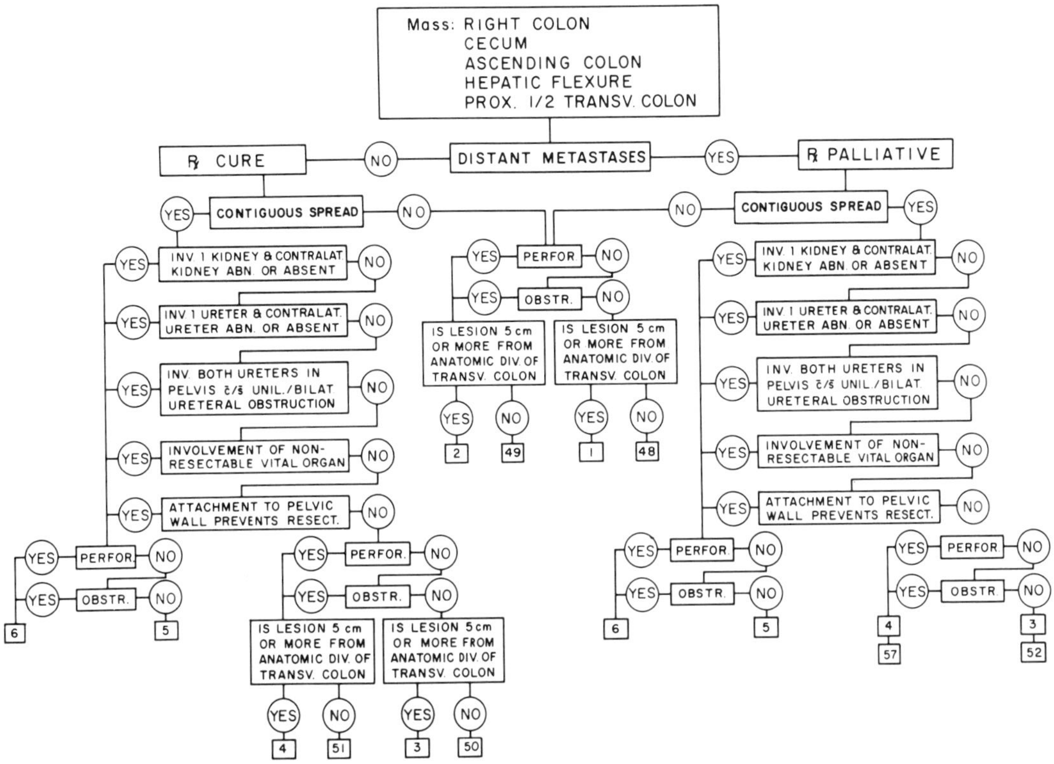

Figure 10–11. Logic diagram for decisions involved in management of adenocarcinomas of the right colon. (From Knutson CO, Watson FR: Preliminary results of a computer logic program for the operative management of colon cancer. Surgery 76:298–308, 1974.)

Figure 10–12. The allocation of cases that preceded the comparison of the distribution of cases by individual variables among cancers with and without histologically confirmed metastases in the regional lymph nodes. (From Spratt JS, Jr, Watson FR, Pratt JL: Characteristics of variants of colorectal carcinoma that do not metastasize to lymph nodes. Dis Colon Rectum 13:243–246, 1970.)

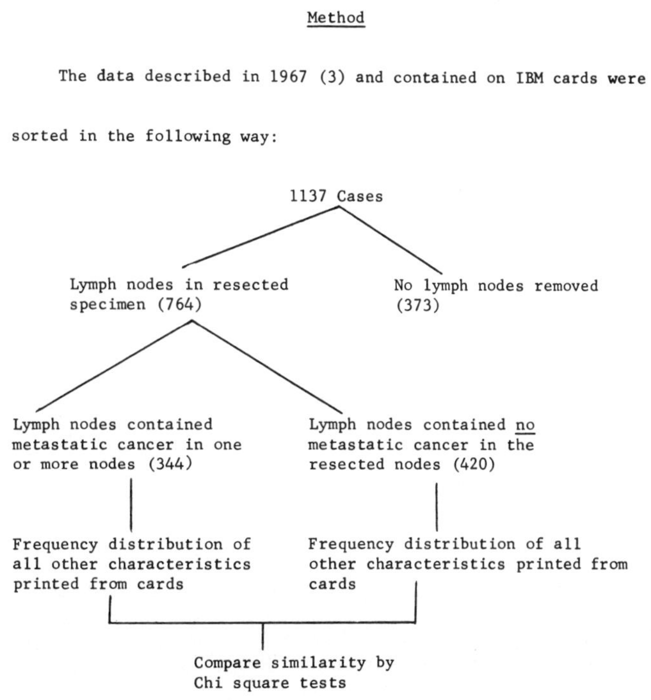
Method

The data described in 1967 (3) and contained on IBM cards were sorted in the following way:

1137 Cases

Lymph nodes in resected specimen (764)

No lymph nodes removed (373)

Lymph nodes contained metastatic cancer in one or more nodes (344)

Lymph nodes contained no metastatic cancer in the resected nodes (420)

Frequency distribution of all other characteristics printed from cards

Frequency distribution of all other characteristics printed from cards

Compare similarity by Chi square tests

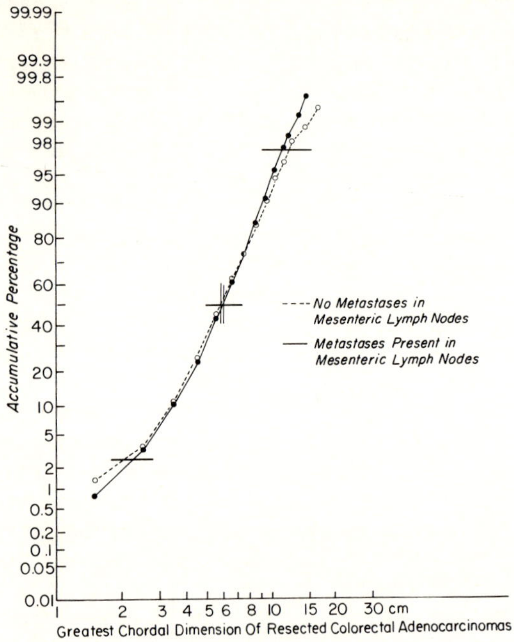

Figure 10–13. The greatest chordal dimension of colorectal adenocarcinomas, with and without metastases in the mesenteric lymph nodes is plotted against the accumulative frequency. The median chordal dimensions for the two distributions are 6.1 and 6.2 cm. The 99 percent confidence range for the size of cancers with metastases was 19.4 to 0.9 cm, and without metastases, 20.3 to 0.9 cm. There was no significant difference between the two means ($p > 0.9$) or between the variances ($p > 0.99$). (From Spratt JS Jr: The lognormal frequency distribution and human cancer. J Surg Res 9:151–157, 1969.)

greatly increased the chance of finding metastatic cancer in lymph nodes. If microscopic examination showed the margin to be of the "pushing" or circumscribed type or if considerable inflammatory cell infiltration surrounded the margin, the cancer was significantly less likely to have metastasized to the lymph nodes.

Neither size nor depth of invasion through the bowel wall or into adjacent organs was a good criterion for predicting the presence of metastases in lymph nodes. In fact, direct extension through muscle into mesenteric fat or direct extension into adjacent organs was more frequently indicative of the absence of metastases in lymph nodes. The nonmetastasizing variant seemed to penetrate the bowel wall and invade adjacent tissues and organs as it continued its progressive local growth but did not metastasize. If the unequivocal diagnosis of a localized, nonmetastasizing variant of colorectal adenocarcinoma could be identified without resection, such a cancer might be cured by local ablation, if this treatment was applied before the cancer penetrated through all layers of the intestine. Localized cancers were still curable even when they had extended into adjacent organs, provided that circumscribing resections were performed (including adjacent organs when necessary for en bloc removal). The 5-year cumulative survival rate of 420 persons with carcinomas of the colon and rectum that had not metastasized to lymph nodes was 48.8 percent, with a standard deviation of 2.8 percent. In the same age group (median 67 years), the survival rate for the base Missouri population was only 76 percent. The difference between expected survival and survival with cancer was 27.2 percent (the difference between 76 percent and 48.8 percent). Theoretically, the difference might be reduced by earlier diagnosis and ablation of the nonmetastasizing cancers because less radical treatment imposes less treatment risk to the patient.

Table 10–25. CHARACTERISTICS SIGNIFICANTLY ($p > 0.95$ BY CHI-SQUARE TEST) ASSOCIATED WITH THE PRESENCE OR ABSENCE OF METASTASES IN THE MESENTERIC LYMPH NODES AMONG RESECTED CANCERS*

No Metastases	Metastases
Absence of proven or suspected metastases outside the field of resection	Past or present association with cancers of the skin
Microscopic margin pushing (well circumscribed) or mixed	Resection done with proven or suspected distant metastases
Deep margin of cancer through inner muscle	Incomplete local resection
Deep margin of cancer into mesenteric fat	Infiltrating tumor margin or microscopic assessment
Direct extension into adjacent organs	Deep margin of cancer into muscle
	Less inflammatory reaction around the periphery of the cancer
	Intravasal cancer near primary

*Adapted from Spratt JS Jr, Watson FR, Pratt JL: Characteristics of variants of colorectal carcinoma that do not metastasize to lymph nodes. Dis Colon Rectum 13:243–246, 1970.

Relationship of Morphologic Characteristics of Colorectal Cancer to Metastasis

The grade or cellular differentiation of the tumors was of no help in predicting the presence or absence of nodal metastasis. The characteristics that might be of most use to the surgeon (those having to do with the tumor-host interface, such as marginal configuration and lymph and blood vascular infiltration) required deep marginal biopsy to ascertain. The tumor-host interface, which is of great significance, is affected by many variables that would be difficult, but not impossible, to measure in the living host. For example, it is not known whether the more favorable tumor margins are due to an immune response, to a complex growth-repressive phenomenon, to variations in local tumor angiogeneses factors, or simply to variable cohesiveness of the cancer cells themselves. It certainly is incompletely known what effect adjunctive therapeutic measures, such as radiotherapy and chemotherapy have on this cancer-host interface. The effect could be adverse. An example of radiotherapeutically induced change in the behavior of a localized cancer is that which occurs with the verrucous cancers. These cancers attain large local bulk and invade adjacent structures. They are amenable to curative surgical ablation, but radiation therapy changes them to highly undifferentiated cancers that are no longer controllable by ablative therapy (Kraus, 1966a).

The observation that skin cancers occur more frequently with colorectal carcinomas that metastasize to lymph nodes than with those that do not is most interesting from the standpoint of comparative pathology. The carcinogen, 3:2′-dimethyl-4-aminobiphenyl, which is reported to produce the full spectrum of histologic variants of colorectal neoplasms in rats, also produced skin cancers on the ears of the rats (see Chapter One).

Progress with Controlled Clinical Trials

Although many more studies on the characteristics of metastasizing and nonmetastasizing cancers could be cited, these studies on historical data obviously need the refinement that controlled clinical trials may provide.

As an example, data from the National Surgical Adjuvant Breast Project (NSABP), in a preliminary trial on data from colorectal cancer, have solidly corroborated the existence of a nonmetastasizing variant of cancer in all size ranges and have confirmed my earlier conclusion that anatomic staging systems in wide contemporary use, such as Dukes' staging system, are simply inadequate for expression of variance in biologic behavior (Wollmark et al., 1983).

Major events in the evolution of a colorectal cancer that were noted included local tumor invasion, metastasis to regional lymphatics, and distant dissemination, in an undefined order. Dukes' clinical-pathologic staging classification along with its variants categorized colorectal cancer utilizing depth of tumor penetration into the bowel wall and presence or absence of regional lymph node involvement. Significantly absent from the Dukes classification was gross tumor size. The long-held impression that gross tumor size was not related to regional lymph node involvement and prognosis might have contributed to this exclusion. Tumor penetration was used rather than tumor size as the morphologic parameter of biologic importance. Clinically, the Dukes system has the shortcoming of being a pathologic classification system that really can be applied accurately to resected specimens only. This deficiency has particularly been evident in relation to carcinoma of the rectum, for which a staging system could be effective in selecting a patient population appropriate for sphincter-saving surgical procedures. The NSABP conducted a reappraisal of the morphologic characteristics of colorectal cancer so that more sensitive prognostic indices not considered in the standard classification schemes could be identified. Included in this reappraisal by the NSABP were many characteristics considered in the EFSCH series, such as histologic differentiation, tumor configuration, tumor location, the presence of gross extramural tumor, and tumor size. Studies were reviewed in which a correlation between tumor size and lymph node status or the incidence of recurrent disease were studied. These studies all challenge the original premise upon which the commonly employed clinical-pathologic staging classifications were based.

In the latter part of 1977, the NSABP began two randomized prospective protocols to ascertain the efficacy of adjuvant therapy in carcinoma of the colon and rectum. A secondary aim was to obtain prospective information on the natural history of colorectal cancer. The data collected permitted an opportunity to corroborate the biologic significance of a number of parameters. In an effort to assess the significance of tumor size as a predictive index of regional lymph node status, an analysis was carried out for both colon and rectal cancers, assessing the frequency distribution of tumor diameter and volume in Dukes' B and C lesions. The analysis was carried out simply to determine the relationship of tumor size to regional node status.

The Dukes classification criteria used in the protocols were those described in 1932 for carcinoma of the rectum and adapted for use in colonic tumors (Dukes, 1932). The criteria for the D category were those described by Turnbull and were characterized by tumors that extended beyond the scope of operative resection as a result of either metastatic disease or contiguous involvement (Turnbull et al., 1967).

Tumor dimensions were recorded by the pathologists. Measurements were carried out in the transverse, longitudinal, and vertical axes of the tumor on the gross specimen. The tumor volume index was determined from the product of the three tumor dimensions. The distribution of the volumes was found to be asymmetric and skewed to the right owing to the presence of a few very large tumors. This asymmetry became a normal distribution by utilizing the logarithm of the index rather than the index itself. Hence, the analysis and comparisons of Dukes' B and C lesions were made in terms of the following variable: $x = \log$ volume index. This tendency conforms with an early observation by the author (J.S.S.) that the sizes of many solid cancers at the time of diagnosis form lognormal frequency distributions (Spratt, 1969) and the specific observation that the sizes of metastasizing (to lymph nodes) and nonmetastasizing colorectal cancers formed two almost identical lognormal frequency distributions (Spratt et al., 1970). The striking homogeneity of these two distributions is discussed earlier in this chapter.

Cumulative frequency distributions of tumor diameter and tumor volume were carried out for Dukes' B and C tumors, and the statistical significance of the differences in these dimensions was calculated using the student t test.

Cumulative frequency distributions of the longest tumor diameter and the log volume index of colon cancers were determined for Dukes' B and C lesions. Two-hundred seventy-five patients with Dukes' B lesions and 395 patients with Dukes' C lesions were available. The mean longest tumor diameter (± standard error) for Dukes' B lesions was 5.7 (± 0.2) cm and 5.2 (± 0.1) cm for Dukes' C tumors. In the analysis of tumor volume, 199 patients with Dukes' B and 261 with Dukes' C lesions were assessed for all three tumor dimensions. The mean log tumor volume index representing the logarithm of the product of the three dimensions was 1.57 (± 0.04) for Dukes' B and 1.49 (± 0.04) for Dukes' C cancers. Although no differences were evident that were statistically significant for either longest tumor diameter or tumor volume index, examination of the frequency distribution curves disclosed that Dukes' C tumors were consistently *smaller* than Dukes' B tumors throughout the distribution. The mean number of lymph nodes examined by the pathologists for Dukes' B and C cancers was not significantly different.

Similar analyses were applied for Dukes' B and C carcinomas of the rectum. The longest tumor diameter for 91 patients with Dukes' B and for 145 patients with Dukes' C tumors was used. Mean longest tumor diameters for B and C lesions were 5.6 (± 0.2) cm and 4.8 (± 0.2) cm, respectively. The difference was not statistically significant. In the analysis of tumor volume, 64 patients with Dukes' B and 95 patients with Dukes' C tumors were compared. The mean tumor volume index for Dukes' B lesions was *larger* than for Dukes' C, 1.52 (± 0.06) versus 1.33 (± 0.05). This difference was statistically significant ($P < 0.02$). In cumulative frequency distributions of volume, Dukes' B tumors were consistently larger than Dukes' C lesions throughout the distribution. The frequency distribution of the number of lymph nodes examined for Dukes' B and C rectal cancers was not significantly different.

The accumulating evidence demonstrating no association between tumor size and regional lymph node status is becoming overwhelming. As a result of relatively recent efforts to increase the predictive index of colorectal classification systems, a number of morphologic parameters were considered.

This challenge to there being an association between tumor size and lymph node status began in 1964 in an analysis by Grinnell (1965). Utilizing a clearing technique for examining regional lymph nodes, 941 colorectal cancers were examined. No positive nodes were found in tumors less than 1.5 cm, and the percentage with positive nodes progressively increased with increasing tumor size and peaked at 53 percent for tumors between 5.0 and 6.9 cm. This correlation between tumor size and nodal status was statistically significant.

In 1975, Godwin and Brown were able to establish an association between size of the primary lesion and depth of penetration, which is an established prognostic indicator. In 1980, Cohen reviewed 205 patients with rectal cancer, taking into account the degree of histologic differentiation, tumor configuration, and tumor size. The results of this study demonstrated that when the primary lesion was ulcerated, 12 percent of patients with tumors less than or equal to 4 cm had positive nodes compared with 42 percent of patients with tumors greater than 4 cm. If the tumors were poorly differentiated and greater than 4 cm, the percentage of positive nodes rose to 77 percent. In two recent reports from the Peter Bent Brigham Hospital, recurrence patterns of over 281 patients undergoing curative resection for colorectal cancer were evaluated (Olson et al., 1980; Malcolm et al., 1981). Histologic differentiation could not be associated with recurrence; however, the size of the primary tumors significantly predicted treatment failure. Twelve percent of the patients with tumors less than or equal to 3 cm had recurrent cancer compared with 29 percent with tumors greater than 3 cm. A logistic regression analysis described in the more recent study suggested that tumor penetration and lymph node status contributed independently to the risk or recurrence (Malcolm et al., 1981).

Although the preceding studies showed that there is little relationship between the total number of lymph nodes removed or the length of the bowel resected and survival, there is an inverse relationship between the number of removed lymph nodes that contain metastatic cancer and survival. To reiterate, the data from Spratt and Spjut (1967) showed that resected cancers with no metastases in the lymph nodes were associated with an accumulative 5-year survival rate of 49 percent, which dropped to 24 percent with the presence of any positive nodes. All patients with 16 or more lymph nodes containing metastases died within 5 years of resection of the cancer. In considering the progression of colon cancers, cancers with a tendency to metastasize to lymph nodes would generally have to be resected while the primary was less than 3 cm, and preferably less than 2 cm if adjacent node-bearing mesentery was present, to optimize chances for cure by surgery alone.

The fact that there is a limit on the probability of cure by surgery alone when extensive lymph nodal metastases are present was confirmed in a different way by Grinnell (1965). He reported that if resected para-aortic lymph nodes contained metastatic cancer, the patient would not survive 5 years. Although the literature contains many retrospective studies supporting marginal improvements in survivorship with various technical modifications, there remains no controlled clinical trial confirming these improvements. Conflicting conclusions in various studies support the need for trials when the potential gains justify a feasible study. As an example of the variable results in historical studies, Enker and associates (1980) reported a series of 216 patients with carcinoma of the large bowel in which patients with positive lymph nodes and full-thickness penetration of the bowel wall by cancer had a 5-year survival rate of 70.5 percent. These researchers systematically performed wide anatomic and radical lymph node dissections as a routine. They also concluded that their patients had a lower local recurrence rate than expected.

The NSABP study represented the first analysis of natural history data using randomized prospective protocols. Cumulative frequency distributions assessing tumor diameter and tumor volume in Dukes' B and C patients failed to demonstrate that tumor size was predictive of regional node status. If any correlation was evident, it was the association of Dukes' C lesions with smaller tumors. This inverse relationship was statistically significant for tumor volume in the case of rectal cancer. For the relationship between tumor size and regional lymph node status to be assessed accurately, a number of other factors must be considered, such as tumor configuration. Preliminary analysis of data relative to tumor configuration indicated that three quarters of the tumors were ulcerating and these were equally distributed to B and C classes in both colon and rectal cancers. In the B and C categories, the depth of penetration was similarly distributed in that transmural involvement was present in all Dukes' B lesions and the majority of Dukes' C tumors. Dukes' A lesions were excluded from this analysis because they were not randomized to a therapeutic regimen. Similar considerations could extend to other prognostic indices such as cancer differentiation.

This NSABP analysis considered tumor size as a single prognostic factor for lymph node involvement. For full evaluation of the importance of tumor size, size was considered in conjunction with other prognostic factors utilizing a multivariate approach. The conclusion was that tumor size as a single factor did not correlate with regional node involvement when the analysis was limited to Dukes' B and C lesions. These findings confirm the unique biologic behavior of colorectal cancer.

Significance of Ovarian Metastases on Prognosis

Other studies have looked at the unique impact of still other variables on prognosis. For example, ovaries are the frequent site of metastases from cancers originating in many different organs, including breast, gastric, pancreatic, and colorectal cancers. This has led to periodic interest in prophylactic oophorectomies. However, controlled clinical trials have never shown that this enhances survivorship. Ovarian metastases have been regarded as a local manifestation of generalized carcinomatosis in most situations. The status of ovarian metastases with respect to colorectal cancers has been the subject of several reviews.

In a review by MacKeigan and Ferguson (1979), only seven patients were found who had ovarian metastases and survived 5 years. Yet, their review documented that from 3 to 8 percent of the ovaries contained metastases at the time of the original laparotomy. Israel and associates (1965) made the general observation that younger women are more prone to have metastatic ovarian cancer than primary ovarian cancer. They surmised that the functioning ovary might be a more fertile site for metastases. Webb and associates (1975) later observed that 50 percent of all women with ovarian metastases were premenopausal.

The prevalence of ovarian metastases is so great that all suspicious appearing ovaries should be removed from any woman past childbearing years. In the same group and in the presence of cancers that have extended to the serosal surfaces, oophorectomies should be performed. This recommendation is not based on any knowledge that survivorship will be enhanced. However, presence of ovarian metastasis provides a useful parameter for assaying the tendency of the colon cancer for transperitoneal metastasis. The inconvenience and morbidity of a pelvic mass secondary to the metastasis will occasionally be avoided.

RELATION BETWEEN THE NO-TOUCH ISOLATION TECHNIQUE AND PROGNOSIS

The primary surgical management (no-touch isolation technique versus conventional technique) of colonic adenocarcinoma was studied in a unique series by Turnbull and associates (1967). Turnbull (1976) provided a separate review of cancer of the sigmoid colon treated by the no-touch technique. The improved results with this technique were apparent in this segmental subset, in which the inferior mesenteric lymphatic bundle was ligated before manipulation of the cancer.

In 1955, Fisher and Turnbull reported cancer cells in the portal venous blood of eight of 25 resected segments (for cancer) of the colon and suggested that the cells had been scattered by operative manipulation. In late 1953, Turnbull adopted a technique of colon resection for cancer wherein the cancer-bearing segment was not manipulated or handled in any manner until after the lymph/vascular pedicles were divided and ligated and the colon was divided at the elected sites for resection. To emphasize the type of technique, the name no-touch isolation was adopted. This method of resection was applied to every cancer of the colon operated on by Turnbull after 1953. During this same time, five staff surgeons at the Cleveland Clinic Hospital continued to perform resections of the colon with the conventional technique, which is characterized by ligation and division of the lymphovascular pedicles after mobilization of the cancer-bearing segment.

Turnbull's first reports were based on a computer analysis of the results of surgical treatment of 896 patients with cancer of the colon treated at the Cleveland Clinic Hospital from 1950 to 1964. The records of 2225 patients with a diagnosis of malignancy of the colon, rectum, and anus recorded at the Cleveland Clinic Foundation from 1950 to 1964 were reviewed. A systematic follow-up study was instituted, and all pertinent data were recorded on individual code sheets. The verified data were subjected to analyses (Turnbull et al., 1967).

Since this report was only on survival rates among patients with cancer of the colon, the following categories were excluded from the study: patients with cancer in a polyp, cancer of the rectum or anus, carcinoid tumors, malignancy other than adenocarcinoma, or operations first done at other hospitals and patients not operated.

Cancers of the colon were defined as those tumors located at or above a point 5.5 in. (14 cm) above the anus, as recorded at the time of proctosigmoidoscopic examination. The level of each tumor was determined preoperatively by the operating surgeon. After the preceding exclusions, there were 1707 patients with cancer of the colon and rectum; 896 patients with cancer of the colon were available for statistical analysis. Twenty-one (2.4 percent) of these patients were lost to follow-up.

Turnbull divided cancer of the colon into four clinicopathologic stages: A (cancer confined to colon), B (cancer extension into pericolic fat), C (cancer metastasis to mesenteric lymph nodes only), and D (metastatic cancer in distant site or not resectable locally).

Calculation of Survival Rates

Survival rates were calculated by the actuarial method, and life tables were prepared to show survival rates with and without correction for age. The median ages of the patients ranged from 60 to 63 years among individual life tables. In regard to survival rates calculated without correction for age, postoperative deaths, death from cancer, and death from natural causes were all considered deaths from cancer. Age-corrected survival rates were calculated in the usual manner, utilizing the life tables for Ohioan white males from the years 1959 through 1961.

Turnbull treated 664 patients using the no-touch isolation technique. Five other staff surgeons operated on 232 patients using the conventional technique. The resectability rates were the same in both groups.

The accumulative 5-year survival rate without correction for age was 46.9 percent for 896 patients. The resectability rate was 84.2 percent. The operability rate was 96.2 percent. Since the 5-year survival rate was unusually high, the rates were compared according to the surgical techniques. The resectability rates were the same in both groups. For all stages, the cumulative 5-year survival rate for the no-touch technique was 50.86 percent compared with 34.82 percent for the conventional technique. The difference was most dramatic for C-stage cancers, the 5-year survival rate being 57.84 percent for the no-touch technique and 28.06 percent for the conventional technique.

The death rate from metastatic cancer was greater during the first 2 years following a conventional resection. Most of these deaths were due to metastasis to the liver. This greater incidence of fatal hepatic metastasis was considered secondary to operative manipulation of the cancer-bearing segment. Although the death rate (from hepatic metastasis) was greater in the first 2 years after conventional resection, the 5-year survival rate of the no-touch isolation group was unusually high.

Ninety percent of stage C cancers extended into the mesenteric fat as well as metastasized to the mesenteric lymph nodes, making this class of colonic cancer most likely to be disseminated by surgical manipulation at the time of resection. The operative mortality was 2.2 percent. The survival rate of 81.6 percent was found to be constant in regard to the right and left sides of the colon. This high survival rate reflects the greatly increased salvage rate of patients with stage C cancers of the colon who underwent resection by the no-touch isolation technique.

Turnbull concluded that operative manipulation of a cancer-bearing segment of colon increased the incidence of fatal metastases, which were predominantly hepatic. With his technique for removal of the cancer-bearing segment in 460 patients who underwent "resection for cure," the age-corrected 5-year survival rate was 81.6 percent.

The evidence suggested that the greatly improved survival rates were due to the use of the no-touch isolation resection method and that conventional manipulative resection techniques for cancer of the colon should be abandoned. Unfortunately, this was not a controlled study, and rigid statistical proof of the value of the no-touch technique is not available. However, the no-touch technique should certainly be one arm of any controlled clinical trial for colonic cancer.

Since 1964, the use of the no-touch technique has been continued, and an updated study, started before Turnbull's death, is now in progress (Fazio, 1982).

DOES DELAY AFTER ONSET OF SYMPTOMS AFFECT PROGNOSIS?

Several investigators have provided studies of the proposition that delay in diagnosis and treatment after the onset of symptoms reduces the chances of cure. There has been a general failure to establish an association between the duration of symptoms from a cancer before treatment and prognosis. It has been noted that some cancers seem to disseminate before they reach the threshold size producing symptoms or permitting discovery.

Lim and associates (1974) assayed the association between end results for colorectal neoplasms and delay in diagnosis. They recognized that biologic properties of these cancers seem to have a profound influence over prognosis that is independent of the size of the neoplasms. If this is true from a very early stage of the neoplasms, perhaps at stages before the cancers are large enough to produce symptoms, delay in diagnosis and treatment after the onset of symptoms might have little impact on prognosis. The coefficients of correlation between survival and patient or doctor delay from the onset of symptoms were determined for various areas, including colon and rectum. None of these was significant at a $p < 0.05$ level. Patients with delay of less than one month showed no improvement in curability. These observations do not negate the value of earlier diagnosis but do show the need for a definition of "early." A diagnosis of 1-cm neoplasm cannot be considered early if the neoplasm contains a billion cancer cells. Slowly growing neoplasms with a long preresection history may still be quite curable. No correlation was found between the length of delay and socioeconomic status. In fact, private patients often presented with longer delays.

Two additional studies provide identical conclusions. Polissar and associates (1981) observed that no single symptom nor the duration of symptoms of up to 1 year was associated with survivorship for 154 colorectal cancer patients studied.

McDermott and associates (1981) surveyed 154 patients with 99 percent follow-up and observed that the proportion of curative and palliative operations was unrelated to the duration of symptoms. Survival was worse when symptoms had been present for less than 3 months.

Sugarbaker (1981), in summarizing a review of the literature on the issue of delay, concluded that patient delay after the onset of symptoms did not affect prognosis. Patients with symptoms tolerable for longer periods often had biologically more favorable cancers. Patients driven to see physicians after only short symptomatic periods often had more aggressive cancers. This should not be construed to mean that any delay after the appearance of suggestive symptoms is justified, since cancers might progress to crisis situations that require treatments associated with higher mortality rates.

RELATIONSHIP BETWEEN FAMILY HISTORY AND PROGNOSIS

Albano and associates (1982) observed such a significant improvement in the survivorship of colon and breast cancer among people with a positive family history of cancer that they concluded that heredity should be considered in the stratification of cases for clinical studies. The characteristics they observed for cases with hereditary colon cancer were a significantly younger age of onset (46 years) and an excess of cancers in the proximal colon (49 percent). The study group consisted of 20 families with nonpolyposis hereditary colon cancer. The families demonstrated an autosomal dominant mode of inheritance. The researchers observed an improved survival rate among the younger patients with hereditary disease compared with a worse survival rate for those afflicted with sporadic nonhereditary colon cancer.

Obviously, adenocarcinomas of the colon and rectum present with a broad spectrum of properties, many of which affect prognosis, along with a great number of properties unique to the host having the cancer. Surgical management provides improvements in end results, and fine points in surgical care have a very significant impact on outcome. The entire history of management contains very few controlled clinical trials but does contain a very large wealth of observations on the relationship between many properties of both the patient and the cancer that are associated with prognosis. For any controlled clinical trial to be fruitful, the impact of these prognostic factors must be corroborated. Matching similar subsets of factors in controlled clinical trials will provide a statistical challenge that is as complicated as the clinical challenge confronting those attempting to further improve the prognosis of patients with these cancers.

Tumors within reach of biopsy forceps or other excisional instruments of a sigmoidoscope should be removed so that the cellular nature of the tumor can be ascertained. Tumors seen on roentgenograms beyond the reach of a sigmoidoscope should be treated as if they were cancers when they are larger than 12 mm in diameter. Tumors larger than this have a greater likelihood of being cancers than is the mortality rate attendant upon resection of the bowel containing the tumor (Spratt and Akerman, 1960b). Tumors smaller than 12 mm in diameter within the segments of the colon that are not directly visible may be observed for a time (3 to 6 months). Those that increase in size within 6 months should be treated as cancers or be biopsied.

This attitude toward smaller tumors is predicated upon the material presented earlier in this chapter. The very low frequency of cancers among small tumors was less than the mortality rate attendant upon transabdominal removal of colonic tumors. With the availability of the flexible endoscope, observation for growth of small tumors seen on barium enema studies is probably no longer justified when biopsy or removal by way of a flexible endoscope is possible (see Chapter Six). However, this is a hypothesis that has not been tested by rigid experimental design.

ASSOCIATION OF STEPS IN THE PRIMARY MANAGEMENT OF COLORECTAL CANCERS AND END RESULTS

Obviously the management of colorectal cancers requires many judgmental decisions and complex technical acts. The impact of many of these decisions and acts has been discussed. A review of the literature confirms the lack of controlled clinical trials needed to determine the best methods for managing the many subsets of colorectal cancers. In an attempt to simplify the complex problem, Knutson and Watson (1974) organized available data into sequential statements of explicit logic. The logic system was computer adapted to expedite access and manipulation. It was a synthesis of many clinical studies referenced by them. It was tested against 304 cases and was found to cover a 96 percent compliance rate in the hospital of origin (EFSCH). The fact that there was such a high compliance rate in the hospital in which the study originated is not unexpected. However, the system was subsequently tested in another city (Louisville, Ky.). Variations from the programmed logic resulted in a statistically significant increase in both the risk of the patient's dying and the risk of failure to control the cancer (Knutson et al., 1978).

Knutson and Watson (1974) made the following assumptions: (1) The patient had to be an acceptable risk for operation and be able to tolerate any procedure deemed necessary to remove the cancer once the intraoperative findings were known; (2) The surgeon had to be qualified to perform any procedure deemed necessary at the time of surgery; and (3) there could not be synchronous tumors.

The importance of technical expertise and a sound knowledge of human anatomy and physiology on the part of the operating surgeon cannot be overemphasized. Many authors have written fine texts on colorectal surgery, i.e., Shackelford and Zuidema (1981). However, the purpose here is to address the *decisions* the surgeon has to make in selecting the most appropriate procedure, not the techniques of these procedures.

Given the limitations noted previously with any combination of intraoperative findings, a sequence of simple questions and answers leads through the entire decision-making process necessary to select the best management method. Following the response to the sequence of questions, the logic software was programmed to display a suggested list of acceptable procedures, in order of preference, based on the operative findings as interpreted by the surgeon and on the most currently available medical knowledge. The program had no provision to "limit" the surgeon in his choice of procedures. However, procedures not generally accepted in specific settings were not listed. For any given set of intraoperative findings, all acceptable management procedures could be listed with only two exceptions: (1) the patient with a cancer of the right colon should not be left with an ileostomy; and (2) if at all possible, any perforated cancer should be removed at the primary laparotomy.

Beyond these two considerations, any currently acceptable operation was included in the list of possible treatments. In addition, other data were displayed, such as potential curability; comparison of initial colostomy plus delayed resection versus primary resection; primary versus delayed anastomosis; abdominal drainage; and delayed versus primary skin closure.

The logic system divided the colon into five segments determined by the colonic blood supply. All neoplasms arising within the same anatomic segment were treated in a similar fashion. For example, the same set of programmed questions and treatment options could be applied for both a cecal tumor and a lesion of the hepatic flexure, providing the intraoperative findings were similar (Fig. 10–14).

Analysis of the surgical decision-making process on an element-by-element basis raised nine basic questions to be answered before a valid management decision could be made (Table 10–26). Various combinations of these basic factors encompassed nearly all conditions encountered intraoperatively. The same basic considerations applied to neoplasms arising in any segment of the colon, but the surgical options differed.

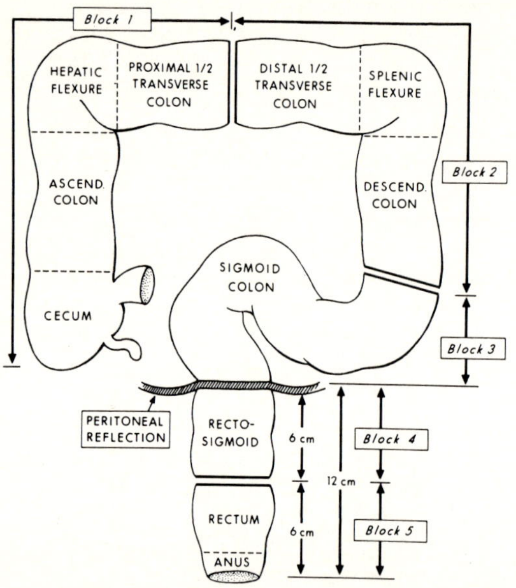

Figure 10–14. Schematic diagram of regional divisions of the colon, such as is used for a computer management logic program. (From Knutson CO, Watson FR: Preliminary results of a computer logic program for the operative management of colon cancer. Surgery 76:298–308, 1974.)

The basic elements of the surgical procedures, combined in various orders, formulated the exact operation to be used (Table 10–27). There were 12 basic surgical procedures commonly used for colon cancer, three types of direct anastomosis, five methods of handling the transected ends of the bowel if direct anastomosis was not desirable, and three additional considerations pertaining to skin closure, perforated bowel, and abdominal drainage.

Although there are 288 possible combinations of the elements listed, only 57 of the

Table 10–26. NINE FACTORS THAT MUST BE CONSIDERED AT THE TIME OF SURGERY BEFORE MAKING A MANAGEMENT DECISION*

1. Tumor location
2. Distant metastasis
3. Perforation
4. Obstruction
5. Contiguous spread (five factors)
   a. Involves 1 kidney and contralateral kidney is abn/abs†
   b. Involves 1 ureter and contralateral ureter is abn/abs†
   c. Involves both ureters in pelvis
   d. Involves nonremovable vital organ
   e. Attachment to pelvic wall prevents resection

*From Knutson CO, Watson FR: Preliminary results of a computer logic program for the operative management of colon cancer. Surgery 76:298–308, 1974.

†Abnormal or absent.

Table 10–27. THE ELEMENTS OF THE OPERATIVE PROCEDURE: OPTIONS*

I. Primary procedure (conventional or en bloc):
   A. Right hemicolectomy
   B. Right hemi- and partial left colectomy
   C. Left hemicolectomy
   D. Left hemi- and partial right colectomy
   E. Anterior sigmoid resection
   F. Abdominoperineal resection
   G. Segmental (sleeve, wedge) resection
   H. Internal intestinal bypass
      1. Ileotransverse
      2. Ileosigmoid
   I. Pelvic exenteration
   J. Delayed colectomy
   K. Nothing
II. Anastomosis:
   A. Direct
      1. End-to-end
      2. End-to-side
      3. Side-to-side
   B. None
      1. Proximal colostomy
         a. Temporary
            1. Diverting
            2. Decompressing
         b. Permanent-end
      2. Distal mucous fistula
      3. Close distal rectal stump
III. Other considerations:
   A. Drain
   B. Delay primary skin closure
   C. Close perforation

*From Knutson CO, Watson FR: Preliminary results of a computer logic program for the operative management of colon cancer. Surgery 76:298–308, 1974.

combinations were acceptable treatments for the surgical management of colonic neoplasms.

The program displayed the options for surgical procedures and optional methods of management of the transected bowel, which were based on the location of the neoplasm and accurate documentation of any combination of nine operative considerations. It also listed the optional procedures in order of preference based on the most current knowledge available.

The logic flow diagrams for each colon segment are illustrated in Figures 10–11 and 10–15 to 10–17.

The corresponding management options are illustrated in Tables 10–14 through 10–17. The numbers in the squares at the bottom or at the end of each logic diagram correspond to the treatment numbers for the respective neoplasm location, which are tabulated in Tables 10–28 through 10–32. By defining the different intraoperative settings, one can follow the logic flow diagrams to the suggested therapy options for any lesion of the colon or rectum.

To establish the validity and practical appli-

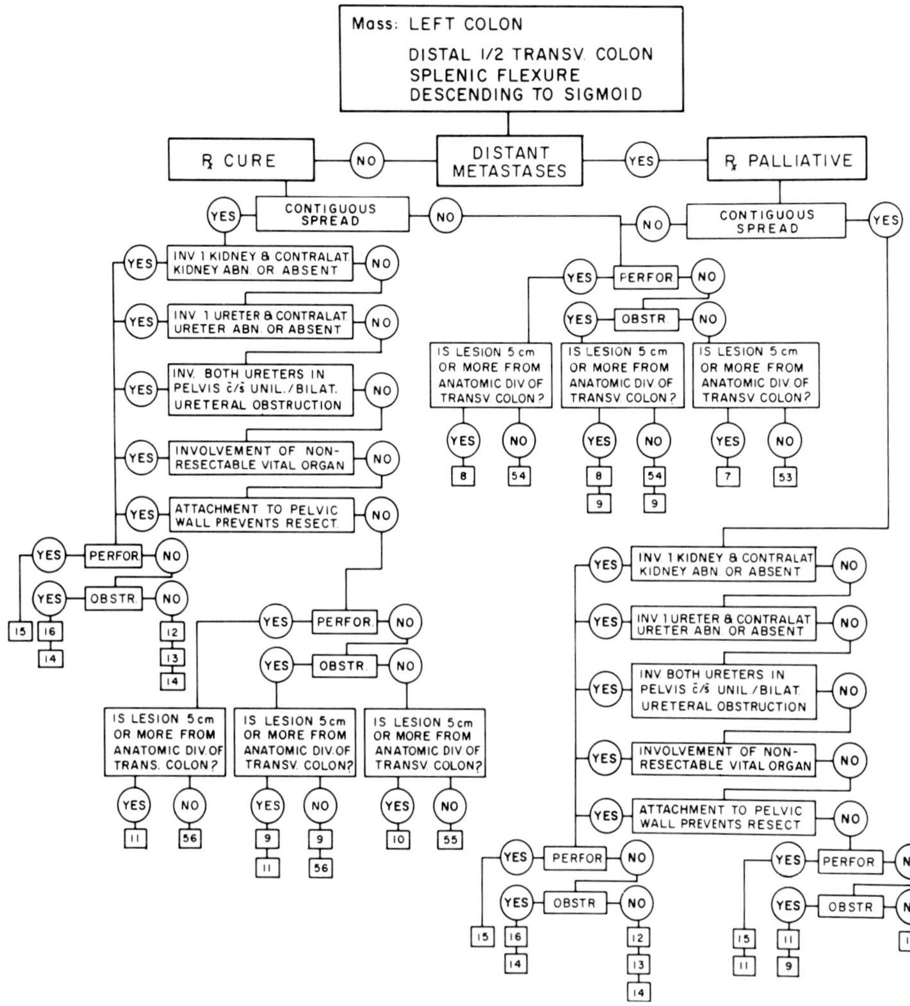

Figure 10–15. Logic diagram for decisions involved in management of adenocarcinomas of the left colon, above the peritoneal reflection. (From Knutson CO, Watson FR: Preliminary results of a computer logic program for the operative management of colon cancer. Surgery 76:298–308, 1974.)

cability of this logic model, 304 cases of colon cancers treated at EFSCH were reviewed retrospectively, with no attempt to preselect cases, other than to assure specific numbers of cancers for possible site (Knutson and Watson, 1974).

The nine intraoperative questions used in the logic program were answered using recorded intraoperative findings. The pathologist's report was not used to answer the nine questions. Only the information available to the surgeon at the time he had to make his decision was considered.

The options displayed on the computer and the procedures actually performed were placed into one of four categories for the purpose of comparing them: (1) The actual treatment was the same as the logic diagram–recommended treatment (96 percent concurrence); (2) the actual treatment was inadequate by the logic diagram (1 percent); (3) the actual treatment proved superior to the logic diagram (0 percent); and (4) the logic diagram did not cover the surgical situation (3.3 percent).

In 291 instances (96 percent), the programmed treatment recommendations correlated well with what was actually done. In three cases (one percent), the tumor was transected to remove some of the neoplasm. These three procedures, performed in the 1950s, were considered inadequate based on current philosophy. In each case, given the operative findings, the program suggested more appropriate and current procedures. In no case was the program's suggested approach inadequate. There were ten situations (three percent) that the computer program did not handle in the preliminary stage of logic development be-

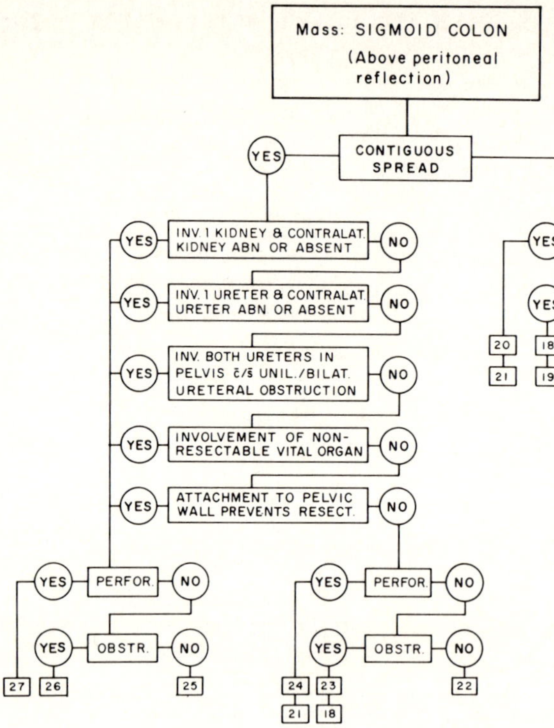

Figure 10–16. Logic diagram for decisions involved in the management of adenocarcinomas of the sigmoid colon, above the peritoneal reflection. (From Knutson CO, Watson FR: Preliminary results of a computer logic program for the operative management of colon cancer. Surgery 76:298–308, 1974.)

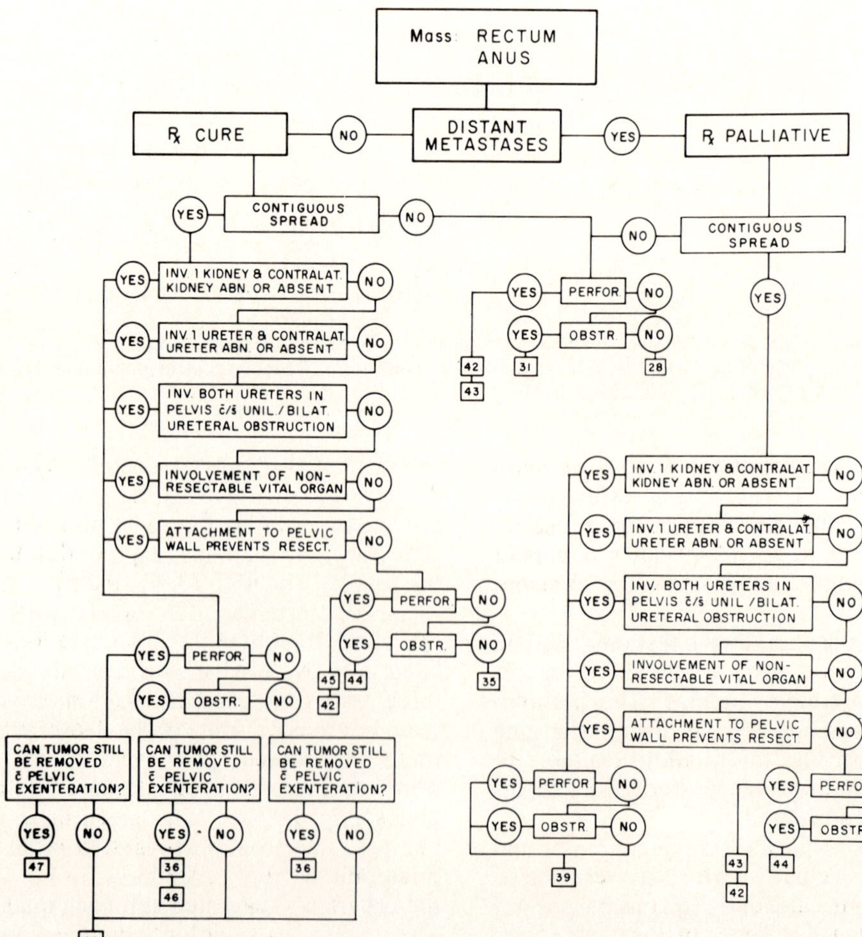

Figure 10–17. Logic diagram for decisions involved in the management of carcinomas of the rectum and anus. (From Knutson CO, Watson FR: Preliminary results of a computer logic program for the operative management of colon cancer. Surgery 76:298–308, 1974.)

Table 10–28. **TREATMENT (T) OPTIONS FOR RIGHT COLON LESIONS***

T1	(A)	Right hemicolectomy with end-to-end ileotransverse colostomy
T2	(A)	Right hemicolectomy with end-to-end ileotransverse colostomy
	(B)	Delay primary skin closure
	(C)	Drain (if indicated)
T3	(A)	En bloc right colon resection with end-to-end ileotransverse colostomy
T4	(A)	En bloc right colon resection with end-to-end ileotransverse colostomy
	(B)	Delay primary skin closure
	(C)	Drain (if indicated)
T5	(A)	Interval ileotransverse colostomy bypass either: (1) end-to-end with two mucous fistula exclusions, (2) end-to-side with one mucous fistula exclusion, or (3) side-to-side
T6	(A)	Internal ileotransverse colostomy bypass either: (1) end-to-end with two mucous fistula exclusions, (2) end-to-side with one mucous fistula exclusion, or (3) side-to-side
	(B)	Delay primary skin closure
	(C)	Drain (if indicated)
T48	(A)	Right hemicolectomy with partial left colectomy with end-to-end ileocoloanastomosis
T49	(A)	Right hemicolectomy with partial left colectomy with end-to-end ileocoloanastomosis
	(B)	Delay primary skin closure
	(C)	Drain (if indicated)
T50	(A)	En bloc right colon and partial left colon resection with ileocoloanastomosis
T51	(A)	En bloc right colon and partial left colon resection with ileocoloanastomosis
	(B)	Delay primary skin closure
	(C)	Drain (if indicated)
T52	(A)	Segmental resection of tumor with end-to-end ileocolo- or colocolostomy
T57	(A)	Segmental resection of tumor with end-to-end ileocolo- or colocolostomy
	(B)	Drain (if indicated)
	(C)	Delay primary skin closure

*Adapted from Knutson CO, Watson FR: Preliminary results of a computer logic program for the operative management of colon cancer. Surgery 76:298–308, 1974.

cause of variance from the basic possibilities. Owing to the limited sophistication of development, the program could not preoperatively evaluate the risks to the patients. For the 10 situations (3 percent) that the program could not handle, the actual procedure performed was of a lesser magnitude than that suggested by the computer program. In addition, had those patients been better surgical risks, the procedures suggested by the program would have been more acceptable.

Even in its infancy, this computer program attained 97 percent reliability in its decisions. Further refinement of the logic and the integration of preoperative evaluation could significantly reduce or eliminate altogether the residual 3 percent of exceptions to the program. Technological changes continue to evolve, often more rapidly than the scientific process of determining their value can proceed.

A system of this nature has unique potential. It represents a uniform, complete, and systematic method for collecting and analyzing data essential to the evaluation of currently used procedures. It can provide physicians with ready access to the most current medical knowledge reduced to terms of the most acceptable modes of therapy for any given set of operative circumstances. The various options

Table 10–29. **TREATMENT (T) OPTIONS FOR LEFT COLON LESIONS**

T7	(A)	Left hemicolectomy with end-to-end anastomosis
T8	(A)	Left hemicolectomy with end colostomy
	(B)	Distal mucous fistula (if possible)
	(C)	Drain pelvis (if indicated)
	(D)	Delay primary skin closure
T9	(A)	Temporary proximal diverting colostomy
	(B)	Delay primary skin closure
	(C)	Definitive colectomy at later date
T10	(A)	En bloc resection with left colectomy and end-to-end anastomosis
	(B)	Proximal colostomy (temporary)
T11	(A)	En bloc resection with left colectomy and end colostomy
	(B)	Distal mucous fistula (if possible)
	(C)	Drain pelvis (if indicated)
	(D)	Delay primary skin closure
T12	(A)	Proximal end colostomy with distal mucous fistula
T13	(A)	Do nothing at this time
	(B)	When symptomatic—do proximal end colostomy
T14	(A)	Ileosigmoid colostomy bypass (end-to-side)
	(B)	Exteriorize proximal colon as mucous fistula
T15	(A)	Proximal end colostomy with distal mucous fistula
	(B)	Close perforation (if indicated)
	(C)	Drain pelvis (if indicated)
	(D)	Delay primary skin closure
T16	(A)	Proximal end colostomy and distal mucous fistula
	(B)	Delay primary skin closure
T53	(A)	Left hemicolectomy and partial right colectomy with end-to-end colocolostomy
T54	(A)	Left hemicolectomy and partial right colectomy with end-to-end colocolostomy
T55	(A)	En bloc resection of left hemi- and partial right colectomy with end-to-end anastomosis
T56	(A)	En bloc resection of left hemi- and partial right colectomy with end colostomy
	(B)	Distal mucous fistula
	(C)	Drain pelvis (if indicated)
	(D)	Delay primary skin closure

*Adapted from Knutson CO, Watson FR: Preliminary results of computer logic program for the operative management of colon cancer. Surgery 76:298–308, 1974.

Table 10–30. **TREATMENT (T) OPTIONS FOR SIGMOID COLON LESIONS ABOVE PERITONEAL REFLECTION***

T17	(A)	Anterior resection with colorectal anastomosis
	(B)	Temporary proximal colostomy (if indicated)
T18	(A)	Temporary proximal decompression colostomy
	(B)	Delay primary skin closure
	(C)	Definitive sigmoid resection at later date
T19	(A)	Anterior resection with proximal end colostomy (Hartmann's procedure)
	(B)	Distal mucous fistula (if possible)
	(C)	Delay primary skin closure
T20	(A)	Anterior resection with proximal end colostomy
	(B)	Distal mucous fistula (if possible)
	(C)	Drain pelvis (if indicated)
	(D)	Delay primary skin closure
T21	(A)	Temporary proximal decompression colostomy
	(B)	Close perforation (if possible)
	(C)	Drain pelvis
	(D)	Delay primary skin closure
T22	(A)	En bloc resection with sigmoid colectomy and colorectal anastomosis
	(B)	Temporary proximal colostomy (if indicated)
T23	(A)	En bloc resection of sigmoid colon and proximal end colostomy
	(B)	Distal mucous fistula (if possible)
	(C)	Delay primary skin closure
T24	(A)	En bloc resection of sigmoid colon and end colostomy
	(B)	Distal mucous fistula (if possible)
	(C)	Drain pelvis (if indicated)
	(D)	Delay primary skin closure
T25	(A)	Permanent proximal end colostomy with distal mucous fistula
T26	(A)	Permanent proximal end colostomy with distal mucous fistula
	(B)	Delay primary skin closure
T27	(A)	Permanent proximal end colostomy with distal mucous fistula
	(B)	Close perforation (if possible)
	(C)	Drain pelvis (if indicated)
	(D)	Delay primary skin closure

*Adapted from Knutson CO, Watson FR: Preliminary results of computer logic program for the operative management of colon cancer. Surgery 76:298–308, 1974.

Table 10–31. **TREATMENT (T) OPTIONS FOR RECTOSIGMOID COLON LESIONS BELOW PERITONEAL REFLECTION***

T17	(A)	Anterior resection with colorectal anastomosis
	(B)	Temporary proximal colostomy (if indicated)
T28	(A)	Abdominoperineal resection
T29	(A)	Proximal end colostomy with distal mucous fistula
	(B)	Delay primary skin closure
	(C)	Definitive colectomy at later date (anterior resection or abdominoperineal resection)
T30	(A)	Anterior resection, oversew rectal stump (Hartmann's procedure)
	(B)	Proximal end colostomy
	(C)	Delay primary skin closure
T31	(A)	Abdominoperineal resection
	(B)	Delay primary skin closure
T32	(A)	Anterior resection, oversew rectal stump (Hartmann's procedure)
	(B)	Proximal end colostomy
	(C)	Drain pelvis (if indicated)
	(D)	Delay primary skin closure
T33	(A)	Proximal end colostomy
	(B)	Drain pelvis (if indicated)
	(C)	Close perforation (if possible)
	(D)	Delay primary skin closure
	(E)	Definitive colectomy at later date (anterior resection or abdominoperineal resection)
T34	(A)	En bloc anterior resection with colorectal anastomosis
	(B)	Temporary proximal colostomy (if indicated)
T35	(A)	En bloc abdominoperineal resection
T36	(A)	Pelvic exenteration
T37	(A)	En bloc anterior resection, oversew rectal stump (Hartmann's procedure)
	(B)	Proximal end colostomy
	(C)	Delay primary skin closure
T38	(A)	En bloc anterior resection, oversew rectal stump (Hartmann's procedure)
	(B)	Proximal end colostomy
	(C)	Drain pelvis (if indicated)
	(D)	Delay primary skin closure
T39	(A)	Permanent proximal end colostomy with distal mucous fistula
	(B)	Close perforation (if present and if possible)
	(C)	Drain pelvis (if indicated)
	(D)	Delay primary skin closure
T40	(A)	Nothing at this time
	(B)	Permanent proximal end colostomy when signs of obstruction appear
T41	(A)	Permanent proximal end colostomy
	(B)	Distal mucous fistula
T46	(A)	Permanent end colostomy
	(B)	Distal mucous fistula
	(C)	Delay primary skin closure
	(D)	Definitive pelvic exenteration at later date
T47	(A)	Permanent end colostomy
	(B)	Distal mucous fistula
	(C)	Treat perforation
	(D)	Drain pelvis (if indicated)
	(E)	Delay primary skin closure
	(F)	Definitive pelvic exenteration at later date

*Adapted from Knutson CO, Watson FR: Preliminary results of computer logic program for the operative management of colon cancer. Surgery 76:298–308, 1974.

can be presented in order of priority based on the continuing accumulation of new data. In addition, each option can be footnoted and referenced for the convenience of the viewer to minimize the amount of time and effort required to obtain the same data. This approach affords the surgeon a reliable checklist for avoiding errors of omission and commission as well as forms a basis for a peer review audit. It can also serve as a cost-effective aid in education. This initial effort is just an indication of the ultimate impact computers could have in refining the "art of medicine" by

Table 10–32. TREATMENT (T) OPTIONS FOR RECTAL OR ANAL LESIONS*

T28 (A)	Abdominoperineal resection
T31 (A)	Abdominoperineal resection
(B)	Delay primary skin closure
T35 (A)	En bloc abdominoperineal resection
T36 (A)	Pelvic exenteration
T39 (A)	Permanent proximal end colostomy with distal mucous fistula
(B)	Close perforation (if present and if possible)
(C)	Drain pelvis (if indicated)
(D)	Delay primary skin closure
T42 (A)	Proximal end colostomy with distal mucous fistula
(B)	Drain pelvis (if indicated)
(C)	Close perforation (if indicated)
(D)	Delay primary skin closure
(E)	Definitive abdominoperineal resection at later date
T43 (A)	Abdominoperineal resection
(B)	Drain pelvis
(C)	Delay primary skin closure
T44 (A)	En bloc abdominoperineal resection
(B)	Delay primary skin closure
T45 (A)	En bloc abdominoperineal resection
(B)	Drain pelvis
(C)	Delay primary skin closure
T46 (A)	Permanent end colostomy
(B)	Distal mucous fistula
(C)	Delay primary skin closure
(D)	Definitive pelvic exenteration at later date
T47 (A)	Permanent end colostomy
(B)	Distal mucous fistula
(C)	Treat perforation
(D)	Drain pelvis (if indicated)
(E)	Delay primary skin closure
(F)	Definitive pelvic exenteration at later date

*Adapted from Knutson CO, Watson FR: Preliminary results of computer logic program for the operative management of colon cancer. Surgery 76:298–308, 1974.

forcing the use of more explicit outcome-oriented logic.

The sample program presented, which incorporates "good" surgical judgment in explicit statements in a logical sequential flow diagram, has potential as a method of teaching. The logic stresses the components of judgmental decisions. It can save time for the student of surgery. The answers remain consistent and reproducible. The fact that logic diagrams can be periodically reviewed by recognized authorities in a particular field can permit such a program to reflect the most current and accepted views. Organization of the management logic to this degree can also permit more scrutiny of the process and the planning of studies to answer points of uncertainty.

The logic diagrams do not accommodate the role of electrocoagulation in the treatment of rectal cancer. The clear demonstration of the existence of a nonmetastasizing variant of colorectal cancer establishes that forms of local ablation should provide excellent results in these cases. Several authors have provided well-studied series reporting excellent results using electrocoagulation in selected cases (Madden and Kandalaft, 1974; Beahrs, 1974; Crile and Turnbull, 1972). Case selection now confines indications to the small, well-differentiated noncircumferential tumors occurring below the peritoneal reflexion and not on the anterior rectal wall in women. Appropriate in-hospital anesthesia and repetitive re-examination and biopsy are necessary for the best results. In this highly selected subset of cases, long-term survivorship has been quite acceptable. Certainly, in a randomized prospective clinical trial, this method should constitute one area for the comparative evaluation of therapy.

A skilled surgeon is essential to make the observations requisite for the program's decisions. The program functions only as a very reliable and rapid recall tool. It can serve as a checklist to ensure thoroughness of an evaluation, consideration of all essential variables, and to keep decisions current with knowledge as it evolves. It offers a quality control mechanism that gives added assurance that one's endeavors are in keeping with the best surgical knowledge. This approach is analogous to process management to improve results through more effective compliance with extant knowledge.

Obviously, improved control of cancer of the colon and rectum requires continued study of all determinants of outcome. Many factors contribute to outcome, imposing a major problem in the stratification of cases and in research design. The number of important variables that exist mandate the broader use of computers in clinical medicine as research, teaching, and accurate recall tools.

VILLOUS ADENOMAS

As a closing entry to this chapter a comment must be made about the villous adenoma because of their close relationship to cancers. Villous adenomas have long been a troublesome problem for surgeons. As reviewed in Chapter Two, they grow at the same rate as adenocarcinomas. They behave as superficial cancers with a tendency to invade. Although the risk of invasive cancer increases with size, the fact remains that very large villous adenomas may be very superficial spreading growths with no invasive cancer. These very large tumors may secrete excessive K^+-rich mucus, producing profound electrolyte disturbances

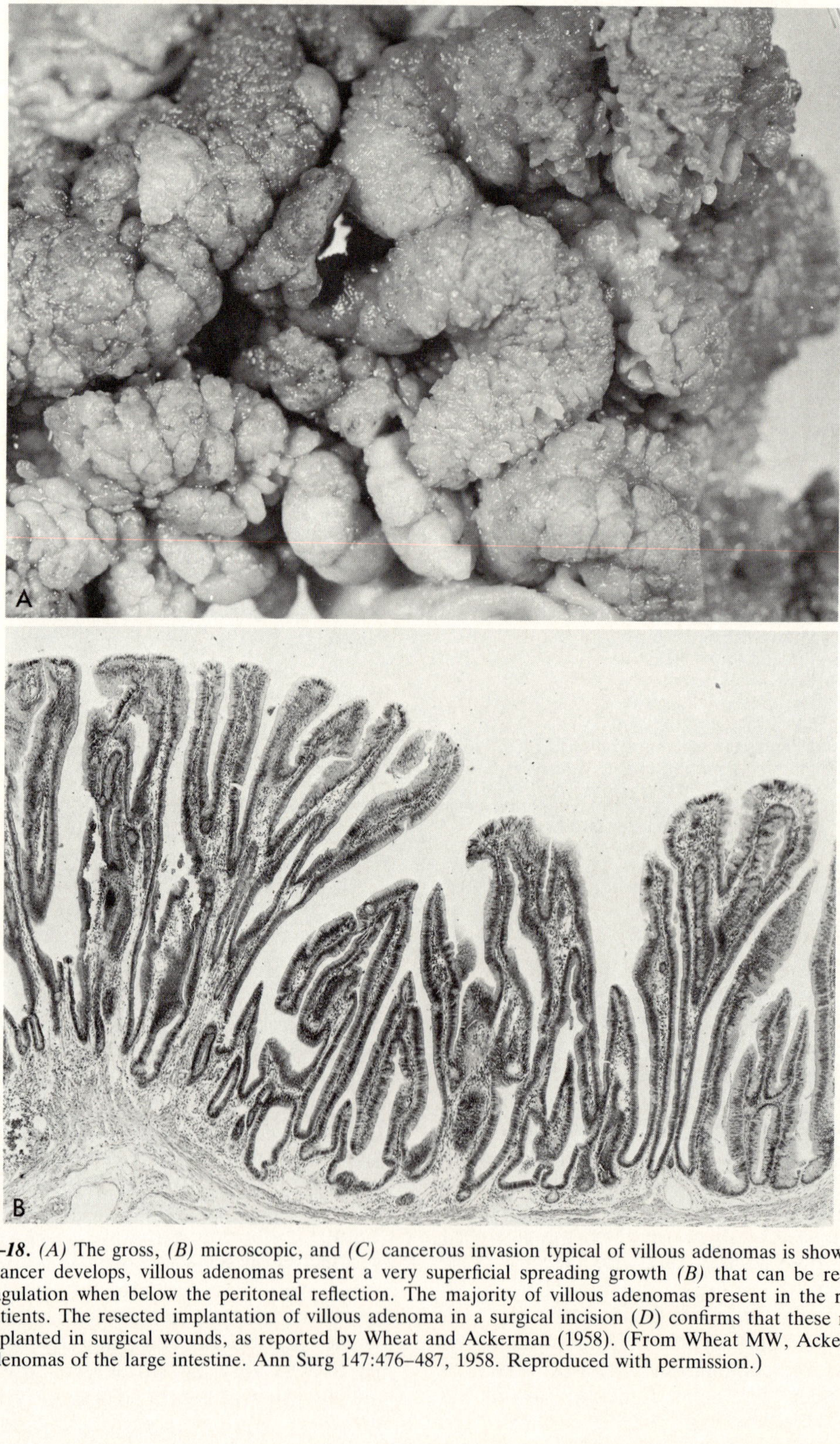

Figure 10–18. *(A)* The gross, *(B)* microscopic, and *(C)* cancerous invasion typical of villous adenomas is shown. Before invasive cancer develops, villous adenomas present a very superficial spreading growth *(B)* that can be removed by electrocoagulation when below the peritoneal reflection. The majority of villous adenomas present in the rectums of elderly patients. The resected implantation of villous adenoma in a surgical incision (*D*) confirms that these neoplasms can be implanted in surgical wounds, as reported by Wheat and Ackerman (1958). (From Wheat MW, Ackerman LV: Villous adenomas of the large intestine. Ann Surg 147:476–487, 1958. Reproduced with permission.)

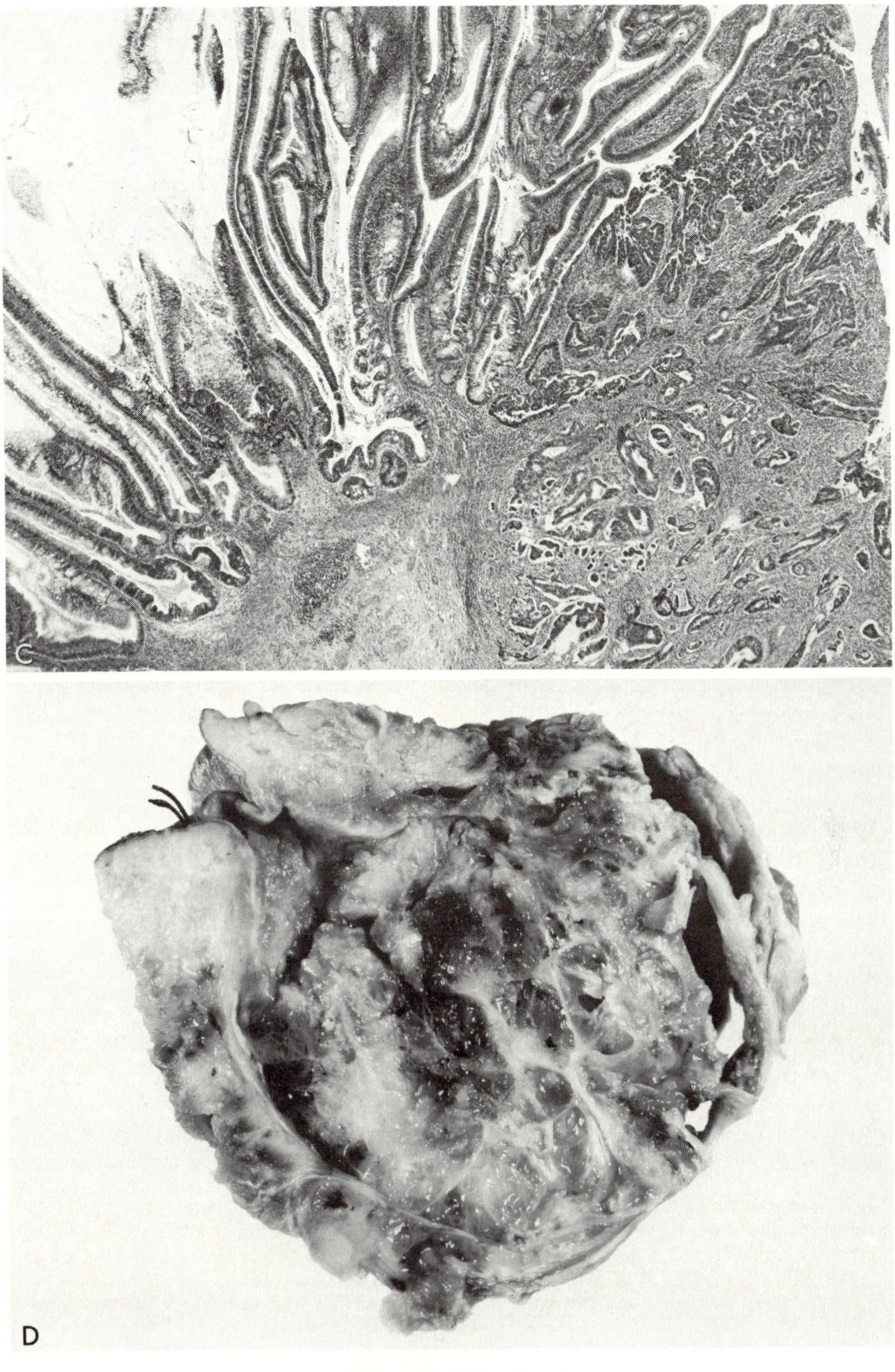

Figure 10–18 Continued.

that may be diagnosed and corrected before any type of surgical intervention (Davis et al., 1962; Findley and O'Conner, 1961; Rudman et al., 1960; Shamblin et al., 1962; Shnitka et al., 1961).

The typical gross, microscopic, and cancerous degeneration and invasion from a villous adenoma are shown in Figure 10–18*A, B,* and *C.* Figure 10–18*D* shows an implantation metastasis from a villous adenoma removed from a posterior proctotomy incision.

For villous adenomas above the peritoneal reflexion, segmental colectomy is an expedient and proper course of action. When they are within the rectum, abdominoperineal resection may be required. However, the lack of proven cancer on biopsy should initiate considerable caution. The noncancerous villous adenoma may be quite large. The average age of presentation is 65 years; therefore, half occur in older people, who are at higher risk for such major operations as abdominoperineal resection. In clean wounds, villous adenomas are implantable, thus caution is required in open resection (Silverman, 1964). Furthermore, their superficial growth pattern lends itself ideally to transanal electrocoagulation. For larger tumors, this can be done in staged procedures with excellent, low-risk control. Less than 10 percent ever invade or metastasize, and, in elderly people, any radical surgical resection would be justified only in the presence of histopathologically proven invasion (Dreese et al., 1962; Jahadi and Baldwin, 1975; Nicoloff et al., 1968; Ramirez et al., 1965; Wheat and Ackerman, 1958). As a curiosity, the development of malignant villous adenoma has even been reported in a colon bypass. It was successfully removed by segmental resection (Goldsmith and Beattie, 1968).

References

Albano WA, Recabaren JA, Lynch HT, Natural history of hereditary cancer of the breast and colon. Cancer 50:360–363, 1982.

American Joint Committee on Cancer. *In* Beahrs OH, Myers MH (eds): Manual for Staging of Cancer. 2nd ed. Philadelphia, JB Lippincott Company, 1983.

Astler VB, Coller FA: The prognostic significance of direct extension of carcinoma of the colon and rectum. Ann Surg 139:846–852, 1954. (Table IX reprinted in AFIP/NCR Fascicle α22, Tumors of the Intestines, Wood DA, 1967.)

Beahrs OH Jr: Status of fulguration and cryosurgery in the management of colonic and rectal cancers and polyps. Cancer 34:965–968, 1974.

Beart RW Jr, van Heerden JA, Beahrs OH: Evolution in the pathologic staging of carcinoma of the colon. Surg Gynecol Obstet 146:257–259, 1978.

Bolt RJ, Mallery OT, Tupper CJ: Appraisal of laboratory procedures in periodic health examinations. Arch Indust Health 13:253–258, 1956.

Brues AM, Weiner AE, Andervont HB: Relation between latent period and growth rate in chemically induced tumors. Proc Soc Exp Biol Med 42:374–377, 1939.

Butcher HR Jr, Spjut HJ: An evaluation of pelvic exenteration for advanced carcinoma of lower colon. Cancer 12:681–687, 1959, and personal communication with the authors.

Chung CK, Zaino RJ, Stryker JA: Colorectal carcinoma: Evaluation of histologic grade and factors influencing prognosis. J Surg Oncol 21:143–148, 1982.

Cohen AM, Wood WC, Gunderson LL, Shinnar M: Pathological studies in rectal cancer. Cancer 45:2965–2968, 1980.

Coller FA, Kay EB, MacIntyre RS: Regional lymphatic metastasis of carcinoma of the rectum. Surgery 8:294–311, 1940.

Coller FA, Kay EB, MacIntyre RS: Regional lymphatic metastases of carcinoma of the colon. Ann Surg 114:56–63, 1941.

Collins VP: Time of occurrence of pulmonary metastasis from carcinoma of the colon and rectum. Cancer 15:387–395, 1962.

Collins VP, Loeffler RK, Tivey H: Observations on growth rates of human tumors. AJR 76:988–1000, 1956.

Cook GB, Margulis AR: Silicone foam diagnostic enema. Surgery 50:513–525, 1961.

Copeland EM: Intravenous hyperalimentation. *In* Surgical Oncology. New York, John Wiley and Sons, 1983, pp. 687–703.

Crile G Jr, Turnbull RB Jr: The role of electrocoagulation in the treatment of carcinoma of the rectum. Surg Gynecol Obstet 135:391–396, 1972.

Davis JE, Seavey PW, Sessions JT Jr: Villous adenomas of the rectum and sigmoid colon with severe fluid and electrolyte depletion. Ann Surg 155:806–816, 1962.

Dorn HF, Cutler SJ: Morbidity from cancer in the United States. Public Health Monograph No. 56, Washington, DC, U.S. Government Printing Office, 1959.

Dreese WC, Gradinger BC, Hellwig CA, et al: Villous tumors of the rectum and sigmoid. Surg Gynecol Obstet 115:182–186, 1962.

Dukes CE: The classification of cancer of the rectum. J Pathol Bacteriol 35:322–332, 1932.

Dukes CE: Cancer of the rectum: An analysis of 1000 cases. J Pathol Bacteriol 50:527–539, 1940. (Note pp. 533–535.)

Dukes CE, Bussy HJR, Lamb GW: The examination and classification of operative specimens of intestinal cancer. Bull Int Assoc Med Mus 27:55–56, 1948. (Note pp. 62–63 re: Stages A, B, C1, C2, and "fourth type.")

Enker WE, Laffer UT, Block GE: Enhanced survival of patients with colon and rectal cancer is based on wide anatomic resection. Ann Surg 190:350–360, 1979.

Fazio V: Personal communication, 1982.

Findley CW, O'Conner TF: Villous adenomas of the large intestine with fluid and electrolyte depletion. JAMA 176:404–408, 1961.

Gabriel WB, Dukes C, Bussey HJR: Lymphatic spread in cancer of the rectum. Br J Surg 23:395–413, 1935.

Gilchrist RK, David VC: Lymphatic spread of carcinoma of the rectum. Ann Surg 108:621–642, 1938.

Godwin JD, Brown CC. Some prognostic factors in survival of patients with cancer of the colon and rectum. J Chronic Dis 28:441–454, 1975.

Goldsmith HS, Beattie EJ Jr: Malignant villous tumor in a colon bypass. Ann Surg 167:98–100, 1968.

Goligher JC: The Dukes' A, B, and C categorization of

the extent of spread of carcinomas of the rectum. Surg Gynecol Obstet 143:793–794, 1976.

Goligher JC, Lee PW, Simpkins KC, Lintott DJ: A controlled comparison: one- and two-layer techniques of suture for high and low colorectal anastomoses. Br J Surg 64:609–614, 1977.

Grinnell RS: The chance of cancer and lymphatic metastasis in small colon tumors discovered on x-ray examination. Ann Surg 159:132–138, 1964.

Grinnell RS: Results of ligation of inferior mesenteric artery at the aorta in resection of carcinoma of the descending and sigmoid colon and rectum. Surg Gynecol Obstet 120:1031–1036, 1965.

Grinnell RS, Lane N: Benign and malignant adenomatous polyps and papillary adenomas of the colon and rectum. An analysis of 1,856 tumors in 1,335 patients. Surg Gynecol Obstet. 106:519–538, 1958.

Harvey WR: Least squares analysis of data with unequal subclass numbers. Washington, DC, U.S. Dept. Agriculture Report No. ARS 20–8, 1960.

Helwig EB: Evolution of adenomas of large intestine and their relation to carcinoma. Surg Gynecol Obstet 84:36–49, 1947.

Higgins GA: Preoperative radiotherapy for colorectal cancer. Ann Surg 181:624–631, 1975.

Israel SL, Helsel EV Jr, Hausman DH: The challenge of metastatic ovarian carcinoma. Am J Obstet Gynecol 93:1094–1101, 1965.

Jaffe BM, Donegan WL, Watson F, Spratt JS Jr: Factors influencing survival in patients with untreated hepatic metastases. Surg Gynecol Obstet 127:1–11, 1968.

Jahadi MR, Baldwin A Jr: Villous adenomas of the colon and rectum. Am J Surg 130:729–732, 1975.

Jenson CB, Shahon DB, Wangensteen OH: Evaluation of annual examination in detection of cancer. JAMA 174:1783–1788, 1960.

Johnson PO: Statistical Methods in Research. New York, Prentice-Hall, 1949, pp. 94–96.

Knutson CO, Fry DE, Barbie RD, Polk HC: Reassessment of intraoperative decisions: why operations for cancer of the large bowel fail. Ann Surg 187:549–554, 1978.

Knutson CO, Watson FR: Preliminary results of a computer logic program for the operative management of colon cancer. Surgery 76:298–308, 1974.

Kraus FT: Verrucous carcinoma: clinical and pathologic study of 105 cases involving oral cavity, larynx and genitalia. Cancer 19:26–38, 1966a.

Kraus FT, PerezMèsa C: Verrucous carcinoma. Clinical and pathologic study of 105 cases involving oral cavity, larynx and genitalia. Cancer 19:26–38, 1966.

Lavery IC, Chiulli RA, Jagelman DG, et al: Survival with carcinoma arising in mucosal ulcerative colitis. Ann Surg 195:508–512, 1982.

Lawrence JC: Gastrointestinal polyps: Statistical study of malignancy incidence. Am J Surg 31:499–505, 1936.

Lim BS, Dennis CR, Gardner B, Newman J: Analysis of survival versus patient and doctor delay of treatment of gastro-intestinal cancer. Am J Surg 127:210–214, 1974.

Lockhart-Mummery JP: Two hundred cases of cancer of the rectum treated by perineal excision. Br J Surg 27:110–124, 1926.

McDermott FT, Hughes ES, Pihl EA, et al: Prognosis in relation to symptom duration in colon cancer. Br J Surg 68:846–849, 1981.

MacKeigan JM, Ferguson JA: Prophylactic oophorectomy and colorectal cancer in premenopausal patients. Dis Colon and Rectum 22:401–405, 1979.

McSherry CK, Cornell GN, Glenn F: Carcinoma of the colon and rectum. Ann Surg 169:502–509, 1969.

McVay JR: Involvement of the lymph nodes in carcinoma of the rectum. Ann Surg 76:755–767, 1922.

Madden JL, Kandalaft S: Electrocoagulation in the treatment of cancer of the rectum. Ann Surg 174:530–540, 1974.

Malcolm AW, Perencevich NP, Olson RM, et al: Analysis of recurrence patterns following curative resection for carcinoma of the colon and rectum. Surg Gynecol Obstet 152:131–136, 1981.

Morson BC, Bussey HJ, Samoorian S: Policy of local excision for early cancer of the colorectum. Gut 18:1045–1050, 1977.

Mottram JC: On correlation between malignancy and rate of growth of tar warts in mice. A J Cancer 22:801–830, 1934.

Mottram JC: On origin of tar tumours in mice, whether from single cells or many cells. J Pathol Bacteriol 40:407–414, 1935.

Nicoloff DM, Cassius ME, Humphrey EW: Management of villous adenomas of the colon and rectum. Arch Surg 97:254–260, 1968.

Olson RM, Perencevich NP, Malcolm AW, et al.: Patterns of recurrence following curative resection of adenocarcinoma of the colon and rectum. Cancer 45:2969–2974, 1980.

Polissar L, Sim D, Francis A: Survival of colorectal cancer patients in relation to duration of symptoms and other prognostic factors. Dis Colon Rectum 24:364–369, 1981.

Polk HC Jr, Spratt JS Jr: Recurrent colorectal carcinoma. Detection, treatment and other considerations. Surgery 69:9–23, 1971.

Polk HC Jr, Spratt JS Jr, Bennett D, et al: Surgical mortality and survival from colonic carcinoma. Arch Surg 89:16–23, 1964.

Portes C, Majarakis JD: Proctosigmoidoscopy: Incidence of polyps in 50,000 examinations. JAMA 163:411–413, 1957.

Ramirez RF, Culp CE, Jackman RJ, Dockerty MB: Villous tumors of the lower part of the large bowel. JAMA 194:863–867, 1965.

Rankin FW, Olson PF: The hopeful prognosis in cases of carcinoma of the colon. Surg Gynecol Obstet 56:366–374, 1933.

Rao CR: Advanced Statistical Methods in Biometric Research. New York, John Wiley and Sons, 1952.

Rider JA, Kirsner JB, Moeller HC: Polyps of colon and rectum. JAMA 170:633–638, 1959.

Rudman I, Otto C, Novota OJ: Villous papilloma of the rectum causing massive electrolyte losses. Arch Surg 81:140–142, 1960.

Scheffe J: The Analysis of Variance. New York, John Wiley and Sons, 1959.

Shackelford RT, Zuidema GD: Surgery of the Alimentary Tract. Philadelphia, WB Saunders Company, 1981.

Shamblin JR Jr, Huff JF, Waugh JM, Moertel CG: Villous adenocarcinoma of the colon with pronounced electrolyte disturbance. Ann Surg 156:318–326, 1962.

Shepherd JM, Jones JS: Adenocarcinoma of the large bowel. Br J Cancer 25:680–690, 1971.

Shnitka TK, Friedman MHW, Kidd EG, MacKenzie WC: Villous tumors of the rectum and colon characterized by severe fluid and electrolyte loss. Surg Gynecol Obstet 112:609–621, 1961.

Silverman JL: Operative implantation on villous adenomas into the soft tissue. Cancer 17:1456–1462, 1964.

Slaney G: Results of treatment of carcinoma of the colon and rectum. Mod Trends Surg 3:69–89, 1971.

Slanetz CA Jr, Herter FP, Grinnell RS: Anterior resection versus abdominoperineal resection for cancer of the rectum and rectosigmoid. An analysis of 524 cases. Am J Surg 123:110–117, 1972.

Smale BF, Mullen JL, Buzby GP, Rosato EF: The efficacy of nutritional assessment and support in cancer surgery. Cancer 47:2375–2381, 1981.

Snedecor GW, Cochran WG: Statistical Methods. 6th ed. Ames, Iowa, Iowa State University Press, 1976.

Sobin LH: Histopathological definition and classification of tumours. WHO Chron 25:363–366, 1971.

Spjut HJ, Spratt JS Jr: Endemic and morphologic similarities existing between spontaneous colonic neoplasms in man and 3:2′-dimethyl-4-aminobiphenyl induced colonic neoplasms in rats. Ann Surg 161:309–324, 1965.

Spratt JS Jr: The lognormal frequency distribution and human cancer. J Surg Res 9:151–157, 1969.

Spratt JS Jr, Ackerman LV: Growth of colonic adenocarcinoma. Am Surg 27:23–28, 1961.

Spratt JS Jr, Ackerman LV: Pathological significance of polyps of the rectum and colon. Dis Colon Rectum 3:330–335, 1960a.

Spratt JS Jr, Ackerman LV: Relationship of the size of colonic tumors to their cellular composition and biological behavior. Surg Forum 10:56–61, 1960b.

Spratt JS Jr, Ackerman LV: Small primary adenocarcinomas of the colon and rectum. JAMA 179:337–346, 1962.

Spratt JS Jr, Ackerman LV, Moyer CA: Relationship of polyps of the colon to colonic cancer. Ann Surg 148:682–698, 1958.

Spratt JS Jr, Butcher HR Jr, Bricker EM: Exenterative Surgery of the Pelvis. Philadelphia, WB Saunders Company, 1973.

Spratt JS Jr, Hoag MG: Mortal diseases among 1000 Ellis Fischel State Cancer Hospital Patients with Comparison to the General Population. Mo Med 63:198–205, 1966.

Spratt JS Jr, Shieber W, Dillard BM: Anatomy and Surgical Technique of Groin Dissection. St. Louis, CV Mosby Company, 1965.

Spratt JS Jr, Spjut HJ: Prevalence and prognosis of individual clinical and pathologic variables associated with colorectal carcinoma. Cancer 20:1976–1985, 1967.

Spratt JS Jr, Spratt TL: Rates and growth of pulmonary metastases and host survival. Ann Surg 159:161–171, 1964.

Spratt JS Jr, Watson FR: The rationale of practice for polypoid lesions of the colon. Cancer 28:153–159, 1971.

Spratt JS Jr, Watson FR, Pratt JL: Characteristics of variants of colorectal carcinoma that do not metastasize to lymph nodes. Dis Colon Rectum 13:243–246, 1970.

Spratt JS Jr, Yuen PF, Sala JM: Preoperative radiotherapy for adenocarcinoma of the rectum (a randomized study). *In* Rush BF Jr, Greenlaw RH (eds): Cancer Therapy by Integrated Radiation and Operation. Springfield, IL, Charles C Thomas, 1968, pp. 102–106.

Stearns MW Jr, Deddish MR: Influence of size on prognosis of operable cancer of rectum and distal sigmoid. Cancer 9:139–140, 1956.

Sugarbaker PH: Carcinoma of the colon—prognosis and operative choice. Curr Probl Surg 18:753–802, 1981.

Susman W: Polypi coli. J Pathol Bacteriol 35:29–333, 1932.

Turnbull RB Jr: Cancer of the sigmoid colon, the influence of the "no-touch" isolation technic on survival. Jpn J Gastroenterol Surg 9:46–60, 1976.

Turnbull RB Jr, Kyle K, Watson FR, Spratt JS Jr: Cancer of the colon: the influence of the no-touch isolation technic on survival rates. Ann Surg 166:420–427, 1967.

Turrell R: Panel discussion, adenomas of large intestine and their malignant potential. Am J Surg 101:97–99, 1961.

Watson FR: A new method for solving simultaneous linear equations associated with multivariate analysis. Psychometrika 29:75–86, 1964.

Watson FR, Spratt JS Jr, LeDuc RJ: Analysis of variance and covariance for colorectal adenocarcinomas in man as a logical prelude to staging. J Surg Oncol 8:155–163, 1976.

Webb MJ, Decker DG, Mussey E: Cancer metastatic to the ovary, factors influencing survival. Obstet Gynecol 45:391–396, 1975.

Wheat MW, Ackerman LV: Villous adenomas of the large intestine. Ann Surg 147:476–487, 1958.

White JE, Enterline JP: Cancer in nonwhite Americans. Curr Probl Cancer 4:3–34, 1980.

Wilson GS, Dale EH, Brines OA: Symposium on early diagnosis of tumors of rectum and colon: Evaluation of polyps detected in 20,847 routine sigmoidoscopic examinations. Am Surg 90:834–840, 1955.

Wittoesch JH, Jackman RJ: Results of conservative management of cancer of rectum in poor risk patients. Surg Gynecol Obstet 107:648–650, 1958.

Wollmark N, Cruz I, Redmond CK, et al: Tumor size and regional lymph node metastasis in colorectal cancer—a preliminary analysis from the NSABP Clinical Trials. Cancer 51:1315–1322, 1983.

Wood DA: The TNM system of classification for gastrointestinal cancer. Proceedings of the Sixth National Cancer Conference. Philadelphia, JB Lippincott Company, 1970, pp. 403–415.

Wood DA: Clinical staging and end results classification: TNM system of clinical classification as applicable to carcinoma of the colon and rectum. Cancer 28:109–114, 1971.

Wood DA: Tumors of the Intestines. Section VI, Fascicle 22, Atlas of Tumor Pathology. Washington, DC, published by the Armed Forces Institute of Pathology under the Auspices of the National Academy of Sciences, 1967.

Wood DA, Robbins GF, Zippin C, et al: Staging of cancer of the colon and rectum. Cancer 43:961–968, 1979.

Young VT: Cited by F. G. Runyeon in Sigmoidoscopy: Its clinical importance to the practitioner. JAMA 147:913–914, 1951.

ELEVEN

Carcinoids

J. S. Spratt, M.D.

Carcinoids occur in the rectum, colon, and appendix as well as in other parts of the gastrointestinal tract, biliary tract, ovaries, pancreas, and lungs. We will restrict our discussion to those carcinoids arising in the appendix, colon, and rectum and to the problems associated with metastatic carcinoid in the liver.

Generally, carcinoids arise from cells that originate from the neural crest of the embryo but that are detached from the central nervous system of the adult. These cells belong to the fascinating group of those endocrine glandular structures having in common amine precursor uptake and decarboxylation (APUD cells). They produce polypeptide hormones and have powerful tissue-response effects (Pearse, 1969). They have features in common with a broad spectrum of "neurocristopathies" (i.e., anomalous developments and neoplasms of neural crest origin).

Of historical note is the fact that the evolving insight into all neurocristopathies began in 1882 with F. von Recklinghausen's classic paper on ". . . den multiplen Neuromen." In commemoration of the centenary year, 1982, an impressive review of progress in the understanding of neurocristopathies was published, including a translation of von Recklinghausen's paper (Riccardi and Mulvihill, 1981).

The complex relationships among neurocristopathies, apudomas, and the function of the intestinal tract present in a wide variety of infrequent forms that can mimic aspects of the carcinoid spectrum. Diarrhea can, for example, be the product of active substances produced by medullary cancers of the thyroid (Norman and Otnes, 1969; Baylin and Wells, 1979). Medullary thyroid cancers originate from the parafollicular cells of the adult thyroid, which are differentiated from neural crest cells that migrate to the ultimobranchial bodies. Medullary thyroid cancers are classified as apudomas because of their mixed output of biologically active polypeptides (Baylin and Wells, 1979).

CARCINOIDS OF THE VERMIFORM APPENDIX

Carcinoids are more prevalent in the vermiform appendix than elsewhere. Often they are discovered incidentally in appendices removed for various reasons. In 1980, Glasser and Bhagavan stated that 1700 cases had been reported in the world's literature during the preceding 100 years. These investigators reported 46 additional cases and confirmed that the most reliable criterion for their behavior is size. In their review, the authors noted that 8.8 percent of the carcinoids metastasized to regional lymph nodes. All those that metastasized were 2 cm in diameter or larger. The authors found that depth of invasion, extension to the serosa, perineural invasion, common histologic features, and location of the carcinoid in the appendix had been reported for both metastasizing and nonmetastasizing carcinoids. Their conclusion was that appendiceal carcinoids with diameters 2.0 cm or greater should be excised via right hemicolectomy, with removal of the lymph node–bearing mesentery.

Moertel and co-workers had earlier come to similar conclusions based on data from the Mayo Clinic (Moertel et al., 1968). Their review covered 144 cases, 137 of which were confirmed with surgery and seven of which were determined by autopsy. Metastasis occurred in only two patients (1.4 percent). Five patients had a synchronous carcinoid in the ileum, and one had a synchronous carcinoid in the rectum. Nineteen (14 percent) with histologically confirmed carcinoids in the appendix had a second primary cancer in another organ. These investigators did not consider that their data justified concluding that carcinoids are associated with an increased tendency to develop cancers in other organs. In this series, metastases occurred in two of three carcinoids measuring 2.0 cm or more. The conclusion of the authors was that appendectomy alone is adequate treatment for appendiceal carcinoids without gross evidence of metastases, with the exception of the rare carcinoid that is larger than 2.0 cm.

Infrequent exceptions to this rule have been reported. In 1979, Syracuse and colleagues reported a series of 92 appendiceal carcinoids among 400,000 surgical pathology specimens accumulated over a period of 70 years. Invasion of the mesoappendix occurred in 13 cases. In two of these cases, ileocolectomy revealed regional lymph node, but no distant, metastases. The primaries measured 1.0 and 1.5 cm. These findings were preceded by two other reports of metastases from 1.0-cm primaries (Dent et al., 1973). The authors recommended that the mesoappendix be thoroughly examined, since a rare small carcinoid may invade the mesoappendix and metastasize. They also advised that ileocolectomy be performed when invasion of the mesoappendix is found, regardless of the size of the primary. In addition, those in Syracuse's group cited scattered references in the literature to distant metastases observed with production of the carcinoid spectrum (see further on), but they found no such cases among the large series they reported. Deceptive morphologic variants of carcinoids also occur in adults, and some can mimic mucin-producing cancers (Olsson and Ljungberg, 1980; Chen and Qizilbash, 1979; Warkel et al., 1978). Warkel and colleagues reported metastases in six of 39 cases but concluded that appendectomy is adequate treatment except for tumors demonstrating atypical foci, a high mitotic count, or spread beyond the appendix, any of which indicates hemicolectomy.

CARCINOIDS IN CHILDREN

Both benign and malignant carcinoids have been reported in children (Chow et al., 1982). Benign carcinoids in children are uncommon, and most are in the appendix. However, Chow and co-workers suggest that malignant carcinoids should be seriously considered in the differential diagnosis of pediatric tumors that have unusual clinical, radiologic, and morphologic characteristics. Ultrastructural studies with electron microscopic examination may be necessary to make the diagnosis. The reported cases were associated with rapid deterioration and only transient response to radiotherapy or chemotherapy.

COLONIC CARCINOIDS

The colon is also the site of rare carcinoids (Brozinsky et al., 1979; Case, 1969; Scott, 1973; MacDonald, 1956). MacDonald reported 26 colonic and 13 rectal carcinoids among 356 gastrointestinal carcinoids found in 450,000 surgical and autopsy specimens. In the colon, 85 percent of the carcinoids were invasive. Metastases were frequent among the larger and more invasive colonic carcinoids. The surgical procedure employed for resection of the primary should be the same as that used for adenocarcinomas in the same segment. These colonic carcinoids have the poorest prognosis of any in the gastrointestinal tract (Morgan et al., 1974).

RECTAL CARCINOIDS

Carcinoids of the rectum occur with no sex or race specificity in the sixth and seventh decades. Most are discovered as submucosal nodules felt on digital rectal examination or seen through a proctoscope. The overlying epithelium will generally be intact. Most are asymptomatic but may produce mild bleeding if they ulcerate. A thorough review by Orloff, published in 1971, confirmed that two findings indicate malignancy: (1) neoplastic invasion into or beyond the muscularis as confirmed on biopsy, and (2) a tumor diameter of 2 cm or more. Thus, all suspected rectal carcinoids should be measured before biopsy, and the biopsy must be deep enough to determine the depth of invasion. The smaller noninvasive carcinoids may be cured by local excision. The larger invasive ones require a more radical

Table 11–1. 3000 CASES OF GASTROINTESTINAL CARCINOID COLLECTED FROM THE LITERATURE*

Site of Origin	Prevalence (%)	Metastases (%)
Appendix	47.0	3
Ileum	27.5	35
Rectum	17.0	12
Stomach	2.5	18
Colon	2.0	60
Jejunum	1.5	35
Duodenum	1.3	16
Meckel's diverticulum	1.0	21
Gallbladder	0.2	25

*Adapted from Orloff, MJ: Carcinoid tumors of the rectum. Cancer 28:175–180, 1971.

extirpation, as can be accomplished by abdominoperineal resection of the rectum. Among 38 patients so managed, Orloff obtained a 5-year survival rate of 76 percent.

Orloff compiled informative comparative data from the literature on 3000 cases of gastrointestinal carcinoids (Table 11–1). These data show a range in malignant behavior. The neoplasms all arise from enterochromaffin cells, which are widely distributed in tissue derived from the primitive gut. As noted previously the cells are thought to reach the primitive gut by migration from the neural crest. However, at this early embryonic stage pleuripotential cells that have the capacity to develop specialized endocrine function have not been totally excluded as progenitors. There is great heterogeneity among carcinoids, and there may exist different types of enterochromaffin cells scattered throughout the gastrointestinal tract that give rise to these neoplasms.

The carcinoids of the rectum arise from the primitive hindgut, where enterochromaffin cells of neural crest origin are histologically different. These histologic differences are also expressed in tumor behavior by the fact that no malignant carcinoid of the rectum has yet been reported to produce a malignant carcinoid spectrum.

METASTATIC CARCINOID SPECTRUM

Carcinoids secrete an array of humoral agents. The components of this array vary with the site of origin of the carcinoid. The result is a spectrum of metabolic effects formerly called "metastatic carcinoid disease," or "metastatic carcinoid syndrome," but correctly renamed "metastatic carcinoid spectrum." As long as the carcinoid is confined to the gut, its humoral products egress via the portal venous circulation and are metabolized in the liver, producing no systemic symptoms. When the liver is the site of metastatic neoplasm, the humoral products have a systemic effect. The products that have been produced by carcinoids include serotonin, 5-hydroxytryptophan, bradykinin, kallikrein, histamine, catecholamines, ACTH, MSH, and insulin. Both kallikrein and bradykinin have been reported to be elevated during flushing attacks. The kinins may be responsible for flushings (Melmon, 1968; Oates and Butler, 1967; Sjoerdsma and Melmon, 1964).

Carcinoids metastatic from the foregut (stomach, pancreas, and bronchus) secrete histamine and 5-hydroxytryptophan, and they are associated with flushing, facial edema, syncopal episodes, Cushing's syndrome, and pluriglandular adenomatosis. Carcinoids metastatic from the midgut (ileum and jejunum) tend to produce the classic "carcinoid syndrome" secondary to serotonin secretion. No active humoral agent has been extracted from carcinoids of the hindgut, except possibly in a case of carcinoid reported by Saegesser and Gross in 1969.

Series large enough to define the full spectrum of behavior in metastatic carcinoid disease are few. In 1979, Dilawari and Douglass reported on the autopsies of patients with metastatic carcinoid. Six of 15 patients had extra-abdominal metastatic carcinoid (most commonly in bone). These were more refractory to therapy.

In 1961, Moertel reported a mean life expectancy of 8.1 years for patients with metastatic carcinoid. In 1970, Martin reported an average life expectancy of 4.3 years, with some patients surviving as long as 23 years. Confronted with such a long-term course, medical professionals have developed various pharmacologic and surgical approaches to help control the neoplasm and its side effects. All these techniques require an understanding of the metabolic consequences of carcinoid secretions.

Carcinoids originate from the enterochromaffin cell precursors in the submucosa and are classified as apudomas. The apudoma neoplasms arise from neuroectodermal cells of the neural crest, and they are drawn into the foregut and its derivatives early in embryologic development. Although they are nerve cells, they exert their effect by secreting neurotransmitter amines locally. They respond to stimulation by other amines, proteins, and polypep-

Table 11–2. **SECRETORY PRODUCTS, HISTOCHEMICAL STAINING PROPERTIES, AND CLINICAL MANIFESTATIONS OF CARCINOIDS ACCORDING TO SITE OF ORIGIN***

Source of Carcinoid	Anatomic Areas	Secretory Products	Staining Properties		Clinical Manifestations
			Argentaffin	*Argyrophil*	
Foregut	Bronchus Stomach Pancreas	5-HTP Myalase Histamine(?)	Negative	Positive	Brightened flush on eating, prolonged flush, facial edema, hypotension, peptic ulcer, Cushing's syndrome, pluriglandular adenomatosis
Midgut	Jejunum Ileum Appendix	Serotonin Bradykinin VIP Motilin(?) Kallikrein	Positive	Positive	Classic malignant carcinoid syndrome
Hindgut	Colon Rectum	No known secretions	Negative	Negative	No known syndrome

*Adapted from Orloff, MJ: Carcinoid tumors of the rectum. Cancer 28:175–180, 1971, and Welbourn, RB, Pearse, AGE, Polak, JM, et al.: The APUD cells of the alimentary tract in health and disease. Med Clin North Am 58:1359–1374, 1974.

tides. APUD cells and most apudomas are characterized by fluorogenic amine content, amine precursor uptake, and aminoacid decarboxylase. Their ultrastructural properties also are typical (see Chapter Four).

The APUD cells develop extensive hormonal specialization. This specialization is found in a variety of forms in apudomas. In Table 11–2, a summary of the variations among carcinoids is given. This list may be incomplete because studies are continuing to yield reports of either confirmed or suspected additional products. As a consequence, before intervention, a rather complete metabolic work-up should be done in suspected cases of metastatic carcinoid. This need is compounded by the occasional existence of apudomas in other organs (multiple endocrine adenopathies) that may also be secreting hormonally active products (e.g., insulinomas, gastrinomas, corticotrophinomas, calcitoninomas, glucagonomas, vipomas, and ACTH-producing apudomas). The apudoma producing only a single hormone is said to produce an orthoendocrine syndrome. The paraendocrine syndrome is produced by the secretion of one or more polypeptides that may be foreign to the cell of origin but that are characteristic of other APUD cells. The products may be measured by radioimmunoassay in the peripheral blood and in the venous blood efferent from the tumor. Normally, most products of APUD cells are destroyed by liver enzymes, and the systemic symptoms occur only with hepatic metastases from which tumor products bypass liver metabolism and directly enter the systemic circulation via the hepatic veins. In the absence of an effective ablative approach to an apudoma, control of secondary symptoms is assisted by accurate knowledge of the apudoma's secretions. Also, control of these effects in the pre-, intra-, and postoperative periods is often essential. Sequential monitoring of products may also provide an accurate method of monitoring response to treatment and suspected relapses. The very prolonged clinical course of many of these cases makes this an important consideration.

The symptoms produced by carcinoids are mechanical as well as humoral. Crampy intestinal pain, distention, partial and complete intestinal obstruction, and palpable mass are some of these. Duration before diagnosis is highly variable. Only local removal for histologic study is required for small carcinoids demonstrating no invasion. However, the larger carcinoids with intramural extension or suspected lymph node metastases should be removed by standard cancer operations that include excision of lymph node–bearing mesentery. Liver metastases must be assessed. Only easily accessible isolated metastases should be touched at the time of initial bowel resection. Nothing is lost by staging the operation. Interval performance of indicated metabolic studies, patient preparation, hepatic scans, and angiograms for definition of the extent and location of metastases and the vascular anatomy of the liver are necessary. Then, when a prepared patient is reentered through an appropriate incision, as complete a removal as possible of all carcinoid metastases in the liver must be done. When excision of the metastases is not possible, massive regression of hepatic carcinoids may be accomplished through hepatic artery ligation (Karakoukis et al., 1979; Dilawari and Douglass, 1979; Gillett and Smith, 1974). Further comments on the surgical management of hepatic metastases are contained in Chapter Fourteen.

Infrequent cases are reported in which the carcinoid spectrum associated with carcinoids of gastrointestinal origin occurs in the absence of hepatic metastases. In 1982, Feldman and Jones reported three patients who had all the symptoms of carcinoid spectrum but no hepatic metastases. Two had intra-abdominal metastases and the third, in whom an ileal carcinoid was present, had large mesenteric lymph node metastases. Hepatic metastases did not appear in any of these patients. Following complete resection of the primaries and metastases, symptoms of the carcinoid spectrum disappeared. The 5-HIAA and platelet serotonin levels returned to normal. The authors concluded that before exploration of patients with carcinoid spectrum, CT scans and ^{99}Tc scans of the liver should be performed. If the presence of hepatic metastases is not suspected or confirmed after these studies, a hepatic artery angiogram should be obtained to rule out hepatic metastases. If none are found, then a cure, or at least long-term control, may be achieved through definitive resection of all intra-abdominal neoplasm. In the 11-year experience of one of the authors (JMF), the appearance of carcinoid spectrum in the absence of hepatic metastases occurred in 6 percent of the patients (3 of 52 serotonin-producing carcinoids with the carcinoid spectrum).

CONTROL OF METABOLIC SYMPTOMS WITH DRUGS

Pharmacologic correction of metabolic symptoms has been partially achieved through administration of metabolic antagonists of specific secretory products and by cytotoxic chemotherapy. Metabolic symptoms can also be aggravated by alcohol, emotional upset, and direct pressure on tumors (Dilawari and Douglass, 1979; Khoury et al., 1979; Gillett and Smith, 1974; Pearse et al., 1977).

Diarrhea has been controlled through administration of the 5-hydroxytryptophan antagonist, methysergide, and by the action of the tryptophan 5-hydroxylase inhibitor, parachlorophenylalanine. Alpha-methyldopa and phenoxybenzamine have been used to control facial flushing. Other drugs of occasional benefit include propranolol, chlorpromazine hydrochloride, promazine hydrochloride, and prednisone. The Isuprel Hydrochloride Mistometer* is of value in treating bronchospasm because it does not provoke facial flushing. Indocin, a prostaglandin inhibitor, has also been helpful in some patients. Antiserotonin drugs cannot control all symptoms because of the diverse nature of the humorally active agents secreted.

The preoperative pharmacologic considerations are critical. Methysergide should be used preoperatively and throughout the procedure for its antiserotonin effect. Agents that induce hypotension are to be avoided, since they can cause release of endogenous epinephrine and norepinephrine. These may stimulate release of large amounts of serotonin from the carcinoid, aggravating the hypotension. Agents and methods that have caused difficulty include thiopental sodium, halothane, and spinal and epidural blocks. If hypotension occurs, methoxamine or angiotensin or both should be administered.

With chronic carcinoid spectrum, right heart damage and failure are well-documented complications. Such failure can be aggravated by norepinephrine and fluid overload. Thus, fluids have to be given with caution during operations, even in the presence of hypotension. The extreme sensitivity of patients with the carcinoid spectrum to epinephrine was well emphasized in 1975 by Levine, who pointed out that doses as small as 0.001 mg may produce a significant response.

Secondary and nonspecific metabolic control of the carcinoid spectrum may also be obtained with chemotherapeutic cytotoxic drugs to which the carcinoid is responsive. In 1979, Dilawari and Douglass reported regression of metastatic carcinoid with 5-fluorouracil (5-FU) and streptozotocin (STZ), with secondary regression of metabolic symptoms. A fall in the daily excretion of 5-HIAA was associated with regression of symptoms, and a rise in 5-HIAA was related to a relapse of symptoms. In all, five of seven patients seemed to have benefited from STZ.

Comments on the surgical aspects of managing bowel cancer metastatic to the liver are to be found in Chapter Fourteen. Extensive resections are now possible, safe, and feasible. A nonspecific regression of hepatic metastases may be obtained, for varying periods of time,

*Isoproterenol hydrochloride aerosol, Breon Labs, New York.

by complete dearterialization of the liver. Various surgical techniques for infusion chemotherapy via the hepatic artery and portal vein continue to show promise. The concept of the liver as a "safe" haven for metastatic bowel cancer, including carcinoid, is under continuing attack. Metastatic cancer and carcinoid strictly confined to the liver are, of course, more amenable to treatment than when the liver is only one of many sites affected by metastatic deposits (Karakoukis et al., 1979; Khoury et al., 1979; Gillett and Smith, 1974; Beaton et al., 1981).

In their comprehensive 1977 review, Foster and Berman reported on a series of 49 partial liver resections performed in 44 patients for carcinoid metastatic to the liver. Palliation was achieved in all but one of the 36 patients for whom follow-up was available. Palliation lasted from a few weeks to over 6 years. Flushing and diarrhea were alleviated promptly, but the cardiac symptoms remained unchanged. The patient who did not benefit died from a perforated peptic ulcer 2 months after the enucleation of several carcinoids. The liver contained numerous foci of metastatic carcinoid at autopsy. Among the 39 patients who survived the first liver resection, 18 were still alive at the time of the review, and these survivors had lived from 2 months to 10½ years. The more gross carcinoid resected, the longer the palliation. The metabolic effects were often reduced, even in the presence of incomplete resection.

The management of carcinoid metastatic to the liver may be subdivided into three areas: (1) suppression of symptoms secondary to the secretions of carcinoids, (2) ablative surgical methods, and (3) ablative chemotherapeutic methods. Selection of therapeutic strategy requires a very careful evaluation of the patient, with particular emphasis given to the anatomic location and size of metastases and to the metabolic consequences of heterogeneous carcinoid secretions. Evaluation and management of the metabolic consequences are the first steps in controlling presenting symptoms and in preparing patients for any type of intervention that might create a flux of secretions.

Symptoms of the secretory products of carcinoids may include watery diarrhea, abdominal cramps, generalized weakness, flushing of the upper face and trunk, progressive telangiectasia, dyspnea with bronchospasm, and right heart failure associated with endocardial fibrosis, with the process involving the tricuspid and pulmonary valves. The symptoms may be aggravated by emotional upset, alcohol, and simple direct pressure on the carcinoid metastases in a wide variety of ways. They may all progress to the advanced states of heart failure. If the carcinoid secretions are allowed to continue their effect too long, the processes initiated may progress even after removal of the carcinoid. The extreme cases of the carcinoid spectrum occur in less than 5 percent of patients with metastatic carcinoid.

SUMMARY

In summary, carcinoids can affect all segments of the large intestine, the rectum, and the appendix. They probably arise from embryologic neural crest cells persisting in the adult, and they belong to the family of neuroendocrine glands classified as apudomas. Their symptoms vary widely, influenced by segment of origin and the hormonal output of the neoplasm. The hindgut carcinoids are less serious than those of the gut proximal to the ileocecal valve. Liver metastases create their own unique set of problems. In all instances, pharmacologic alleviation of symptoms and definitive surgery can be highly beneficial either for cure or for the protracted alleviation of symptoms of neoplasms that often have very prolonged courses.

References

Baylin SB, Wells SA Jr: Management of medullary thyroid cancer. *In* Greenfield LD (ed): Thyroid Cancer. West Palm Beach, FL, CRC Press, 1979, pp. 151–163.

Beaton H, Homan W, Dineen P: Gastrointestinal carcinoids and the malignant carcinoid syndrome. Surg Gynecol Obstet 152:268–272, 1981.

Brozinsky S, Wapnick S, Grosberg SJ: Large colonic carcinoid—report of a case. Am J Proctol Gastroenterol Colon Rectal Surg 30:26–28, 1979.

Case TC: Large carcinoid tumor of the transverse colon. J Am Geriatr Soc 17:1113–1117, 1969.

Chen V, Qizilbash AH: Goblet cell carcinoid tumor of the appendix. Report of five cases and review of the literature. Arch Pathol Lab Med 103:180–182, 1979.

Chow CW, Sane S, Campbell PE, Carter RF: Malignant carcinoid tumors in children. Cancer 49:802–811, 1982.

Dent TL, Batsakis JG, Lindenauer SM: Carcinoid tumors of the appendix. Surgery 73:828–832, 1973.

Dilawari RA, Douglass HO Jr: Gastrointestinal carcinoids; extrahepatic metastases and symptomatology following resection. J Surg Oncol 11:243–248, 1979.

Feldman JM, Jones RS: Carcinoid syndrome from gastrointestinal carcinoids without liver metastases. Ann Surg 196:33–37, 1982.

Foster JH, Berman MM: Solid liver tumors. Major Probl Clin Surg 22:209–234, 1977.

Gillett DJ, Smith RC: Treatment of the carcinoid syndrome by hemihepatectomy and radical excision of the primary lesion. Am J Surg 128:95–99, 1974.

Glasser CM, Bhagavan BS: Carcinoid tumors of the appendix. Arch Pathol Lab Med 104:272–275, 1980.

Karakoukis CP, Douglass HO Jr, Holyoke ED: Technique of infusion chemotherapy, ligation of the hepatic artery and dearterialization in malignant lesions of the liver. Surg Gynecol Obstet 149:403–407, 1979.

Khoury GA, Devine T, Bolt DE: Complete liver dearterialization and the carcinoid syndrome. Br J Surg 66:253–256, 1979.

Levine RJ: Letter: Diagnosis and treatment of malignant carcinoid syndrome. JAMA 231:914–915, 1975.

MacDonald RA: A study of 356 carcinoids of the gastrointestinal tract. Am J Med 21:867–878, 1956.

Martin RG: Management of carcinoid tumors. Cancer 26:547–551, 1970.

Melmon KL: Kinins—one of many mediators of the carcinoid spectrum. Gastroenterology 55:545–548, 1968.

Moertel CG, Dockerty MB, Judd ES: Carcinoid tumors of the vermiform appendix. Cancer 21:270–278, 1968.

Moertel CG, Sauer WG, Dockerty MB, Baggenstoss AH: Life history of the carcinoid tumor of the small intestine. Cancer 14:901–912, 1961.

Morgan JG, Marks C, Hearn D: Carcinoid tumors of the gastrointestinal tract. Ann Surg 180:720–727, 1974.

Norman T, Otnes B: Intestinal ganglioneuromatosis, diarrhoea, and medullary thyroid carcinoma. Scand J Gastroenterol 4:553–559, 1969.

Oates JA, Butler TC: Pharmacologic and endocrine aspects of carcinoid syndrome. Adv Pharmacol 5:109–128, 1967.

Olsson B, Ljungberg O: Adenocarcinoid of the vermiform appendix. Virchows Arch (Pathol Anat) 386:201–210, 1980.

Orloff MJ: Carcinoid tumors of the rectum. Cancer 28:175–180, 1971.

Pearse AG: The cytochemistry and ultrastructure of polypeptide hormone–producing cells of the APUD series, and the embryologic, physiologic and pathologic implications of the concept. J Histochem Cytochem 17:303–313, 1969.

Pearse AG, Polak JM, Bloom SR: The newer gut hormones. Cellular sources, physiology, pathology and clinical aspects. Gastroenterology 72:746–761, 1977.

Riccardi VM, Mulvihill JJ: Neurofibromatosis (von Recklinghausen disease): genetics, cell biology, and biochemistry. (Advances in Neurology, Vol 29) New York, Raven Press, 1981.

Saegesser F, Gross M: Carcinoid syndrome and carcinoid tumours of the rectum. Am J Proctol 20:27–32, 1969.

Scott JE: Carcinoid tumors of the colon. Br J Surg 60:684–685, 1973.

Sjoerdsma A, Melmon KL: The carcinoid spectrum. Gastroenterology 47:104–107, 1964.

Syracuse DC, Perzin KH, Price JB, et al.: Carcinoid tumors of the appendix. Mesoappendiceal extension and nodal metastases. Ann Surg 190:58–63, 1979.

von Recklinghausen F: (On multiple fibromas of the skin and their relationship to multiple neurofibromas). Festschrift in commemoration of the twenty-fifth anniversary of the founding of the Pathological Institute of Berlin, presented to Prof. Rudolf Virchow Berlin, August Hirschwald, 1882. Crump T, trans. Adv Neurol 29:259–275, 1981.

Warkel RL, Cooper PH, Helwig EB: Adenocarcinoid, a mucin-producing carcinoid tumor of the appendix: a study of 39 cases. Cancer 42:2781–2793, 1978.

Welbourn RB, Pearse AGE, Polak JM, et al: The APUD cells of the alimentary tract in health and disease. Med Clin North Am 58:1359–1374, 1974.

TWELVE

Advances in the Surgery of Rectal Carcinoma Utilizing the Circular Stapler

V. W. Fazio, M.D.

Since the description by Miles in 1908 of abdominoperineal resection and permanent colostomy, a variety of operative procedures for the definitive management of rectal cancer have appeared. In general, the controversies concerning surgical technique center on the advantages and disadvantages of sphincter preservation versus total resection with permanent colostomy. It is claimed by some that sphincter preservation is "not radical enough" as a cancer operation and that this form of treatment will lead to a higher rate of pelvic malignant recurrence than rectal exenteration. Moreover, the quality of life for some patients with low colorectal anastomosis can be poor because of poor or indifferent bowel function. Incapacitating diarrhea; urgency and incontinence; and anastomotic complications, such as pelvic abscess, fecal fistula, and stricture, can occur, necessitating a future (or concurrent) temporary colostomy, which sometimes remains permanent. The proponents of anastomotic procedures for carcinoma of the upper and midrectum point out, however, that survival rates with sphincter-preserving techniques are at least as good as those with the Miles operation, provided that the principles of cancer surgery are followed. For example, an en bloc resection of the rectum and sigmoid that encompasses a distal line of clearance of the bowel and mesorectum of 5 cm or more should be performed.

The en bloc resection of adjacent fat, lymph nodes, and vessels is performed with the resection, and the inferior mesenteric vessels are ligated "high" at the origin of the inferior mesenteric artery from the aorta. Although anastomotic complications can occur, they are sometimes predictable and, therefore, partly preventable, at least in terms of their consequences, by the addition of temporary fecal diversion. For many, if not most patients, this is a relatively small price to pay to avoid a permanent colostomy. Frequently, bowel function is poor or imperfect in the early postoperative period, but again, the patient, the final arbiter of the value of the sphincter-preserving operation, invariably is prepared to endure considerable bowel dysfunction temporarily in his quest for ultimate continence and avoidance of a stoma.

At present, a group of factors occurring in the patient and in the biology of the cancer remains that influences the surgeon in the decision to perform a sphincter-preserving operation. Additionally, the skills, training, and bias of the surgeon will play a role in the decision to perform this operation as well as in the choice of a particular technique to be used. Although no single factor always influences the surgeon to preserve sphincter function, patient characteristics that incline the surgeon to do so include the following: lack of obesity, a wide pelvis (females), no history of pelvic irradiation, "reasonable" general good health and freedom from attendant serious cardiovascular disease, and good sphincter tone. The site of the tumor is the most important of these factors when deciding whether to perform the Miles operation or anterior resection of the rectum. Tumors in the upper one third of the rectum (11 to 15 cm from the anal verge) can invariably be treated by anterior resection, unless fixed to other structures. On occasion it may be undesirable despite its feasibility to perform an anastomosis, such as when a patient has widespread malignancy, carcinomatosis, or is a prohibitive surgical risk. In such cases an extended Hartmann procedure may be more suitable. For tumors located in the middle one third of the rectum (7 to 11 cm from the anal verge), a variety of sphincter-preserving operations can be performed, such as the conventional anterior resection with end-to-end colorectal anastomosis. In difficult situations in which access and visibility are diminished, other procedures can be used, such as the Baker side-to-end anastomosis, the abdominal-transsacral approach (Allgöwer et al., 1982; Kraske, 1885; Localio et al., 1980; Marks, 1976; Mason, 1970), the coloanal pull-through operation (Cutait and Figliolini, 1961; Turnbull and Cuthbertson, 1961), the trans-sphincteric operation (Mason, 1974), and the end-to-end transanal coloanal anastomosis (Parks, 1982). Most patients and surgeons find that the functional results of all these alternatives are usually superior to those of colostomy. Each of the procedures, notwithstanding the bias, enthusiasm, and skills of the individual surgeons who champion them, has certain drawbacks, mostly with respect to the technical difficulties associated with these sophisticated operations. The advent of circular stapling devices as a means of facilitating the fashioning of a low colorectal anastomosis has made many, if not all, of the preceding alternatives obsolete. Experienced colorectal surgeons claim (rightly) that staplers do not extend the indications for sphincter preservation. The constraints of location of the tumor, the need to encompass a sufficient distal margin of bowel and mesorectum, and the consideration of the tumor biology affect the outcome of the operations independently of techniques of anastomosis. For many surgeons, however, the stapling technique allows a speedier and usually better anastomotic construction than other methods, and this is especially seen when low anastomoses are made (Beart and Kelly, 1981).

For tumors located in the lower one third of the rectum, traditional curative procedures include abdominoperineal resection of the rectum and permanent colostomy. Yet with the emphasis being placed on sphincter preservation, there is in certain medical centers a willingness to accept something less than the traditional 5 cm of distal clearance. The emphasis seems more on clearing all of the mesorectum so that the superior aspect of the levators are cleared. Provided the tumor is well-differentiated, local recurrence rates are not increased when a distal margin of the bowel of 2 to 3 cm is obtained (Heald et al., 1982). Also, the tumor should not be fixed or significantly tethered and should occupy one third or less of the rectal circumference.

In special situations, local treatment by excision, fulguration, or contact radiotherapy is suitable. For conditions to be optimal, these situations require that the tumor is located posteriorly, the level of the tumor is below peritoneal reflection (7 to 8 cm from the anal verge), the tumor has mobility on palpation, there are no palpable presacral lymph nodes, and the tumor is less than 3.5 cm in size, well-differentiated, and nodular rather than ulcerated in appearance.

The end-to-end (EEA) anastomotic stapler was used by the author in a series of patients undergoing anastomosis of proximal intestine to the rectum or anal canal. The techniques, pitfalls, and immediate postoperative complications using this method in this series are discussed in this chapter. Although these procedures were performed for a variety of pathologic processes, rectal cancer constituted the major indication for operation.

PREPARATION OF PATIENT

Mechanical

Colon preparation of all patients undergoing elective surgery included a liquid-only diet for 48 hours; magnesium citrate, 450 ml orally on the day before surgery; and a tap water rectal washout on the day before surgery and on the morning of surgery. For certain patients who had inflammatory bowel disease or who were unable to tolerate catharsis, the preparation was modified. After induction of anesthesia, a rectal tube was placed in the rectum and a further washout was performed. Povidone-iodine 10 percent was introduced into the rectum (about 100 ml) and the rectal tube was removed. (More recently our unit has dispensed with enemas entirely and now uses mannitol, 10 percent, 1 L the day before surgery instead of magnesium citrate.)

Antibiotic Preparation

The combination of erythromycin base and neomycin, 1 gm of each, taken orally at 1 PM, 2 PM, and 10 PM on the day before surgery, was used, as advocated by Nichols and associates, 1973. Systemic antibiotics, given preoperatively and for 24 hours postoperatively, were used throughout this study period. Various antibiotics were employed in the period from July 1978 to February 1981 as a part of a series of prospective randomized trials.

Although the use of staplers in surgery requires a completely new discipline for those who have not used them before, the same principles apply as for the construction of conventional anastomoses. There should be assurance of a good blood supply to the bowel ends, lack of tension on the anastomosis, equilibration of the bowel openings, an inverting closure, and a well-prepared colon.

DESCRIPTION OF THE INSTRUMENT

The EEA stapler consists of a central barrel (E) enclosing a shaft. The cartridge is advanced over the central shaft along a grooved track, referred to as the guide (G), and is then locked into position on the "shoulder" that forms the cartridge carrier (F) at the distal end of the instrument (Fig. 12–1). The anvil (H) is screwed onto the tip of the central shaft. Within the cartridge there are two staggered rows of stainless steel staples surrounding an inner circular cutting blade, which in turn surrounds an inner plastic cushion that accommodates the "doughnut" rings of tissue produced when the instrument is fired. At firing, grooves within the anvil direct the staples into a B form.

Normally, the blade and staples are not ejected from the cartridge except when the instrument is closed on the bowel ends during the firing procedure. Rarely a "burr" developing on the central shaft may trigger premature firing during loading. Dr. Frank L. Weakley at the Cleveland Clinic has designed a simple loading cylinder that prevents this problem.

At the proximal end of the instrument, the wing nut (A) controls separation and approximation of the anvil and cartridge. The gauge at (D) indicates readiness to fire. By removing the safety catch (B) and firing the trigger mechanism (C), the staples are driven through the full thickness of the bowel ends while the circular knife trims the inverted bowel ends. The safety catch should be in place at all times, except during the actual firing.

Cartridges are available in three sizes: 31 mm, 28 mm, and 25 mm. For colonic anastomoses, the largest head is usually appropriate. Anastomoses involving the small intestine commonly require the smaller head sizes. Templates allow the surgeon to decide which size cartridge is appropriate.

Another instrument, a modified Furniss clamp, provides a fairly rapid method of placing purse-string sutures to the bowel ends. Its series of interlocking serrations grip the bowel end and provide two channels through which the sutures are readily run.

The EEA instrument may be introduced

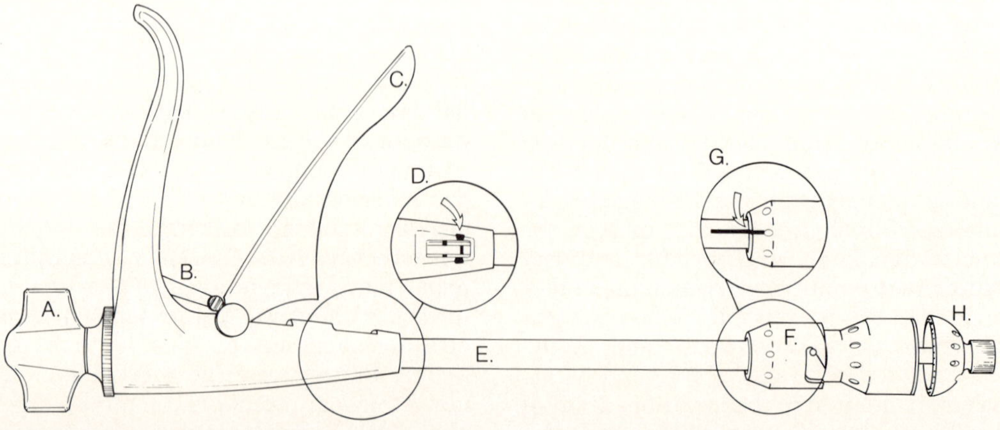

Figure 12–1. The end-to-end anastomosis stapler (EEA). A = wing nut; B = safety pin; C = firing lever; D = gauge indicates readiness for firing when slashes are aligned; E = shaft; F = cartridge carrier; G = guide to loading cartridge onto carrier; H = anvil.

either transanally or by way of a proximal colotomy that will subsequently be closed by sutures placed by hand or autosuture. My preference is the transanal route for all colorectal anastomoses because it obviates the need for making and closing a separate opening on the bowel. The use of this instrument presupposes excellent mechanical preparation of the colon and rectum.

OPERATIVE TECHNIQUE

Resection of the Tumor-Bearing Segment

The patient is placed in the semilithotomy position with slight head-down tilt, using Lloyd-Davies stirrups. A midline incision is used, which is extended up to the xiphoid process if required to mobilize the splenic flexure.

After examination of the intra-abdominal organs and viscera, the small intestine is reflected upward and to the patient's right side with sponges and malleable self-retaining retractors. An incision is made along the line of peritoneal reflection of the left paracolic gutter extending over Gerota's fascia and the prerenal fat. With medial traction on the left colon, a retroperitoneal approach is made to the origin of the inferior mesenteric lymphovascular pedicle, identifying and preserving in turn the left gonadal vein and ureter.

A high ligation of the pedicle is made with doubled No 1. chromic catgut, and the pedicle is divided between ties. The left colic artery is ligated twice just distal to its origin from the inferior mesenteric artery and just proximal to its bifurcation; this preserves the arcade between the ascending and descending branches of the left colic artery, allowing for a conduit in addition to the marginal artery and thus assuring a good blood supply to the chosen site of colonic transsection.

The mobilized left colon mesentery just inferior to the descending branch of the left colic artery is incised across to the junction of the sigmoid and descending colon. With tape tied around the proximal colon to minimize operative contamination, the bowel is divided between clamps.

Incisions are made on either side of the rectosigmoid mesentery down to the approximate level of distal transsection of the rectum. Anterior retraction on the tumor-bearing segment allows for dissection immediately posterior to the distal inferior mesenteric and superior rectal arteries. At this point, the bloodless plane between the investing layer of fascia of the rectum (anteriorly) and Waldeyer's fascia (posteriorly) is entered and traced down to the elected site of rectal transsection. The mesentery of the rectum is ligated, allowing for a margin of clearance of 5 cm or more from the lower border of the tumor. The tumor-bearing segment is irrigated with a cytotoxic agent (my preference is 40 percent ethyl alcohol), the rectum is transsected, and the bowel ends are prepared for the anastomosis.

Further colonic mobilization may be achieved by a second ligation and division of the inferior mesenteric vein at the lower border of the pancreas. In most cases of high anterior resection, the proximal descending colon can be mobilized easily from the prerenal fat and Gerota's fascia without a full takedown of the splenic flexure.

Preparation of the Bowel Ends

At the chosen line of resection, adjacent fat is cleared 2 cm proximal to the resection line. Care is taken to avoid incision of an adjacent diverticulum. A Kocher clamp is placed on the specimen side of the resection line. Proximal to this, the purse-string suture device is placed. Two 0 Proline sutures on a straight Keith needle are used to traverse the channels of the purse-string clamp. This suture is placed so that the ends appear on the antimesenteric border. This method is sometimes time-saving. Commonly, the suture "picks up" opposing mucosa or "misses" some of the serosa, necessitating close inspection of the completed purse-string and correction of any inadequacies. This is probably the procedure of choice for the rectal stump preparation, especially for low anastomoses. Other surgeons choose to place all purse-string sutures by conventional techniques. I have enjoyed some success with the purse-string device (PSD) even for low anastomoses, since the availability of the double-armed Proline suture. Usually access to the cuff of a low-lying rectal stump is suboptimal and use of the former single-armed needle suture allowed only one pass of the needle through the grooves of the PSD. After this, the needle would commonly be bent and not allow for the second traverse. The double-armed needle suture has largely overcome this problem.

When using hand-sutured methods for placement of the purse-string, the technique must be meticulous. In few other areas does the success of the anastomosis construction depend as much on technique. Incorporation of too much tissue in the bites of bowel edge leads to a bulk of tissue with excessive eversion around the central shaft of the instrument. I prefer to take minimal bites of the seromuscular layer, approximately 2 to 3 mm deep, with as little of the mucosa as will accept a stitch. The sutures are placed 7 mm apart. When tied around the central shaft, little or no eversion of tissue should be seen. This is especially important when using the smaller cartridges, such as the EEA 28- or 25-mm sizes. After firing the instrument, the "doughnuts" of proximal and distal bowel are bunched into the housing or hollow chamber of the cartridge. There is little latitude for excessive tissue being crammed into a confined space. In such circumstances, the surgeon will find that the staples are driven through four thicknesses of the bowel wall instead of two, the B form of the staple is not assumed, and/or the blade does not completely cut through the thicknesses of the bowel. There is then difficulty in extracting the instrument, and disruption of part of the anastomosis upon withdrawal of the instrument is likely.

Introduction of the Instrument

The rectum is drained of residual mucus or lavage material by placing a catheter in the rectum. The anal canal is dilated to two fingerbreadths. The lubricated instrument is inserted into the rectum by the assistant, and the direction and angle of the instrument's course is directed by the abdominal operator. During this time, rectal content (usually mucus) can be pushed ahead of the instrument; therefore, packs are strategically placed to obviate the effects of any spill. The sucker is kept handy to aspirate any material as it emerges from the rectal stump. Once the anvil appears, the wing nut of the instrument is opened (counterclockwise) to separate the anvil from the cartridge. The surgeon will have already chosen the size of cartridge to be used. For most rectal anastomoses, the EEA 31 mm or the intraluminal stapler (ILS) 29 mm are appropriate. If any doubt exists, sizers are available to check on the bowel caliber. My preference has been to use rubber dilators graduated every 2 mm from 20 French to 34 French. These serve the extra purpose of producing slight dilatation of the bowel ends (especially the proximal end) that can mean the difference between an easy or a difficult extraction of the instrument after firing. This is especially true if the dilatation is carried out immediately before advancement of the proximal bowel over the anvil. At this point the rectal purse-string is tied around the shaft. After advancing the proximal bowel over the anvil using three Babcock clamps (some surgeons prefer four guy sutures, especially for a low anastomosis), the purse-string is tied. Breaking of the tie is particularly frustrating at this point, so care should be taken, using a surgeon's knot, to prevent slippage. In most cases this will be the most difficult area to assess in terms of adequacy of the tie because it is located deep in the pelvis, and visibility of the mesenteric aspect of the upper tie is poor. During this procedure of tying, the assistant exerts slight traction on the proximal colon mesentery to avoid entrapment of fat in the tie. This traction is maintained as the assistant brings the anvil and cartridge into apposition by clockwise rotation of the wing nut. When the slashes on the instrument are aligned, indicating a satisfactory tissue gap setting, the instrument is ready for firing. The safety catch is released and the trigger is fired using a forceful movement. A distinct feel or, in the case of the ILS, an audible "crunch" is detected with satisfactory firing.

Extraction of the Instrument

After firing, the assistant replaces the safety catch, and the anvil and cartridge are separated by two or three turns of the wing nut. The instrument is rotated slowly 360 degrees, with a downward and lateral or tilted motion to facilitate the passage of the anvil through the anastomosis. If the abdominal operator notes undue tension or descent of the anastomosis during extraction of the instrument, two or three stay sutures are placed on the anterior part of the anastomosis. Educated counter traction will help "lift" the anastomosis over the anvil.

Checking the Integrity of the Anastomosis

After withdrawal of the instrument, the circular pieces of tissue, or "doughnuts," are checked for integrity. I believe all anastomoses should be checked also by instillation of air or Betadine (povidone-iodine) into the rectum until anastomotic distension commences. The reason for this is that even though the "doughnuts" may be intact, forcible extraction of the instrument may disrupt the anastomosis. This is especially likely when a difficult extraction occurs or a very snug fit of the proximal colon over the anvil was noted. Occasionally, "doughnuts" may appear to be intact, but in reality, are held together by the purse-string suture. If any doubts exist, careful dissection of the purse-string from the "doughnuts" will demonstrate the real situation. In the case of incomplete "doughnuts," the location of the inadequacy can be identified by orientating the defect in relation to its location on the anvil or cartridge. If the anastomosis is deficient, then, by hand, suitably placed sutures are made. In the case of a low anastomosis this may be very difficult to do. In such cases, I have used transanal placement of sutures, using No. 30 chromic catgut. Occasionally, this method is also not feasible. Provided the defect is not massive, one can employ sump suction irrigation/drainage of the presacral space with an added temporary loop transverse colostomy. After repair of a suture line defect, the anastomosis is rechecked with Betadine. If any question of the security of the anastomosis remains, then a covering colostomy is used.

Protection of the Low Anastomosis

A number of factors acting singly or in concert lead to degrees of dehiscence of an anastomosis. Aside from constitutional factors, such as the patient's age, nutritional status, use of immunosuppressive agents, and history of vascular disease and previous pelvic irradiation, other factors occurring at operation may serve to produce an undesirable result. Tension on suture lines, degrees of vascular impairment to the cut ends of bowel, fecal loading of the colon or intraoperative contamination, and presence of established intra-abdominal sepsis are factors unrelated to anastomotic technique that favor dehiscence. These errors result from faulty assessment of conditions favoring the performance of an anastomosis. Further colonic mobilization, avoidance of an anastomosis at that operation, or at least construction of a temporary diverting stoma are appropriate corrective maneuvers.

Eversion techniques of anastomosis have been roundly condemned by most surgeons as a result of the clear evidence of the superiority of inversion techniques provided by Goligher and associates in a controlled trial of the two methods. However, as Goligher pointed out, anastomotic leak can still occur in the otherwise low-risk patient, even when the surgeon is satisfied that a technically sound anastomosis has been made. The following factors may serve to produce dehiscence in such circumstances: the presence of excessive collagenase activity in the anastomosis itself; the relative lack of supportive structure in the extraperitoneal rectum, where the vertical muscle fibers have no covering serosa; the presence of obligatory exudate that accumulates around the anastomosis after deep pelvic surgery, the suppuration of which drains through the adjacent suture line.

These factors or their effects may be minimized by the use of: (1) omental wrap, (2) sump suction of the presacral space, and (3) temporary fecal diversion.

Omental Wrap

When feasible, using strategically placed sutures, omentum may be used to wrap the anastomosis. This procedure has been shown to be of value in a canine model (McLachlin et al., 1976) and may exert its effect by facilitating absorption of exudate in the pelvis, by occupying "dead" space and supporting the anastomosis, or by neovascularization of an anastomosis when borderline ischemia is present. When the omentum is short, extra length can be obtained by using a pedicle based on the left gastroepiploic vessels. Further length is obtained and chances of an internal volvulus reduced by drawing this pedicle through a defect made in the root of the transverse mesocolon.

Sump Suction of the Presacral Space

There is still controversy among surgeons as to the value of drainage of the presacral space. There is general agreement among those who have used sump suction for drainage of the presacral space that the amounts of fluid aspirated postoperatively are impressive. Since this medium of serosanguineous fluid seems particularly suitable to nurture any contaminant in the pelvic field, logically, its removal would lessen the likelihood of pelvic abscess formation, especially since the raw surfaces resulting from deep pelvic surgery do not promote clearance of this material. I reported the technique of the Cleveland Clinic Foundation (Fazio, 1978) of applying irrigation to the pelvis as well as suction, since any accumulation of blood clot is not easily aspirated. Three liters of saline per 24 hours are used via a single or two sump drains with suction applied to two more Shirley sump drains for a period of 2 to 3 days until the aspirate is clear. After this, suction only is applied for 1 to 2 more days.

Temporary Fecal Diversion

Temporary fecal diversion may be accomplished either by loop transverse colostomy or loop ileostomy. The latter procedure is especially worth consideration if there is difficulty in exteriorizing the transverse colon after the splenic flexure has been fully mobilized. Furthermore, bowel function and care of the appliance is usually easier for patients with loop ileostomy than with loop colostomy. Incisional hernia is less frequently seen after ileostomy closure than after colostomy closure. There are specific situations when temporary fecal diversion should be used and others when it is desirable to do so. After stapled anastomosis, if intact "doughnuts" are not obtained (even if the suture line is reinforced) or if a leak is present after infusion of the rectal segment with irrigative material, then fecal diversion is provided. The surgeon will frequently judge that diversion is desirable if there has been undue contamination during the anastomosis, if there is excessive fecal loading of the colon, if previous pelvic irradiation has been given (above 3000 or 4000 rad), if a coloanal anastomosis has been made, or if the patient has some deleterious condition.

Prior to closure of the temporary stoma, usually 8 to 12 weeks from the time of anastomosis, proctoscopic and barium contrast roentgenographic evaluation of the anastomosis is done.

METHODS TO FACILITATE CONSTRUCTION OF THE STAPLED LOW COLORECTAL ANASTOMOSIS

With the low colorectal anastomosis, visibility in the pelvis is usually restricted and access is often limited by the narrow nature of the pelvis. This is particularly true in obese and male patients. At times transsection of the rectum below the cancer can lead to the virtual disappearance of the rectal stump as it retracts to the level of the levator muscles.

Access and visibility can be improved by using an incision extending from the xiphoid to the pubic bone. Reflecting the small intestine, outside of the abdomen, upwards and to the right of the patient provides further exposure. A fiberoptic lighted Dever retractor, in addition to a conventional self-retaining retractor, is also useful, especially for a retroprostatic anastomosis. An experienced assistant is invaluable.

Despite having the optimum conditions described previously, difficulties may still be encountered. However, a number of techniques can be used to overcome them.

END-TO-END ANASTOMOSIS

Use of Stay Sutures on the Rectal Cuff

To facilitate placement of the distal purse-string suture, it is desirable to keep tension on the cut edge of the rectum with proximal traction. Long Babcock clamps are useful but may get in the way, especially if only one assistant is available. Placement of four sutures around the circumference of the cut edge is particularly useful as an alternative (Fig. 12–2). As the surgeon places the over-and-over Proline suture, traction on individual stay sutures replaces the need for tissue forceps (Fig. 12–3).

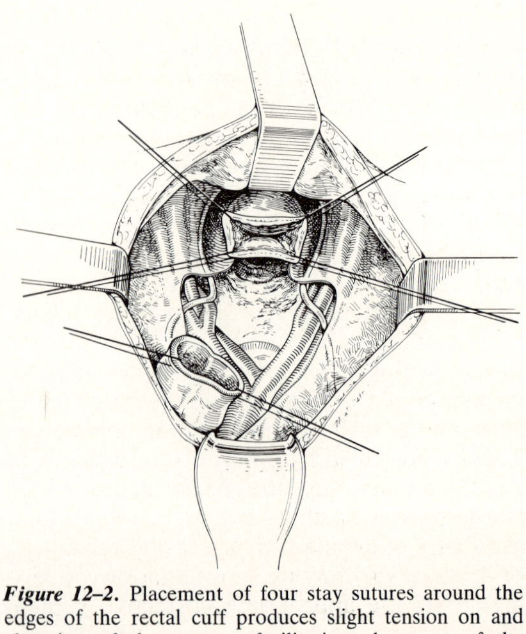

Figure 12–2. Placement of four stay sutures around the edges of the rectal cuff produces slight tension on and elevation of the rectum, facilitating placement of the purse-string suture.

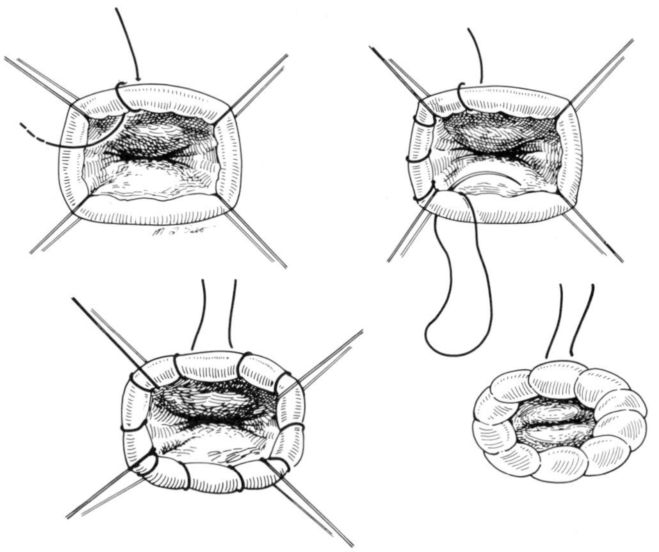

Figure 12–3. Using an over-and-over suture of No. 20 Proline, the surgeon takes minimal bites of the bowel edge to complete the purse-string. Traction on two of the stay sutures obviates the need for tissue forceps. The ends of the suture emerge at the anterior aspect of the rectal cuff. With tension applied *before* making a surgeon's knot, the bowel edge is gathered evenly around the shaft of the instrument.

Perineal Pressure

Blunt perineal pressure, applied by an assistant's gloved fist, may improve access for placing the distal purse-string in critical situations by elevating the rectal segment an inch or two more than previously possible.

Traction of the Specimen

As an alternative to the use of stay sutures on the rectal cuff, the surgeon may choose to use the mobilized sigmoid and rectum as tractors. A linen tape is placed below the cancer so that the lumen is occluded. At the chosen line of resection, the anterior wall of the rectum is incised, leaving the posterior wall intact. This keeps the rectal cuff elevated, providing access to purse-string placement. With continued encirclement of the cuff with the Proline suture, the posterior rectal wall is further incised until separation is completed. A Babcock clamp, stay suture, or tissue forceps may then be used to complete the last centimeter or so of the purse-string closure.

END-TO-END ANASTOMOSIS THROUGH THE STAPLED END OF RECTUM (FIG. 12–4)

In recent years Knight and Griffin (1980) have reported the results of their use of end-to-end anastomosis through the stapled end of the rectum and have promoted interest in this technique. After preliminary mobilization of the rectum, it is stapled across below the rectal cancer using the TA55 or TA30 linear stapler. The bowel is divided above the staple line. The EEA is then introduced into the rectum after first removing the anvil. The instrument

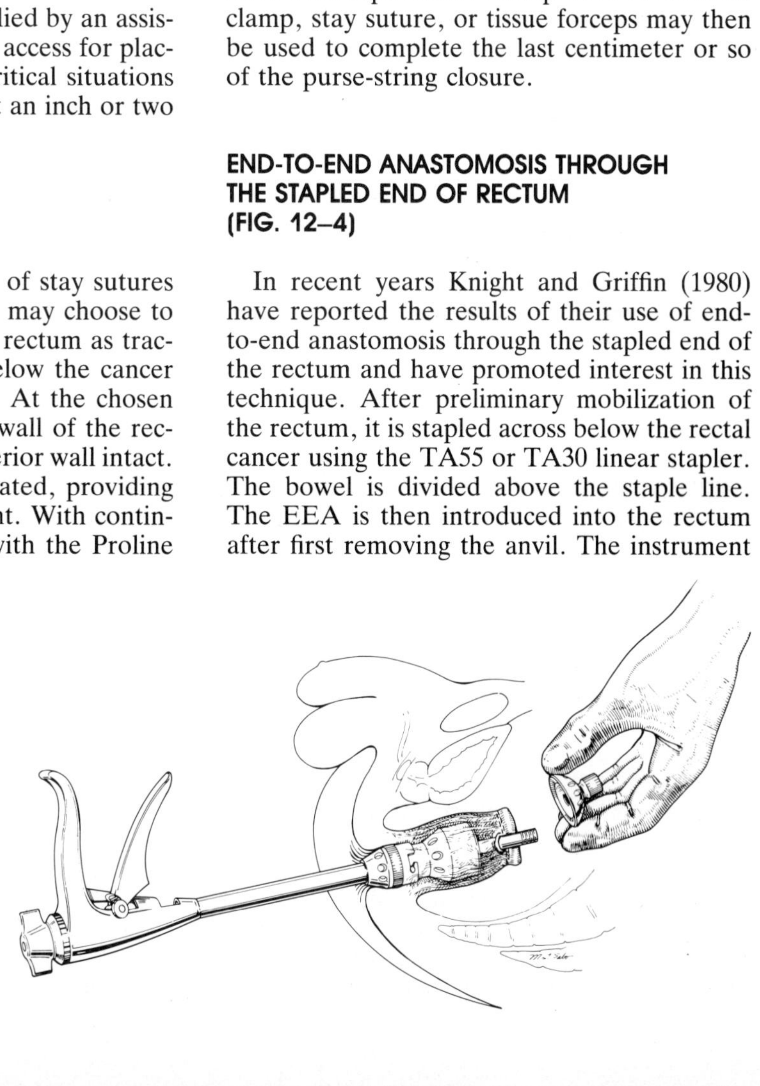

Figure 12–4. Modified end-to-end anastomosis using the EEA. After closure of the rectal segment with the TA55 stapler, the instrument *without the anvil,* is inserted into the prepared rectum. The shaft is brought through or immediately adjacent to the stapled suture line and the anvil is reattached. The colon segment is then drawn over the anvil and its purse-string is tied. The technique obviates the need for placement of a rectal purse-string.

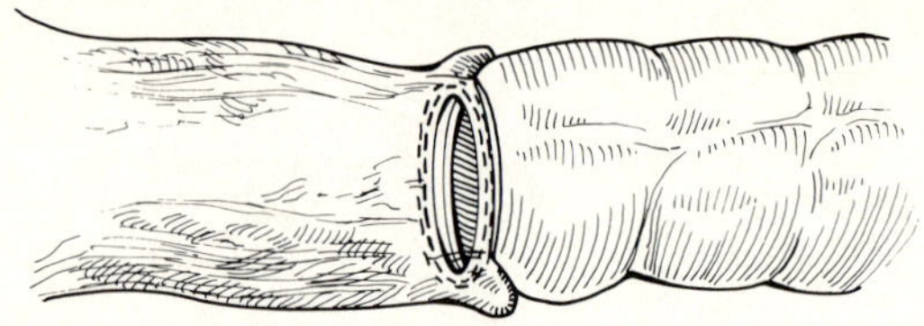

Figure 12–5. The anastomosis is completed. The major drawback of this technique is the need to cut through and staple across an existing staple line. Furthermore, it is sometimes very difficult to gain access to the distal rectum with a linear stapler.

is advanced until the shaft of the instrument abuts against the staple line of the rectal cuff. From the abdomen an incision is made over the shaft; the shaft is pushed through and the anvil is applied. The colon is then tied over the anvil in the usual way. No rectal purse-string is used, and the anastomosis is made as described in the previous section (Fig. 12–5).

The attraction of this operation is that the need for a distal purse-string is obviated and contamination is minimized. There are problems with this technique; for example, it is at times difficult to place a linear stapler deep in the pelvis. However, the major concern is that the EEA blade is required to cut across a row of steel staples; this maneuver is contrary to surgical principles and lacks the endorsement of the manufacturer. Notwithstanding this, continued favorable experiences using this technique are being reported. However, at present I would counsel against this practice, although the use of absorbable staples in the linear staplers may make this a popular alternative to conventional or stapled end-to-end anastomosis.

END-TO-END ANASTOMOSIS USING TRANSANAL PLACEMENT OF THE PURSE-STRING SUTURE ON THE RECTAL CUFF

Following anterior proctosigmoidectomy, the rectal cuff may come to lie at the level of the levator muscles, and despite perineal pressure or other maneuvers, the surgeon may have difficulty placing the distal purse-string suture to his satisfaction. Following anal dilatation (four fingers for two to three minutes) and introduction of an anal speculum, provided the anorectal segment is not particularly long, the purse-string suture may be applied transanally. With this method it is critical that the purse-string suture is placed with exactitude so that the bites incorporate very little tissue and are so placed that the suture will "run" evenly on applying tension and gaps will not be left between the sutures. A fiberoptic light attached to the retractor or speculum is very useful. Adequate mobilization of the rectal cuff is critical. The entire head of the instrument is then advanced through the rectal purse-string, and the proximal colon is tied down over the anvil. The instrument is withdrawn until the shaft between the anvil and the cartridge is visible. The rectal purse-string is tied using a surgeon's knot from the rectal luminal aspect. (Short retractors are used to check that the tie is satisfactory.) Breakage of the tie at this point is particularly frustrating, therefore "educated" tension in the purse-string is used. The method for completion of the anastomosis is outlined in a previous section.

This technique is useful for patients with bulky tumors or with a narrow pelvis. It can be difficult to apply this technique in certain male patients in whom there may be a long anal canal or pronounced sphincter tone.

END-TO-END ANASTOMOSIS USING THE TRANSSACRAL APPROACH

End-to-end anastomosis using the transsacral approach is a modification of the operation of Localio and associates (1980) and is used to facilitate placement of the distal purse-string suture. Certainly, the exposure with this technique is excellent. Lazorethes of Toulouse has also added a modification, in which a partial division of the sphincters is done (somewhat similar to the York-Mason operation). This further facilitates placement of the distal purse-string. The sphincters are repaired after the anastomosis is made.

These variations have not been used in our unit because they seem somewhat excessive and require considerable care in positioning the patient to allow both abdominal and perineal exposure. Furthermore, breakdown of the sphincter repair is a potential risk. Nevertheless, Lazorethes has described excellent results and minimal morbidity with the use of this technique.

SIDE-TO-END ANASTOMOSIS

The hand-sutured side-to-end colorectal anastomosis (Baker, 1950) offers considerable advantages to the surgeon by providing rea-

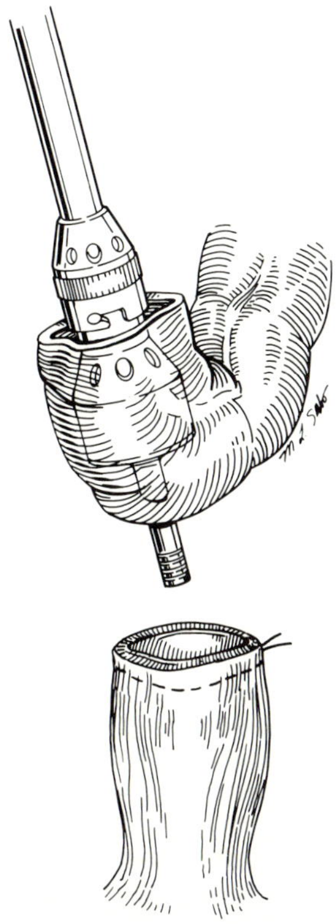

Figure 12–6. Side-to-end anastomosis using the EEA. The shaft of the instrument is advanced into the open colon end and brought through the antimesenteric aspect of the colon. The anvil is then attached.

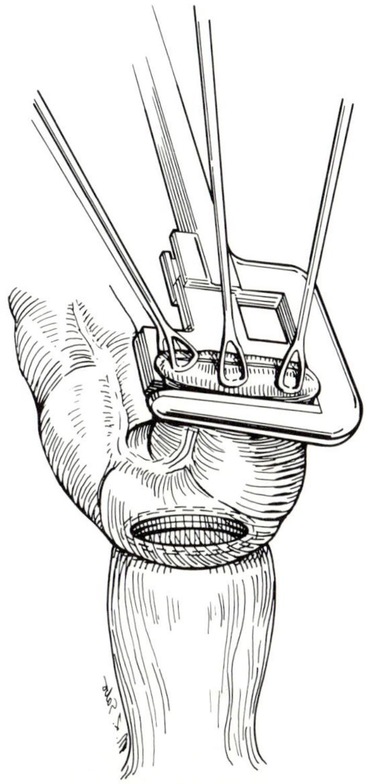

Figure 12–8. After constructing the stapled anastomosis, the end of the colon is closed with the TA55 or TA90 linear stapler, and redundant bowel beyond the stapler is excised.

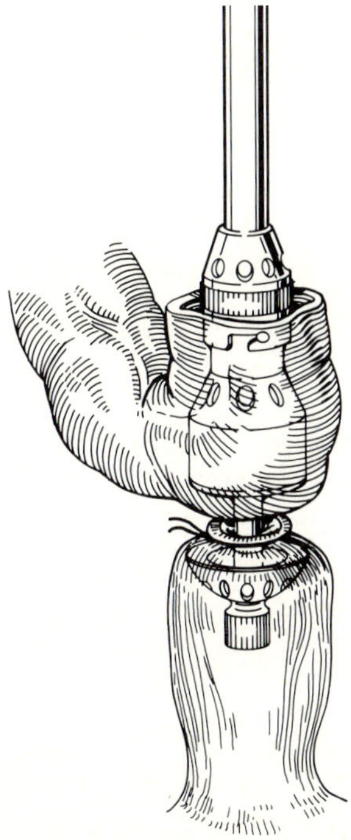

Figure 12–7. The rectal purse-string is tied, and the anvil and cartridge are approximated.

sonable visibility while he is placing individual sutures. In certain circumstances, this technique has value when using the circular stapler, especially when the proximal colon is bulky or the lumen is considerably dilated.

After placing the distal (rectal) purse-string suture, the circular stapler is inserted through the open end of the colon after first removing the anvil. The shaft is brought through the antimesenteric border of the colon (Fig. 12–6), and the anvil is reattached to the shaft. The anvil is placed into the open rectal cuff and the purse-string is tied (Fig. 12–7). The instrument is fired without the need for a colonic purse-string. The instrument is withdrawn, the tissue rings are checked, and the open colonic end is closed with the TA55 linear stapler (Fig. 12–8).

END-TO-SIDE ANASTOMOSIS

End-to-side anastomosis is useful when there is limited access to the pelvis, such as occurs in the narrow male pelvis. This method has an obvious advantage over the one outlined in the section on end-to-end anastomosis using

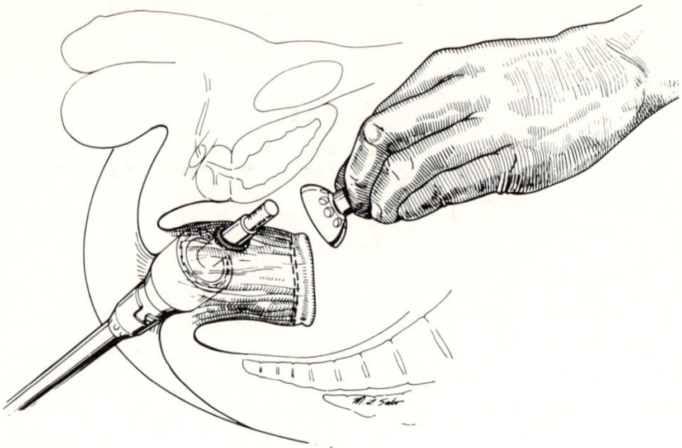

Figure 12–9. End-to-side anastomosis using the EEA. The shaft is advanced through the anterior rectal wall after closure of the rectal segment with the stapler. The anvil is reapplied.

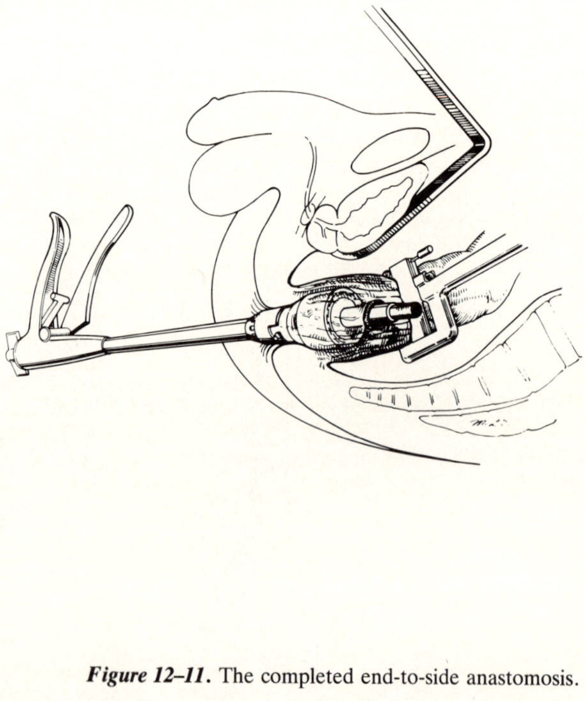

Figure 12–10. In a variation of the method seen in Figure 12–9, the linear stapler is left attached to allow slight upward traction on the specimen. (For clarity, the shaft is depicted coming through the lateral wall of the rectum.)

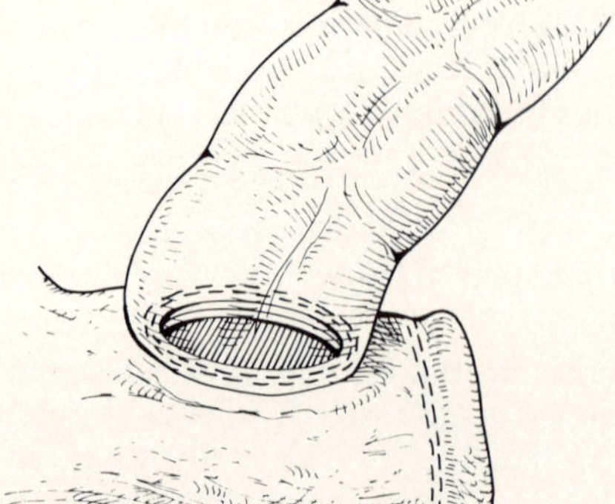

Figure 12–11. The completed end-to-side anastomosis.

the Knight-Griffin approach because the surgeon does not have to cut across steel staples. However, there is a need for a greater length of rectum than in the latter case and clearly a coloanal or ultra low colorectal anastomosis could not be constructed in this way. The other major use for this anastomosis is the establishment of bowel continuity after a previous Hartmann operation, especially one done for diverticular disease. In that situation, identification and mobilization of the rectal stump can be quite difficult. With this technique, minimal mobilization of the rectum is required, but good clearance of the anterior rectal wall is needed.

The instrument is introduced without the anvil per rectum (a plastic condom over the anvil will minimize trauma to the bowel mucosa), and the abdominal operator determines the optimal place for the shaft to penetrate (Fig. 12–9). The anvil is then reapplied to the shaft. A variation of this method is to leave the TA55 instrument attached to the rectal segment after firing (Fig. 12–10) so that cephalad traction may be applied. The proximal colon can then be advanced over the anvil, after resecting the specimen, and the anastomosis is completed (Fig. 12–11).

THE PULL-THROUGH TECHNIQUE

As pointed out previously, the problems with low anastomoses, using staple techniques, lay mainly in placing the purse-string suture on the rectal cuff in an exact manner. Despite all the maneuvers listed, the shape of the pelvis

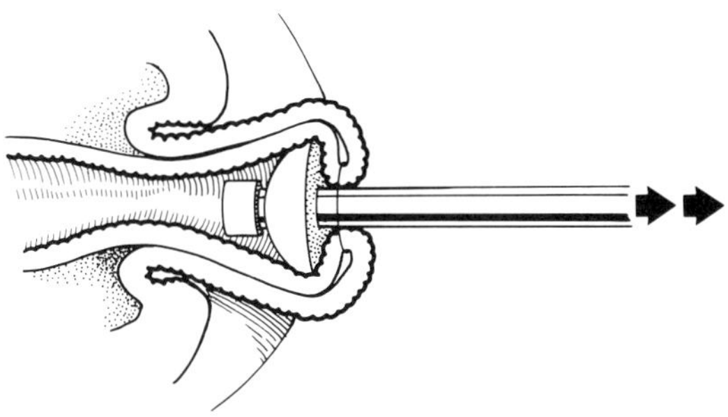

Figure 12–13. Traction on the obturator produces eversion of the lower rectal segment, simulating procidentia of the rectum.

may make the construction of such an anastomosis very difficult indeed. This may be deduced by the operator after full mobilization of the rectum has been carried out. The pull-through technique is particularly useful in the male patient with a very narrow pelvis and in whom transsection of the rectum below the cancer leaves a rectal cuff of 1 to 2 cm above the anorectal ring.

This operation is performed with the patient placed in Lloyd-Davies stirrups in the modified lithotomy-Trendelenburg position. The perineum is separately prepared and draped. After full rectal mobilization is carried out by the abdominal operator, a heavy silk or linen tie is used to occlude the rectum below the cancer. An obturator, such as one used with a rigid sigmoidoscope, is inserted into the prepared rectum (Fig. 12–12). (Shown in diagram is an obturator with a design similar to that of the shaft and anvil of the EEA instrument.) A stout silk ligature is tied around the rectum below the head of the obturator. Traction on the obturator (Fig. 12–13) produces eversion of the lower rectal segment, simulating a full-thickness rectal procidentia.

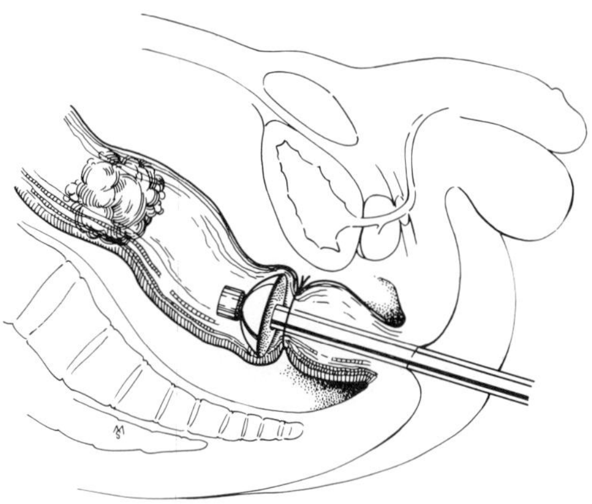

Figure 12–12. The pull-through operation using the EEA stapler. After full mobilization of the rectum, a linen tie (not shown) occludes the rectal lumen below the cancer. A stout silk ligature is tied below the head of the obturator.

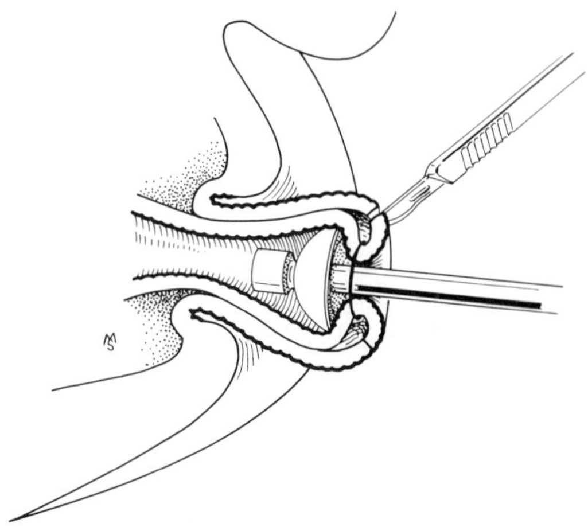

Figure 12–14. Incision of prolapsed rectum through all layers until underlying rectal serosa is seen.

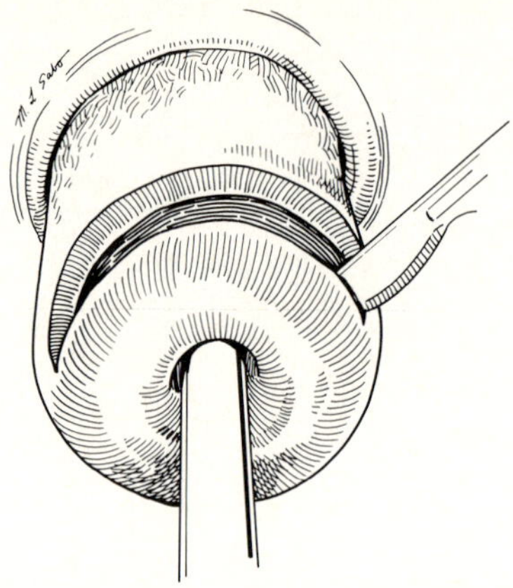

Figure 12–15. After about half the circumference of the everted bowel incised, a No. 20 Proline purse-string suture is applied.

The perineal operator then incises the mucosal aspect of the everted rectum just below the head of the obturator. The incision is carried through all layers of the outer (lower) rectal segment for about half of the circumference of the everted bowel. The serosal aspect of the rectum at the level of the obturator is exposed (Figs. 12–14 and 12–15).

At this point, the surgeon places the purse-string suture of No. 20 Proline into the cut edge of the everted rectum under direct vision while an assistant maintains gentle traction on the stem of the obturator. Continued circumferential sectioning of the everted rectum is performed, placing more Proline sutures as visibility improves until the purse-string is complete (Fig. 12–16).

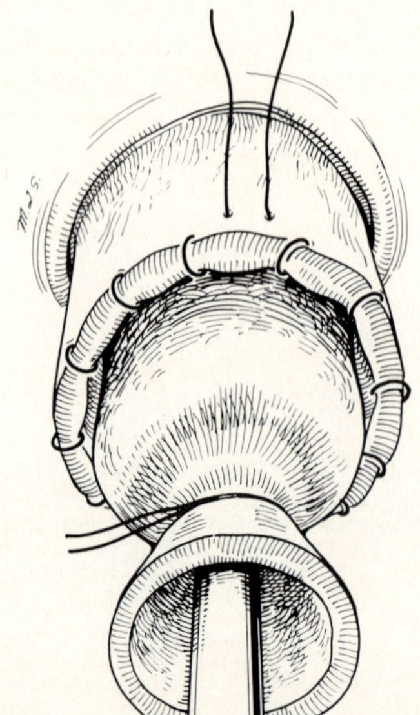

Figure 12–16. Sutures are placed at intervals around the bowel edge, serially sectioning the lower rectal segment. Visibility for exact placement of sutures is excellent.

The surgeon now has two alternatives with respect to the next phase of the operation. If the cancer or mesorectum is not particularly bulky, the specimen may be delivered through the rectal stump by continued traction on the obturator stem. This is done until a point corresponding to the junction of the sigmoid colon and descending colon has been reached. (A previously placed identifying suture is useful.) The specimen may then be transsected, leaving the pulled-through colon segment protruding beyond the everted rectum. This open end is prepared as for a "conventional" stapled anastomosis, and the second purse-string suture is placed.

This purse-string is tied down over the shaft of the EEA after the anvil has been inserted into the open colon (Fig. 12–17). The instrument is advanced into the pelvis, guidance being provided by the abdominal operator (Fig. 12–18). The anvil and the cartridge are then approximated by clockwise rotation of the wing nut (Fig. 12–19). This is continued until the tissue gap setting is appropriate, and then the instrument is fired and withdrawn (Fig. 12–20).

The second alternative may be used when tumor bulk or other circumstances indicate that a problem may occur when the specimen is pulled through the everted rectum (Fig. 12–21). Instead of resecting the tumor segment from below, the specimen (with the obturator) is delivered into the abdomen. The obturator is removed (in the case shown in Figure 12–21, this is simply achieved by unscrewing the anvil from the obturator stem). The specimen is resected. The proximal colon is prepared and a purse-string suture placed. The EEA is then introduced transanally and the proximal colon is tied down over the anvil. The instru-

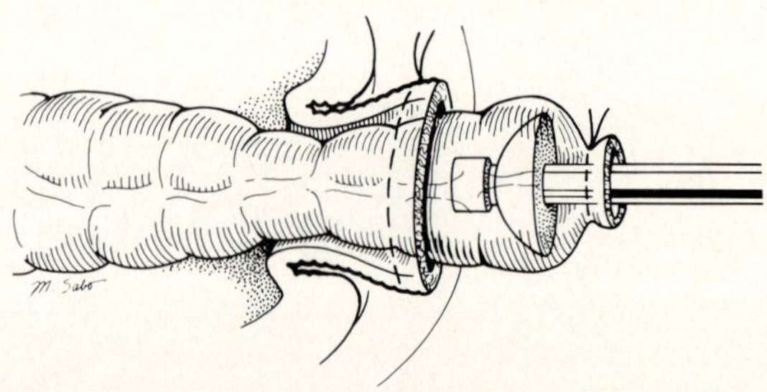

Figure 12–17. After delivery through the everted rectum, the specimen is resected, a purse-string suture is applied to the protruding colon segment, and the anvil of the EEA is introduced into the colon. The purse-string is tied.

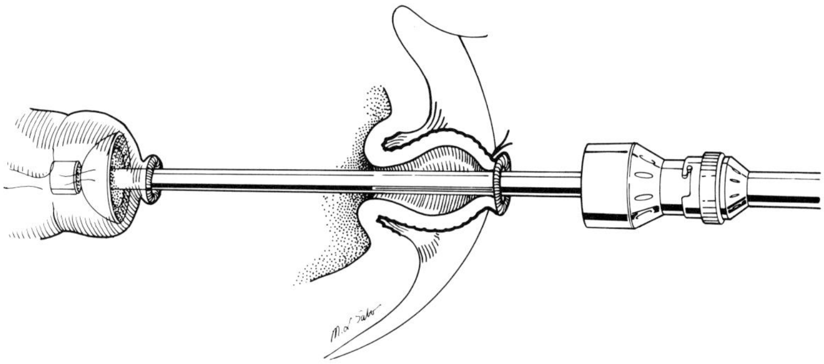

Figure 12–18. The EEA is advanced into the pelvis, and the rectal pursestring is tied around the shaft. (For clarity, the shaft is depicted as excessively long.)

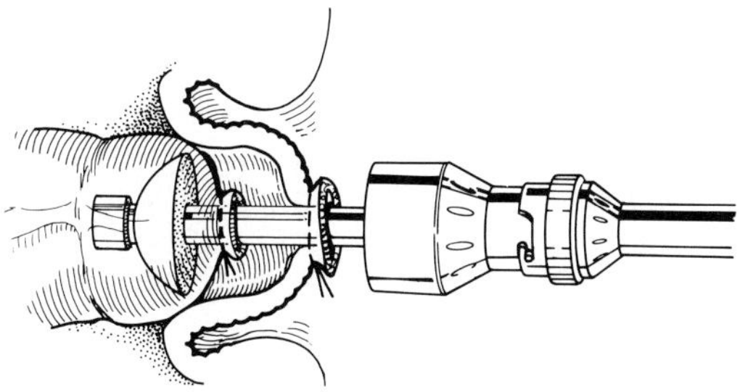

Figure 12–19. The anvil and the cartridge are approximated.

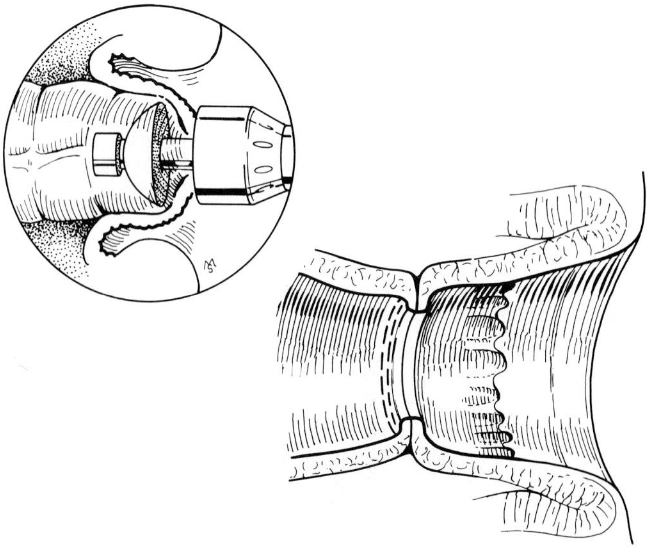

Figure 12–20. The tissue gap setting is checked, the instrument is fired and withdrawn. The anastomosis "rises" into the pelvis.

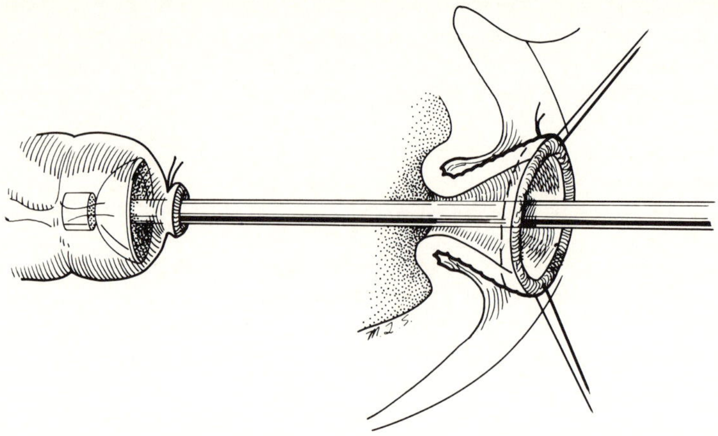

Figure 12–21. When tumor bulk prevents delivery of the specimen through the everted rectum, the following method is used. The obturator stem and the attached specimen are delivered into the abdomen, and the specimen is resected from above. The EEA is advanced into the abdomen through the everted rectum, and the proximal purse-string is tied over the anvil. The instrument is withdrawn until the cartridge emerges. The rectal purse-string is tied, and the procedure outlined in Figure 12–19 is followed.

ment is withdrawn until the cartridge is seen emerging beyond the everted rectum. The distal purse-string is tied. The anastomosis is completed in the usual way.

Dr. Frank L. Weakley in our department has had considerable experience with this stapled pull-through operation. His preference has been to use the first of the two alternatives listed. Although my own experience has been considerably less, only five cases, I have chosen to use the second of the two alternatives in the instances previously described. The procedure is somewhat reminiscent of the Maunsell-Weir operation in which a primary hand anastomosis is done after initial mobilization and resection, instead of a delayed anastomosis, as in the case of the Turnbull-Cutait operation (Cutait and Figliolini, 1961; Turnbull and Cuthbertson, 1961). I believe that there is a place for this pull-through operation in the occasional situation when the experienced surgeon believes that an anastomosis will be difficult to construct even with the use of alternative maneuvers.

PITFALLS, PROBLEMS, AND POSSIBLE SOLUTIONS WHEN USING THE CIRCULAR STAPLING DEVICE

Several pitfalls and problems with the use of the circular stapling device have been discussed or alluded to already. Premature firing of the staples while the cartridge is being advanced onto the instrument has not been seen in our department in several years. There is no risk of this occurring at all if disposable instruments are used. The surgeon must confirm that the knurled knob on the anvil is screwed down flush with the end of the shaft; otherwise, an excessive tissue gap occurs at the time of firing the instrument. The problems with the use of modified Furniss clamp have already been discussed. Clearance of the mesentery must be adequate without allowing for possible ischemia to the bowel end. In practice this amounts to a clearance of only 1 to 2 cm of the mesenteric margin. Specifics of placement by hand and tying of the purse-string suture were outlined previously. Other difficulties are now discussed.

Difficulty in Advancing the Instrument

With transanal use of the EEA, difficulty in advancing the instrument is encountered more when constructing the high than the low anastomosis. Also, the flat nature of the anvil of the EEA is not well suited to allow negotiation of the instrument through intestine. Recently, however, this has been modified. When the rectal lumen is somewhat contracted, such as when there has been a previous colonic diversion, use of the circular stapler may be impossible altogether or may require a smaller cartridge size, which in turn has its own set of disadvantages. Previous pelvic surgery may produce considerable tethering of the rectum to the sacrum, which is caused by fibrosis. There may be an advantage then in using the curved circular stapler. This is the only indication for the use of this type of stapler in pelvic surgery. It is the responsibility of the abdominal operator to guide the instrument in its cephalad course. Occasionally, I have worn a second glove at this point, placed the index finger into the open rectum and, after palpating the anvil, directed the assistant in advancing the instrument. The second glove is then discarded.

When using the instrument by way of a proximal colotomy, it is important to make the colotomy fairly close to the end of the colon, that is, about 7 to 8 cm away. This is done so that the colonic traverse, and the likelihood of mucosal trauma, are limited. This option may indeed be chosen if the rectal lumen is somewhat narrowed but the rectal cuff itself is reasonably large. The colotomy is then closed in two layers in the transverse axis.

Difficulty in the Extraction of the Instrument

There is difficulty extracting the instrument when the bites on the bowel edge by the purse-string suture have been excessive, leading to an excessive bulk of tissue between the purse-string and the shaft. Incomplete severing of this tissue and the bowel wall by the circular blade prevents instrument withdrawal. Attempts at withdrawal produce intussusception of the anastomosis into the rectal segment. If the sectioning of bowel ends is nearly complete, firm withdrawal of the instrument with countertraction on the anastomosis may complete the section, sometimes leaving a tongue of mucosa on one of the "doughnuts." In other circumstances, the entire anastomosis may have to be redone.

Difficulty in the extraction of the instrument may be encountered in a more benign form when there has been a snug fit of the bowel end over the anvil. Extraction is then facilitated by using a lateral and downward rotatory motion in withdrawing the instrument. This is a special advantage of the ILS instrument because a metal rim on the anvil surface may be used to gently "lever" the anastomosis away from the instrument. Guy sutures on the quadrants of the anastomosis also facilitate extraction under these circumstances. Some of these difficulties may be minimized by preliminary dilatation of the proximal colon end. Glucagon and topical lidocaine (Xylocaine) have not been useful in my experience.

Incomplete "Doughnuts" and Anastomotic Leakage

Following withdrawal of the instrument, the "doughnuts" are orientated in relation to their respective positions on the anastomotic line. Defects in the "doughnuts" can then indicate where the anastomosis is deficient. Even if the anastomosis does not leak after insufflation with Betadine, it should be regarded as deficient if the "doughnut(s)" are incomplete. For the high colorectal anastomosis there is little difficulty in placing sutures by hand to turn in this defect. For the low anastomosis, this can also be attempted. If access prevents placement of these sutures, then transanal placement of No. 30 chromic catgut on a ¾ circle needle may be possible. Betadine testing should then be repeated. When neither method is possible, provided the leak on Betadine testing is small, temporary colostomy and sump drainage of the presacral space are advised. If there is a major leak or obvious major dehiscence, then the surgeon must judge the respective merits of performing abdominoperineal excision of the rectum; redoing of the stapled anastomosis; or using another method, such as the conventional pull-through operation. I have on two occasions followed the last course.

It must be stressed that the finding of intact "doughnuts" in no way assures that the anastomosis is intact. Forcible extraction of the instrument can produce considerable anastomotic trauma. In the final analysis, anastomotic leaks and incomplete "doughnuts" result from faulty surgical technique with respect to placement of the purse-string suture.

Bleeding

Bleeding rarely occurs with stapled colonic anastomoses. In fact, I have not encountered one case. Smith (1981) reported 19 cases (0.5 percent) in a poll of members of the American Society of Colon and Rectal Surgeons.

Stricture

It is difficult to define the term stricture because all anastomoses (of the inversion type) produce a degree of narrowing after operation. Furthermore, most cases of stricture, even with "significant" narrowing of the lumen, eventually dilate so that proctoscopic recognition of the problem is difficult after six months have passed from the time of operation. "Stricture" has arbitrarily been defined as a narrowing that does not allow easy passage of a pediatric proctoscope (15-mm diameter). Only two pa-

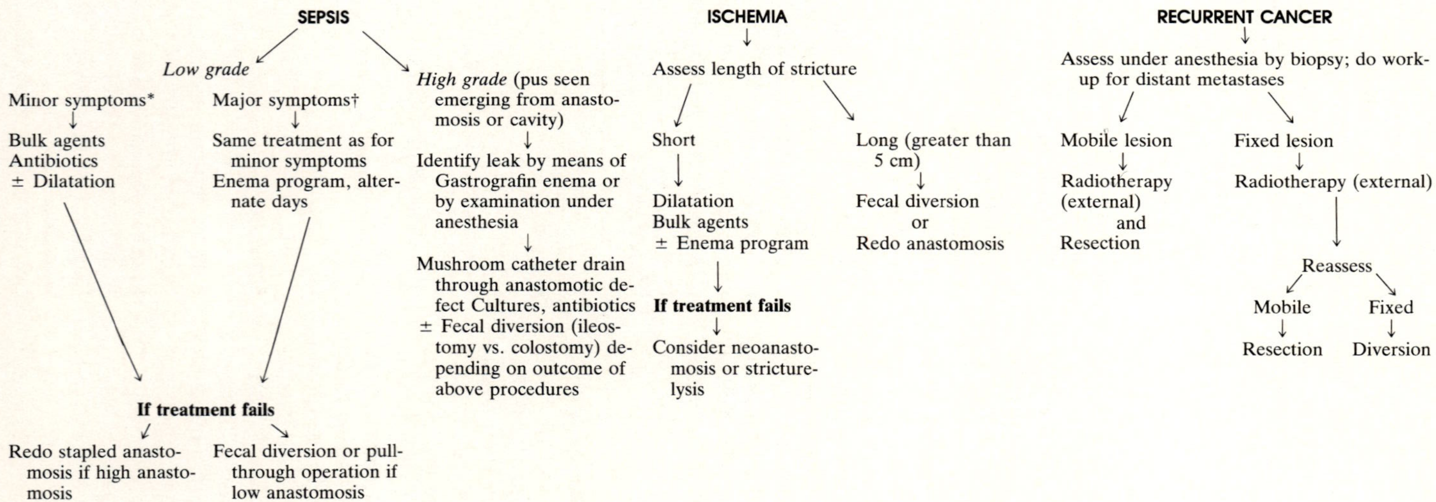

*Minor symptoms: Some disability due to diarrhea/constipation, urgency, tenderness, incontinence
†Major symptoms: Major disability due to diarrhea/constipation, urgency, tenderness, incontinence, pain

Figure 12–22. Guidelines for management of anastomotic stricture following stapled colorectal anatomosis.

tients of 183 undergoing rectal anastomoses in the author's series had evidence of this. One of these required dilatation on one occasion. Smith (1981), however, reported 315 strictures in 3594 cases (8.8 percent); it is probable that the definitions of stricture used by the surgeons polled in that survey varied. Nevertheless, it is probable that most of those cases did pose some problems for the surgeons involved.

Ischemia, sepsis, and recurrent cancer constitute the major causes of stricture. In the early postoperative period, edema of the anastomosis is usual, and it is uncommon that an adult-sized rigid proctoscope can be passed through the anastomosis without difficulty until a month or more has passed by. Digital palpation of the anastomosis may indicate that a "fin" stricture or web has formed. This is fairly easily broken down by the surgeon's finger. The occurrence of this web is related to the fact that the B form of the staples provides excellent inversion of the anastomosis and good serosal apposition of the bowel ends but poor mucosal apposition. The raw surface of the mucosa can abut against another segment of mucosa, producing a partial web, or granulation tissue may become exuberant on the exposed edge of the mucosa. This profuse growth of tissue, along with neo-epithelialization, may produce an exaggerated mucosal fold.

After one or several months, anastomotic narrowing is usually consequent upon sepsis or a degree of ischemia. Sepsis results from an occult or overt suture line leak. In this situation, the anastomosis is not only strictured but also considerably indurated. Treatment depends on a number of factors. The length of the stricture is assessed by barium or Gastrografin contrast studies or alternatively by endoscopy, using the pediatric gastroscope. Other factors are outlined in Figure 12–22, along with guidelines for management.

Bowel Function after Low Anterior Resection

Following construction of a low anastomosis (or coloanal anastomosis), the reservoir or storage capacity of the rectum is essentially removed. Bowel actions increase in number from four to ten per day. Continence is almost always preserved provided that there is reasonable access to toilet facilities.Urgency remains a problem for several weeks to months, depending on the amount of rectal reservoir remaining. When urgency is a problem, the patient is advised to use enemas every second or third day for 8 to 10 weeks. This acts in a way similar to colostomy irrigation, except that in this case the patient is able to "hold" an enema. Lane and Parks (1977) studied the anal sphincters of 12 patients in whom a coloanal anastomosis had been made. They determined that receptors for distention and "rectal sensation" lay not in the rectal wall, which was surgically removed, but probably in the levator muscles themselves. Provided that the sphincter mechanism itself was not disturbed at operation or subsequently by sepsis, then good functional results could be expected. In a study by Smith (1981), 124 patients (3.5 percent) had variable degrees of incontinence. Of the 124 patients, 79 were incontinent of gas, 40 of liquid, and only five of stool. Most patients, however, had undergone construction of a high anastomosis.

Local Recurrence of Cancer

One of the major concerns with respect to stapled anastomoses has been that with this "new" facility to perform more sphincter-saving operations, surgeons may "cheat" in obtaining an adequate margin of clearance distally. There is good evidence that more sphincter-preserving operations for cancers located in the upper and middle thirds of the rectum have been performed by surgeons in the United States in the late 1970s than in the early 1970s (Mettlin et al., 1981). The increasing rate of such operations cannot be ascribed only to the use of stapling instruments. At present the number of patients for study (i.e., those having anterior rectal resection with stapled anastomosis for cancer with 5 or more years of follow-up) are too few for critical analysis. Nevertheless, local recurrence rates at 2 years after operation have been reported by Heald and associates (1982). When operating for cure, Heald and associates found that not one of 50 patients had local recurrence. Eight percent had liver metastases and a further 4 percent had distant metastases elsewhere. In our own series, in which the Turnbull-Cutait pull-through operation was used, pelvic recurrence of cancer was noted in 5.5 percent of patients (Kirwan et al., 1978). In this operation, the extent of rectal resection is the same as that in low-stapled anastomosis.

In the end analysis, I suspect that the frequency of local recurrence of cancer will remain the same whether a hand-sutured or stapled anastomosis is used. Other things being equal, any increase in pelvic recurrence rates with autosuture methods would indicate that the surgeons are not performing adequate cancer operations. Establishment of intestinal continuity is a secondary concern.

METHODS OF STUDY AND RESULTS OF RECTAL ANASTOMOSES USING THE EEA

From July 1978 to February 1982, the author performed 241 stapled intestinal anastomoses using the EEA in 232 patients. Of these, 183 anastomoses were made involving the rectal segment. The cases were consecutive. As part of a prospective study to determine leak rates from the anastomosis, a Gastrografin enema was given to each patient between the eighth and 12th postoperative day to radiographically assess the integrity of the anastomosis. Additionally, at this time proctoscopic evaluation was done in the first 36 patients to provide further information concerning the status of the anastomosis. Since this evaluation provided no more information of value than that obtained from contrast roentgenography alone, this practice of early postoperative proctoscopy was abandoned.

There were 21 patients with ileorectal anastomoses in whom the diagnoses were as follows: carcinoma of the colon, six patients; polyposis coli, four patients; Crohn's disease, seven patients; and ulcerative colitis, four patients. High colorectal anastomoses were made in 67 patients and low colorectal or coloanal anastomoses were made in 95 patients. A low colorectal anastomosis was defined as one in which the anastomosis is made to the extra peritoneal rectum, where the lateral ligaments of the rectum have been divided and the supralevator fascia has been displayed. In the group with high colorectal anastomoses, the following diagnoses were made: cancer, 37 patients; diverticulitis, 20 patients; Crohn's disease, six patients (ileorectosigmoid fistulae); villous adenoma, two patients; and one patient with teratoma and one with sigmoid volvulus. Almost all patients underoing low colorectal anastomosis or coloanal anastomosis had a diagnosis of cancer.

Table 12–1. **PROPORTION OF PATIENTS WITH RADIOLOGIC OR CLINICAL LEAKS***

Anastomosis	No. of Patients	Radiologic Leak	Clinical Leak
Ileorectal	21	1 (4.8%)	0
High CRA*	67	1 (1.5%)	0
Low CRA*	95	8 (8.4%)	5 (5.3%)
Total	183	10 (5.5%)	5 (2.7%)

*CRA = Colorectal anastomosis.

The proportion of patients with radiologic evidence of a leak or a clinical leak from their rectal anastomoses is indicated in Table 12–1. Most leaks occurred within the first year after the use of the circular stapler. As expected, the problems, determined both radiologically and clinically, were greatest with low colorectal anastomoses. A clinical leak was defined as one associated with signs of sepsis (leukocytosis, tachycardia, pyrexia) or evidence of pelvic abscess (ileus) or purulent discharge from the rectum or fecal fistula. One of the five patients with a clinical leak had a rectovaginal fistula following combined radiotherapy and total hysterectomy for carcinoma of the endometrium. Subsequently, a separate primary carcinoma of the midrectum was found for which resection and a low colorectal anastomosis were done. There were no patients with an abdominal wall fecal fistula. Four of the five patients with clinical leaks had had 3000 rad or more delivered to the pelvis prior to surgery, which indicates that irradiation may have contributed to the leaks. Nevertheless, it is my belief that, in general, a major factor was that of surgeon error in making purse-string sutures that took excessively large bites on the bowel edge.

Results from this experience in relation to anastomotic integrity compare well with those from other reports. Goligher and associates (1979) reported radiologic leak rates of 0 and 25 percent in 38 high and 24 low colorectal anastomoses, respectively. In the latter group, there was an 8 percent clinical leak rate. This was much lower than the 16 percent clinical leak rate reported by the same author, when hand-sutured techniques were used (Goligher et al., 1977). Heald and Leicester (1981) reported a 25 percent clinical leak rate in 61 patients undergoing colorectal anastomosis. Other reports of radiologic leak rates for stapled colorectal anastomoses have been in the 20 to 28 percent range (Dorricott et al., 1982; Taggart, 1981).

It is clear from this report and others that stapled anastomoses to the rectum can be done with relatively low rates of anastomotic breakdown. Most reports, including the present one, stress that a learning period is needed, during which difficulties in the use of the instrument can be encountered and a higher than expected rate of anastomotic complications may be seen.

To an extent, these difficulties can be minimized for surgeons new to stapling by gaining experience in stapling workshops, by using the technique initially in constructing high anastomoses, in which a technical error can be easily corrected, and by performing temporary colostomy more frequently if any concern is present about the integrity of an anastomosis. Interestingly, in seven of my patients in whom incomplete "doughnuts" necessitated reinforcement of the suture line and temporary colostomy, only one patient had a radiologic leak.

There are no clear guidelines one can offer with respect to the use of the optional techniques available to facilitate the construction of a stapled anastomosis, but the various considerations have been outlined in this chapter. There is the occasional patient in whom the rectal edge is so thin, friable, or short that a stapled anastomosis should not be attempted. In such a situation, a conventional pull-through operation should probably be performed.

For patients who have had extensive pelvic irradiation or whose colon and rectal calibers are small by virtue of longstanding diversion or if the surgeon is inexperienced with the use of autosuture, then the use of circular staples is contraindicated.

The concern expressed by some surgeons that resident training in hand-sewn anastomoses will suffer if circular stapling becomes the order of the day, can be partially dismissed by the fact that, to my knowledge, no teaching surgeon *always* uses staples for anastomotic construction. In the proximal colon and small intestine, hand-suturing is still the commonest method of joining bowel ends. It is true, however, that experience for residents in low colorectal anastomoses may well be limited with the use of the stapler in modern practice. However, one could argue that the use of the colonoscope has reduced the amount of experience that radiology residents get in barium enema examinations.

The more pressing concern regarding the possibility of increased rates of pelvic recurrence with the use of the circular stapler has been partially addressed in this chapter. In essence, only time will tell, and until then, the intellectual honesty of the surgeon in obtaining an adequate margin of pararectal tissue and bowel wall clearance will determine the propriety of a low anastomosis versus a Miles operation.

In 1978, in an elegant and eloquent editorial, Professor Hugh Dudley, Director of the Academic Surgical Unit of St. Mary's Hospital, London, England, argued persuasively for sphincter-preserving operations for cancer of the middle third of the rectum:

> And so, if I had a cancer of the midthird of the rectum which I hoped was Dukes' A or B but had to fear was Dukes C, what would I do? I am absolutely certain—and this I am sure will bring the wrath of most colorectal surgeons on my head, but no matter I would not have an abdomino-perineal resection with a colostomy. However managed, however much we delude ourselves, a permanent potentially incontinent abdominal anus is an affront difficult to bear, so that I marvel that we and our patients have put up with it so long. It says much for the social indifference of the one and the social fortitude of the other.
>
> Given my combination of rational and emotional antagonism to a colostomy, what would I have? If the surgeon (carefully selected, of course) thought it feasible, I would have as low an anterior resection as possible, asking him to preserve the posterior and lateral fascia of the pelvic wall as far as he could because my fast declining virility is transmitted through there and, though I want above all to live, I do not think a radical extrafascial dissection is going to make much difference except to the comfort and dignity of my dying days. If he can reconstruct, good luck to him and good hope for me. I would not press him to ensure an arbitrary 4 cm. of bowel distal to the tumour edge. I can, with appropriate techniques, hope for a very low incidence of complications from a properly performed anastomosis deep in the pelvis and, more recently, there is the prospect of either an endoanal procedure, or even perhaps some clever stapling manoevre.

Acknowledgement

I would like to thank Mark L. Sabo and Kathleen Jung, Department of Medical Illustration, Cleveland Clinic, for the artwork in this chapter. I would also like to thank Eleanor Stanton and Carol Fazio for their secretarial and editorial assistance in preparing the manuscript.

References

Allgöwer M, Durig M, Hochstetter AV, et al: The parasacral sphincter-splitting approach to the rectum. World J Surg 6:539, 1982.

Baker JW: Low end to side rectosigmoidal anastomoses: Description of a technique. Arch Surg 61:143–157, 1950.

Beart TW, Kelly KA: Randomized prospective evaluation of the EEA stapler for colorectal anastomosis. Am J Surg 141:143–147, 1981.

Cutait DE, Figliolini FJ: A new method of colorectal anastomosis in abdomino-perineal resection. Dis Colon Rectum 6:335–342, 1961.

Dorricott NJ, Baddeley RM, Keighley MR et al: Complications of rectal anastomoses with end-to-end anastomosis (EEA) stapling instrument. Clinical and radiological leak rates and some practical hints. Ann R Coll Surg Engl 64:171–174, 1982.

Dudley HAF: If I had carcinoma of the middle third of the rectum. Br J Surg 1:1035–1037, 1978.

Fazio VW: Sump suction and irrigation of the presacral space. Dis Colon Rectum 21:401–405, 1978.

Goligher JC, Lee PWR, Macfie J, et al: Experience with the Russian Model 249 suture gun for anastomosis of the rectum. Surg Gynecol Obstet 148:517–524, 1979.

Goligher JC, Lee PWR, Simpkins KC, Lintott DJ: A controlled comparison one- and two-layer techniques of suture for high and low colorectal anastomoses. Br J Surg. 64:609–614, 1977.

Goligher JC, Morris C, McAdam WA, et al: A controlled trial of inverting vs. everting intestinal suture in clinical large bowel surgery. Br J Surg 57:817–822, 1970.

Heald RJ: Towards fewer colostomies—the impact of circular stapling devices on the surgery of rectal cancer in a district hospital. Br J Surg 67:198–200, 1980.

Heald RJ, Husband EM, Ryall RD: The mesorectum in rectal cancer surgery—the clue to pelvic recurrence? Br J Surg 69:613–616, 1982.

Heald RJ, Leicester RJ: The low stapled anastomosis. Br J Surg 68:333–337, 1981.

Kirwan W, Turnbull RB Jr, Fazio VW, Weakley FL: Pull-through operation with delayed anastomosis for rectal cancer. Br J Surg 65:685–689, 1978.

Knight CD, Griffin FD: An improved technique for low anterior resection of the rectum using the EEA stapler. Surgery 88:710–714, 1980.

Kraske P: Zur extirpation hochsitzender mastdarmkrebse. Verh Dtsch Ges Chir 14:464, 1885.

Lane RH, Parks AG: Function of the anal sphincters following coloanal anastomosis. Br J Surg 64:596–599, 1977.

Localio SA, Eng K, Ransom JHC: Abdomino-sacral approach for retrorectal tumors. Ann Surg 191:555, 1980.

McLachlin AD, Olsson LS, Pitt DF: Anterior anastomosis of the rectosigmoid colon. An experimental study. Surgery 80:306–311, 1976.

Marks G: Combined abdominotranssacral reconstruction of the radiation-injured rectum. Am J Surg 131:54–59, 1976.

Mason AY: Surgical access to the rectum: a transsphincteric exposure. Proc Soc of Med (Suppl) 63, 91–94, 1970. Presented at International Conference on Proctology, June, 1969.

Mason AY: Trans-sphincteric surgery of the rectum. Prog Surg 13:66, 1974.

Mettlin C, Mittelman A, Nataraian N, et al: Trends in the United States for the management of adenocarcinoma of the rectum. Surg Gynecol Obstet 153:701–706, 1981.

Miles WE: A method of performing abdomino-perineal excision for carcinoma of the rectum and the terminal portion of the pelvic colon. Lancet 2:1812–1813, 1908.

Nichols R, Broido P, Condon RE: Effectiveness of preoperative neomycin-erythromycin intestinal preparation on the incidence of infectious complications following colon surgery. Ann Surg 178:453–462, 1973.

Parks AG: Per-anal anastomosis. World J Surg 7:531, 1982.

Smith LE: Anastomosis with EEA stapler after anterior colonic resection. Dis Colon Rectum 24:236–242, 1981.

Taggart RE: Colorectal anastomosis: factors influencing success. J Soc Med 74:111–118, 1981.

Turnbull RB JR, Cuthbertson AM: Abdomino-rectal pull-through resection for cancer and for Hirschsprung's disease. Cleve Clin Q 28:109–115, 1961.

THIRTEEN

Immunology and Immunotherapy of Colorectal Tumors

M. K. Wallack, M.D.
J. A. Wolf, M.D.
M. C. Michaelides, Ph.D.

Although there has been an unprecedented explosion of knowledge in basic immunology since the 1960s, very little has found practical application in the diagnosis and treatment of human cancer. Even the basic premise, that the cancer patient benefits from the stimulation of immune response, will not remain unchallenged. Although this point of view has been widely held, opposing views have been expressed by respected investigators (Prehn and Outzen, 1980). The crucial question is whether stimulation of immune responses in a tumor-bearing host will result in tumor regression or tumor enhancement. A related controversial issue concerns the immunogenicity of human tumors. It is generally agreed that viral and chemical carcinogen-induced animal tumors are immunogenic but that spontaneous animal tumors are not immunogenic. Is human cancer analogous to the spontaneous or to the carcinogen-induced malignancies? Facts supporting each point of view exist. This should be kept in mind as tumor immunity and immunotherapy are reviewed.

Human colorectal tumors are likely to be carcinogen-induced, and their antigenicity will be discussed. Furthermore, results from investigations of syngeneic animal colon cancer models will be presented. The development of hybridoma technology has permitted the production of monoclonal antibodies directed to colorectal tumors; their properties will be reviewed. Finally, an update on the status of clinical immunotherapy for colorectal cancer will be provided.

IMMUNOBIOLOGY OF EXPERIMENTAL COLON TUMORS

The syngeneic animal colon tumor models include rat and mouse models. These chemically induced colon tumors were developed following the description of colon tumor induction in rats with 1,2-dimethylhydrazine (DMH) by Druckrey in 1967. The rat colon tumors have been investigated most extensively. They have been used in research on primary colon tumors, on serially transplanted tumors, and on cultured lines derived from primary tumors. Reports on the murine colon tumors are fewer, and most of them refer to serially transplanted tumors from the parental primary malignancy or to cultured colon cancer lines.

Rat Colon Tumor Model

The chemically induced rat colon tumors are histologically similar to human colon tumors but are more likely to develop in multiple areas of the colon. Furthermore, liver metastases are very rare in the rat model, and there is no evidence for circulating oncofetal antigens in the cancer-bearing hosts, analogous to carcinoembryonic antigen (CEA) in humans. Most extensive investigations on the rat tumor model have been reported by Sjögren and his colleagues Bansal and Steele. Others have made significant contributions as well, and the findings obtained with this model will be reviewed.

Evidence for Existence of Specific Tumor-Associated Antigens (TAAs)

Rats bearing colon tumors develop both cell-mediated and humoral immunity to these tumors. Cell-mediated immunity was first demonstrated by tests in which lymphocytes from rats bearing colon tumors were cytotoxic for the colon carcinoma cells in vitro (Steele and Sjögren, 1974). This is analogous to the findings described by the Hellströms for patients with colorectal cancer. Such lymphocytes could be obtained from rats bearing primary or isografted colon tumors or immunized with rat colon tumor cells. This cytotoxicity was specific for rat colon cancer cells and fetal gut cells and was not observed with normal kidney, normal adult colon mucosa, polyoma tumor, mammary carcinoma, or fibroadenoma. The TAAs involved in the microcytotoxicity assay in vitro were cross-reactive among rat colon carcinomas induced by three different chemical carcinogens in two distinct rat strains. This cell-mediated immunity was maintained for a long time after tumor removal.

Cell-mediated immunity was investigated in vivo by isograft rejection. Results from this study have suggested the presence of strong "unique" antigens and of weak "common" tissue-type antigens. These conclusions were drawn from experiments in which groups of rats were immunized with rat colon cancer (Steele and Sjögren, 1977; Sjögren, 1981). All the unimmunized control animals developed tumors after subsequent challenge with colon cancer cells; none of the animals immunized with homologous cells developed any tumors, indicating the presence of strong transplantation antigens. All rats immunized with heterologous colon cancer cells succumbed to the challenge, although their tumors were smaller than those of the untreated group, suggesting the presence of weak tissue-type antigens. Animals immunized with fetal gut also developed smaller tumors upon challenge, as did multiparous females, suggesting that embryonic antigens may also act as weak tissue-specific antigens. These protection experiments in vivo do not support the in vitro finding of extensive cross-reactions among rat colon tumors.

Humoral responses developed in colon tumor–bearing rats, since their sera could block lymphocyte cytotoxicity specifically (Sjögren, 1978). Again, this is analogous to the Hellströms' findings with sera from patients with colorectal carcinoma. This blocking activity of rat serum disappeared rapidly after tumor excision (Sjögren and Steele, 1975; Martin et al., 1976). Furthermore, sera from carcinogen-treated rats, obtained before the development of colon tumors, showed antitumor antibodies to be reactive in a complement-dependent cytotoxicity test; these sera demonstrated embryonic antigens as well (Sjögren, 1978; Martin et al., 1976). Antibodies could be detected at a relatively high titer only for a short period after DMH treatment and before tumor appearance, after which the activity disappeared or was drastically reduced.

Immunologic Manipulation of Colon TAAs Affecting Tumor Induction by Carcinogens

Enhanced DMH-induced carcinogenesis was reported for immunosuppressed rats. The propensity for developing multiple bowel cancers was increased in rats treated with antithymocyte globulin (ATG), from 17 to 61 percent in one experiment and from 20 to 73 percent in another (S. Bansal et al., 1978b; Sjögren, 1978). The frequency of tumor metastases was also significantly increased for the experimental group.

Inhibition of DMH-induced carcinogenesis was observed under three experimental conditions. In one experiment, inhibition was observed following immunization of rats with transplantable syngeneic colon cancers. Groups of rats were preimmunized with one of three syngeneic colon tumors or with mammary carcinoma or were left untreated as controls, and they were then exposed to carcinogen. Tumor incidence was the same for the group preimmunized with mammary tumor as for the untreated control, whereas it was 20 percent for the group pretreated with one of the colon tumors as compared with 46 percent for controls. Tumorigenesis was not significantly inhibited in groups pretreated with either of the other two colon carcinomas (Sjögren, 1978). These data support the conclusion that immunization against certain TAAs may form the basis for immunopreventive intervention. In a second set of experiments, inhibition of tumorigenesis was observed following preimmunization with fetal tissue. Tumor incidence was 100 percent for control rats but only 38 percent for rats immunized with liver and gut tissues from 12- to 13-day-old embryos (B. Bansal et al., 1978a; Sjögren, 1980). When newborn liver and gut tissues were used for immunization, all rats developed tumors.

These findings provide supportive evidence for the presence on rat colon tumors of antigens that are shared with fetal tissues. In a third experiment, inhibition was also observed when multiparous rats were used for DMH treatment. Tumor incidence was significantly reduced when compared with that among age-matching virgin female controls (30 percent versus 65 percent). This suggests that multiparous females may be analogous to rats immunized with fetal tissues (Sjögren, 1978).

Immunotherapy of Rat Colon Tumors

One approach to the treatment of rat colon carcinoma requires the surgical excision of primary tumors that develop following carcinogen treatment. In some studies, the effect of surgical excision alone on the development of subsequent tumors has been described, whereas in other studies the animals were subjected to immunotherapy following primary tumor excision.

Bansal and co-workers reported in 1979 that excision of primary colon tumors in DMH-treated rats led to significantly reduced frequency of additional subsequent tumors, two tumors in ten excised rats versus 13 in ten control rats (B. Bansal, 1979). Similar experiments were conducted in 1982 by Steele and co-workers, who reported that 75 percent of the animals developed local or regional recurrences following resection of their primary tumors (Harte et al., 1982). This was used as a baseline, and rats were divided into three groups following resection of their primary tumors: Recurrence rate was 80 percent for the first group, which served as untreated controls; 36 percent for the second group, which was immunized postoperatively with irradiated rat colon tumor cells; and 75 percent for the third group, which was immunized with irradiated rat non–colon tumor cells as a specificity control.

Another approach to the treatment of rat colon carcinoma involves adjuvant immunotherapy without primary tumor resection. In one study conducted by Bansal, rats undergoing treatment with DMH were subjected to multimodal therapy with agents that affect immune responses (*Corynebacterium parvum,* levamisole, transfer of sensitized lymphocytes, and "unblocking" serum); four of ten experimental animals remained tumor-free, whereas all ten control animals developed tumors (B. Bansal, 1978b). In this study, multimodal therapy was superior to any single-agent treatment tested. Passive transfer of sensitized lymphocytes and unblocking serum, combined with nonspecific immunotherapy, significantly reduced tumor development in DMH-treated rats.

Enker has employed rat colon isografts in immunotherapy experiments. Following intraperitoneal inoculation of viable rat colon tumor cells, animals were divided into groups that were immunized with irradiated homologous rat colon carcinoma (Enker and Jacob, 1976; Enker, 1978b). For some groups, these immunizing cells had also undergone surface modification with either concanavalin A (ConA) or neuraminidase or both. The results showed that 80 percent of unimmunized controls died of cancer but that 50 to 70 percent of the experimental rats survived with apparent cure. The best results were obtained when neuraminidase-treated cells were used with or without ConA.

Immunotherapy has also been evaluated in the rat colon model after excision of isografted tumors. Following excision, rats were challenged intraperitoneally with homologous rat colon cancer cells and were then randomized to each of 12 groups (Enker, 1978a and b). Treatments varied from nonspecific immunotherapy alone, to tumor-specific immunotherapy with irradiated unmodified or neuraminidase-treated tumor cells, to a combination of both treatment modalities. The survival rate was 27 percent in untreated control rats, whereas the best experimental group exhibited a 70 percent survival rate. Optimal results were obtained from less intensive immunization with neuraminidase-modified tumor cells and with the addition of nonspecific adjuvant therapy (methanol extraction residue of bacille Calmette Guérin).

Immunoprophylaxis and immunotherapy of isografted rat colon carcinoma were also reported in 1977 by M. Martin and co-workers, who used two independent lines of chemically induced rat colon cancer. They studied various forms of treatment, including immunizations with neuraminidase- and mitomycin-treated tumor cells as well as nonspecific adjuvant treatment alone. Significant tumor enhancement occurred in most cases, although inhibition was observed in one experiment. In that case, tumor incidence was reduced from 100 percent in the control group to 25 percent in the experimental group, in which nonspecific adjuvant (bacille Calmette Guérin, BCG) was used with viable tumor cells to inoculate the rats.

Different results were reported when BCG was injected into the colon lumen in rats exposed to DMH for colon-tumor induction. Tumor incidence and rate of growth were similar for both the experimental and control groups (Rogers and Gildin, 1975).

Murine Colon Tumor Model

In 1975, Griswold and Corbett reported the development of colon tumors C26, C36, and C51 in BALB/C mice and C38 in C57BL/6 mice exposed to chemical carcinogens. Most of the research that has been carried out on these tumors has focused on the effects of chemotherapeutic agents in controlling tumor growth. Research on the immunobiology of murine colon tumors has not involved primary tumors that develop following carcinogen induction. Instead, it has focused on the use of the murine colon tumors either as transplantable isografts or as cultured lines from the parental tumors.

Goldrosen reported in 1980 that orthotopic transplantation of colon tumor C38 into the submucosa of the cecum results in a tumor that metastasizes readily (65 percent) to the liver. In this study, the host's specific antitumor response was monitored with the leukocyte adherence inhibition (LAI) assay. The systemic antitumor response was monophasic, appearing at 4 weeks and disappearing at 8 weeks after implantation, prior to the development of liver metastases. The local and regional antitumor response was biphasic, developing at 4 weeks, disappearing at 6 weeks, reappearing at about 7 weeks, and disappearing permanently at 8 weeks after implantation.

The transplantable colon tumors of BALB/C mice (C26, C36, and C51) have been examined in vivo to assess their immunogenicity. All three tumors were immunogenic, with C36 the most immunogenic, followed by C26 and then C51 (Brattain et al., 1980). Immunization with one colon tumor conferred resistance to challenge with the other colon tumors. The authors concluded that each of these tumors contains "unique" tumor-specific transplantation antigens. An in vitro serologic examination of these and other BALB/C tumors (in which an ^{125}I protein-A assay was used) demonstrated that C51 was most immunogenic, followed by C26, whereas C36 was weakly immunogenic, if at all. This serologic investigation indicated the presence of "unique" TAAs on C51 and C26 in addition to murine leukemia virus antigens, fetal antigens, and shared tissue-type antigens (Cleveland et al., 1979).

Results from various immunotherapy experiments with C26 colon tumor cells have been reported. Growth retardation or regression of established tumor transplants was observed following the sequential administration of three agents (normal spleen cells, xenogeneic "immune" RNA, and tumor antigen) (Fukushima et al., 1982a and b). Optimal doses for these agents were established (1×10^7 spleen cells, 0.5 to 1.0 mg "immune" RNA, and 0.4 mg tumor antigen); higher or lower doses decreased the antitumor effect. These data suggest that DNA synthesis or lymphocyte proliferation or both are essential to the action of immune RNA in sensitizing lymphocytes. Host factors may also be necessary for the interaction of immune RNA–sensitized lymphocytes with tumor antigen, since this was ineffective in vitro.

From the parental tumors C26, C36, and C51, cell lines have been established in vitro and characterized by Belnap and co-workers (Belnap et al, 1979). Both the parental and the cultured colon tumors C26 and C51 grew faster and were more metastatic to the lungs than C36.

The colon tumors C26 and C36 were also adapted to grow in vitro by Sato (Sato et al., 1981) as C-C26 and C-C36 and were characterized. Although these two lines are similar to their parental tumors (C26 and C36) in tumorigenicity, tumor growth, and associated mortality, they differ from them in their metastatic potential. In Sato's study, C-C36 metastasized readily to the lungs (78 percent), whereas C-C26 was poorly metastatic (9 percent). Splenomegaly, which has not been described for any of the parental tumors, developed in mice bearing the C-C36 tumors. Sato's group additionally characterized the immunogenicity of these lines in vivo by immunizing mice with one colon tumor and challenging them with the same or the other colon tumor. Both tumors were immunogenic, and mice immunized with one colon tumor resisted challenge from the same ($P < .0001$) or the other colon tumor ($P < .0001$) (Sato et al., in press). These are the only reports from transplantation experiments in rodents that suggest the presence of strong cross-reactive TAAs among colon tumors.

Summary

Research with the rat colon tumor model has provided evidence for the existence of colon TAAs that are also expressed in fetal liver and gut tissues. According to in-vitro experiments, these appear to be tissue-specific antigens that are shared among rat colon tumors. However, results from transplantation experiments in vivo favor the existence of strong TAAs, "unique" for each rat colon tumor, and of weak TAAs that may be shared between colon tumors. There is data supporting the idea that immunologic manipulation of TAAs may affect the induction of colon tumors by carcinogens. Enhanced tumorigenesis can be observed in immunosuppressed rats. Tumorigenesis has been inhibited specifically in rats preimmunized with certain colon tumors or with fetal tissue and in multiparous rats. Immunotherapy experiments hold some promise for future investigation.

Murine colon tumors have been assessed for immunogenicity by transplantation resistance. Results from these experiments indicate the presence of strong "unique" transplantation antigens on parental tumors and on some of their cultured lines. However, other cultured lines from the parental tumors appear to share strong "common" antigens.

MONOCLONAL ANTIBODIES (MoAb's)

The development of hybridoma techniques by Köhler and Milstein in 1975 provided a method for the production of virtually unlimited amounts of monoclonal antibodies. This approach has opened new avenues for research in tumor immunology and has offered hope for future clinical applications. Most hybridomas currently result from the fusion of immunized mouse splenocytes with non–protein-producing mouse myeloma cells; the resulting hybridomas secrete mouse immunoglobulin. For clinical application, it would be desirable to produce hybridomas secreting human immunoglobulin, and although success has been reported in some cases (Olsson and Kaplan, 1980; Croce et al., 1980; Schlom et al., 1980), technical problems have prevented widespread application of this approach. Most of the research on MoAb's to colorectal tumors has been conducted at the Wistar Institute in Philadelphia and involves a xenogeneic system. Cultured human colon cancer lines are used to immunize BALB/C mice, whose spleens are subsequently fused with murine myeloma cells. Successful hybridomas secrete mouse immunoglobulins that react specifically with human colorectal tumor cells.

In the early studies, only two of 104 hybridomas were reported to be specific for human colorectal tumors (M. Herlyn, 1979). Since then, 15 additional specific hybridomas have been described (Koprowski et al., 1979). In the early reports, no MoAb's showed reactivity with normal human tissue or with other tumors, and only two of them were directed to CEA. However, when MoAb's from this group were characterized further, reactivity was found with gastric and pancreatic carcinoma cells in addition to colorectal tumors (M. Herlyn et al., 1982). There are four areas in which MoAb's to colorectal tumors could be useful: (1) identification of tumor surface antigens; (2) diagnosis of malignancy; (3) tumor localization; and (4) immunotherapy.

Identification of Tumor-Surface Antigens

Although the question of tumor-specific surface antigens on human cancers has been extensively discussed in the literature, their existence must still be considered uncertain (Oettgen and Old, 1980). The critical issue is specificity, and on the basis of current knowledge it is probably more realistic to refer to such antigens as "tumor-associated" rather than "tumor-specific" antigens. Tumor-associated antigens (TAAs) appear to be fetal antigens that are re-expressed on neoplastic cells. MoAb's should prove useful for the isolation and biochemical characterization of TAAs, and such information is forthcoming.

Some of the MoAb's to human colorectal tumors are directed against surface antigens that are shed into the tissue culture medium, whereas other MoAb's recognize antigens that remain confined to the tumor cell surface. Of the antigens that are released into the tissue culture medium, some are glycolipids that react with three of the MoAb's. Two other MoAb's recognize a different type of antigen, which is also shed and which has been identified by autoradiography as a monosialoganglioside (MSG) (Steplewski et al., 1981). It is in fact a sialylated blood group (Le^a) antigen. The sialic acid at the nonreducing terminal of MSG is the immunodominant determinant, since exposure to neuraminidase destroys the ability of MSG to react with the MoAb's. The only normal tissue in which Steplewski's group could detect this antigen was columnar epithelium of secretory ducts, such as those found in pancreas, liver, and bronchi. They also observed it in human meconium, a rich source of human glycolipids, suggesting that MSG may be a fetal antigen that is re-expressed by colon carcinoma. It may be appropriate to mention the 1982 report by Miyauchi and co-workers, who found that rabbit antiserum to 3-fucosyllactose reacts with human colon adenocarcinoma and murine teratocarcinoma cells and only with severely restricted regions in normal tissues. The relationship between this antigen, the MSG antigen, and the specific antigen in colorectal patient sera described by Shochat and co-workers in 1982 has not been determined.

Diagnosis of Malignancy

The same two MoAb's that recognize MSG also react with an antigen present in the sera of some patients who have advanced colorectal carcinoma. Magnani and colleagues have developed a binding-inhibition radioimmunoassay to detect such antigens in patient sera. These investigators initially reported in 1981 that 72 percent of patients with advanced colorectal carcinoma were positive in this assay and that no false-positives were detected among sera from healthy volunteers. Furthermore, no significant cross-reactions were observed with sera from patients having nonmalignant bowel diseases or noncolon malignancies, except those patients with gastric and pancreatic carcinomas. It is unlikely that CEA was involved in this inhibition assay, since there was no correlation between the level of CEA in the patient sera and the ability of the sera to inhibit binding of the MoAb's to the colorectal tumors. When these studies were extended (M. Herlyn et al., 1982) to include larger numbers of patients, serum-binding inhibition was observed most frequently in patients with pancreatic cancer (92 percent) or gastric cancer (72 percent) and less frequently (64 percent) in the sera of patients with colon cancer. False-positive results were reported for two of 108 (1.8 percent of the group) healthy controls, but both individuals came from high-risk families. Sera from seven of 89 patients (8 percent) with other malignancies were positive. In a longitudinal study (Sears et al., 1982b), sera from patients in whom resection of primary colorectal cancer was performed were evaluated using these two MoAb's. Preoperatively, sera from 66 of 85 of these patients (78 percent) demonstrated circulating antigen that was detected by at least one of the two MoAb's. Malignancy recurred postoperatively in ten of the patients (12 percent), and in eight of these individuals (9.4 percent), these recurrences were predicted serologically.

Tumor Localization

The first question to be addressed is whether MoAb's, which have demonstrated specificity to colorectal tumors in vitro, bind specifically to such tumors in vivo. In several studies conducted by Sears and co-workers, resected human colon, containing colorectal carcinoma and normal intestinal mucosa, was perfused for an hour through the mesenteric vessels with medium containing either MoAb's to colorectal tumors or MoAb's with other reactivities as a control for nonspecific binding (Sears et al., 1981; Sears et al., 1982a). Thirty specimens and five different MoAb's were tested: three IgG1, one IgG2a, and one IgM. Specific binding was observed only with the IgG2a MoAb, which had also suppressed tumor growth in nude mice. This antibody bound specifically to colorectal tumor in three of ten trials; in four trials, the antibody bound both tumor and normal colon, in one trial it bound normal colon preferentially, and in the remaining two trials no binding took place. These experiments suggest that further evaluation is necessary before MoAb's can be considered for clinical use. The authors argue, with some justification, that IgM MoAb's cannot be evaluated in this perfusion system, since they do not appear to cross the capillary endothelium in the one-hour perfusion period, probably because of their size. Furthermore, two of the three IgG1's used in these perfusion experiments recognize the MSG antigen that is shed from the tumor cell surface. This shedding may account for, or at least contribute to, the lack of specific binding observed in these studies. The colon perfusion model may prove useful for "typing" primary bowel tumors for reactivity with a given MoAb out of a panel of MoAb's with different specificities. If specific binding is demonstrated in this model, consideration could be given to the use of the MoAb for localization of any future metastases or for immunotherapy.

The most commonly employed technique for

tumor localization involves radiolabeling of immunoglobulin with ^{131}I. Many investigators have conducted experiments on the localization of colorectal tumors using ^{131}I anti-CEA, with variable success. An example is Hedin's 1982 study, in which three IgG1 monoclonal mouse anti-CEA were radiolabeled with ^{131}I. Excellent tumor localization was observed with one of these antibodies and good localization was seen with a second, but the third antibody did not exhibit any preferential localization to the tumor. These findings could not be explained by differences in the binding constants for CEA among these antibodies, since the MoAb that did not localize had a higher association constant than the MoAb with excellent tumor localization characteristics ($K_{assoc.}$ 7.4×10^8 M^{-1} versus 1.2×10^8 M^{-1}). Since all three antibodies are of the same isotype, and since the results cannot be explained by differences in methodology or technique, it is evident that much remains to be understood about tumor localization in which MoAb's are used in vivo.

Immunotherapy with MoAb's

The problems associated with tumor localization must be addressed before immunotherapy can be considered. In two studies conducted by Herlyn and co-workers, the effectiveness of MoAb's in suppressing tumor growth in vivo was evaluated, and an interesting correlation with immunoglobulin isotype was observed. Only IgG2a MoAb's effectively suppressed human colon tumor growth in nude mice; MoAb's of other isotypes were ineffective (Herlyn et al., 1980, 1982). These experiments also provided evidence for the involvement of macrophages as effector cells in tumor suppression. In another, more promising approach to immunotherapy, toxic molecules covalently bound to MoAb's could be guided by the exquisite specificity of the antibodies to destroy the tumor. Although many toxic agents could be used, the α-chain of ricin appears best at this time. It has been used successfully in the treatment of experimental murine leukemia (Vitetta et al., 1983) both in vitro and in vivo. Steplewski (1981) of the Wistar Institute has covalently coupled an anticolon MoAb to the α-chains of diphtheria toxin and of ricin (Gilliland et al., 1980). In these studies, both conjugates were effective in killing tumor cells in vitro. The MoAb used in these experiments was the same IgG2a (1083–17–1a) that has demonstrated tumoricidal activity in nude mice. It will be interesting to evaluate the efficacy of such conjugates in vivo, especially with the use of MoAb's that are not tumoricidal by themselves.

Summary

Murine MoAb's to human colorectal tumors have been created. Their usefulness for antigen characterization, diagnosis of malignancy, tumor localization, and immunotherapy was reviewed. Two of these MoAb's are IgG1's, reactive with a monosialoganglioside shed from human colorectal lines. These same two antibodies react with an antigen present in the sera of patients with colorectal, gastric, or pancreatic carcinoma. When researchers evaluated MoAb's to colorectal tumors for tumor suppression in vivo using nude mice, they found that only IgG2a MoAb's caused suppression. Moreover, when five different MoAb's were tested for tumor localization in perfused human colon, specific binding was observed in only 10 per cent of the trials and was restricted to the same IgG2a MoAb that was able to suppress colorectal tumors in nude mice.

ANTIGENICITY OF HUMAN COLORECTAL CANCER

The rationale for clinical cancer immunotherapy depends on the proposed existence of distinctive surface properties of neoplastic cells, which enable a host to distinguish them from their normal counterparts. As previously described, numerous researchers have attempted to delineate such surface differences in animal models. Genetic heterogeneity complicates the corresponding work in humans; although a human tumor may elicit an immune response in an experimental setting, it is rarely clear whether the response is mounted to a discrete tumor-specific antigen or to a coincidental species-, tissue-, or individual-specific determinant.

Building on earlier work in xenogeneic systems, Gold demonstrated antigens common to human adenocarcinomas derived from digestive tract epithelium but not found in corresponding normal tissues (P. Gold and Freedman, 1965a and b). The finding of cross-reacting antigens in fetal digestive epithelium lent support to the initial view of these substances as tumor- and tissue-specific oncofetal antigens, labeled "carcinoembryonic antigen" (CEA). Subsequent investigations revealed the presence of CEA not only in sera of gastrointestinal cancer patients but also in various other benign and malignant conditions, identifying it more accurately as a tumor-associated antigen. Naturally occurring humoral activity directed against CEA variably has been found and thought to be specific (P. Gold, 1967; J. Gold, 1972); found and thought to be nonspecific (Collatz et al., 1971; MacSween, 1975); or not found at all (LoGerfo et al., 1972). When found, anti-CEA titers failed to correlate with the clinical status of the patient (P. Gold, 1967). Investigators could not demonstrate naturally occurring cell-mediated immunity to CEA (Lejtenyi et al., 1971). In all likelihood, CEA does not play a significant role in host response to colorectal adenocarcinoma; circulating levels of CEA have some value in diagnosis, clinical monitoring, and prediction of prognosis in colon cancer.

The notion of tumor-specific oncofetal antigens has received support from the demonstrated ability of colon cancer patients to mount a delayed cutaneous hypersensitivity response to preparations of autologous tumor or fetal digestive tissue (Hollingshead et al., 1970). Hellström and co-workers published a series of classic articles describing cell-mediated immunity in autologous colon cancer systems; lymphocytes from colon cancer patients inhibited in vitro colon cancer cell colony formation and were cytotoxic to cultured autologous tumor cells as well as to cells of fetal gut and liver (I. Hellström and coworkers, 1970a and b, 1971a, 1972; Hellström and Hellström, 1974). Tumors of similar histologic origins shared cross-reactive antigens, although individually unique tumor antigens could also have been present (I. Hellström et al., 1971a). Other investigators have confirmed and extended this work (Nairn et al., 1971; Nind et al., 1975; Pihl et al., 1975). Additional methods have been studied that avoid the difficulties of tissue culture and its associated risks of introducing artifactual antigens. Elias and his associates report the ability of colon tumor homogenates to inhibit migration of autologous leukocytes, indicating a specific cellular response (Elias, 1977). Evidence for a specific humoral antitumor response is less clear. Workers at the National Cancer Institute found complement-dependent cytotoxicity in the sera of colorectal cancer patients, albeit in an allogeneic tissue-culture assay (Schultz et al., 1975).

Obviously, the ability of native lymphocytes to respond to autologous tumor does not suffice to prevent clinical disease. One possible explanation is the presence of circulating factors in cancer patients' sera that can abrogate lymphocyte reactivity to the tumor. The Hellström group has found that autologous or allogeneic sera can block the action of sensitized lymphocytes against tumor cells in colony-inhibition and lymphocyte-cytotoxicity assays (I. Hellström et al., 1970b, 1971b; Hellström and Hellström, 1974). Under various in-vitro conditions, antibodies, tumor antigen preparations, or antigen-antibody complexes can produce this effect (Alexander, 1974; Baldwin et al., 1972, 1973; Bull et al., 1973; I. Hellström et al., 1971b; Sjögren et al., 1971, 1972; Witz, 1973). A general correlation of serum blocking activity with host tumor burden suggests that circulating tumor antigen may be an important ingredient (I. Hellström et al., 1971b; Elias et al., 1977). In addition to specific blocking factors, various nonspecific inhibitors of lymphocyte function may be produced by colon tumors (Edwards, 1973; Remacle-Bonnet, 1978; Whitehead, 1980). To complicate matters further, Hellström and co-workers described naturally occurring "unblocking" serum factors that can alter the ability of other "blocking" sera to interfere with specific lymphocyte action (I. Hellström et al., 1971c).

A discussion of tumor-associated antigens might include reference to Oettgen and Old's classification of surface antigens, based on autologous typing of astrocytoma, malignant melanoma, and renal cell carcinoma (Oettgen and Old, 1980). "Class 1" antigens are peculiar to an individual tumor, whereas "class 2" antigens may be found in tumors of a given tissue type (e.g., in adenocarcinomas of the colon); and "class 3" antigens include a diverse group of tumor-associated markers, some of which may be alloantigens. Structural (Kahan et al., 1976) and immunologic investigations suggest that human colorectal adenocarcinomas bear recognizable class 3 and class 2 determinants and, perhaps, class 1 as well. The relationship of such antigens to afferent and efferent immune responses in the natural host remains to be elucidated.

Although it seems likely that adenocarcinomas derived from human colonic epithelium express characteristic antigenic determinants, the situation is far more complex than that seen in syngeneic animal models. These antigens bear an unclear relationship to histocompatibility markers, blood group antigens, and other normal cell surface components. The complexity of the host response to the tumor confounds the situation still further:

". . . While cancer-bearing patients . . . may be capable of recognizing the presence of a tumor, the tumor-bearing state is associated with a failure in the interpretation of this recognition into an effective tumoricidal response. Thus, the detection of various circulating tumor antigens, or of fetal antigens, is no guarantee that the presence of cellular immunity reflects an appropriate effector response" (Enker, 1978a).

ASSESSMENT OF IMMUNOCOMPETENCE

The ability of colorectal cancer patients to mount local inflammatory responses to their tumors bears an important relationship to prognosis (Spratt and Spjut, 1967). Regional lymph nodes draining colon tumors remain competent to respond to a variety of immune stimuli, even when partially replaced by metastatic tumor (Fisher et al., 1972); hyperplasia, predominantly of T-lymphocyte compartments and perhaps also of B-lymphocyte compartments, has an especially favorable implication (Patt et al., 1975; Pihl et al., 1976). Not all authors agree (Tsakraklides et al., 1975). Some investigators suggest that local factors may interfere with regional immune defenses (Edwards et al., 1973; Nind et al., 1973; Pihl et al., 1975).

The complexity of the host-tumor relationship frustrates attempts to monitor systemic immunocompetence in a clinically meaningful way. Generally, host immunocompetence has a favorable implication for clinical status (Eilber et al., 1975). Most authors agree that advancing malignant disease has a deleterious effect on immunocompetence, owing to both specific and nonspecific factors (Kahan et al., 1977). However, particular assays for measuring immunocompetence may be heavily influenced by the timing of the test with respect to clinical course (I. Hellström et al., 1973; House, 1975) as well as by such coincidental host factors as surgery (Cochran et al., 1972; Greco et al., 1978), nutrition, and general health. Extrapolations from animal models and available information in humans suggest that measures of cell-mediated immunity have the greatest relevance to antitumor response, although this is by no means certain (Oettgen and Old, 1980).

Relatively crude indices of cell-mediated immunity (e.g., peripheral blood lymphocyte counts) have some correlation with clinical course. Pretreatment lymphocyte counts relate significantly to stage of disease at presentation (Bone and Lauder, 1974) and perhaps to post-treatment disease-free interval and statistical survival (Kim et al., 1976; Mavligit et al., 1978b). Not all researchers agree (Panettiere and Chen, 1982). In an extensive immunologic survey of patients with colon cancer, Evans and co-workers demonstrated that the fraction of circulating B-lymphocytes (by EAC rosette formation) pertained to the extent of disease and possibly to later disease recurrence, whereas the fraction of circulating T-lymphocytes declined with advanced disease (Evans et al., 1977) Mitogen-induced lymphocyte blastogenesis is a more sophisticated, albeit nonspecific, measure of cell-mediated immune function. Depressed blastogenic response to such mitogens as phytohemagglutinin generally correlates with extent of disease and perhaps with survival (Lauder and Bone, 1973; Wanebo and Pinsky, 1978), although again some authors disagree (Kaplan et al., 1975; Waller et al., 1980).

The use of delayed cutaneous hypersensitivity responses to recall antigens as a means of monitoring cell-mediated immunocompetence has generated a great deal of inquiry. Several investigators have demonstrated a relation among the ability of patients to respond to dinitrochlorobenzene (DNCB), the extent of their disease (Kronman et al., 1972; Bone and Lauder, 1974; Wanebo et al., 1976; Rao et al., 1977), and their prognosis (Bone et al., 1973; Wanebo et al., 1976; Rao et al., 1977). Unfortunately, the relationship is not consistent (Panettiere and Chen, 1982), and it may be more of a function of the patient's general condition than of disease stage. Patients may occasionally show good skin-test reactivity, even in the presence of obviously advancing malignancy (Falk et al., 1975; Enker, 1978a). ". . . Skin tests for recall antigens, skin tests to new sensitizing antigens, and mitogen stimulation assays are crude measurements which may ultimately have no direct bearing on the role of immunology in the host's response to cancer" (Enker, 1978a). Until better information becomes available, the most productive approach may be to monitor a broad battery of indices of immunocompetence (Sjögren, 1974). Thus, although Waller and co-workers found no significant differences between colon cancer patients and controls in a wide range of immunologic assays, they could demonstrate a significant improvement in immune function after surgical resection of evident disease (Waller et al., 1980). Likewise, Evans and colleagues related a set of immune parameters to tumor recurrence after surgery (Evans et al., 1977). At least two groups of investigators have suggested immunologic profiles appropriate for monitoring the immunocompetence of colorectal cancer patients (Lurie et al., 1975; Ichiki et al., 1978).

Host immunocompetence may be affected by a number of agents and conditions, such as nutrition, drugs, intercurrent disease, and specific and nonspecific tumor-associated factors. Generalized immunologic impairment as well as specific derangements in any of the limbs of the immune response may result. Until such deficits can be better characterized, immunologic monitoring must be as broad as possible and therefore will remain relatively unsophisticated.

CLINICAL IMMUNOTHERAPY

Early surgical intervention remains the only modality with proven curative efficacy in treatment of adenocarcinoma of the colon and rectum. A significant number of patients will suffer recurrent disease after attempted surgical cure, especially in those instances in which the primary tumor penetrates the bowel wall or spreads to the regional lymph nodes. Few options exist for effective palliation; systemic 5-fluorouracil may offer some benefit in a small percentage of cases. Consequently, a pressing clinical necessity drives the search for additional means of treatment.

Immunotherapy has been attempted in a surprising number of patients with colorectal cancer, often in cases of advanced disease after traditional therapies have failed. Available published studies confuse as often as they enlighten because of wide variations in the types of patients treated, inadequate control of the multitude of clinical and experimental variables, mingling of therapeutic modalities, and inadequate or premature processing of results (Enker et al., 1981). Experimental evidence suggests that spontaneous tumors express only a weak immunogenicity in the natural host and that hosts with large tumor burdens react poorly to antigenic stimuli of all kinds. Patients most likely to benefit from immunologic manipulation are relatively well-nourished, functional patients from whom all evident disease has been removed but in whom there is a high risk of tumor recurrence; these are the so-called "minimal residual disease" patients. Patients should be classified according to known major prognostic variables prior to randomization into prospective trials (Kissner et al., 1979). The variable results of primary surgical therapy and the modest improvements in disease-free interval and survival expected from immunotherapy indicate the need to study fairly large numbers of patients along with carefully matched concurrent controls. Existing data in animal models and in clinical trials with other malignancies point out the sensitivity of results to different dosage schedules and routes of agent administration; immunotherapeutic agents may be effective only in a narrow dosage range, with insufficient stimulation at lower dosages and immune paralysis at higher dosages (Humphrey, 1972; Kahan, 1977; Enker, 1978b). Specific immune response against tumor cells may persist for only a limited time (Kahan et al., 1977), so that dosage may need to be repeated over a protracted period, perhaps in a manner related to the cell kinetics of the tumor (Enker et al., 1978b). Assays for monitoring specific and nonspecific immune responses in the subjects should be chosen carefully, and attention should be paid to the additional caveat that even placebo therapy may occasionally result in an improvement in immunologic parameters (Moertel et al., 1978). The possibility of enhancing tumor growth rather than inhibiting it continues to haunt the minds of immunotherapy researchers; no convincing evidence of tumor enhancement has manifested itself in trials with colorectal cancer so far.

Published trials of immunologic intervention in colon cancer fall into two broad groups, nonspecific and specific immunotherapy. Nonspecific immunotherapy consists of the administration of various adjuvant substances, often bacterial products, in an attempt to stimulate immune and reticuloendothelial systems in general and, possibly, to repair subliminal deficits in specific response through "shotgun" treatment (Falk et al., 1976b; Kahan et al., 1977). Some experimental models have shown a benefit from this approach, and it has had modest success in the treatment of a few human tumors. Opponents cite experimental evidence that the tumor-bearing host is already maximally stimulated (Burk et al.. 1975) and argue that further nonspecific stimulus is as likely to activate tumor-protective blocking mechanisms as it is to activate an antitumor response (Enker and Jacobitz, 1976). Falk has found preliminary results using synthetic nonspecific agents that stimulate selective components of the immune response (Falk et al., 1981). Bansal and co-workers have described another novel approach, achieving some clinical improvement with extracorporal serum processing to remove blocking activity from a patient with advanced metastatic colon cancer (S. Bansal et al., 1978a).

Concurrent use of chemotherapeutic and immunotherapeutic agents in clinical trials remains controversial. Trials of this type attempt to combine "the debulking capability of chemotherapy with the potential for control of microscopic disease by immunotherapy" to produce a synergistic response (Macdonald, 1976). In limited doses, chemotherapeutic drugs may selectively depress humoral immunity, which is believed to be responsible for some immune blocking activity (Heppner et al., 1974); alternatively, chemotherapy may enhance serum cytotoxicity for tumor cells (Segerling et al., 1975). Appropriately timed stimulation might enhance immunologic "rebound" after chemotherapy (Kahan et al., 1977). Unfortunately, none of these theoretical considerations has proved clinically useful in colon cancer trials to date. Commonly employed methods of cancer treatment—including surgery, irradiation, and chemotherapy—may actually suppress responses to immunotherapy. In any case, the employment of multiple therapeutic modalities in clinical trials serves to obscure the factor responsible for any benefit noted; some single-agent advantage of an immunotherapeutic treatment should be demonstrated before it is included in combination trials.

Trials with Nonspecific Agents

Bacille Calmette Guérin

The attenuated mycobacterium, bacille Calmette Guérin (BCG), has had wide application as an immune adjuvant in animal systems. Preliminary results in human malignant melanoma and other tumors prompted clinical trials in adenocarcinoma of the colon. The best known work on this topic is the widely published study conducted by investigators at M. D. Anderson Hospital in Houston, Texas (Mavligit et al., 1974, 1975, 1976, 1977a and b, 1978a to d; Gutterman et al., 1976a and b; Valdivieso and Mavligit, 1978). Mavligit and co-workers performed a randomized trial of patients treated with BCG by dermal scarification, with or without concomitant oral 5-fluorouracil. The study groups consisted of patients with Dukes' C carcinoma resected for cure; an additional stratification for number of involved lymph nodes was included. Altogether, 121 patients were studied. With a maximum follow-up of 50 months, analysis revealed no significant difference between the two arms of the trial, although both arms showed prolongation of median disease-free interval and survival compared with a group of historical controls. This study received extensive criticism regarding the use of historical controls, and some commentators disputed the efficacy of 5-fluorouracil given by mouth. In an interesting side light, serial skin tests to recall antigens during the trial could not be correlated with disease progression. Another clinical trial worthy of mention came from Canada. McPherson and co-workers initiated a protocol with patients who had colon cancer that had penetrated the bowel wall with or without nodal involvement—modified Dukes' staging B_2 and C—and who had undergone resection for cure (McPherson et al., 1979). After stratification for stage, patients were randomly divided into three groups: patients receiving oral BCG therapy alone (36 patients altogether), patients receiving oral BCG plus oral methyl-CCNU and intravenous 5-fluorouracil (32 patients), and untreated concurrent control patients (43 patients). After approximately 30 months' follow-up, the researchers found no significant improvement in disease-free interval among the concurrent randomized treatment groups; results in the Dukes' B_2 patients receiving chemoimmunotherapy were significantly poorer than those in the control group. Interpretation of these findings deserves some caution in view of their preliminary nature. Oral administration of BCG was the route originally used for tuberculosis prophylaxis in humans. Several researchers have chosen this route in colon tumor immunotherapy trials because of improved patient acceptance and the theoretical advantage of delivering the immune stimulant more directly to the tumor-involved area (Panettiere and Chen, 1982). The efficacy of oral BCG in this context remains controversial (Mavligit et al., 1978b).

The literature contains several investigations of the concurrent use of BCG and chemotherapy. After preliminary work suggested that such work was associated with a possible advantage (Falk, 1975), Falk and co-workers conducted a randomized trial of intraperitoneal and oral BCG given with 5-fluorouracil in advanced colon cancer; they found that this method had no significant benefit over chemotherapy alone (Falk et al., 1976a and b,

1977). Likewise, Engstrom and colleagues found no advantage in adding intradermal BCG to chemotherapy in advanced bowel cancer (Engstrom et al., 1975, 1978). The ability of advanced cancer patients to respond to immune manipulation has been questioned repeatedly. Using patients with minimal residual disease, workers in the Southwestern Oncology Group discovered a slightly significant improvement in disease-free interval with the addition of oral BCG to chemotherapy; this study is still being conducted (Panettiere, 1977; Panettiere and Chen, 1982).

Methanol-Extracted Residue of BCG

Methanol-extracted residue of BCG (MER-BCG) is a nonviable fraction of extracted mycobacteria and does not include those moieties responsible for tuberculin skin reactivity (Moertel et al., 1975). Advantages of MER-BCG over usual preparations of BCG pertain mostly to its greater facility for dose standardization and response quantitation and its inability to cause systemic infection in impaired hosts (Enker, 1978a). The Gastrointestinal Tumor Study Group (GITSG) reported in 1979 a prospective randomized trial testing immunotherapy with intradermal MER-BCG versus chemotherapy (methyl-CCNU and 5-fluorouracil), versus chemotherapy plus MER-BCG, and versus an untreated concurrent control group (Lokich, 1979). A total of 394 patients, resected for cure of Dukes' B_2 and C colon carcinoma, were classified according to stage and site of primary lesion. The patients experienced significant local toxicity from MER-BCG treatments, and after median follow-up of 13 months, they demonstrated no statistically significant differences among the treatment arms in recurrence or survival.

Results of a smaller study performed in Israel contrasted with the GITSG findings. After curative resection, 53 patients with Dukes' B_2 and C colon cancer were randomly classified into two therapeutic groups. One group received radiotherapy (4000 rads, lower abdomen) and chemotherapy (5-fluorouracil); the other group received identical treatment with the addition of intradermal MER-BCG (Robinson, 1979a and b, 1980, 1982). Criteria for classification included age, sex, and stage of disease. Analysis at 24 and 36 months' follow-up suggested significant improvements in disease-free interval, recurrence rate, and survival for the MER-BCG group; later analysis showed this improvement only in female patients. This protocol suffered from the lack of a concurrent control. It also differed from the GITSG study in its use of radiotherapy and in the timing of immunotherapy with respect to chemotherapy. Graduated dose adjustments for individual patients decreased the local toxicity of MER-BCG.

In several trials, including the Veterans Administration Surgical Oncology Group, patients with recurrent or metastatic disease encountered significant toxicity and derived little benefit from the addition of MER-BCG to chemotherapy (Moertel et al., 1975, 1978; Richards et al., 1979; Higgins et al., 1981).

Levamisole

The antihelminthic agent, levamisole, weakly potentiates general immune reactivity to a variety of antigens, probably via macrophage stimulation (Nystrom et al., 1977). In an admirably straightforward study from Belgium, levamisole was tested as a single agent in a nonrandomized, concurrently controlled population (Verhaegen et al., 1982). Thirty treated patients, matched with controls for age, sex, and disease stage, received oral levamisole for up to 2 years and were followed for 5 years. Patients with Dukes' B_2 and C cancer manifested a survival advantage. The nonrandomized nature of the study prevents any confident conclusions.

Several investigators have found no benefit from adding levamisole to chemotherapy (Valdivieso et al., 1977; Bedikian et al., 1978a and b; Bancewicz, 1980). Curiously, one group did find an advantage of this method in patients with advanced disease but not in patients with small tumor burdens; the significance of this finding is unclear (Borden et al., 1982).

Corynebacterium parvum

A nonviable derivative of the bacterium *Corynebacterium parvum* has shown some effectiveness as an adjuvant agent in animal systems and in preliminary human experiments (Israel et al., 1975; Nystrom et al., 1977). A few inquiries have been made into its use in colorectal cancer. A British group attempted to administer *C. parvum* intravenously as a single agent to patients with minimal residual disease (Souter et al., 1982a and b). Although they detected no significant benefit, protocol difficulties and substantial dosage variations due to toxicity compromise their results. An Australian team combined intramuscular *C. parvum* with chemotherapy in patients with advanced disease (Bolton, 1977; Gough et al.,

1978, 1979), without apparent advantage; their inability to detect antibodies to *C. parvum* raises doubts as to the systemic efficacy of the intramuscular route.

Despite tantalizing sporadic reports of success, clinical trials of nonspecific adjuvant immunotherapy for colorectal cancer have yielded no firm evidence of significant benefit. New adjuvant agents may come to light; larger, more carefully designed studies might discover advantages previously overlooked. However, from the present perspective, nonspecific immune stimulation appears to offer little gain over traditional therapies.

Specific Immunotherapy

Malignant cells, probably bearing recognizable surface aberrations, proliferate with impunity in otherwise immunocompetent hosts. The implied malfunction in immune surveillance could occur at any of a multitude of discrete steps in afferent or efferent mechanisms. The ultimate goal of specific therapy would be to correct the essential deficiencies, allowing normal function to resume. Although current science lacks the sophistication for such a task, earnest efforts continue in the attempt to provoke a specific antitumor response.

Most investigators who have conducted specific immunotherapeutic programs have employed tumor vaccines, using modified or unmodified tumor cells, in an attempt to provoke cell-mediated responses to tumor antigens. A few researchers have undertaken work not involving tumor vaccines (e.g., the experiments of Pilch and coworkers with "immune RNA") but without any concrete results as yet (Pilch et al., 1977). Most tumor vaccines depend on the presence of "helper" moieties to magnify the response to weakly immunogenic tumor antigens; such moieties might include histocompatibility antigens, chemically modified cell surface components, or exogenous antigens from viral infection (Oettgen and Old, 1980). After results from experimental animal models are obtained, vaccines are given intradermally or subcutaneously in repeated doses, over the period of greatest risk for tumor recurrence (Kahan et al., 1977). Researchers encounter some difficulty in devising appropriate assays to monitor specific responses (Oettgen and Old, 1980).

Humphrey, Griffen, and associates at several institutions immunized patients with crude, homogenized, presumably allogeneic, tumor preparations (Humphrey et al., 1971, 1972; Griffen et al., 1972a and b). In these early studies, all patients had advanced colorectal cancer and were not randomized. Following vaccination, some patients underwent a series of partial exchange transfusions of plasma and leukocytes with blood-group–matched patient partners. Approximately one third to one half of treated patients showed some clinical response. Many patients manifested enhanced specific antitumor activity as measured by serum assays and delayed cutaneous hypersensitivity.

In a "minimal residual disease" model, tumor-bearing syngeneic rats demonstrated significantly improved survival following immunization with surface-modified tumor cells (Enker and Jacobitz, 1976; Enker, 1978a; Enker et al., 1978b). Cells were modified using concanavalin A or *Vibrio cholerae* neuraminidase. An Austrian team is applying these concepts in a human trial. Rainer and co-workers have initiated a randomized trial using neuraminidase-modified allogeneic tumor vaccine, compared with chemotherapy (cytosine arabinoside, mitomycin, and 5-fluorouracil) or with concurrent controls (Rainer et al., 1981). The patient population consists of people resected for cure of Dukes' B or C colon cancer, classified according to stage and operative procedure. Vaccinated patients show enhanced reactivity to tumor cells, tested by delayed cutaneous hypersensitivity; there are notable differences in reactivity between stages. The immunotherapy group appears to have a prolonged disease-free interval compared with the other groups, although results are still too preliminary to allow definite conclusions.

Experiments in a murine model suggested the feasibility of inducing virally augmented oncolytic immunity; viral antigens expressed on the surface of infected tumor cells seem to intensify the immunogenicity of tumor-associated antigens. Wallack and colleagues at the Wistar Institute in Philadelphia and at Washington University in St. Louis have pioneered the application of these ideas in human colon cancer (Wallack et al., 1977; Wallack, 1980, 1981). Preliminary work in patients with advanced disease indicated the safety and possible clinical efficacy of a vaccine composed of allogeneic colon tumor cells infected with vaccinia virus. A prospective randomized trial is in progress, involving patients resected for cure of Dukes' B and C colorectal cancer. Preliminary analysis supports a slight advantage in disease-free interval for Dukes' B patients and in survival for Dukes' C patients, although these early findings have not yet achieved statistical significance. Results are sufficiently encouraging to justify an expanded trial of more prolonged treatment at several dosage levels.

Honesty compels investigators to admit that specific immunotherapy has not yet given any more concrete results than nonspecific immunotherapy for adenocarcinoma of the colon and rectum. Clinical trials continue while more elegant approaches await further advances of basic research into the host-tumor relationship. One author has expressed the situation succinctly: "Initial enthusiasm must be tempered by results until clinical science can approach the subject in a more sophisticated manner" (Enker et al., 1981).

SUMMARY

Investigations with syngeneic animal models indicate that carcinogen-induced colon carcinomas possess distinctive surface antigens. The existence of analogous antigens in "spontaneous" human colorectal cancer is supported by indirect evidence. The genetic heterogeneity of human hosts forms a substantial barrier to clear delineation of human tumor-specific antigens. Even though a tumor-bearing host may immunologically recognize neoplastic cells, blocking factors and other undefined aberrations of immune function can prevent an effective response. The host-tumor relationship is a complex interaction that researchers' inquiries have not yet deciphered. New techniques involving the use of monoclonal antibodies offer some unique advantages in studying tumor antigens and possibly have clinical promise as well.

Despite encouraging results in animal systems, no effective immunologic adjuvant therapy has come from empirical trials. Further work needs to be done in devising appropriate means to assess patient immunocompetence and to monitor results of specific therapy. Most clinical studies have utilized nonspecific adjuvant immunotherapy without results of major importance. Specific immunotherapy offers more hope from a theoretical standpoint; barring some fortuitous discovery, clinical specific immunotherapy will remain relatively unsophisticated until basic investigations light the way to more advanced methods.

References

Alexander PA: Escape from immune destruction by the host through shedding of surface antigens. Cancer Res 34:2077, 1974.

Baldwin RW, Embleton MJ, Price MR: Inhibition of lymphocyte cytotoxicity for human colon carcinoma by treatment with solubilized tumour membrane fractions. Int J Cancer 12:83, 1973.

Baldwin RW, Price MR, Robins RA: Blocking of lymphocyte mediated cytotoxicity for rat hepatoma cells by specific antigen-antibody complexes. Nature New Biol 238:185, 1972.

Bancewicz J, MacPherson SG, McVie JG, et al: Adjuvant chemotherapy and immunotherapy for colorectal cancer. J Roy Soc Med 73:197, 1980.

Bansal BR, Mark R, Rhoads JE, Bansal SC: Effect of embryonic tissue immunization on chemically induced gastrointestinal tumors in rats. I. Can embryonic antigens act as rejection antigens? J Natl Cancer Inst 61:189, 1978a.

Bansal BR, Mark R, Mobini J, et al: Demonstration of effective anti-tumor immunity in an autochthonous host bearing primary colon tumors induced by 1,2-dimethylhydrazine dihydrochloride. J Natl Cancer Inst 63:127, 1979.

Bansal BR, Mobini J, Bansal SC: Multimodal immunotherapy of primary gastrointestinal tumors in rats. Cancer 42:2079, 1978b.

Bansal SC, Bansal BR, Thomas HL, et al: Ex vivo removal of serum IgG in a patient with colon carcinoma. Cancer 42:1, 1978a.

Bansal SC, Mark R, Bansal BR, Rhoades JE: Immunologic surveillance against chemically induced primary colon carcinoma in rats. J Natl Cancer Inst 60:667, 1978.

Bedikian AY, Valdivieso M, Mavligit GM, et al: Sequential chemoimmunotherapy of colorectal cancer. Cancer 42:2169, 1978a.

Bedikian AY, Valdivieso M, Mavligit GM, et al: Sequential chemoimmunotherapy of colorectal cancer. Proc Am Assoc Cancer Res 19:418, 1978b.

Belnap LG, Cleveland PH, Colmerauer MEM, et al: Immunogenicity of chemically induced murine colon cancer. Cancer Res 39:1174, 1979.

Bolton PM: Chemotherapy, immunotherapy, and chemoimmunotherapy of colorectal cancer. Aust Radiol 21:328, 1977.

Bone G, Appleton DR, Venables CW: Cutaneous delayed hypersensitivity responses to 2,4-dinitrochlorobenzene—A prognostic guide in malignant disease. Br J Surg 60:906, 1973.

Bone G, Lauder I: Cellular immunity, peripheral blood lymphocyte count, and pathological staging of tumors in the gastrointestinal tract. Br J Cancer 30:215, 1974.

Borden EC, Davis TE, Crowley JJ, et al: Interim analysis of a trial of levamisole and 5-fluorouracil in metastatic colorectal carcinoma. *In* Terry WE (ed): Immunotherapy of Human Cancer. New York, Elsevier, 1982, p. 231.

Brattain MG, Strobel-Stevens J, Fine D, et al: Establishment of mouse colonic carcinoma cell lines with different metastatic properties. Cancer Res 40:2142, 1980.

Bull DM, Leibach JR, Williams MA, et al: Immunity to colon cancer assessed by antigen-induced inhibition of mixed mononuclear cell migration. Science 181:957, 1973.

Burk MW, et al: Refractoriness of lymph node cells from tumor-bearing animals. Int J Cancer 15:49, 1975.

Cleveland PH, Belnap LG, Knotts FB, et al: Tumor-associated antigens of chemically induced murine tumors: the emergence of MuLV and fetal antigens after serial passage in culture. Int J Cancer 23:380, 1979.

Cochran AJ, Spilg WGS, Mackie RM, et al: Postoperative depression of tumor-directed cell-mediated immunity in patients with malignant disease. Br Med J 4:67, 1972.

Collatz E, Von Kleist S, Burtin P: Further investigations of circulating antibodies in colon cancer patients: on the autoantigenicity of the carcinoembryonic antigen. Int J Cancer 8:298, 1971.

Croce CM, Linnenbach A, Hall W, et al: Production of human hybridomas secreting antibodies to measles virus. Nature 288:488, 1980.

Druckrey H, et al: Selektiverzeugung von darmkrebs bie ratten durch 1,2 dimethylhydrazin. Naturwissenschaften 54:285, 1967.

Edwards AJ, Rowland GF, Lee MR: Reduction of lymphocyte transformation by a factor produced by gastrointestinal cancer. Lancet 1:687, 1973.

Eilber FR, Nizze JA, Morton DL: Sequential evaluation of general immune competence in cancer patients: correlation with clinical course. Cancer 35:660, 1975.

Elias EG, Elias LL, Didolkar MS, et al: Cellular immunity in patients with colorectal adenocarcinoma measured by autologous leukocyte migration inhibition. Cancer 40:687, 1977.

Engstrom PF, Catalano RB, Creech RH, et al: Chemoimmunotherapy of colorectal carcinoma with 5-FU plus BCG. Proc Am Assoc Cancer Res 16:234, 1975.

Engstrom PF, Paul AR, Catalano RB, et al: Fluorouracil versus fluorouracil plus BCG in colorectal adenocarcinoma. *In* Terry WD (ed): Immunotherapy of Cancer. New York, Raven Press, 1978, p. 587.

Enker WE: Adjuvant immunotherapy for large bowel cancer: experimental studies in a relevant pre-clinical model. *In* Enker WE (ed): Carcinoma of the Colon and Rectum. Chicago, Year Book Medical Publishers, 1978a, p. 259.

Enker WE, Jacobitz JL: The definitive value of active-specific immunotherapy for experimental carcinoma of the colon. Surgery 80:164, 1976.

Enker WE, Jacobitz JL, Craft K, et al: Surgical adjuvant immunotherapy for colorectal cancer. J Surg Oncol 10:389, 1978b.

Enker WE, Kemeny N, Shank B, et al: Defining the needs for adjuvant therapy of rectal and colonic cancer. Surg Clin North Am 61:1295, 1981.

Evans JT, Goldrosen MH, Han T, et al: Cell-mediated immune status of colon cancer patients. Cancer 40:2716, 1977.

Falk RE, Landi S, Cohen F, et al: Use of oral and intraperitoneal BCG in the treatment of malignant melanoma and adenocarcinoma. *In* Crispen, RG (ed): Neoplasm Immunity: Theory and Application. Chicago, ITR, 1975, p. 169.

Falk RE, MacGregor AB, Ambus U, et al: The use of adjuvant therapy with BCG combined with chemotherapy in the treatment of gastrointestinal cancer. *In* Lamoureux G (ed): BCG in Cancer Immunotherapy. New York, Grune and Stratton, 1976a, p. 217.

Falk RE, MacGregor AB, Ambus U, et al: Combined treatment with BCG and chemotherapy for metastatic gastrointestinal cancer. Dis Colon Rectum 20:215, 1977.

Falk RE, MacGregor AB, Landi S, et al: Immunostimulation with intraperitoneally administered bacille Calmette Guérin for advanced malignant tumors of the gastrointestinal tract. Surg Gynecol Obstet 142:363, 1976b.

Falk RE, Makowka L, Rotstein LE, et al: Clinical evaluation of NED 137 in gastrointestinal cancer. *In* Hersh EM (ed): Augmenting Agents in Cancer Therapy. New York, Raven Press, 1981, p. 313.

Fisher B, Saffer EA, Fisher ER: Studies concerning the regional lymph node in cancer. Cancer 30:1202, 1972.

Fukushima M, Colmerauer EM, Nayak SK, et al: Immunotherapy of a murine colon cancer with syngeneic spleen cells, immune RNA and tumor antigen. Int J Cancer 29:107, 1982a.

Fukushima M, Colmerauer EM, Nayak SK, et al: Antitumor effect of syngeneic spleen cells treated with immune RNA and tumor antigen. Int J Cancer 29:113, 1982b.

Gilliland DG, Steplewski Z, Collier RJ, et al: Antibody-directed cytotoxic agents: use of monoclonal antibody to direct the action of toxin A chains to colorectal carcinoma cells. Proc Natl Acad Sci 77:4539, 1980.

Gold JM, Freedman SO, Gold P: Human anti-CEA antibodies detected by radioimmunoelectrophoresis. Nature New Biol 239:60, 1972.

Gold P: Circulating antibodies against carcinoembryonic antigens of the human digestive system. Cancer 20:1663, 1967.

Gold P, Freedman SO: Demonstration of tumor-specific antigens in human colonic carcinomata by immunological tolerance and absorption techniques. J Exper Med 121:439, 1965a.

Gold P, Freedman SO: Specific carcinoembryonic antigens of the human digestive system. J Exper Med 122:467, 1965b.

Goldrosen MH: Murine colon adenocarcinoma. Immunobiology of metastases. Cancer 45:1223, 1980.

Gough IR, Bolton PM, Clunie GJA, et al: Chemoimmunotherapy in disseminated melanoma and colorectal carcinoma. Aust NZ J Surg 48:296, 1978.

Gough IR, Clunie GJA, Bolton PM, et al: A trial of 5-fluorouracil and *Corynebacterium parvum* in advanced colorectal carcinoma. Dis Colon Rectum 22:223, 1979.

Greco RS, Salvati E, Rubin R, et al: Cell-mediated immunity in adenocarcinoma of the colo-rectum. J Surg Res 24:253, 1978.

Griffen WO, Jewell WR, Meeker WR, et al: Newer concepts of cancer of the colon and rectum: immunotherapy for patients with cancer of the large intestine. Dis Colon Rectum 15:116, 1972a.

Griffen WO, Meeker WR: Colon carcinoma and immunologic phenomena. Surg Clin North Am 52:839, 1972b.

Griswold DP, Corbett TH: A colon tumor model for anticancer agent evaluation. Cancer 36:2441, 1975.

Gutterman JV, Mavligit GM, Blumenschein G, et al: Immunotherapy of human solid tumors with bacille Calmette Guérin. Ann NY Acad Sci 277:135, 1976a.

Gutterman JV, Mavligit GM, Hortobagyi G, et al: BCG immunotherapy of disseminated breast cancer and colorectal cancer. *In* Lamoureux G (ed): BCG in Cancer Immunotherapy. New York, Grune and Stratton, 1976b, p. 227.

Harte PJ, Steele G, Rayner AA, et al: The effect of "tissue-type" specific immunotherapy on colon cancer recurrence in a minimal residue disease model. Curr Surg 39:21, 1982.

Hedin A, Wahren B, Hammarström S: Tumor localization of CEA-containing human tumors in nude mice by means of monoclonal anti-CEA antibodies. Int J Cancer 30:547, 1982.

Hellström I, Hellström KE: Newer concepts of cancer of the colon and rectum: cellular immunity to human colonic carcinomas. Dis Colon Rectum 15:100, 1972.

Hellström I, Hellström KE, Pierce GE, et al: Cellular immunity to colonic carcinomas in man. *In* Burdette WJ (ed): Carcinoma of the Colon and Antecedent Epithelium. Springfield, IL, Charles C Thomas, 1970a, p. 176.

Hellström I, Hellström KE, Shepard TN: Cell-mediated immunity against antigens common to human colonic carcinomas and fetal gut epithelium. Int J Cancer 6:346, 1970b.

Hellström I, Hellström KE, Sjögren HO, et al: Demonstration of cell-mediated immunity to human neoplasms of various histological types. Int J Cancer 7:1, 1971a.

Hellström I, Hellström KE, Sjögren HO, et al: Serum factors in tumor-free patients cancelling the blocking of cell-mediated tumor immunity. Int J Cancer 8:185, 1971c.

Hellström I, Sjögren HO, Warner G, et al: Blocking of cell-mediated tumor immunity by sera from patients with growing neoplasms. Int J Cancer 7:226, 1971b.

Hellström I, et al: Sequential studies on cell-mediated tumor immunity and blocking serum activity in ten patients with malignant melanoma. Int J Cancer 11:280, 1973.

Hellström KE, Hellström I: Lymphocyte-mediated cytotoxicity and blocking serum activity to tumor antigens. Adv Immunol 18:209, 1974.

Heppner GH, Griswold DE, DiLorenzo J, et al: Selective immunosuppression by drugs in balanced immune responses. Fed Proc 33:1882, 1974.

Herlyn D, Koprowski H: IgG2a monoclonal antibodies inhibit human tumor growth through interaction with effector cells. Proc Natl Acad Sci 79:4761, 1982.

Herlyn D, Steplewski Z, Herlyn MF, Koprowski H: Inhibition of growth of colorectal carcinoma in nude mice by monoclonal antibody. Cancer Res 40:717, 1980.

Herlyn M, Sears HF, Steplewski Z, Koprowski H: Monoclonal antibody detection of a circulating tumor-associated antigen. I. Presence of antigen in sera of patients with colorectal, gastric, and pancreatic carcinoma. J Clin Immunol 2:135, 1982.

Herlyn M, Steplewski L, Herlyn D, Koprowski H: Colorectal carcinoma-specific antigen: detection by means of monoclonal antibodies. Proc Natl Acad Sci 76:1438, 1979.

Higgins GA, Donaldson RC, Humphrey EW, et al: Adjuvant therapy for large bowel cancer. Surg Clin North Am 61:1311, 1981.

Hollinshead A, Glen D, Bunnag B, et al: Skin-reactive soluble antigen from intestinal cancer-cell-membranes and relationship to carcinoembryonic antigens. Lancet 1:1191, 1970.

House AK, Wisniewski S, Woodings B: Immunity in colonic tumor patients after operation. Dis Colon Rectum 18:100, 1975.

Humphrey LJ, Boehm B, Jewell WR, et al: Immunologic response of cancer patients modified by immunization with tumor vaccine. Ann Surg 176:554, 1972.

Humphrey LJ, Murray DR, Boehm OR, et al: Immunotherapy of cancer in man. Studies of patients with cancer of the alimentary tract. Am J Surg 121:165, 1971.

Ichiki AT, Collmann IR, Wenzel KL, et al: Immunologic studies of colonic cancer: evaluation of immunocompetence. South Med J 71:271, 1978.

Israel L, Edelstein R, Depierre A, et al: Daily intravenous infusions of *Corynebacterium parvum* in twenty patients with disseminated cancer. J Natl Cancer Inst 55:29, 1975.

Kahan BD, Rutzky LP, Berlin B, et al: Cell surface alterations on colon adenocarcinoma cells. Cancer Res 26:3526, 1976.

Kahan BD, Pellis NR, Rutzky LP, et al: Active specific immunotherapy potential for treatment of large bowel cancer. Cancer 40:2740, 1977.

Kaplan MS, Mino FO, Summerfeld KB, et al: Phytohemagglutinin-stimulated immune response. Arch Surg 110:1217, 1975.

Kim JS, et al: Prognostic significance of peripheral lymphocyte counts and carcinoembryonic antigens in colorectal carcinoma. J Surg Oncol 8:257, 1976.

Kisner DL, Davis HL, Muggia FM: Current adjuvant trials in colorectal cancer. Front Gastrointest Res 5:102, 1979.

Köhler G, Milstein C: Continuous cultures of fused cells secreting antibody of predefined specificity. Nature 256:495, 1975.

Koprowski H, Steplewski L, Mitchell K, et al: Colorectal carcinoma antigens detected by hybridoma antibodies. Somatic Cell Genet 5:957, 1979.

Koprowski H, Herlyn M, Steplewski Z, Sears HF: Specific antigen in serum of patients with colon carcinoma. Science 212:53, 1981.

Kronman BS, Shapiro HM, Localio SA: Delayed hypersensitivity responses of patients with carcinoma of the colon and other related tumors. Dis Colon and Rectum 15:106, 1972.

Lauder I, Bone G: Lymphocyte transformation in large bowel cancer. Br J Cancer 28:78, 1973.

Lejtenyi MC, Freedman SO, Gold P: Response to lymphocytes from patients with gastrointestinal cancer to the carcinoembryonic antigen of the human digestive system. Cancer 28:115, 1971.

LoGerfo P, Herter FP, Bennett SJ: Absence of circulating antibodies to carcinoembryonic antigen in patients with gastrointestinal malignancies. Int J Cancer 9:344, 1972.

Lokich JJ: Adjuvant therapy for surgically curable colon cancer: a controlled study of chemo and immune therapy. Proc Ann Soc Clin Oncol 20:423, 1979.

Lurie BB, Bull D, Zamchek N, et al: Diagnosis and prognosis in colon cancer based on profile of immune reactivity. J Natl Cancer Inst 54:319, 1975.

Macdonald JS: The immunobiology of colorectal cancer. Semin Oncol 3:421, 1976.

McPherson TA, Young D, Lim C, et al: Adjuvant chemoimmuno- and immunotherapy in B_2 and C colorectal cancer. *In* Jones SE (ed): Adjuvant Therapy of Cancer. II. New York, Grune and Stratton, 1979, p. 603.

MacSween JM: The antigenicity of carcinoembryonic antigen in man. Int J Cancer 15:246, 1975.

Magmani JL, Brockhaus M, Smith DF, et al: A monosialoganglioside is a monoclonal antibody-defined antigen of colon carcinoma. Science 212:55, 1981.

Martin F, Martin M, Lagneau A, et al: Circulating antibodies in rats bearing grafted colon carcinoma. Cancer Res 36:3039, 1976.

Martin MS, Martin F, Justrabo E, et al: Immunoprophylaxis and therapy of grafted rat colon carcinoma. Gut 18:232, 1977.

Mavligit GM, Gutterman JV, Burgess MA, et al: Immunotherapy: its possible application in the management of large bowel cancer. Am J Dig Dis 19:1047, 1974.

Mavligit GM, Gutterman JV, Burgess MA, et al: Adjuvant immunotherapy and chemoimmunotherapy in colorectal cancer of the Dukes' C classification. Cancer 36:2421, 1975.

Mavligit GM, Gutterman JV, Burgess MA, et al: Prolongation of postoperative disease-free interval and survival in human colorectal cancer by BCG or BCG plus 5-fluorouracil. Lancet 1:871, 1976.

Mavligit GM, Gutterman JV, Malahy MA, et al: Adjuvant immunotherapy and chemoimmunotherapy in colorectal cancer. Cancer 40:2726, 1977a.

Mavligit GM, Gutterman JV, Malahy MA, et al: Systemic

adjuvant immunotherapy and chemoimmunotherapy in patients with colorectal cancer. *In* Salmon SE (ed): Adjuvant Therapy of Cancer. Amsterdam, Elsevier, 1977b, p. 279.

Mavligit GM, Gutterman JV, Malahy MA, et al: Systemic adjuvant immunotherapy and chemoimmunotherapy in patients with colorectal cancer. *In* Terry WD (ed): Immunotherapy of Cancer. New York, Raven Press, 1978a, p. 597.

Mavligit GM, Malahy MA, Gutterman JV, et al: Clinical immunotherapy as adjuvant therapy for colon and rectal cancer. In Enker WE (ed): Carcinoma of the Colon and Rectum. Chicago, Year Book Medical Publishers, 1978b, p. 133.

Mavligit GM, Malahy MA, Hersh E: Systemic adjuvant therapy with BCG versus BCG plus 5-FU in colorectal cancer Dukes' Class C. Proc Am Assoc Cancer Res 19: 212, 1978c.

Mavligit GM, Malahy MA, Zatopek N, et al: Adjuvant immunotherapy for colorectal cancer. *In* University of Texas System Cancer Center Immunotherapy of Human Cancer. New York, Raven Press, 1978d, p. 355.

Miyauchi T, Yonezama S, Takamura T, et al: A new fucosyl antigen expressed on colon adenocarcinoma and embryonal carcinoma cells. Nature 299:168, 1982.

Moertel CG, O'Connell MJ, Ritts RE, et al: A controlled evaluation of combined immunotherapy (MER-BCG) and chemotherapy for advanced colorectal cancer. In Terry WD (ed): Immunotherapy of Cancer. New York, Raven Press, 1978, p. 573.

Moertel CG, Ritts RE, Schutt AJ, et al: Clinical studies of methanol extraction residue fraction of bacille Calmette Guérin as an immunostimulant in patients with advanced cancer. Cancer Res 35:3075, 1975.

Nairn RC, Nind AP, Guli EP, et al: Immunological reactivity in patients with carcinoma of the colon. Br Med J 4:706, 1971.

Nind AP, Matthews N, Pihl EAV, et al: Analysis of inhibition of lymphocyte cytotoxicity in human colon carcinoma. Br J Cancer 31:620, 1975.

Nind AP, Nairn RC, Rolland JM: Lymphocyte anergy in patients with carcinoma. Br J Cancer 28:108, 1973.

Nystrom JS, Bateman JR, Weiner J: Adjuvant treatment of colorectal cancer. West J Med 126:95, 1977.

Oettgen HF, Old LJ: Immunotherapy of colon cancer. Cancer 45:1218, 1980.

Olsson L, Kaplan H: Human-human hybridomas producing monoclonal antibodies of predefined antigenic specificity. Proc Natl Acad Sci 77:5629, 1980.

Panettiere FJ: Adjuvant chemotherapy and chemoimmunotherapy for locally advanced large bowel adenocarcinoma. *In* Salmon SE (ed): Adjuvant Therapy of Cancer. Amsterdam, Elsevier, 1977, p. 265.

Panettiere FJ, Chen TT: SWOG study of adjuvant chemotherapy with and without oral BCG in the postoperative treatment of cancer of the colon. *In* Terry WE (ed): Immunotherapy of Human Cancer. New York, Elsevier, 1982, p. 207.

Patt DJ, Brynes RK, Vardiman JW, et al: Mesocolic lymph node histology is an important prognostic indicator for patients with carcinoma of the sigmoid colon: an immunomorphologic study. Cancer 35:1388, 1975.

Pihl E, Hughes ESR, Nind APP, et al: Colonic carcinoma: clinicopathological correlation with immunoreactivity. Br Med J 3:742, 1975.

Pihl E, Nairn RC, Nind AP, et al: Correlation of regional lymph node in vitro antitumor immunoreactivity histology with colorectal carcinoma. Cancer Res 36:3665, 1976.

Pilch YF, Ramming KP, Dekernion JB: Preliminary studies of specific immunotherapy of cancer with immune RNA. Cancer 40:2747, 1977.

Prehn RT, Outzen HC: Fourth International Congress of Immunology; Immunology 80. New York, Academic Press, 1980, p. 651.

Rainer H, Kovats E, Lehmann HG, et al: Effectiveness of postoperative adjuvant therapy with cytotoxic chemotherapy or immunotherapy in the prevention of recurrence of Dukes' B and C colon cancer. Recent Results Cancer Res 79:41, 1981.

Rao B, Wanebo HJ, Pinsky CM, et al: Delayed hypersensitivity reactions in patients with carcinoma of the colon and rectum. Surg Gynecol Obstet 144:677, 1977.

Remacle-Bonnet MM, Pommier GJ, Luc C, et al: Nonspecific suppressive and cytostatic activities mediated by human colonic carcinoma tissue or cultured cell extract. J Immunol 121:44, 1978.

Richards F, Muss HB, Cooper MR, et al: Chemotherapy versus chemoimmunotherapy in advanced adenocarcinoma of the colon and rectum. Cancer 43:91, 1979.

Robinson E, Bartal A, Cohen Y, et al: Adjuvant therapy in colorectal cancer. Bio Med 31:8, 1979a.

Robinson E, Bartal A, Cohen Y, et al: Adjuvant therapy in colorectal cancer. Proc Am Assoc Cancer Res 20:408, 1979b.

Robinson E, Bartal A, Cohen Y: Treatment of radically operated colorectal cancer patients with combined adjuvant therapy. *In* Terry WD (ed): Immunotherapy of Human Cancer. New York, Elsevier, 1982, p. 217.

Robinson E, Bartal A, Mekori T: Results of postoperative treatment of colorectal cancer by radiotherapy, chemotherapy and immunotherapy. Recent Results Cancer Res 75:80, 1980.

Rogers AE, Gildin J: Effect of BCG on dimethylhydrazine induction of colon tumors in rats. J Natl Cancer Inst 55:385, 1975.

Sato N, Michaelides MC, Wallack MK: Characterization of tumorigenicity, mortality, metastasis, and splenomegaly of two cultured murine colon lines. Cancer Res 41:2267, 1981.

Sato N, Michaelides MC, Wallack MK: Transplantation immunity and cross-protection of two cultured murine colon lines. J Natl Cancer Inst (in press, 1983).

Schlom J, Wunderlich D, Teramoto YA: Generation of human monoclonal antibodies reactive with human mammary carcinoma cells. Proc Natl Acad Sci 77:6841, 1980.

Schultz RM, Woods WA, Chirigos MA: Detection in colorectal carcinoma patients of antibody cytotoxic to established cell strains derived from carcinoma of the human colon and rectum. Int J Cancer 16:16, 1975.

Sears HF, Herlyn M, Del Villano B, et al: Monoclonal antibody detection of a circulating tumor-associated antigen. II. A longitudinal evaluation of patients with colorectal cancer. J Clin Immunol 2:141, 1982b.

Sears HF, Herlyn D, Herlyn M, et al: Ex vivo perfusion of a tumor-containing colon with monoclonal antibody. J Surg Res 31:145, 1981.

Sears HF, Herlyn D, Herlyn M, et al: Ex vivo perfusion of human colon with monoclonal anticolorectal cancer antibodies. Cancer 49:1231, 1982a.

Segerling M, Dhanian S, Borsos T: Chemotherapeutic drugs increase killing of tumor cells by antibody and complement. Science 188:55, 1975.

Shochat D, Pant KD, Goldenberg DM: Colon-specific antigen-p (CSAP) 11: further characterization in colorectal and pancreatic cancer. Cancer 50:927, 1982.

Sjögren HO: Section meeting on immunology and immunotherapy. Am J Dig Dis 19:1064, 1974.

Sjögren HO: Immunology of experimentally induced large

bowel cancer. *In* Enker WE (ed): Carcinoma of the Colon and Rectum. Chicago, Year Book Medical Publishers, 1978, p. 247.

Sjögren HO: Immunoprevention of large bowel cancer: an animal model. Cancer 45:1229, 1980.

Sjögren HO: Immunoprevention. *In* Ledeck MS (ed): Inhibition of Tumor Induction and Development. New York, Plenum Press, 1981, p. 203.

Sjögren HO, Hellstrom I, Bansal SC, et al: Suggestive evidence that blocking antibodies of tumor-bearing individuals may be antigen-antibody complexes. Proc Natl Acad Sci USA 68:1372, 1971.

Sjögren HO, Hellstrom I, Bansal SC, et al: Elution of "blocking factors" from human tumors capable of abrogating tumor cell destruction by specifically immune lymphocytes. Int J Cancer 9:274, 1972.

Sjögren HO, and Steele G: The immunology of large bowel carcinoma in a rat model. Cancer 26:2469, 1975.

Souter RG, Gill PG, Morris PJ: A trial of nonspecific immunotherapy using systemic *C. parvum* in treated patients with Dukes' B and C colorectal cancer. Br J Cancer 45:506, 1982a.

Souter RG, Gill PG, Morris PJ: Adjuvant immunotherapy with *corynebacterium parvum* in colorectal cancer. In Terry WD (ed): Immunotherapy of Human Cancer. New York, Elsevier, 1982b, p. 221.

Spratt JS, Spjut HJ: Prevalence and prognosis of individual clinical and pathologic variables associated with colorectal carcinoma. Cancer 20:1976, 1967.

Steele G, Harte PJ, Rayner AA, et al: The effect of adjuvant immunotherapy on tumor recurrence after segmental resection of carcinogen-induced Wistar/Furth primary bowel adenocarcinomas. J Immunol 128:7, 1982.

Steele G, Sjögren HO: Cross-reacting tumor-associated antigens among chemically induced rat colon carcinomas. Cancer Res 34:1801, 1974.

Steele G, Sjögren HO: Cell surface antigens in a rat colon cancer model: correlation with inhibition of tumor growth. Surgery 82:164, 1977.

Steplewski Z, Chang TH, Herlyn M, Koprowski H: Release of monoclonal antibody-defined antigens by human colorectal carcinoma and melanoma cells. Cancer Res 41:2723, 1981.

Tsakraklides VT, Wanebo HJ, Sternberg S, et al: Prognostic evaluation of lymph node morphology in colorectal cancer. Am J Surg 129:174, 1975.

Valdivieso M, Bedikian A, Burgess MA, et al: Chemoimmunotherapy of metastatic large bowel cancers. Cancer 40:2731, 1977.

Valdivieso M, Mavligit GM: Chemotherapy and chemoimmunotherapy of colorectal cancer. Surg Clin North Am 58:619, 1978.

Verhaegen H, Decree J, Decock W, et al: Levamisole therapy in patients with colorectal cancer. *In* Terry WD (ed): Immunotherapy of Human Cancer. New York, Elsevier, 1982, p. 225.

Vitetta ES, Krolick KA, Miyama-I-naba M, et al: Immunotoxins: a new approach to cancer therapy. Science 219:644, 1983.

Wallack MK: A new approach in the immunotherapy of carcinoma of the colon and rectum. J Surg Oncol 13:29, 1980.

Wallack MK, Steplewski Z, Koprowski H, et al: A new approach in specific active immunotherapy. Cancer 39:560, 1977.

Wallack MK: Immunotherapy in colorectal cancer. Missouri Med 78:23, 1981.

Waller CA, Gill PG, MacLennan ICM: Enhancement of lymphocyte-mediated cytotoxicity after tumor resection in patients with colorectal cancer. JNCI 65:223, 1980.

Wanebo HJ, Rao B, Pinsky C, et al: Delayed hypersensitivity reactions in patients with colorectal cancer. *In* Crispen R (ed): Neoplasm Immunity: Mechanisms. Chicago, ITR, 1976, p. 157.

Wanebo HJ, Pinsky CM: A review of immunologic reactivity in patients with colorectal cancer. *In* Enker WE (ed): Carcinoma of the colon and rectum. Chicago, Year Book Medical Publishers, 1978, p. 227.

Whitehead JS, Kim YS: An inhibitor of lymphocyte proliferation produced by a human colonic adenocarcinoma cell line in culture. Cancer Res 40:29, 1980.

Witz IP: The biological significance of tumor-bound immunoglobulins. Curr Top Microbiol Immunol 61:151, 1973.

FOURTEEN

Hepatic and Pulmonary Metastases

J. S. Spratt, M.D.

HEPATIC METASTASES

Hepatic metastases from bowel cancer are a major cause of increased morbidity and mortality in victims of this type of cancer. The author and associates studied the natural history of a series of largely untreated hepatic metastases seen at the Ellis Fischel State Cancer Hospital (Jaffe et al., 1968). In the period before 1966, effective therapy for most hepatic metastases was rare; in fact, the only treatments offered were diagnosis, supportive care, and follow-up. The follow-up, fortunately, was complete, thanks to the perseverance of the social service director, Miriam G. Hoag.

In all, 390 cases of proven or suspected hepatic metastases were seen between 1940 and 1966. Of these, 177 were from the colon and rectum. Biopsy was performed on 75 to confirm the histology of the metastasis. In 102, diagnosis was based on intraoperative examination of the liver. However, the survival curves for the two groups were identical.

The median survival time, from the time of diagnosis of the metastatic colon cancer to the liver, was 146 days, with only 37 patients (9.5 percent) surviving more than 10 months. The survival time for patients with hepatic metastases from rectal cancer was similar to that of patients with hepatic metastases from colon cancer. Survival rates were greater for patients with well-differentiated cancers and for those with cancers not so far advanced as to create abnormal hepatic function studies.

According to uncontrolled data, if resection intended to be curative for colorectal cancer was performed in a patient who later developed hepatic metastases, the cumulative survival rate for these patients was only 47 percent 10 months after the diagnosis of hepatic metastases. This rate dropped to 28 percent at 10 months for patients who had resections done when the surgeon knew residual cancer existed (palliative resection). For patients with only colostomy diversions, the cumulative survival rate was 15 percent at 10 months and for patients with laparotomies, only 7 percent at 10 months. The operative mortality rate in the presence of hepatic metastases was 15 percent. Only two of 45 patients with advanced metastases confirmed by percutaneous needle biopsy died in the hospital.

The longest survival time in this series was 3762 days (10 years and 3 months). This was a patient in whom hepatic metastases were described at laparotomy but were not biopsied. The longest survival time with histologically proven hepatic metastases was 1052 days or 2 years and 11 months. The longest survivorship reported after proven hepatic metastases was nearly 15 years from the time of biopsy confirmation of the metastases (Levine et al., 1982).

Fifty-six cases in the Ellis Fischel series (14 percent) had only a solitary metastasis, as determined by inspection at laparotomy. Data for this series were accumulated during the period of time when resection of metastases was rarely done. Even though this figure is low, the suspected presence of limited metastases that might be resectable as the only residual disease mandates a thorough evaluation of each patient, including a general workup for metastases. Isolated metastases can be resected with long survivorship.

From a review of the literature and the results of the Solid Liver Tumor Survey (SLTS), Foster and Berman (1977) concluded that from 10 to 30 percent of patients with primary cancer of the gastrointestinal tract can be expected to have hepatic metastases present at first laparotomy for cancer. They estimated that about one-quarter of these patients will have metastases limited to a single lobe or segment. Their end result data confirmed that occasional benefit from resection can be obtained for patients with bowel cancer, particularly colon cancer. Carcinoids that metastasize to the liver produce an array of unique metabolic problems (see Chapter Eleven), but after these are addressed, the surgical problems of carcinoids metastatic to the liver are similar to those found with most other hepatic metastases from colonic cancer.

Knowledge of the surgical anatomy of the liver affords an understanding of hepatic resections and their associated pitfalls. Foster and Berman (1977) have documented the array of complications that occur as a result of hepatic resections and have described the learning experience that has resulted in the reduction of the frequency of these complications. A progressive increase in hepatic resectability and a reduction in mortality rates were confirmed.

The SLTS identified those points pertinent to the surgical management of hepatic metastases. The greatest overall success was with cancers of the colon and rectum, including both cancers with or without metastases to mesenteric lymph nodes. Of 16 5-year survivors, nine had synchronous and seven had metachronous hepatic metastases. A "disease-free interval" was of little prognostic value once metastases had occurred. Survival after resections for synchronous or metachronous metastases was similar.

Before 1974, many of the complications that were documented were those one would expect, considering that resective techniques were not well developed at that time. Among 82 operative deaths, 15 occurred within the first 30 postoperative days owing to failure to control hemorrhage. There were only three intraoperative deaths, which were caused by air emboli. The remaining deaths were due to a variety of causes, e.g., liver failure (technical), liver failure (cirrhotic), cardiopulmonary failure, upper gastrointestinal hemorrhage, sepsis, recurrent cancer, and "judgment error."

The student of the history of surgery can obtain a fascinating review of the "state of the art" through 1974 by reading the classic studies in physiology, anatomy, pathology, diagnostic aids, and operative techniques (including pre- and postoperative care). My purpose here is to comment selectively on later studies relevant to the management of hepatic metastases from neoplasms of the colon and rectum.

A hepatic computed axial tomography (CAT) scan and hepatic artery angiogram are indicated for preoperative evaluation, in the absence of extrahepatic metastases but with known or suspected hepatic metastases. Even with nonresectable metastases, benefit may still be obtained from dearterialization of the liver and perfusion of the liver by means of the hepatic artery or portal vein.

Hepatic Metastases from Squamous Cancer of the Anus

Squamous cell carcinoma of the anus also metastasizes to the liver, although infrequently. In 1962, MacLean and associates reviewed the literature during a period of time when anal cancer was more prevalent than it seems to be now. Of 869 reported squamous cell cancers of the anus, only 24 (2.7 percent) had metastasized to the liver, even though these cancers have a potential ingress into the portal venous system by way of the superior hemorrhoidal veins. More virulent squamous cancers of the anus could metastasize to the liver by way of the systemic circulations, just as squamous cell cancers of the head and neck do.

These older case reports largely provide descriptive statistics, rather than methods for controlling the metastases. There are no reports of hepatic metastases from squamous cell cancer of the anus that were controlled by resection of the liver.

Resection

Preoperative planning is essential for a safe and effective resection of hepatic metastases. Such planning must include delineation of the extent of hepatic involvement, preoperative mass of functioning liver, and probable postoperative mass of functioning liver. The histologic type of hepatic metastases needs to be confirmed. The primary cancer should either be controlled or controllable. Preoperative patient preparation and postoperative metabolic support are essential. This kind of assessment is also necessary before dearterialization of the liver or hepatic artery and portal vein perfusion. In the case of carcinoids, there occasionally exists an indication for the palliative resection or even enucleation of large tumor masses to relieve symptoms of the carcinoid spectrum. The inevitable side effects of carcinoid secretions should be controlled preoperatively and intraoperatively (see Chapter Eleven).

As discussed in Chapter Eleven, Gillett and Smith (1974) have confirmed the value of extensive resection of both the involved liver and of the primary carcinoids.

Determining Anatomic Extent

Determining the anatomic extent of hepatic metastases and their relation to the vascular anatomy of the liver is an essential step in the work-up. A flat film of the abdomen can provide an estimation of liver size. Liver contour can be determined by the liver shadow and the direction of organ displacement.

Other roentgenographic diagnostic techniques of value in these cases include hepatic arteriograms, venograms (splenoportograms and inferior venacavograms with retrograde hepatic venograms) and cholangiograms. Radioisotope scanning differentiates between functional and nonfunctional metastases. Both ultrasound imagery and CAT scans can define the extent of liver involvement and permit the measurement of the dimensions of metastases. Of greatest value to the surgeon is the hepatic artery angiogram, which can determine the relationship of metastatic cancer to the vascular anatomy of the liver. Knowledge of the anatomy of the hepatic artery is essential if the option of dearterialization of the liver is elected in lieu of resection. A number of aberrant arrangements of the hepatic arterial system can occur. With modern arteriography, the specific vascular anatomy of each patient can be determined.

An occasional adenocarcinoma of the colon will grow contiguously and invade the liver, in the absence of true metastases. In fact, the presence of a colon cancer large enough to invade the liver by contiguous growth and the absence of any discontiguous deposits of cancer should suggest that the surgeon has encountered a nonmetastasizing variant of colon cancer (Spratt et al., 1970). In this instance, all the involved structures must be resected en bloc, including the primary colon cancer and a margin of tissue proved to be histologically free of cancer. The favorable prognosis associated with quite large but nonmetastasizing colon cancers is discussed in Chapter Ten. Foster and Berman (1977) identified 15 patients with right colon cancer adherent to the liver who had undergone wedge resection of the contiguously involved liver. There were no operative deaths. Six died of recurrent cancer and a seventh was alive with persistent cancer 52 months after resection. Seven lived cancer-free for prolonged periods. Wedge resections in these cases can usually be done without entering the hilum of the liver.

Since SLTS, reported by Foster and Berman (1977), others have verified the safety and benefit of selected partial hepatectomies for cancers of the colon and rectum metastatic to the liver. Fortner and associates (1978) reported their experience with 25 colorectal cancers metastatic to the liver among 108 patients with liver metastases. The 3-year survival rate after resections for metastatic colorectal cancer reached 72 percent. Postoperative hospital stay was reduced to 13 days and the operative mortality rate fell to 4 percent. The standard preoperative evaluation included a detailed history and physical examination, technetium and frequently a rose bengal liver scan, selective celiac and superior mesenteric arteriograms, blood chemistries including alpha fetoprotein and carcinoembryonic antigen levels, chest x-ray, and gastrointestinal radiologic examinations, as indicated. Computed transaxial tomography was done in the more recent cases. Percutaneous needle biopsy and peritoneoscopy were performed only in patients thought unsuitable for laparotomy.

Percutaneous biopsy, an encouragingly exact and low-risk procedure, can provide histologic confirmation of metastatic cancer in the liver before laparotomy. Schwerk and Schmitz-Moormann (1981) reported that the percutaneous biopsy had an overall accuracy of 91.6 percent, a sensitivity of 92.2 percent, a specificity of 88.9 percent, and a high predictive value of positive results, i.e., cytology, 97.8 percent; histology, 100 percent. A correlation between echo patterns and histology was not found.

Techniques for Resection

Fortner and associates (1978) have reduced operative techniques for hepatic resection to standard routines. The abdomen is explored through a subcostal incision. If the tumor is resectable, the incision is extended to a bilateral subcostal incision with a paraxiphoid extension. Alternatively, since all vital structures are midline, an exploratory upper midline incision may be performed. This may be extended to the pubis if necessary or into the chest if required. The chest is rarely opened, except when diaphragmatic involvement or massive tumor is present, requiring more exposure for resection. Biopsy of the liver is not done if it is believed that the patient can potentially be cured by hepatic lobectomy.

For a right hepatic lobectomy, the falciform ligament is incised to the vena cava. The triangular and coronary ligaments of the right lobe of the liver are severed. The liver is retracted upward and to the left, exposing the right kidney, right adrenal gland, and vena cava. Dissection continues, exposing the bare area of the liver to the suprahepatic vena cava. Laparotomy pads are then placed in the hepatic fossa. The liver is thus brought up to a more convenient level for hilar dissection. Dissection to expose the right and left hepatic arteries is then performed. The right hepatic artery is ligated and divided, after which the right hepatic duct and the cystic duct are ligated and divided. The right branch of the portal vein is dissected free, ligated, and divided. Care must be taken to avoid injury to posterior branches. Isolation and ligation of the major hepatic veins prior to incising the liver capsule are not necessary. The dissection is time-consuming and potentially dangerous. The capsule is incised with cautery along the line of demarcation that extends from the gallbladder fossa inferiorly to the right of the suprahepatic vena cava. The liver parenchyma can then be separated using the handle of the knife to gently spread by fracturing. Identified intrahepatic vessels and periportal structures are doubly hemoclipped as they are encountered and are divided between the clips. Larger vessels and structures are ligated individually. Control of major hepatic veins can be obtained with pressure from the left hand, which holds the specimen as it is resected. Bleeding points are identified and are transfixed with catgut sutures, and the anterior and posterior lips of the transected surface can be approximated using interrupted No. 1 horizontal mattress sutures. The raw area of the liver can thus be covered, preventing oozing and bile leakage. Coverage may also be obtained with omentum. A Shirley sump* is placed in the right upper quadrant, and the abdomen is closed.

*Anpro-anproline Shirley sump catheter: H. W. Anderson Products, New York.

For a left hepatic lobectomy, the approach is similar. Mobilization of the liver is obtained by dividing the triangular ligament. The right lobe of the liver is not dissected. The left lobe is mobilized toward the inferior vena cava, taking care to avoid injury to the inferior phrenic vein and any collateral vessels. The lesser omentum is divided between clamps at the hepatic portal after identification of the major arterial supply. The left hepatic artery, left branch of the portal vein, and left hepatic bile duct are individually identified, ligated, and divided. If the tumor is confined to the lateral segment of the left lobe, a left lateral segmentectomy can be performed. This procedure is the same as that described for the total left hepatic lobectomy, except that the blood supply to the medial segment of the left lobe must be preserved. Transection of the liver must be made just to the left of the falciform ligament.

For an extended right hepatic lobectomy, the techniques of dissection of structures in the hepatic portal, mobilization of the right lobe, and resection of the liver parenchyma are the same as those for right hepatic lobectomy. However, in the extended right hepatic lobectomy, care must be taken to preserve the gastrohepatic ligament because it frequently contains an anomalous collateral artery from the celiac axis or left gastric artery to the lateral segment of the left lobe. The bile duct to the lateral segment can be very superficial and small. Therefore, particular attention should be given to identifying and preserving the biliary ducts to the lateral segment in the early stage of the resection. The resection line should be about 1 cm to the right of the falciform ligament, since the structures in the portal triad branch extensively in the umbilical fissure. Branches to the left lobe are located at the base of the umbilical fissure. These are readily apparent on the transection of the fused lips of medial and lateral left lobe segments overlying the area.

Unless contraindicated by the extent of tumor, it is safer and easier to leave some of the posterior portion of the caudate lobe. The hepatic vein to the left lobe of the liver usually has medial and lateral branches. The medial branch of the left hepatic vein can be identified, ligated, and divided inside the liver parenchyma at the final stage of hepatic resection. The resected liver surface is sutured as described previously. The lateral segment may be anchored in position by suturing the falciform ligament to the anterior abdominal wall if extensive distortion of the structures in the hepatic portal is anticipated after liver resection.

A catheter can be placed in the hepatic artery or portal vein in some patients for postresection chemotherapy (Fortner and Pahnke, 1976; Kim et al., 1977).

Results of Resection

The resectability rate in the series by Fortner and associates (1978) for malignant disease was *33 percent* (95 of 289). Duration of the operation and postoperative hospital stay was longer, and estimated blood loss was greater, for patients treated with the isolation perfusion technique compared with those treated with the standard resection. Operating time for resection ranged from 2.25 to 9.75 hours, with an average time of 5 hours, and there was an average blood loss of 3000 ml. The median postoperative hospital stay was 15 days. Hypoglycemia or hypoalbuminemia was prevented by administration of 5 or 10 percent glucose solutions, plasma, or albumin.

The 30-day operative mortality was 9 percent overall for the 108 patients, with a rate of only 4 percent when the standard type of resection was performed. An operative mortality rate of 17 percent for the isolation-perfusion technique was a reflection of the technique and the advanced stage of disease of many patients who were resected before 1975. With extended right hepatic lobectomy, the operative mortality rate was 14.2 percent (4/22); with right hepatic lobectomy, 2.7 percent (1/36); with left hepatic lobectomy, 23.8 percent (5/21); and with segmentectomy 0 percent (0/24). The operative mortality was similar for curative and palliative resections; it was 10 percent (4/40) and 12.5 percent (6/48), respectively.

In 1980, Hanks and associates reported on a series of hepatic resections that included seven patients with metastases from colonic adenocarcinomas. They came to the conclusion that major and beneficial hepatic resections could be performed in the small subset of patients who have a limited number of metastases.

In 1982, Logan and associates updated UCLA experience with hepatic resection for metastatic colorectal carcinomas. In the UCLA series, 19 patients had undergone partial hepatectomy for metastatic colorectal carcinoma, including five trisegmentectomies, eight lobectomies, and six segmentectomies, with only one (5.3 percent) mortality. Twelve lesions were solitary and seven multiple. Mean survival was 27.4 months, with three patients surviving over 5 years and one nearly 8 years. Better mean survival existed for patients with solitary (33.2 months) rather than with multiple (15.8 months) lesions. For various subsets, mean survivorships were as follows: segmentectomies (44.7 months), lobectomies (24.3 months), and trisegmentectomies (11.0 months). For patients in whom the appearance of hepatic metastases was delayed more than two years, mean survivorship was 40.5 months; less than one year, 24.8 months. For patients with synchronous metastases, mean survivorship was 23.1 months. None of the 12 surviving patients had evidence of recurrent disease, but many had short follow-up. This experience further supports the value of definitive surgical treatment of resectable colorectal carcinoma metastatic to the liver. Systemic therapy seems markedly less effective in this resectable subset.

Adson and Van Heerden (1980) reported matched-pair historical controls in an effort to confirm the benefit of resecting colorectal cancer metastatic to the liver. They reported only two hospital deaths and 32 surviving patients, with an 82 percent 1-year survival rate and a 41 percent 3-year survival rate. At the time that the report was written, three patients were still alive 10 to 22 years after resection. Their conclusions were that from 20 to 30 percent of their patients had indeed benefited from resection.

Ryan and associates (1982) reported their experience using the Lin hepatic compression clamp in major hepatic resections. By using the Lin clamp in conjunction with the fracture technique, blood loss was markedly reduced. These authors also used the Hepco Upper Hand retractor and an extended subcostal incision. Complications, operative mortality rates, and operative time were also significantly reduced. Their experience was based on 52 patients ranging in age from 3 days to 77 years and included 19 trisegmentectomies and 23 right lobectomies. Wedge and segmental resections were excluded from the report.

Metabolic Management with Hepatic Resection

With the aid of serum electrophoresis, the changes in different protein fractions were studied in patients following liver resection (Almersjö and Bengmark, 1969). Albumin catabolism and synthesis were studied with the aid of ^{131}I- and ^{125}I-tagged human albumin in 5 of 12 patients. The total protein concentration was within normal limits during the whole postoperative period. There was a continuous decrease in the albumin concentration during the first 3 postoperative weeks and a simultaneous increase in globulin during the same period. The catabolism of albumin was found to be the same after liver resections as it was after other types of major surgery. The synthesizing capacity of albumin was decreased during the first postoperative week in all patients who had liver resections and during the first 3 weeks in those who had more than 70 percent of the liver resected. The findings were in agreement with the results of studies of changes in different liver-produced coagulation factors. The requirement of albumin substitution was calculated to be 40 to 70 gm per day during the first week and 10 to 20 gm per day during the following 2 weeks. The serum albumin had to be monitored frequently during this critical period when liver regeneration was restoring its capacity to synthesize albumin at a rate that would stay abreast of catabolism. Exogenous albumin must be provided intravenously to make up the deficit during the period of regeneration.

Dearterialization of the Liver for Metastases

Regression of cancer in the liver (primary and metastatic) occurs following dearterialization of the liver because malignant tumors of the liver are supplied almost exclusively by arterial blood (Breedis and Young, 1954). Normal liver is supplied both by arterial and portal venous blood. Necrosis of cancers in dearterialized livers occurs very rapidly but is generally incomplete. Also, the effect is short lived because the rearterialization of the liver occurs in a matter of days.

Complete dearterialization of the liver should be reserved for low-risk patients with unresectable metastases. Surgery for dearterialization of the liver is aided by celiac artery angiography and selected angiograms that delineate the variegated anatomy of the hepatic artery, its origin, and its branches.

Dearterialization requires the ligation of the right, left, and common hepatic arteries and the right gastric and duodenal arteries and the division of all peritoneal attachments of the liver, taking care to avoid injury to the large veins. The gallbladder may become ischemic and require removal after ligation.

Many of the changes produced by the massive surgical resection of the liver are also produced by dearterialization, as a result of the partial but recoverable necrosis. The same pattern of close postoperative support required for massive resection is also required for dearterialization. Dearterialization offers transient benefit for both large bowel adenocarcinomas and carcinoids (Khoury et al., 1979; Karakousis et al., 1979).

Catheters may be inserted at the time of ligation. The independent or simultaneous methods and the results of hepatic artery or portal vein infusion are covered in the next section.

Hepatic Perfusion

The technologic ability to deliver long-term, controlled-dose chemotherapy to hepatic metastases has improved steadily. The very slow growth of many colonic cancers and their metastases insures that only a very small percentage of total cellular composition will be replicating at any one time. For cycle-specific drugs, this is a major disadvantage. To counter this, it is necessary to evaluate the administration of drugs over long periods of time, at effective dosage levels and in subtoxic amounts.

The treatment of colorectal cancers metastatic to the liver, by both hepatic arterial and portal venous perfusion, has been the subject of a number of reports since the early 1960s, when interest first arose in this approach. The rationale for early efforts to control hepatic metastases evolved, in part, from a study by Willis (1952). He reported that, among 59 patients who had died from cancer of the colon, residual cancer found at autopsy was in the liver in only 19 percent of the series. Reciprocally, 81 percent of the patients had extrahepatic metastases contributing to death.

Donegan and associates (1969) reported an early series in which treatment for hepatic metastases using hepatic artery infusion confirmed the susceptibility of metastases from colonic cancers to sustained infusion. In that report, there were 8 patients with hepatic metastases from colonic cancers and two with metastases from rectal cancers. About half of the metastases responded with reduction in size to the daily infusion of 500 mg of 5-fluorouracil. For maintenance, this dosage was reduced to infusion of 250 mg daily. Low-volume Watkins chronometric infusion pumps were used (Watkins and Khazei, 1966; Sullivan et al., 1967). The study was uncontrolled but matched-pair analysis showed a significant increase in survivorship at 300 days.

Implantable perfusion pumps have been developed, which have the potential for overcoming the inconvenience of earlier systems. In 1980, Buchwald and associates described preliminary results using a totally implantable, percutaneously refillable infusion pump, which feeds a catheter cannulated into the hepatic artery at laparotomy. The pumps were implanted in subcutaneous pockets. They were well tolerated and permitted the delivery of chemotherapy on a long-term outpatient basis.

Bland and Polk (1983) reported on their review of 15 major series that described the various infusion methods for treating hepatic metastases and the end results. The patients treated by infusion survived an average of 10.2 months and the controls survived an average of 5.4 months, with considerable variance. This was a very mixed group of 904 patients; there were no reports of dramatic improvement. However, it was documented that the technology for infusion chemotherapy of the liver, by a variety of methods, was well advanced. The limits on progress for the treatment of hepatic metastases by hepatic infusion chemotherapy are limited by Willis' (1952) observation that only 19 percent of the metastases from colon cancer involved only the liver. Also, the need for more effective drugs or drug combinations was confirmed. There is a continuing need to determine: (1) the ideal drug combination and dosage schedule, (2) whether the advantage of perfusion delivery over systemic delivery is great enough to justify the use of perfusion, and (3) if those patients at high risk who develop only hepatic metastases can be identified with sufficient accuracy to justify an adjuvant trial of perfusion therapy.

PULMONARY METASTASES

Colorectal adenocarcinomas occasionally produce metastases with the lung as the only remote site. Long-term survivors from the resection of these metastases have been reported (Habein et al, 1959). Polk and Spratt (1971) reported on the effectiveness of follow-up after resection of colorectal cancers. The thoracic roentgenogram was useful in the identification of unsuspected pulmonary metastases. In their series, one long-term survivor after resection of pulmonary metastases was reported.

In 1970, Mountain provided a major contribution to the management of pulmonary metastases. His criteria, still valid, for the surgical resection of pulmonary metastases were the following: (1) The patient must be able to tolerate the necessary operation. (2) Cancer must be absent at the primary site. (3) Other cancer must not exist beyond the scope of the pulmonary resection. Bilateral metastases were not excluded by these criteria. His reported results were very acceptable, although uncontrolled.

In one series, the natural history of untreated pulmonary metastases was used as the basis for understanding this problem (Spratt and Spratt, 1964). Spratt and Spratt reported a log normal frequency distribution for the net tumor volume doubling times for ten cases of pulmonary metastases from colorectal adenocarcinoma. The mean was 109 days, with 95 percent confidence range of 9 to 1300 days. These data, reviewed extensively in Chapter Two, provided an estimate of the extreme variance in the percentage of cells in mitosis, which must be taken into account when cycle-specific chemotherapy is considered.

An example of the selected resection of pulmonary metastases is provided by the case of S. B., a 57-year-old woman who underwent a left hemicolectomy in March 1980 for a Duke's A cancer, with no metastases in the mesenteric lymph nodes. She was completely asymptomatic on all follow-up visits, but pulmonary metastases were seen on chest x-rays in August 1980, September 1981, and in retrospect on her preoperative chest x-ray of March 1980. A complete work-up showed no other signs of cancer. The metastases were doubling their volume about every 173 to 199 days, and their size 17 months after the colon resection ranged from 7 to 10 mm. In September 1981, separate metastases were resected, by means of a median sternotomy, from the left upper lobe, the right upper lobe, and the right lower lobe.

Charles Moertel, M.D., was consulted to see if there was a chemotherapeutic option to surgical resection in this case. He stated, "All randomized controlled trials of adjuvant chemotherapy in colorectal cancer have failed to demonstrate a significant advantage for treated patients over controls" (Moertel, 1981).

The residual survivorship of the patient was estimated not to exceed 1384 days, or about

3.7 years, based on a rate of growth of the largest metastasis present in September 1981 (Spratt and Spratt, 1964). An extenuating circumstance in her case was the presence of a cardiac problem that could have been aggravated by cardiotoxic chemotherapeutic drugs.

Four hundred and two days after resection of her pulmonary metastases, her chest radiograph remained clear, but her carcinoembryonic antigen (CEA) had risen and the presence of bilateral hepatic metastases was confirmed at laparotomy. A hepatic arterial catheter was inserted and a subcutaneously implanted Infusaid perfusion pump was attached. On 5-fluoro-2′-deoxyuridine (5 FUDR) her CEA fell and she remained asymptomatic 673 days after the pulmonary metastases were resected. This projection of survivorship by the use of actual doubling time ($Dt_{(ACT)}$) suggests that she has definitely benefited from and continues to benefit from the treatment, 1231 days after pulmonary resection at the time of this writing.

The optimum strategy for the performance of chest x-rays, as part of the follow-up in patients who have had resected colorectal cancers is not known. Most patients will not meet Mountain's criteria (Mountain, 1970). Those who do will appear over an ill-defined time span. At this time, we believe that patients should have a chest x-ray every 3 to 6 months during the first 48 postresection months (Polk and Spratt, 1971). This effort will be rewarded by the discovery of the occasional patient who will benefit from surgical resection. Contemporary pulmonary imaging methods permit a remarkably accurate assessment of the extent of metastases and have now become an integral part of preoperative evaluation. Those who do not meet Mountain's criteria will not derive benefit from resection.

A series of 14 patients undergoing resection of pulmonary metastases from large bowel cancer were reported by Hughes and associates (1982). Two patients lived disease free for 6 and 12 years, and a third patient was doing well 2 years after resection of metastases. Six of the remaining 11 patients developed pulmonary metastases from 74 to 136 months after resection of the colonic primaries. They survived from 9 months to 11 years after the pulmonary resections. In eleven patients death was eventually caused by systemic metastases in the brain, the spinal cord, or bone. This pattern is characteristic of cancers that grow slowly but still disseminate.

SUMMARY

Metastases to the lung or liver vary widely, from single or limited metastases to miliary metastases. They also exhibit a wide range of growth rates, from very slow to very rapid. Selected metastases are resectable with favorable results. Controlled clinical trials have yet to be conducted for the best management of many of the morbid presentations of these metastases. Encouraging results merit continuing study.

References

Adson MA, Van Heerden JA: Major hepatic resections for metastatic colorectal cancer. Ann Surg 191:576–583, 1980.

Almersjö O, Bengmark S: Changes in serum protein fractions after 20–80 percent liver resections in man—especially albumin changes. A study with electrophoresis and 131-I and 125-I tagged human albumin. Acta Chir Scand 135:311–319, 1969.

Bland KI, Polk HC Jr: Therapeutic measures applied for curative and palliative control of colorectal carcinoma. Surg Annu 15:123–161, 1983.

Breedis C, Young G: The blood supply of neoplasms in the liver. Am J Pathol 30:969–977, 1954.

Buchwald H, Grage TB, Vassilopoulos PP, et al: Intraarterial infusion chemotherapy for hepatic carcinoma using a totally implantable infusion pump. Cancer 45:866–869, 1980.

Donegan WL, Harris HS, Spratt JS Jr: Prolonged continuous hepatic infusion. Results with fluorouracil for primary and metastatic cancer in the liver. Arch Surg 99:149–157, 1969.

Fortner JG, Kim DK, Maclean BJ, et al: Major hepatic resection for neoplasia: personal experience in 108 patients. Ann Surg 188:363–371, 1978.

Fortner JG Pahnke LD: A new method for long-term intrahepatic chemotherapy. Surg Gynecol Obstet 143:979–980, 1976.

Foster JH, Berman MM: Solid liver tumors. *In* Ebert PA (ed): Major Probl Clin Surg 22:209–234, 1977.

Gillett DJ, Smith RC: Treatment of the carcinoid syndrome by hemihepatectomy and radical excision of the primary lesion. Am J Surg 128:95–99, 1974.

Habein HC Jr, Clagett OT, McDonald JR: Pulmonary resection for metastatic tumors. Arch Surg 78:716–723, 1959.

Hanks JB, Meyers WC, Filston HC, et al: Surgical resection for benign and malignant liver disease. Ann Surg 191:584–592, 1980.

Hughes ES, McConchie IH, McDermott FT, et al: Resection of lung metastases in large bowel cancer. Br J Surg 69:410–412, 1982.

Jaffe BM, Donegan WL, Watson F, Spratt JS Jr: Factors influencing survival in patients with untreated hepatic metastases. Surg Gynecol Obstet 127:1–11, 1968.

Karakousis CP, Douglass HO Jr, Holyoke ED: Technique of infusion chemotherapy, ligation of the hepatic artery and dearterialization in malignant lesions of the liver. Surg Gynecol Obstet 149:403–407, 1979.

Khoury GA, Divine T, Bolt DE: Complete dearterialization and the carcinoid syndrome. Br J Surg 66:253–256, 1979.

Kim DK, Watson RC, Pahnke LD, Fortner JG: Tumor vascularity as a prognostic factor for hepatic tumors. Ann Surg 185:31–34, 1977.

Levine AW, Donegan WL, Irwin M: Adenocarcinoma of the colon with hepatic metastases: fifteen year survival. JAMA 247:2809–2810, 1982.

Lin TY: A simplified technique for hepatic resection: The crush method. Ann Surg 180:285–290, 1974.

Logan SE, Meier SJ, Ramming KP, et al: Hepatic resection of metastatic colorectal cancer. A ten-year experience. Arch Surg 117:25–28, 1982.

MacLean MD, Murray FH, Bacon HE: Hepatic metastasis of squamous cell carcinoma of the anal canal: review of literature and case report. Dis Colon Rectum 5:51–55, 1962.

Moertel C: Personal communication, December 1981.

Mountain CF: Surgical management of pulmonary metastases. Postgrad Med 48:128–132, 1970.

Polk HC Jr, Spratt JS Jr: Recurrent colorectal carcinoma: detection, treatment, and other considerations. Surgery 69:9–23, 1971.

Ryan WH, Hummel BW, McClelland RN: Reduction in the morbidity and mortality of major hepatic resection. Am J Surg 144:740–743, 1982.

Schwerk WB, Schmitz-Moormann P: Ultrasonically guided fine-needle biopsies in neoplastic liver disease: cytohistologic diagnoses and echo pattern of lesions. Cancer 48:1469–1477, 1981.

Spratt JS Jr, Spratt TL: Rates of growth of pulmonary metastases and host survival. Ann Surg 159:161–171, 1964.

Spratt JS Jr, Watson FR, Pratt JL: Characteristics of variants of colorectal carcinoma that do not metastasize to lymph nodes. Dis Colon Rectum 13:243–246, 1970.

Sullivan RD, Watkins E Jr, Oberfield RA, Khazei AM: Current status of protracted arterial infusion cancer chemotherapy for the treatment of solid tumors. Surg Clin N Am 47:769–784, 1967.

Watkins E Jr, Khazei AM: Arterial infusion chemotherapy of liver cancer. Bull Soc Int Chir 25:279–292, 1966.

Willis RA: The Spread of Tumors in the Human Body. 2nd ed. London, Butterworth, 1952, p.181.

FIFTEEN

Pseudomyxoma Peritonei

J. S. Spratt, M.D.
H. Wald, M.D.
R. Adcock, B.S.

Pseudomyxoma peritonei is a syndrome characterized by mucinous ascites and is usually produced by peritoneal surface growth of low-grade mucin-producing adenocarcinomas. Most of the neoplasms arise from the appendix or the ovary, but occasionally they may arise from mucin-producing neoplasms in other parts of the gastrointestinal tract. The syndrome is infrequent, and large series (50 cases) have not been reported in the literature. In one of the larger series, 2 cases of appendiceal, 12 of ovarian, and 3 of uncertain origin were reported (Long et al., 1969). This study, supported by a review of the literature, documented the chronicity of these cases, the importance of avoiding overtreatment, and the importance of several basic treatment principles to minimize morbidity. The best results were obtained by initial laparotomy with (1) resection of all gross neoplasm, the organs of origin, both ovaries, the appendix, and the omentum; (2) complete evacuation of the mucinous ascites; and (3) the administration of mild intracavitary chemotherapy. The use of thiotepa with this surgical approach was associated with protracted remissions.

An important histologic feature correlated well with prognosis—the growth pattern on the peritoneum of the mucin-producing adenocarcinoma. When the growth was one cell thick and noninvasive, the prognosis was improved. When the growth pattern consisted of multiple cell layers, especially with islands of mucin in the subperitoneal tissues, the prognosis was worse. Thus, a careful review of the histologic growth pattern can be of great value to the clinician in predicting the aggressiveness of the neoplastic process in a case of pseudomyxoma peritonei and the potential responsiveness to intracavitary chemotherapy (Long et al., 1969). The results of this series are shown in Figure 15–1 (Long et al., 1969).

Long's 1969 study stimulated a continuing interest in this infrequent but morbid syndrome. Performance specifications for a delivery system for the safe administration of intracavitary hyperthermic chemotherapeutic perfusion of the peritoneal cavity with a filtered perfusate from which free cells and other debris were removed on recirculation were formulated. A pilot unit was designed and constructed. This system is referred to as the *thermal infusion filtration system* (TIFS) (Spratt et al., 1980a and b).

A review of the pathophysiology of peritoneal carcinomatosis and ascites will be presented before the discussion of this system and its effects.

PATHOPHYSIOLOGY AND LABORATORY EVALUATION OF MALIGNANT ASCITES

In 1977, Bronskill and co-workers reported the quantitative determination of peritoneal drainage rates in malignant ascites. Whenever the outflow rate of ascitic fluid was less than 50 ml per hour, diaphragmatic and mediastinal lymphatics were generally abnormal, most frequently from tumor permeation. Potential sources of ascites included the tumor, excess production of ascitic fluid from peritoneum not involved with tumor, and the oncotic pressure of the exudate. With intractable ascites, the

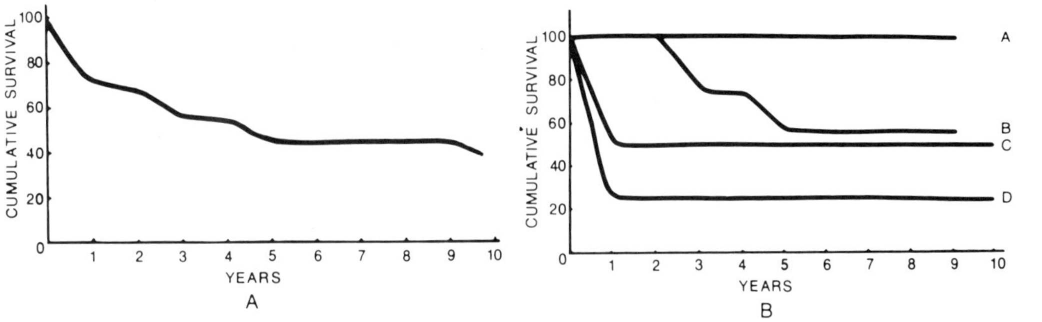

Figure 15–1. *A,*1 Cumulative survival for all patients with pseudomyxoma after intial treatment. The five-year rate of 45 percent is superior to that of patients with ovarian cancer. *B,* Cumulative survival for all patients with pseudomyxoma after initial treatment. Survival after various treatment regimens are compared. A, multiple operative procedures combined with alkylating agents (five patients); B, multiple operative procedures (five patients); C, paracenteses only (two patients); D, single operative procedure, including oophorectomy (five patients). Testing for clinical significance of these data at five years, we obtain $\chi^2 = 7.89$, $p < .05$. (From Long RT, Spratt JS Jr, Dowling E: Pseudomyxoma peritonei. Am J Surg 117:162–169, 1969.)

lymphatic drainage was often blocked by neoplasm. This could often be demonstrated by the failure of intraperitoneal radiocolloids to make the diaphragmatic and mediastinal lymphatics visible. An additional but incompletely studied factor is the possibility that the viscosity of the ascites associated with pseudomyxoma peritonei may simply be too great for adequate lymph egress.

In parallel flow rate studies involving a two-compartment model (plasma and peritoneal cavity) and radioactive iodinated serum albumin (RISA), Bronskill and colleagues showed that the radiocolloids failed to fill these lymphatics when the flow rate between the compartments was less than 50 ml per hour (Bronskill et al., 1977). An important measurement of the effect of any treatment was the ability to demonstrate that this flow, if subnormal, increased after treatment.

In 1973, Meyers reviewed the anatomic locus of peritoneal seeding of cancer and the dynamics of flow of peritoneal fluid. The four major sites of seeding were (1) the pouch of Douglas at the rectosigmoid level; (2) the right lower quadrant at the lower end of the small bowel mesentery; (3) the left lower quadrant along the superior border of the sigmoid mesocolon and colon; and (4) the right paracolic gutter lateral to the cecum and ascending colon. These were all sites at which the flow of peritoneal fluid was preferentially and repeatedly arrested. The dynamic flow of peritoneal fluid was confirmed by fluoroscopic roentgen contrast studies. The flow pattern was determined by mesenteric reflections and peritoneal recesses. Fluid pooled in dependent recesses. Upward flow from these dependent recesses was an active process proceeding along both lateral gutters to the subphrenic spaces. The lower hydrostatic pressure in the subphrenic space that accompanies respiration was considered the driving force for this pattern. These observations are potentially pertinent to determination of the most effective anatomic site for placement of catheters used in intracavitary perfusion and chemotherapy. They also indicate the need for designing effective input and output catheters that will facilitate a thermal equilibrium within the peritoneal cavity.

Work by Cailleau and colleagues in 1974 confirmed that malignant cells derived from effusions in humans are viable in tissue culture. Whether the patient gains a therapeutic advantage from the mechanical removal of neoplastic cells from malignant effusions has not been determined. There is, however, sound evidence that free-floating malignant cells are viable. In fact, effusions provide a fertile source of tumor cell lines. The rate of shedding of these cells has not been measured accurately. Useful experimental objectives in the study of tumor cell kinetics in effusions are evaluation of the type and number of cells removed by a filtration system and determination of the rate of removal. The latter would be helpful in assessing optimal lengths of recycling time and the effect of agents that might increase the rate of shedding (e.g., heparin, mucolytic agents, proteolytic agents, and hyaluronidase).

In 1974, Chandrasekhar and Buehler considered the diagnostic significance of various laboratory tests performed on malignant effusions. Their clinical laboratory evaluation of the malignant effusions was directed toward

(1) verifying or refuting previous studies, (2) providing a multifactorial characterization of the effusions, and (3) verifying the diagnosis that an effusion is indeed associated with malignant cells. The differential diagnosis of fluids in body cavities was found feasible on the basis of many of these factors. There are additional important methods in cytologic studies, including block smears, staining techniques, and enzyme studies (Backman and Pasila, 1974). A more certain method is actual biopsy of all serosal surfaces associated with effusions (Bakalos et al., 1974). Carcinoembryonic antigen (CEA) in both serum and ascites may reach extremely high levels in cases of pseudomyxoma peritonei and serum CEA levels may often be used to monitor response to treatment (JSS, personal cases).

Both computed tomography and sonography have been used to evaluate the extent of pseudomyxoma peritonei (Mayes et al., 1981; Seshul and Coulam, 1981). Reported findings are nonspecific and are seen with other problems. One usually finds peritoneal scalloping of the lower margin or ascitic septation or both. "Scalloping" refers to extrinsic pressure on the liver margin by adjacent implants that occurs in the absence of parenchymal hepatic metastases. The "septation" is thought to represent mucinous nodules in the ascites.

THERAPEUTIC APPROACHES

Hyperthermia

Physiologic Effects. Although hyperthermia can be induced by heated intracavitary fluid, the hyperthermic effect will, in many ways, be similar in its physiologic effect to systemic hyperthermia induced by other methods. In 1977, Larkin and colleagues reviewed these effects. They induced hyperthermia with a water blanket modified to sustain a water temperature of 49 degrees C. The patients were warmed under sedation, and core temperature was measured with rectal and esophageal probes. Core temperature was elevated to 42 degrees C and maintained at that level for 2 hours during each treatment. Vital signs were monitored every 15 minutes along with continuous EKG monitoring throughout the procedure. Urine output was constantly monitored by indwelling catheter. Intravenous solutions were administered at a rate adequate to maintain urinary output. Electroencephalographic monitoring was performed in early cases but later proved unnecessary and was discontinued. Each treatment was administered under light nitrous oxide (60 percent) and oxygen (40 percent) anesthesia supplemented by intravenous narcotics and barbiturates as needed. Premedication consisted of atropine, morphine, and a barbiturate.

With this therapy alone, over 50 percent of the patients treated by Larkin and coworkers experienced objective regression of their neoplasms. The blanket-warming system required 90 to 120 minutes to raise the core temperature to 42 degrees C, with temperature rising about 0.5 degree C every 15 minutes. Pulse rates climbed steadily, ranging between 130 and 207, with an average of 162. The systolic blood pressure increased slightly, but the diastolic pressure dropped. About 15 percent of the patients developed mild cardiac arrhythmias—PVCs and bigeminy—that occasionally proved difficult to control with antiarrhythmic agents (e.g., xylocaine). Sweating became profuse. Large quantities of crystalloid solutions (alternating D5RL and D51/2NS) were required to replace losses. Arterial blood gases showed mild metabolic acidosis compensated for by hyperventilation during and after the hyperthermia.

Electrolytes were monitored serially with the following results:

1. There was no change in Na^+ or Cl^-.
2. K^+ increased immediately following treatment and then dropped.
3. Bicarbonate dropped during and after treatment in response to a mild metabolic acidosis.
4. Serum Ca^{++}, Mg^{++}, and PO_4 fell but returned to pretreatment levels 3 to 4 days after treatment without supplementation.

Hyperglycemia developed during and after treatment, and diabetic patients required supplementary insulin. Hemolysis did not occur, and hemoglobin and hematocrit did not drop. Central nervous system changes did not occur, determined by either clinical observation or EEG. Renal function, as measured by BUN and creatinine levels, remained constant. Serum enzymes sometimes increased markedly after treatment whenever any signs of liver or heart disease coexisted. The values returned to normal within several days. Coagulation parameters (PT and PTT) remained constant. The polymorphonuclear cell counts rose regularly after treatment, but lymphocytes decreased. Uric acid levels rose mainly in those patients exhibiting a tumor response. Pulmonary function studies were inconclusive. Mild diarrhea occurred regularly after each treatment and lasted 1 to 2 days.

Two patients died in Larkin's series. One was a debilitated 32-year-old man with massive melanoma who died from unknown cause 24 hours after treatment. At autopsy, massive necrosis in the melanoma was confirmed. The second patient was a 59-year-old debilitated woman with lymphoma who exhibited a similar pattern of demise. About 20 hours after treatment, she became drowsy, tachypneic, hypotensive, and oliguric. She died within 5 hours following cardiorespiratory failure. The common factors in these two patients were poor physiologic condition, large amounts of thermally sensitive neoplasm, and massive liver involvement.

The necrosis of tumors is related to both temperature and duration of exposure of tumor to hyperthermia. In 1980, Storm and coworkers reaffirmed that hyperthermia from 42 to 50 degrees C could be tolerated with virtually no normal tissue damage. The range of necrosis obtained supported the use of higher temperatures for longer periods of time. Storm's group concluded that thermal death could occur after 30 hours at 42 degrees C, after 3 to 4 hours at 45 degrees C, and after minutes at 50 degrees C. Much work is needed to define the optimal time-temperature-frequency schedules for all types of visceral cancers, including those producing pseudomyxoma peritonei.

Hyperthermic Potentiation of Radiation Therapy. In addition to potentiating effects of drugs on cancer, hyperthermia differentially enhances the effect of radiotherapy. Intracavitary hyperthermia can be used in conjunction with radionuclides that concentrate on serosal surfaces (Leith et al., 1977). Hyperthermia may potentiate the effect of radiation in several ways: destruction of cells (which does not appear to be oxygen-dependent), inhibition of recovery of sublethally radiated cells, and improvement in the therapeutic ratios of the radiotherapy.

In 1961, Shingleton and colleagues developed a method of enhancing the efficacy of the chemotherapeutic agents added to the reentry spigot by cycling ascitic fluid through a warmer, raising its temperature to 41 to 42 degrees C. In parallel, total body hypothermia was induced, lowering body temperature to between 31 and 32 degrees C. This technique has been used successfully on the extremities and might be feasible for intracavitary treatment.

Proteolytic Enzymes

In 1974, Titscher and co-workers compared Au^{198}, proresid (podophyllinic acid 2-ethylhydrazide), cyclophosphamide, and Wobe-Mugos in the local management of effusions. These investigators found Wobe-Mugos to be the most effective single agent in the control of malignant effusions.* The theory is that tumor cells are more effectively penetrated and degraded by proteolytic enzymes than normal cells are. The authors' findings served as evidence of enhanced cell degradation.

These results suggested that commercially available proteolytic enzymes that can be used in the recycled fluid either alone or with other therapeutic agents require further study. The preparation selected should be sterile, of low antigenicity, miscible in water, and optimally effective in lysing tumor cells but not normal mesothelial cells.

Corynebacterium parvum and Cyclophosphamide

In 1975, Fisher and colleagues demonstrated in C3H tumors in mice that, of various combinations tried, the intraperitoneal administration of *C. parvum* and cyclophosphamide was most effective in suppressing tumor growth. These investigators observed that "a marked desmoplastic reaction characterized those tumors exhibiting the greatest inhibition of tumor growth." With this finding plus other evidence cited in their article, Fisher's group concluded that there is "a rationale for investigation of such combined therapy in human malignancy."

Chemotherapy by Dialysis

In 1978, Myers and associates studied the effects of administering chemotherapy by peritoneal dialysis alone. Although the agent crossed the peritoneum and entered the blood stream, the drug levels in the plasma were 50 to 100 times lower than those in the peritoneal fluid. Myers's group used methotrexate in the

---

*Wobe-Mugos is the trade name for a proteolytic enzyme combination distributed by the Scientific Department of Messrs. MUCOS Emulsionsgesellshaft mbH, 8022 Grünewald/Munich. It had not been approved by the FDA for distribution in the United States at the time of this writing.

dialysate and administered citrovorum factor 40 hours after dialysis. The treatment plans were based on computer simulation. The authors employed a permanent indwelling Tenckhoff catheter and treated patients with dialysis, 2 to 6 hours per week, using methotrexate concentrations of 1 to 7 $\times$ 10^{-5} ng per ml for 5 weeks. This method was used to treat ovarian cancers in which residual tumor masses were less than 0.5 cm in diameter.

The Thermal Infusion Filtration System (TIFS)

Design and Methods

Thermal infusion filtration system was designed to provide a delivery system for evaluating intracavitary hyperthermic chemotherapy for malignant ascites and neoplasms on serosal surfaces producing pseudomyxoma peritonei. With respect to the management of malignant effusions, the increased dynamics of flow with TIFS are both physiologically tolerable and important in achieving the optimal distribution of heat, fluid, and chemotherapeutic agents at doses that can be obtained by systemic administration. Furthermore, the hyperthermic conditioning prior to chemotherapy is potentially beneficial alone for the preferential destruction of neoplastic cells. These two performance characteristics, along with the potential of mechanical filtration of malignant cells, distinguish TIFS as a unique integrated unit.

Results have encouraged additional inquiry into specific physiologic and pharmacokinetic combinations, and they have emphasized the need to continue exploration into cell removal rates, anticipated percentage of cell recovery, and fluid distribution relative to intracavitary surface exposure. Developmental research with TIFS is still in progress (see below).

The TIFS was designed to recirculate intracavitary effusions aseptically through the combined actions of dynamic fluid flow, free-cell and debris filtration, hyperthermia, and adjunctive chemotherapy. TIFS incorporates components of several methods of treatment. Two units form the basic system: (1) the transport unit, which consists of medical-grade tubing, connectors, and filters; and (2) the mechanical unit, which is composed of a pump, a heat exchanger, and temperature-monitoring devices. The system infuses and recirculates variable volumes of isotonic solution at controlled levels of hyperthermia through operatively placed infusion catheters, through which a prewarmed (> 41.5 : < 50 degrees C, but variable temperature) volume of sterile solution flows to the peritoneal cavity. Next, the transport unit circulates the fluid through a dual filter component and a warming coil, from which the fluid is returned to the peritoneal cavity. This process is repeated for the entire treatment period.

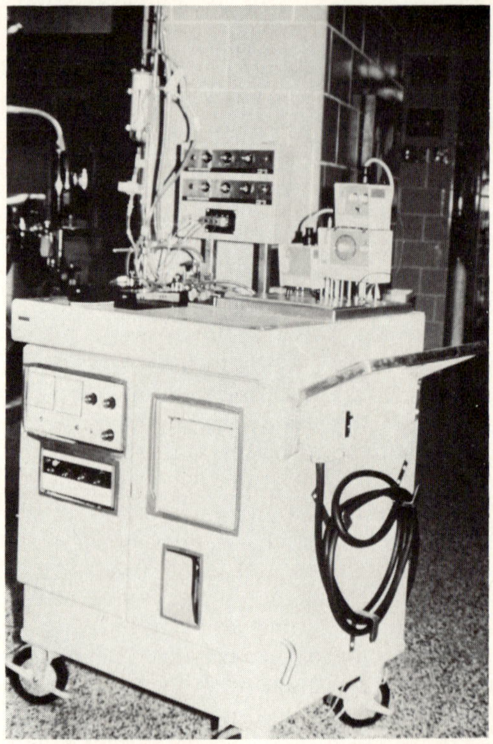

Figure 15–2. The thermal infusion-filtration system is designed to recirculate intracavitary effusions or substituted solutions, such as Ringer's lactate. The system provides a dynamic fluid flow, filtration of cells and debris with each cycle, and controlled intracavitary hyperthermia and allows for the administration intracavitary chemotherapy. With specially designed intracavitary catheters, the system provides intracavitary hyperthermia to 50° C, ± 0.5. Further details on this delivery system are provided in the text and in works by Spratt and associates (1980a and b).

The prototypic design (Figs. 15–2 to 15–4) was described by Palta and associates in 1979. It utilizes a Masterflex* variable-speed rotor pump accommodating a medical-grade tubing having a ¼-in. (0.952-cm) outside diameter. In this unit, the heat input and monitoring devices incorporate into an integrated system. A more versatile system can be obtained with

*Model number 7555-40, Cole-Parmer Instrument Co., Chicago, IL.

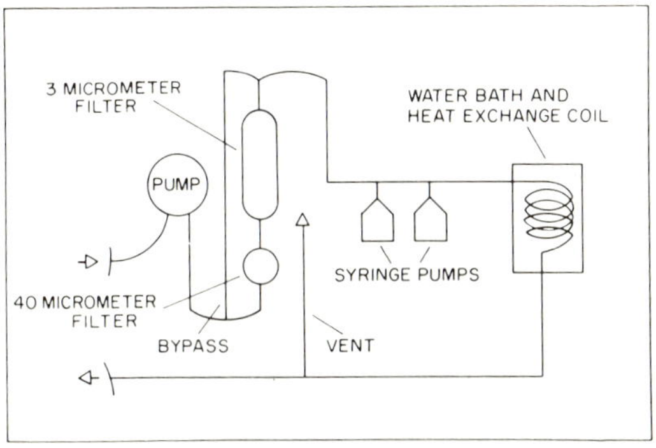

Figure 15–3. Fluid flow schematic of the thermal infusion filtration system. Arrows show the direction of the fluid flow. (From Spratt JS, Adcock RA, Muskovin M, et al: Clinical delivery system for intraperitoneal hyperthermic chemotherapy. Cancer Res 40:256–260, 1980.)

cardiac perfusion pumps but requires peripheral equipment for heating the perfusate. The unit is shown in Figures 15–3 and 15–4.*

The prewarmed solution is infused until the abdominal wall is distended. When the peritoneal cavity is full, the fluid is pumped from the peritoneal cavity through the exit catheter. The fluid continues through the transport unit and flows back into the patient through entry catheters. A temperature probe (Sarns 12100) is located on the entry line just proximal to the patient. A second temperature probe is located just distal to the patient at the exit line. Fluid traveling through the transport unit passes through a dual set of filters (45-μm Pall EC3840 and 5-μm Delta Medical PB-005, respectively). These filters will effectively remove both debris and free cells in the perfusate. A bypass of these filters is also incorporated into TIFS to permit filter changes. Heat exchange occurs across a coil placed in a Thermomix 1460-BKU immersion water bath.*

The anatomic complexity of the peritoneal cavity has required the design of special catheters for the intraperitoneal delivery systems. These are essential to rapid, wide diffusion and uniform hyperthermia. Dual pumps on both inflow and outflow sides are being added. The changes in design permit a uniform, very rapid delivery and evacuation of perfusate throughout the peritoneal cavity. Tubes of varying length, accommodating different sizes of peritoneal cavities, have been devised to deliver and evacuate perfusate equally throughout their length. The delivery tubes are now placed in the medial side of the posterior gutter, one on each side of the root of the dorsal mesentery. The removal tubes are placed ventrolaterally near the abdominal wall. Trials in rabbits indicate that control of temperature is now more concise and uniform, as has been confirmed by placement of thermistors in the peritoneal cavity of the rabbit in upper, middle, and lower abdominal areas varying from dorsal to ventral. This permits maintenance of closely controlled temperatures in excess of 41.5 degrees C for periods longer than 1 hour. Higher temperatures are attainable with the system. With the long uniform flow and suction catheter and minimal surgical intervention, similar controlled uni-

*Sarns model numbers 5M6008 and 5M6002, Sarns, Inc., Ann Arbor, MI.

*B. Braun Melsungen A.G., W. Germany. Available from Cole-Parmer Instrument Co., Chicago, IL.

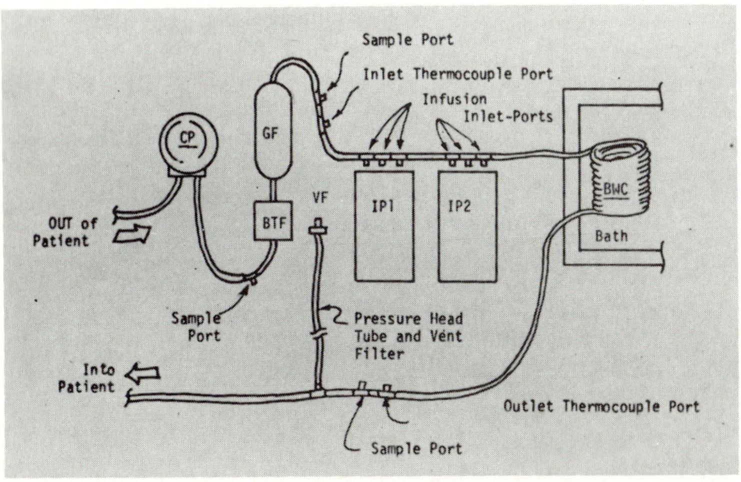

Figure 15–4. Electrical diagram of the thermal infusion filtration system. Arrows show the direction of the fluid flow.

formity of temperature should be attainable in humans. Both the phrenogastric ligament and the gastrocolic ligament must be opened to allow free flow into the lesser sac. The inlet catheters should be placed through the transverse mesocolon to perfuse both colic spaces adequately. The end of one catheter goes to the pelvis along each side of the rectum. The removal catheters must be placed in anterolateral or ventrolateral positions. Thermistors are placed at scatter sites throughout the cavity to verify temperature control.

TIFS in Animals

The preliminary assessment of the TIFS performed with the prototypic model in simulated cavities has provided a good approximation of mixing dynamics and steady-state time that might be expected in the animal model. A preclinical experimental protocol involving the dog model was designed to assess TIFS (Spratt et al., 1980b).

In the preclinical trials of TIFS, surgical application, temperature control, fluid dynamics, and physiologic effects were evaluated. Fifteen female mongrel dogs weighing from 17.2 to 25.4 kg were subjected to hyperthermic peritoneal perfusion. Only the circulating fluid was used to induce the hyperthermia.

In the first trials, ten acutely affected dogs were used. The relationship of animal mass to the time required to elevate core temperature (measured rectally) to 41 degrees C at 10 liters per hour was studied. The flow dilution dynamics at various flow rates were studied with 0.5 percent Evans blue solution. Nembutal anesthesia (60 mg per kg) was used in each dog. Peritoneal dialysis catheters* were placed at both the right and left lateral gutters of the peritoneal cavities. A small incision was required for each placement. The catheters were held in place by a purse-string suture. The infusing catheter was oriented to infuse toward the diaphragm. The sump catheter, in the opposing lateral gutter, was directed into the pelvic cavity. An artificial effusate (350 to 400 ml dog plasma and 1650 to 1800 ml sterile 0.9 percent NaCl solution) was introduced intraperitoneally in all dogs to provide a pseudoexudate.

Five chronically affected dogs were perfused at 41 degrees C (peritoneal cavity temperature) for 2 hours under physiologic monitoring and were kept under observation for 2 weeks, with subsequent evaluation of adhesions, peritonitis, and histologic changes. Tissue specimens were then taken from liver, spleen, kidney, pancreas, stomach, adrenal, bowel, mesentery, and aortic nodes.

During the TIFS runs, thermistor probes* were placed in the rectum and peritoneal cavity of each animal. An esophageal probe was also placed. All probes were calibrated at 45 ± 0.5 degrees C (S.D.) in the constant temperature bath of the unit and were accurate to ± 0.2 degrees C.

All 15 dogs survived the hyperthermic perfusion without noticeable distress. The chronically affected animals were fully recovered within 24 hours and survived the 2-week observation period without behavioral or physiologic changes. Small amounts of chronic intraperitoneal bleeding were noted but apparently resulted from incision bleeding. Some leakage of perfusate at insertion sites occurred in early runs but was corrected with refinement of placement technique and change of catheters.

Each infusion resulted in a fully distended abdomen. Following injection of 0.5 percent Evans dye solution (2 ml) in eight acutely affected animals peritoneal equilibrium was reached in 7 minutes at 10 liters per hour and in 9 minutes at 6.0 liters per hour. Samples were taken at 1-minute intervals for the first 10 minutes and then at 5-minute intervals for the remainder of a 2-hour interval. Percentage of transmittance was read at 540 nm on a Beckman DB spectrophotometer.†

The time necessary to heat the mass of each animal to 41 degrees C varied. Generally, the greater the weight of the dog, the longer the time required. Exceptions occurred, but the reasons are not known. Each trial was standardized at a flow rate of 10 liters per hour and a water bath temperature of 45 degrees C, and a 6-ft line distance from water bath to infusion site was used. Because of the weight versus time variability, an equation enabling the prediction of the time required to induce total body hyperthermia by the weight of the subject has not been developed. Initially, 45 degrees C bath temperature and 10 liters per hour circulation rate for 1.5 to 2.0 hours were sufficient, in most cases, to bring rectal temperatures (used as a measure of core temperature) to 41 degrees C. At flow rates of less than 8

*McGaw Laboratories, Glendale, CA.

*Yellow Springs Instrument Co., Yellow Springs, OH.

† Beckman Instruments, Inc., Fullerton, CA.

liters per hour, there was failure to reach 41 degrees C in 100 percent of the trials, with perfusion periods up to 3.5 hours. Increasing bath temperature to 55 degrees C was tolerated and shortened the time needed to heat each animal.

Evaluation of the chronically affected dogs at the end of 2 weeks revealed minimal peritoneal adhesions and no gross defects in the peritoneum, omentum, or abdominal organs. Gram-positive wound-site infections were prevalent but were restricted to cutaneous tissue. No peritoneal, abdominal, or organ infection was noted.

The animal studies did not reveal undesirable effects due to the TIFS perfusion procedure over 1.5 to 2 hours.

The temperature-controlled shut-down system, which prevented excess hyperthermia, was 100 percent reliable when the thermostat was set at ± 0.5 degrees C. TIFS was determined to be safe for clinical application. The surgical procedure for placement of the dialysis catheters was unremarkable. Hyperthermia was induced at a steady increase without a significant temperature differential between the heat exchange bath and the body mass (rectal probe) or peritoneal effusate (direct peritoneal temperature probe). Placement of the probe directly into the peritoneal cavity was considered the most conservative approach for monitoring and controlling hyperthermia in routine procedure.

Temperature in the rectum lagged behind that of the peritoneal cavity by approximately 0.4 degrees C. There was a difference of 2.1 degrees C between esophageal and intraperitoneal temperature readings. This lower temperature in the esophagus is due to airway cooling. Such differences are relatively insignificant at these nonlethal temperatures.

Dilution studies suggested that a dynamic equilibrium was established between the intracavitary compartments within minutes when the cavity was fully distended with a fluid reserve. Blood pressures, heart rates, and cardiac indices were expected to be elevated under hyperthermic conditions. These expectations were confirmed, but the elevations were not as great as expected.

In the animal experiments, the TIFS unit met design expectations for controlled intracavitary hyperthermia. The dynamics of flow were essential to achieving the rapid uniform distribution of perfusate and chemotherapeutic agents. Hyperthermic conditioning prior to chemotherapy was obtainable. These characteristics, along with the mechanical filtration of malignant cells, distinguish TIFS as a unique integrated delivery system.

A basic need since the beginning of the TIFS studies has been an animal model that develops peritoneal carcinomatosis with ascites similar to that seen in man. After an exhaustive search of the veterinary literature and consultation with many veterinary pathologists the statement can be made that no truly analogous system exists in animals. The closest thing found was the VX-2 carcinoma implanted in the peritoneum of the Australian white rabbit. Progress with the rabbit has led to an improvement in intraperitoneal catheters in relation to both design and placement to ensure a more rapid and uniform attainment of desired levels of hyperthermia, reducing the risk of unequal levels of hyperthermia and streaming of flow. Increased knowledge of thermolethality confirms that thermal resistance rapidly develops and that thermolethal levels must be attained quickly and uniformly. We can now quickly and uniformly attain a desired therapeutic temperature window at 41.5 to 43 degrees C throughout the peritoneal cavity and maintain it for over an hour without damage to the rabbit's viscera. The control system on TIFS allows for quick fluxes of higher temperatures if desired. The distribution of temperature was confirmed by six intraperitoneal thermistors.

Four catheters (two inflow and two outflow) were found to provide more rapid and complete peritoneal fluid mixing. They consist of simple Silastic tubes, with an inside diameter of ¼ inch and an outside diameter of ½ inch. Multiple holes are placed in the catheters with an 18-gauge needle used as a punch on a motorized drill after removal of the needle point. A perforated ½-inch Penrose drain covers the intraperitoneal length of each catheter. A hole in a Y-connector is used for placing the thermistors.

The inlet catheter on the right is tacked to the posterior peritoneum and is carried up behind the liver. The inlet catheter on the left extends under the stomach to the lesser sac. The outlet catheters egress through the lower abdomen. Incisions are all closed with running locked sutures. Further technical details are to be found in the thesis by Perez (1983).

The improved system has now been well-tested in the rabbit and we have transferred to our laboratories the ability to induce and maintain V2-X cancers in the peritoneum of the rabbit. This places us in the position to do controlled trials in the rabbit using hyperthermic intraperitoneal chemotherapy for a series of promising adjuvants. Considering the high dosage from chemotherapy obtainable for intraperitoneal tumors with this system with respect to systemic drug levels, the feasibility of the rapid exposure to multiple agents as suggested by the chemotherapy model of Goldie (1979) and the close and uniform control of the level of hyperthermia obtainable with TIFS, we will be in a position to evaluate thermolethality synergistic with chemotherapy, if such synergism exists at all, using the Goldie model.

Critical issues in obtaining a synergistic lethal effect from hyperthermia are the absolute tissue temperature, duration of tissue exposure to hyperthermia, and tissue resistance to the effects of heat initially and after exposure. Storm and associates (1980) heated neoplasms from 40 to 50 degrees C from one to ten times for periods varying from 13 to 600 minutes. They then did several biopsies to assay the percentage of necrosis. Several treatments at 40 to 50 degrees C produced 70 to 100 percent necrosis. Lower temperatures had progressively less effect. The improved TIFS catheters permit more diffuse and rapid fluxes at higher temperatures and also permit parallel evaluation of electrolyte and pH modifications intraperitoneally.

In summary, progress has been made in the technical design and testing of a delivery system that has many potential useful clinical features. However, delay in finding an animal model and the cost have slowed progress. At this point, we are in a position to proceed with controlled clinical trials evaluating the synergism of hyperthermia with a spectrum of drug combinations that are administered intraperitoneally with a dynamic fluid flow system. Further slow progress is anticipated because of deficiencies in funding.

TIFS in Humans

Continued developmental research concerned with thermal infusion filtration therapy as it pertains to the conditions defined by the TIFS unit and aimed at refining TIFS for clinical application appears to be highly warranted.

The first human patient treated with TIFS was a 35-year-old man with a 2-year history of early satiety and abdominal distention (Spratt et al., 1980a). After a nondiagnostic examination, he underwent an exploratory laparotomy. After his abdomen was opened, extensive mucin was evacuated, and an omental biopsy was performed. A limited exploration revealed no primary tumor. Histopathologic examination disclosed a low-grade adenocarcinoma with many mucin-containing cysts lining the peritoneum. The surgery provided some symptomatic relief. However, in less than 1 year, the patient's abdominal girth began to increase and his symptoms recurred. His admitting examination was completely within normal limits, except for obvious moderate abdominal distention (girth at umbilicus, 80 cm; weight, 63 kg) and a CEA value of 126.5 ng/ml. His preoperative evaluation included an exercise tolerance test that was used to evaluate his tolerance to hyperthermia. The decision had been made not to allow the tachycardia produced by hyperthermia to exceed the heart rate induced at the patient's exercise tolerance test.

Surgeons reoperated on the patient, using TIFS, in February of 1979. After a thorough preoperative evaluation, including mechanical bowel preparation, general endotracheal anesthesia was induced. A Swan-Ganz catheter was inserted to monitor cardiac output. Thermal probes were placed in the esophagus and rectum. At closure of the abdominal incision, a third probe was placed directly into the peri-

Table 15–1. **LABORATORY VALUES***

	Sodium (mEq/liter)	Potassium (mEq/liter)	Chlorine (mEq/liter)	Carbon Dioxide (mEq/liter)	Alkaline Phosphatase (gm/dl)	Total Protein (gm/dl)	Albumin (gm/dl)
Preoperative†	145	5.1	105	29	71	8..5	4.4
Postoperative range‡	133–134	3.6–4.3	97–106	21–31	66–84	4.2–6.2	2.1–2.9
Discharge‖	143	4.2	98	29	107	6.1	2.8

*From Spratt, J. S., Adcock, R. A., Sherrill, W., and Travathen, S.: Hyperthermic peritoneal perfusion system in canines. Cancer Res. 40:253–255, 1980.

†Values at 1 day before surgery.

‡Value range 13 days after surgery.

§Value at 5 days after surgery.

‖Values at 21 days after surgery.

toneal cavity. A Foley catheter was inserted to monitor urinary output. The laparotomy was carried out through the midline, excising en bloc the patient's previous laparotomy scar.

The peritoneal cavity was again found to contain extensive mucin. The omentum was thickened. The extensive mucin and peritoneal seeding obscured visibility, and the exploration proceeded cautiously. The appendix was found to be grossly normal but demonstrated neoplasm on its serosal surface. The mesentery of the transverse colon was thickened. Multiloculated mucin-filled cysts were extensively present in the omentum, transverse mesocolon, hilus of the spleen, distal pancreas, splenic flexure, and peritoneal cavity. The gelatinous sites contained numerous cancer cells on cell block. When the entire distribution of tumor was reviewed, the pathologist concluded that the pancreas was the organ of origin and that the primary cancer was a cystadenocarcinoma of the pancreas (Compaguo and Oertel, 1978). The gross distribution of tumor was such that the bulk could be resected by removing the ascending colon, the transverse colon, and the omentum. Upon entering the lesser peritoneal sac and attempting to mobilize the splenic flexure, extensive involvement by mucin and mucinous tumor cysts was encountered in the lesser peritoneal sac, distal pancreas, splenic pedicle, and left subphrenic space. The surgical resection was then extended to include the spleen and the distal pancreas. The intestine was anastomosed by an end-to-end ileo-descending colostomy with approximation of the adjacent mesentery. On completion of this resection, the peritoneum was still studded extensively with neoplasm, although all the gross masses were removed. Glisson's capsule was involved superficially, but no metastasis to the hepatic parenchyma was evident.

Two Argyle Saratoga Model 28 sumps* were inserted through the smallest incision that would accommodate them, and an 0-chromic catgut purse-string suture† was placed around their peritoneal entry point to minimize leakage. One catheter was placed in the upper left quadrant with the end laid into the left subphrenic region. The second was placed in the lower right quadrant with the end placed on the pouch of Douglas. The midline abdominal incision was then closed to the peritoneum with continuous 0-chromic catgut and to the fascia with figure-of-eight No. 28 stainless steel wire sutures.† The skin was closed with interrupted 4-0 silk.†

The two catheters were then attached to TIFS for immediate peritoneal perfusion with filtration. The peritoneal cavity was primed with lactated Ringer's solution (2.5 liters), and the temperature of the cycling fluid was conservatively elevated every 15 minutes for 1.5 hours, until the thermal probe directly in the peritoneal cavity reached 42 degrees C. The patient's rectal temperature reached 39.5 degrees C at the same time. During a remaining 15-minute interval, the filter unit was bypassed, and 105 mg of N,N′,N″-triethylenethiophosphoramide (thiotepa)‡ were administered (1175 m^2 × 60) in the line going directly to the peritoneal cavity. After perfusion, the catheters were left in place. The patient's postoperative course was uncomplicated.

A second run with amethopterin (methotrexate)‡ was performed 5 days later. Under light general anesthesia, the Saratoga sumps were reattached to the TIFS. The system was again primed with 2.5 liters of lactated Ringer's

*Sherwood Medical Industries, Inc., St. Louis, MO.
†Ethicon, Inc., Somerville, NJ.
‡Lederle Laboratories, Pearl River, NY.

Table 15–1 **LABORATORY VALUES** *(Continued)*

	Glucose (mg/dl)	CEA (ng/ml)	Hemoglobin (mg/dl)	Hematocrit (vol. %)	Platelets (× 10^5/cm)	Weight (kg)	5-min exercise tolerance (beats/min)
Preoperative†	98	126.5	15	43.9	4.8	65.3	170
Postoperative range‡	93–137	105§	2.7–37.9	24.7–13.1	2.0–5.9	55.8–70.3	—
Discharge ‖	112	22.6	11.7	36.2	7.6	55.8	102

solution, and the temperature was steadily elevated. When the temperature of the peritoneal fluid stabilized at 42 degrees C, methotrexate (75 mg) was administered. The perfusion was then continued for 30 minutes, and methotrexate levels in the perfusate and in the serum were measured at 5, 15, and 30 minutes. After treatment, the peritoneal cavity was drained of residual fluid, and the Saratoga sumps were removed.

The design of the chemotherapy protocol called for administration of a cell cycle–nonspecific agent (thiotepa), followed 5 days later with a cell cycle–specific agent (methotrexate). Thiotepa was chosen because of its previously demonstrated safety for intraperitoneal use (Dedrick et al., 1978). A full systemic dose of 60 mg per m^2 was infused. Methotrexate, 40 mg per m^2, was administered on the fifth day, followed by citrovorum rescue. Mild hematologic suppression was seen on the fourth day, but the blood counts returned to normal by day 5. No systemic effects were noted with the methotrexate.

Laboratory Values and Results. Pertinent laboratory data were obtained before, during, and after the surgical and perfusion procedures (Table 15–1). Preoperative values were obtained the day before surgery. Postoperative ranges are those values recorded for 13 days after the first hyperthermic treatment. The discharge values are those observed 21 days after surgery.

No satisfactory method for determining differential concentrations of thiotepa in the perfusate and the serum was available. However, the differential methotrexate concentrations were determined during the second hyperthermic treatment and are presented in Table 15–2. There was a 1000-fold difference between the two compartments (peritoneal fluid and serum) at each 5-minute interval up to 30 minutes.

Table 15–2. **METHOTREXATE CONCENTRATION DURING HYPERTHERMIC PERFUSION*,†**

Time After Administration (minutes)	Concentration of Methotrexate (ng/ml)	
	Blood ($\times 10^{-7}$)	*Perfusate* ($\times 10^{-4}$)
5	2.4	1.76
15	7.5	1.59
30	9.9	1.08

*Adapted from Spratt, J. S., Adcock, R. A., Muscovin, M., et al.: Clinical delivery system for intraperitoneal hyperthermic chemotherapy. Cancer Res. 40:256–260, 1980.

†Seventy-five mg of methotrexate were instilled into perfusate at 0 time. The time at which chemotherapy was administered was approximately 1.5 hour after perfusion began in both the first and second treatments.

The patient's postoperative course was uneventful except for a minor pulmonary atelectasis with bacteremia following the second hyperthermic treatment. He was normothermic 48 hours after each treatment.

In spite of the extensive intra-abdominal resection, the patient's body weight after the first perfusion (63.0 kg) was the same as on admission. His weight increased to 69.8 kg after the second perfusion. This increase suggested edema. His weight then dropped to 55.3 kg by the time of discharge. Several units of serum albumin were administered during the postoperative period to return the serum albumin levels to normal and to mobilize peritoneal edema. Albumin levels dropped acutely during both runs.

During the 1.5-hour period of hyperthermia, intraperitoneal debris was filtered by the sequential 40- and 3-micron filters in the system. These filters were bypassed during chemotherapy. Significant debris accumulated in both the 40-micron prefilter and 3-micron cell filters. There was no effort to quantify the recovery of cells at this time. No attempt was made to culture cells on this run, but cell cultures have been obtained in subsequent cases for chemosensitivity evaluation.

The pulsatile flow of the circulating fluid during both treatments was 15 liters per hour. This rate appeared to be well tolerated by the patient. There was no hemorrhage. The hyperthermia did not induce any shock or hyperpyrexia.

This treatment plan consisted of the administration of cell cycle–nonspecific agent (thiotepa) followed 5 days later by the cell cycle–specific agent methotrexate with intraperitoneal hyperthermia. Methotrexate had been used by Dedrick and colleagues in 1978, adjunctive to peritoneal dialysis. Since low-grade cancers such as pseudomyxoma peritonei generally show poor response to systemic chemotherapy, this chemotherapeutic rationale was considered feasible and at least as effective as systemic treatment. The presence of methotrexate in the serum during the procedure indicated absorption from the peritoneal perfusate. The concentration of the peritoneal perfusate, however, was 1000 times greater than that of the serum. This indicated a margin of safety to the patient with regard to the toxic effects of methotrexate.

Larkin and colleagues in 1977 confirmed that no undesirable effects occurred at 42 degrees

C for up to 2 hours. No ill effects became apparent. Prior exercise tolerance determined that the patient could withstand a stress pulse of 170 beats per minute for 5 minutes. The maximum cardiac rate induced during the procedure was 145 beats per minute, well below his stress tolerance. Preoperative stress tests must be done routinely before hyperthermia is induced to determine the maximum pulse rate tolerable to the cardiovascular conditioning of the individual patient. In this patient, the planned level of hyperthermia was attained at a safe cardiac rate. The patient's postoperative course was uncomplicated. He remained fully functional and at work until slow reaccumulation of ascites necessitated re-exploration in March of 1981. The patient insisted on hyperthermic Ringer's lactate alone in the TIFS unit with no chemotherapy. This was done for 30 minutes at 42.5 degrees C. The patient did well for another year, requiring only a laparotomy to remove mucin in March of 1982. As of November 1983, he has been actively engaged in setting up a foundation for the study of rare diseases and continues to work without discomfort although he is known to have residual neoplasm.

Therapeutic Efficacy. The question of therapeutic efficacy of TIFS is at present the subject for a controlled clinical trial on these infrequent cases. Our preference is a protocol for periodic retreatment as indicated by rising CEA values. However, the first patient remained active, comfortable, and at work with recurring symptomatology 49 months after treatment. Although his laboratory chemistry and hematologic parameters remained normal, his CEA value remained consistently higher than normal.

As experience with the TIFS unit increases, models of treatment may be developed to provide effective hyperthermic chemotherapy of other neoplasms of the abdominal cavity that are known to have a high probability for local or regional recurrence. The immediate postoperative period in these high-risk cases might even be the optimal time for its use, since the tumor burden would be minimal during this period.

Aside from the potential cytotoxicity of hyperthermia, two mechanical capabilities of TIFS make its potential appealing for the treatment of intraperitoneal cancers: (1) The fluid dynamics of the system provide maximal fluid-surface contact with the peritoneal compartments with minimum irritation; and (2) the mechanical filtration process permits the removal of malignant cells that may be free-floating or shed from the surface of the serosa by virtue of fluid momentum with passage through the peritoneal cavity. Free-floating neoplastic cells are viable in ascitic fluid. This is especially true in pleural effusions.

Related Studies and Systems. In 1978, Dedrick and co-workers took a more studied look at the administration of intraperitoneal chemotherapy. They noted that pharmacokinetic calculations indicate that hydrophilic anticancer drugs administered intraperitoneally in large volumes may be expected to maintain a significantly greater concentration in the peritoneal space than in the plasma. They considered that this concentration difference was adequate to offer a potentially exploitable biochemical advantage in the treatment of patients with presumed microscopic residual ovarian cancer confined to the peritoneal cavity.

Their model has many of the characteristics of TIFS. Tumors treated must be of small thickness. Large volumes of drug-containing solution must be used to ensure exposure of the entire peritoneal surface. Care must be exercised to avoid the coadministration of drugs that might lessen either hepatic or renal clearance of the chemotherapeutic agent. The ratio of plasma clearance to peritoneal permeability should be high. The added impact of hyperthermia to such a system requires further study.

Considerable developmental research is in progress. TIFS represents a step. Other sources of clinical hyperthermia that are potentially effective for treating pseudomyxoma peritonei are now being marketed and are under active clinical investigation, with FDA approval. The annular phased array system (APAS)* is one. The APAS consists of 16 radiating apertures operating in phase. It can achieve uniform heating at the center of the abdomen. The frequency range of output is 55 to 110 MHz, delivering 1000 watts maximum per quadrant through an aperture 50 cm across. This system, used with indwelling heat-resistant dialysis catheters, has a potential for intracavitary hyperthermia equivalent to that achieved with TIFS.

TISSUE CULTURE AND DRUG SENSITIVITY STUDIES

Tseng reviews in Chapter Seventeen progress in tissue culture assays that can be per-

*BSD Medical Corporation, Salt Lake City, Utah.

formed to measure the rate of growth, effect of chemotherapeutic agents on the culture (percentage of cell-kill or cell–growth enhancement), and estrogen-receptor content. Heterogeneity of cultures is uniformly present in cancer cell cultures. The correlation of this new source of information with clinical behavior and response to treatment is in progress. Pending these correlations, data from tissue cultures need to be classified as experimental findings.

In the case of cell cultures from patients with pseudomyxoma peritonei, cell cultures have been readily established from the ascitic fluid. The cell lines from pseudomyxoma peritonei have exhibited very slow cell replication. Thus, a large sample must be taken to increase the chances that a cell culture line of a volume adequate for further tests will be established. Fresh, sterile effusions from both the peritoneal and pleural cavity may be used as a source of viable cells for tissue culture. When cells grow more slowly, weeks may pass before information is received from the laboratory, creating a delay in the accessibility of the chemosensitivity data for clinical use. Treatment plans based on these new data require correlation with clinical response.

ADVERSE EFFECTS ASSOCIATED WITH PERITONEOVENOUS SHUNTS USED FOR PSEUDOMYXOMA PERITONEI

The peritoneovenous shunts can result in catastrophic consequences when used for pseudomyxoma peritonei. In 1981, Smith and coworkers reported a case in which peritoneovenous shunts produced massive embolization of neoplasm to the pulmonary vasculature. Secondarily, the embolization induced pulmonary hypertension, persistent hypoxia, intravascular coagulation, and partial thrombosis of the superior vena cava. Small fragments of mucinous neoplasm were entrapped in the thrombi. The lung contained numerous gelatinous emboli in the small arteries and arterioles of all lobes, and occlusion was confirmed at autopsy. Although tumor cells in the emboli appeared viable, vascular wall invasion was not identified. The authors concluded, on the basis of their case and a review of the literature, that peritoneovenous shunts are contraindicated in the presence of pseudomyxoma peritonei.

REPRESENTATIVE CASE STUDIES

Because of the infrequency of pseudomyxoma peritonei, some observations about representative cases merit inclusion as a basis for further study.

A 46-year-old man contacted the author (JSS) in July 1982, saying he had pseudomyxoma peritonei. The patient had searched the literature and found articles on the syndrome. He had been treated in Toronto by R.E. Falk, whose methodology and results have been reported (Falk et al., 1983). The patient was concerned because of some residual abdominal distention. He was re-explored as a possible candidate for TIFS, and a small amount of fluid was discovered. Multiple biopsies showed no residual cancer, although the patient did have residual mucin in the tissues. He did well for sixteen additional months after that laparotomy. His original tumor was a villous mucus-secreting papilloma of the appendix, extensively involving visceral and parietal peritoneum. The diagnosis was confirmed at laparotomy in October of 1980 in Toronto.

By November 1983, he was complaining of anxiety and some abdominal discomfort. His abdominal girth had increased and a CAT scan suggested recurrent fluid. A repeat laparotomy was performed and on this occasion, he had extensive mucinous ascites associated with scattered mucin-containing cysts. Extensive evacuation and irrigation were performed and a dialysis catheter was inserted for instillation of thiotepa, followed 5 days later by methotrexate without hyperthermia. The histopathologic examination showed all cysts to be lined with a single layer of noninvasive cuboidal mucin-producing cells. Throughout, the patient has continued productive work.

A second case involved a 62-year-old woman with biopsy-proven papillary mesothelioma, myxoid type, first confirmed at laparotomy in March 1980. She was treated with systemic chemotherapy involving an array of agents but showed no response. Repetitive paracenteses were required with increasing frequency for pseudomyxomatous ascites.

In July of 1982, a second laparotomy was done. Extensive nodular involvement of the omentum and peritoneal seeding were noted. An omentectomy, representative peritoneal biopsies, and a cholecystectomy were performed, and the common duct was explored for symptomatic gallstones. An Ash column disk catheter was inserted for postoperative infusion and drainage.

The patient tolerated this procedure well and experienced an uncomplicated postoperative course. Histopathologic confirmation of the same neoplasm was reported. At laparotomy, a sample of the patient's myxomatous ascitic fluid was mixed with equal parts of 5 percent dextrose in water. The myxomatous material was completely miscible in the 5 percent dextrose solution, as is generally the case with mucopolysaccharides composing the myxomatous material found with pseudomyxomatous peritonei.

Both the biopsy material of solid tumor from the omentum and ascitic fluid were submitted to Tseng (see Chapter Seventeen) for tissue culture and chemosensitivity testing. Abundant tissue growth occurred from both sources. The cultured cells were insensitive to vincristine, 5-fluorouracil, Adriamycin, and tamoxifen.

The patient remained asymptomatic for 4 months on intermittent irrigation with 5 percent dextrose and water via the dialysis catheter. However, after 4 months, fluid flowed in but did not return. In November of 1982, the patient was given 0.8 mg per kg of thiotepa intraperitoneally via the catheter. During that same month, she was re-explored. The interstices of the disk had become clogged with fibrin clots, which, on histologic examination, contained no neoplasm. The peritoneum proved grossly normal. Several peritoneal biopsies were obtained, and no neoplasm was found. The catheter was left in place but has not been used further, and the patient's abdomen has remained free of ascites. As of November of 1983, the patient has been completely asymptomatic. Whether cured or not, she has experienced remarkable palliation from this very simple procedure.

According to the 1975 report of Green and co-workers, whenever repetitive accumulation of mucinous ascites continues in spite of treatment, the instillation of intraperitoneal 5 percent dextrose solution makes the mucopolysaccharides in the ascites less viscous and easier to remove by paracentesis, which perhaps simplifies palliative evacuation. Green's group claims that celiotomies are therefore less frequently needed. The author (JSS) has confirmed the complete miscibility of the mucopolysaccharides associated with pseudomyxoma peritonei in 5 percent dextrose and water.

SUMMARY

In conclusion, cancers that induce pseudomyxoma peritonei by their slow growth on the peritoneal surface and on the omentum produce a chronic disorder that merits continuous study. These rare cases are not hopeless. Something new can be learned from each that might lead to the eventual control of this problem. Collectively, a controlled clinical trial with the participation of many investigators will be necessary to accumulate a sufficient number of cases to test hypotheses concerning optimal management. Many of the principles and techniques may ultimately be useful as an adjuvant form of treatment for visceral neoplasms known to be associated with a high risk for intraperitoneal recurrence.

References

Ash SR: Hemodialysis laboratory, Purdue University, 1982. Personal communication.

Backman A, Pasila M: Pleural biopsy in the diagnosis of pleural effusion. Scand J Resp Dis 89 (suppl):155–157, 1974.

Bakalos D, Constantakis N, Tsicricas T: Recognition of malignant cells in pleural and peritoneal effusions. Acta Cytol (Baltimore) 18:118–121, 1974.

Bronskill MJ, Bush RS, Ege GN: A quantitative measurement of peritoneal drainage in malignant ascites. Cancer 40:2375–2380, 1977.

Cailleau R, Mackay B, Young RK, Reeves WJ Jr: Tissue culture studies on pleural effusions from breast carcinoma patients. Cancer Res 34:801–809, 1974.

Chandrasekhar AJ, Buehler JH: Diagnostic evaluation of pleural effusions. Geriatrics 29:116–119, 1974.

Compagno J, Oertel JE: Mucinous cystic neoplasms of the pancreas with overt and latent malignancy (cystadenocarcinoma and cystadenoma). A clinicopathologic study of 41 cases. Am J Clin Pathol 69:573–580, 1978.

Dedrick RL, Myers CE, Bungay PM, DeVita VT Jr: Pharmacokinetic rationale for peritoneal drug administration in the treatment of ovarian cancer. Cancer Treat Rep 62:1–11, 1978.

Falk RE, Calhoun K, Langer J, et al: The effect of radiofrequency hyperthermia on experimental and clinical neoplasms when used with metronidazole. Presented at Central Surgical Association, 1983.

Fisher B, Wolmark N, Saffer E, Fisher ER: Inhibitory effect of prolonged *Corynebacterium parvum* and cyclophosphamide administration on the growth of established tumors. Cancer 35:134–143, 1975.

Goldie JH, Coldman AJ: A mathematical model for relating the drug sensitivities of tumors to their spontaneous mutation rates. Cancer Treat Rep 63(11–12):172, 1979.

Green N, Gancedo H, Smith R, Bernett G: Pseudomyxoma peritonei—nonoperative management and biochemical findings—a case report. Cancer 36:1834–1837, 1975.

Larkin JM, Edwards WS, Smith DE, Clark PJ: Systemic thermotherapy: description of a method and physiologic tolerance in clinical subjects. Cancer 40:3155–3159, 1977.

Leith JT, Miller RC, Gerner EW, Boone MLM: Hyperthermic potentiation, biological aspects and application to radiotherapy. Cancer 39 (suppl 2):766–779, 1977.

Long RT, Spratt JS Jr, Dowling E: Pseudomyxoma peritonei. Am J Surg 117:162–169, 1969.

Mayes GB, Chuang VP, Fisher RG: CT of pseudomyxoma peritonei. AJR 136:807–808, 1981.

Meyers MA: Distribution of intraabdominal malignant seeding: dependency on dynamics of flow of ascitic fluid. Am J Roentgenol Radium Ther Nucl Med 119:198–206, 1973.

Myers CE, Jones R, Londer H, et al: Pharmacology of high-dose methotrexate (MTX) administered in a peritoneal dialysis. Am Soc Clin Oncol Abstr 1978:390.

Palta JR, Spratt JS, Bull SR, Dunlap CE: Design and testing of a thermal infusion filtration system. Unpublished manuscript. School of Engineering, University of Missouri, Columbia, MO, 1979.

Perez AJ: Uniform hyperthermic perfusion of the peritoneum of rabbits. Master of Science Thesis. Department of Anatomy, University of Louisville, 1983.

Rosato FE, Wallach MW, Rosato EF: The management of malignant effusions from breast cancer. J Surg Oncol 6:441–449, 1974.

Rudman D, Chawla RK, DelRio AE, et al: Orosomucoid content of pleural and peritoneal effusions. J Clin Invest 54:147–155, 1974.

Safa AR, Tseng MT: Response to methotrexate of cultured cells of the 7,12-dimethylbenzanthracene-induced mammary tumors of rats: a kinetic and ultrastructural study. IRCS (Int Res Commun Syst) Med Sci Libr Compend 9:522–523, 1981.

Seshul MB, Coulam CM: Pseudomyxoma peritonei: computed tomography and sonography. Benzanthracene 136:803–806, 1981.

Shingleton WW, Parker RT, Mahaley S: Abdominal perfusion for cancer chemotherapy with hypothermia and hyperthermia. Surgery 50:260–265, 1961.

Smith RRL, Sternberg SS, Paglia MA, Golbey RB: Fatal pulmonary tumor embolization following peritoneovenous shunting for malignant ascites. J Surg Oncol 16:27–35, 1981.

[1]Spratt JS, Adcock RA, Muskovin M, et al: Clinical delivery system for intraperitoneal hyperthermic chemotherapy. Cancer Res 40:256–260, 1980(g).

[2]Spratt JS, Adcock RA, Sherrill W, Travathen S: Hyperthermic peritoneal perfusion system in canines. Cancer Res 40:253–255, 1980(b).

Storm FK, Harrison WH, Elliott RS, Morton DL: Hyperthermic therapy for human neoplasms: Thermal death time. Cancer 46:1849–1854, 1980.

Titscher R, Kokron O, Letnansky K: Local therapy of malignant pleural effusions. Neoplasma 21:465–469, 1974.

Tseng MT, Capuco AV: Estrogen receptor content in enzymatically dispersed, gradient enriched cell subpopulations of the DMBA–induced mammary tumors in the rat. IRCS (Int Res Commun Syst) Med Sci Libr Compend 9:595–596, 1981.

SIXTEEN

Epithelial Tumors of the Large Intestine in Children

J. J. Buchino, M.D.
D. B. Groff, M.D.

Epithelial tumors of the large intestine in children can be divided into three major categories, i.e., polyps, carcinoids, and carcinomas. Most physicians involved in the care of children are quite familiar with juvenile polyps. However, frequently they do not have much experience with many of the polyposis syndromes. Also, they often fail to recognize that both carcinoids and carcinomas occur in childhood. The purpose of this chapter is to examine these entities and their interrelationships.

POLYPS

Polyps in childhood have the same histologic classification as polyps in adults (see Chapter Nine). However, the frequency of occurrence is significantly different. Juvenile polyps occur most frequently, accounting for approximately 98 percent of all childhood polyps. Adenomatous polyps and hamartomatous polyps usually occur only in association with the various polyposis syndromes. Villous polyps are extremely rare and are usually seen in the older adolescent with multiple polyposis.

Juvenile polyps have a characteristic gross appearance. They are oval, with a smooth surface, and most commonly have a narrow pedicle (Fig. 16–1). The cut surface usually contains numerous cystic spaces filled with a mucinous material. Microscopically, these polyps typically have a fibrous stroma that contains an intense inflammatory infiltrate composed of neutrophils, eosinophils, and plasma cells (Figs. 16–2 and 16–3). This stroma surrounds mucus-filled, dilated cystic spaces of various sizes, which are lined by mucus-secreting, columnar epithelium. The surface of these polyps is made up of a single layer of columnar epithelium, which is frequently ulcerated. These lesions have alternatively been designated as inflammatory polyps and retention polyps. We believe that neither term is totally appropriate. Although these polyps do contain significant inflammatory infiltrates, the term inflammatory polyp may cause confusion with reference to polyps resulting from inflammatory bowel disease. The term retention polyp implies a pathogenesis that is by no means certain.

Numerous theories have been proposed to explain the pathogenesis of juvenile polyps. Horrileno and associates (1957) were the first to question the neoplastic nature of these polyps. They postulated that these polyps resulted from hyperplastic changes secondary to persistent mechanical irritation and that this, coupled with a chronic active inflammatory infiltrate, led to the formation of retention cysts. Roth and Helwig (1963) supported this concept in their review of juvenile polyps. Morson (1962) considered juvenile polyps to be hamartomatous malformations and clearly not neoplastic. This view is supported by studies in which fibroblasts, but no epithelial elements, are shown to grow in tissue culture (Romer et al., 1971). It has been postulated that juvenile polyps result from altered cell kinetics and are therefore true neoplasms (Lipper et al., 1981). Other theories have implicated factors such as allergies, intestinal mucosal angiomatous changes, and diet in the pathogenesis of these tumors (Alexander et al., 1970).

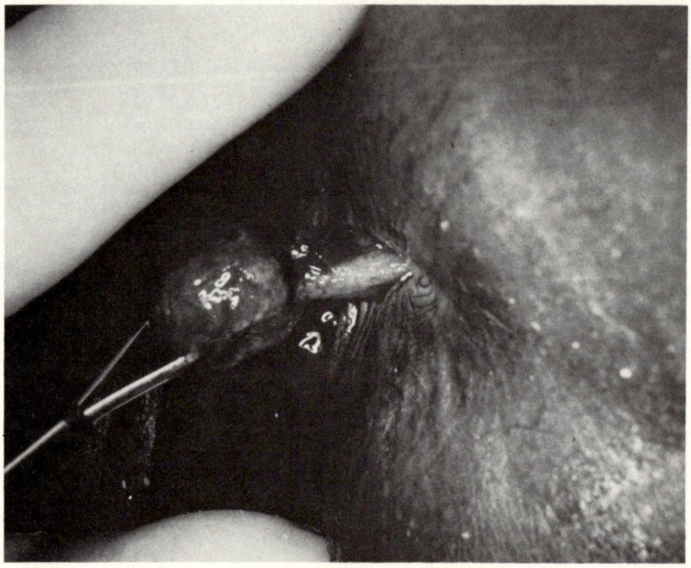

Figure 16–1. Prolapsed juvenile polyp. Note smooth surface and substantial narrow pedicle.

Sixty to 75 percent of juvenile polyps will occur in patients during the first decade of life (Franklin and McSwain, 1972). Juvenile polyps are seldom found on routine physical examination because the rectal exam is usually not part of the standard childhood physical. The most common symptom associated with juvenile polyps is bright red blood passed per rectum (80 to 90 percent) (Franklin and McSwain, 1972; Holgersen et al., 1971). Protrusion of the polyp through the rectum is the second most common complaint. Nonspecific complaints of abdominal pain or change in bowel habits is seen in about one quarter of

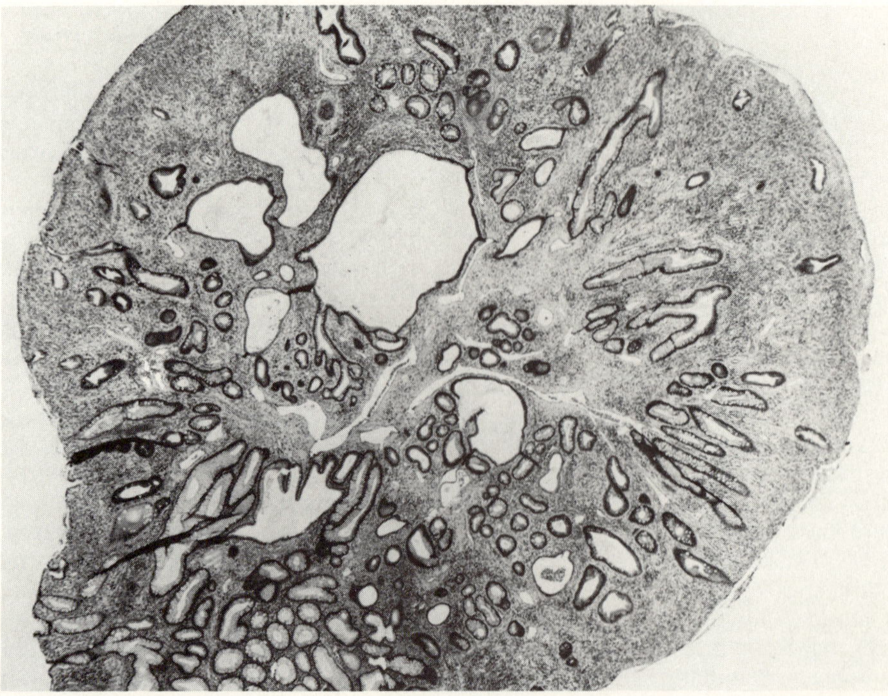

Figure 16–2. Low-power micrograph of a juvenile polyp with mucous-filled cystic spaces and fibrous stroma with inflammatory infiltrate. (H & E ×25)

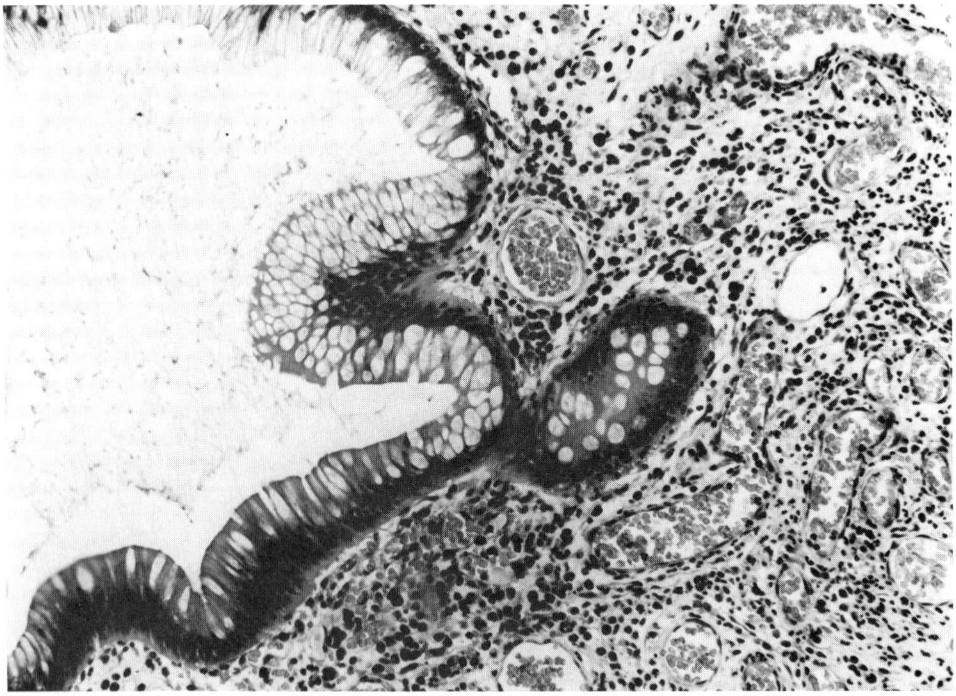

Figure 16–3. High-power view of juvenile polyp demonstrating inflammatory infiltrate composed of neutrophils, eosinophils, and plasma cells. (H & E ×250)

the patients. The distribution of juvenile polyps within the large intestine is similar to that of adenomatous polyps or carcinoma in adults. Forty percent occur within the rectum. The rectosigmoid and sigmoid regions of the colon are the next most frequent sites of involvement. These three regions account for approximately 70 percent of juvenile polyps. Although most patients will have only a single lesion, multiple polyps can occur in up to 30 percent of patients. The condition known as juvenile polyposis coli is not well defined but usually designates patients with more than 10 juvenile polyps and as high as several hundred (Veal et al., 1966). However, juvenile polyposis occurs in only 3 to 5 percent of children with juvenile polyps (Erbe, 1976).

Since significant bleeding rarely occurs with juvenile polyps, emergency management is seldom required. Up to one year of age, blood in the stool is almost always due to a fissure in ano; other causes of bleeding, such as intussusception or enterocolitis, usually have associated findings that exclude consideration of polyps. The initiation of an intussusception by a polyp is exceedingly rare (Holgerson et al., 1971). Bleeding from a Meckel's diverticulum is perhaps the only common differential diagnosis that warrents consideration, and this tends to occur in a younger age group than do rectal polyps. In addition, bleeding from polyps is usually bright red, whereas that from a Meckel's diverticulum is more melanotic. Patients with multiple polyps in the colon located above the rectosigmoid almost always have at least one polyp that can be palpated on rectal examination or visualized through the sigmoidoscope.

History is significant because even asymptomatic children who have a family history of juvenile polyposis should be examined by barium enema. If the barium enema shows polyps, sigmoidoscopy should be performed to obtain histologic confirmation of the diagnosis. If such children have bleeding, the yield of positive findings will be high.

The bleeding in an average patient with juvenile polyps consists of bright red blood in the stool or passed after the stool with each bowel movement over a period of 3 to 4 days. Initial evaluation must include a rectal examination, which should reveal the polyp in over half the patients. It is important to be alert for the presence of anal fissures, even in older children in whom a constipated stool may be the cause of this condition. Since many of the polyps are on a pedicle or stalk, the unskilled examiner may miss them when the polyp moves ahead of the examining finger. An appropriate technique of examination includes careful palpation along the rectal wall so that the polyp can be trapped between the examining finger and the sacrum.

If no polyp is found on skillful rectal examination, the management should be conservative. It is our preference to have the patient's parents document, in writing, the number of stools each day and whether there is blood in the stools. This record is kept for 3 weeks. Most often all bleeding ceases after 3 to 7 days and no further diagnostic measures need to be taken. The presumptive diagnosis is bleeding from a sloughed juvenile polyp. Juvenile polyposis and familial polyposis will not be missed by conservative management, since patients with these disorders will continue to have bleeding episodes, necessitating further examination. If bleeding continues, the patient should be scheduled for a sigmoidoscopy. This is best performed under general anesthesia when the patient is under 6 years of age. Colonoscopy need not be performed at this time because of the increased risk of morbidity and mortality and the knowledge that 90 percent of all polyps can be treated through the sigmoidoscope. Any polyp found on sigmoidoscopy is removed using the snare and electrocautery.

If no polyps are seen on sigmoidoscopy, a barium enema with air contrast is performed on the same day because the colon has been prepared for the sigmoidoscopy. One should be aware that lymphoid hyperplasia, not unusual in this age group, may give the appearance of multiple polyps. If a polyp located beyond the reach of the sigmoidoscope is seen on barium enema or if rectal bleeding continues in the absence of the visualization of any polyps, colonoscopy is performed and the polyps removed if found. Celiotomy and colotomy for the removal of polyps in childhood are never performed unless bleeding is severe. The rare presentation of juvenile polyposis in infancy may be life threatening because it results in intraluminal protein loss with subsequent hypoalbuminemia and malnutrition. These patients may require total colectomy, with a sphincter-preserving pull-through procedure. A Soave-type muscularis sleeve pull-through procedure, as performed for the treatment of Hirschsprung's disease, is very satisfactory (Soper and Kent, 1971). Patients with juvenile polyposis need to be counseled that they will be at higher risk for carcinoma as adults. The adult relatives of a child with juvenile polyposis also need to be told that they may be at more risk than the average person for colon cancer.

Gelb and associates (1962) suggested that juvenile polyps have as much premalignant potential as adenomatous polyps. However, for the most part this has not proved to be the case. There have been several cases reported of colonic carcinoma occurring in adults who had multiple juvenile polyposis as children (Goodman, 1979; Restrepo et al., 1978; Smilow, 1966; Stemper et al., 1975). This potential association of juvenile polyposis with carcinoma requires further elucidation, but for the present it seems reasonable that these patients should have careful follow-up with frequent evaluations.

Adenomatous polyps, common in adults, rarely occur in children, unless they are associated with either familial polyposis or Gardner's syndrome. Unlike the juvenile polyp, the adenomatous polyp is clearly neoplastic. It is characterized grossly by a velvety or fine papillary surface on a knotlike mass, which may or may not have a pedicle. Microscopically, there is a proliferation of glands with numerous mitotic figures. In contrast to juvenile polyps, adenomatous polyps produce scanty amounts of mucus.

Familial adenomatous polyposis is an autosomal dominantly inherited disorder that has an estimated incidence of one in 8000 in the general population. This syndrome is characterized by numerous adenomatous polyps, varying from 100 to a few thousand distributed throughout the large bowel. Although these polyps are benign, they are associated with the development of colonic adenocarcinoma. Approximately 80 percent of untreated patients with familial polyposis will develop colonic carcinoma (Bussey, 1975). Although the initial diagnosis of familial polyposis is usually made during the proband's fourth decade of life, other family members may be diagnosed well within the first decade. Because of the high tendency of patients with familial polyposis to develop carcinoma, familial polyposis in adults is treated by either total colectomy or total proctocolectomy. However, in a growing child, total colectomy represents a serious impediment to normal growth and development. Fortunately, the average age for the development of colonic carcinoma in these patients is 39; its occurrence during the first two decades of life is exceedingly rare (Erbe, 1976). This has led to management by early identification of familial polyposis, close follow-up of the patient, and colectomy after the pubertal growth spurt is complete, which is late in the second decade of life.

In 1953, Gardner described a family with multiple intestinal polyps, osteomas, and soft-tissue abnormalities. Epidermoid cysts, fibromas, dermoid tumors, mesenteric fibromatosis, lipomas, and wound fibromatosis are now also considered soft-tissue manifestations of Gardner's syndrome (Watne et al., 1977). Like familial polyposis, the polyps of Gardner's syndrome are adenomatous. Although the polyps are predominately in the large bowel, they may rarely involve small intestine. Initially, the development of adenomatous polyps in the colon before the age of 10 in children with this syndrome was thought to be rare. However, Naylor and Lebenthal (1979) reported a kindred with Gardner's syndrome, in which polyposis was detected in children 18 months, 6 years, and 9 years of age. Like familial polyposis, there is a marked tendency for patients with Gardner's syndrome to develop adenocarcinoma of the colon. In addition, these patients have a tendency to develop pancreatoduodenal carcinoma as well.

Gardner's syndrome is inherited as an autosomal dominant pattern, with variable expressivity (Erbe, 1976). Many patients within a kindred may manifest only one or two features of the triad. The syndrome actually has many features in common with the neurocrestopathies, although no reference so designating it could be found. A number of anomalies seen with Gardner's syndrome are of neural crest origin, such as fibromatosis, pigmentation, and developmental anomalies. An alternate explanation for the phenomena of Gardner's syndrome may lie with the fibroblasts rather than with cells of the neural crest. Growth abnormalities in fibroblasts from cutaneous biopsy specimens of patients with this syndrome can be regularly demonstrated in tissue culture. The fibroblasts, unlike the fibroblasts from unaffected individuals, display a lack of contact inhibition, have decreased requirements of serum for growth, have elevated levels of plasminogen activator, and show alterations in the intracellular distribution of actin cables. The cells grow without anchorage. They do not form palpable tumors in athymic mice (BALB/C nu/nu). They are much more susceptible to conversion to sarcoma. Observations such as the preceding may potentially enable the earlier identification of individuals susceptible to colon neoplasia.

Peutz-Jeghers syndrome consists of gastrointestinal polyposis and abnormal mucocutaneous pigmentation (Jeghers et al., 1949). The polyps may be found throughout the entire gastrointestinal tract but are most commonly found in the proximal small intestine and less commonly in rectum, colon, and stomach, respectively. The gross appearance is basically the same no matter where in the intestine they occur. They resemble adenomatous polyps with a lobulated surface. Microscopically, these lesions are easily differentiated from other polyps by their distinctive hamartomatous appearance (Fig. 16–4) consisting of an arborization of muscularis mucosae, underlying a mucosa composed of normal glands and lamina propria.

An extraintestinal manifestation of this syndrome is the appearance of melanin spots, which may be found on the face, lips, buccal mucosa, digits, or perianal region. These spots usually occur in infancy or early childhood. Although the lesions on the skin tend to fade at puberty, those of the buccal mucosa remain.

Patients with these polyps most frequently present with recurrent colicky abdominal pain (Erbe, 1976). Both intussusception and obstruction may result from these polyps, particularly when they are located in the small intestine. Rectal bleeding is a more common presentation in those children with colonic polyps. The syndrome is inherited in an autosomal dominant fashion. Although the polyps are non-neoplastic, several reports have indicated a 2 to 3 percent risk of gastrointestinal cancer in these patients (Matuchansky et al., 1979; Ryo et al., 1978; Cochet et al., 1979). This potential predisposition to malignancy has been viewed with skepticism by some authors (Linos et al., 1981). In any event, because of the widespread distribution of polyps with this syndrome, surgical management for either polyposis or prophylaxis for neoplasia must be conservative.

CARCINOID

Carcinoid tumors are rare in children. They are most commonly found incidentally in the vermiform appendix. From 1935 to 1980, the Hospital for Sick Children in Toronto had 13 cases, with a reported incidence of 1 in 446 appendices (Rubin et al., 1981). Ryden and associates (1975) were able to identify 26 cases of appendiceal carcinoid in children under 15 years of age in a retrospective review of cases at the Armed Forces Institute of Pathology. Rectal carcinoids, not uncommon in adults, are exceedingly rare in children, with only a few scattered cases reported (Gold et al., 1971;

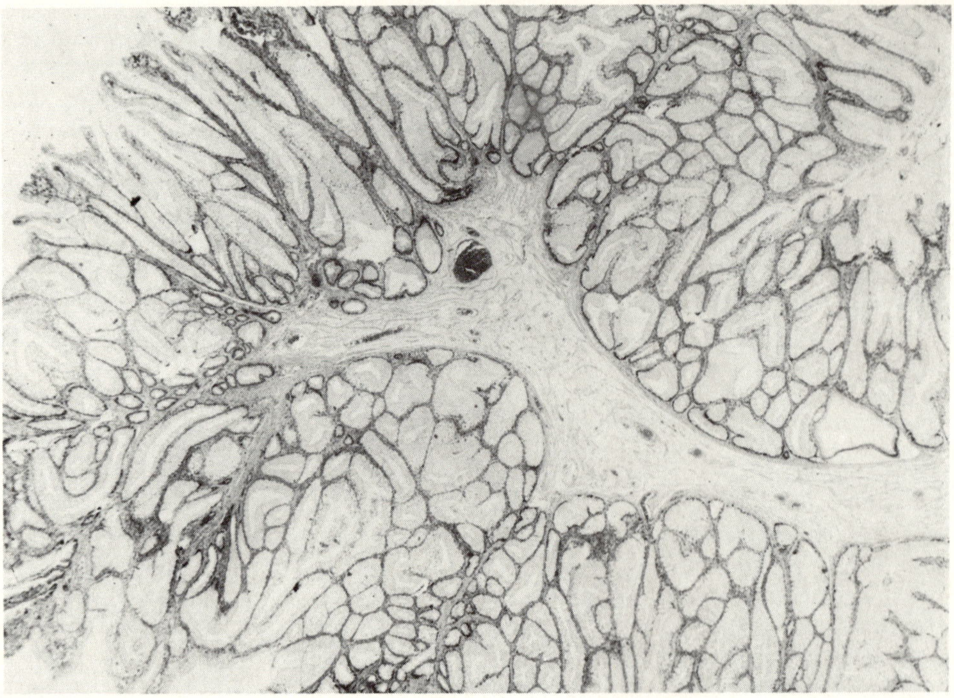

Figure 16–4. Peutz-Jeghers syndrome polyp (hamartomatous), with muscularis mucosae extending into the polyp and surrounding the glands in several areas. (H & E ×25)

Bates, 1962; Caldarola et al., 1964; Root et al., 1959; Rubin et al., 1981).

Carcinoid tumors in children have the same histologic appearance as those seen in adults (see Chapter Eleven). They are composed of Kulchitsky's cells and are considered part of the amine precursor uptake and decarboxylation (APUD) system, as designated by Pearse in 1954. Differentiating carcinoids that will behave in a benign manner from aggressive ones is frequently difficult. Criteria such as microscopic invasion of muscle coats, lymphatic and vascular invasion and size greater than 2 cm in diameter have been used to designate malignancy (MacDonald, 1956; Moertel et al., 1968). However, none of these criteria can be viewed as absolute. In the 30 cases of appendiceal carcinoid in children reviewed by Ryden and associates (1975), none were found to behave in a malignant fashion, regardless of size, depth of invasion, or perineural invasion. It should be noted, however, that three ranged from 1 to 2 cm and only one of the 30 tumors was greater than 2 cm in diameter. The median duration of follow-up of these patients was 13.1 years. A marked preponderance (77 percent) in females was found in this series, as has been similarly noted in adults. Treatment was simple appendectomy in all cases. We agree with the authors' conclusion that small appendiceal carcinoids in children do not behave aggressively, and therefore, more extensive surgery after appendectomy is not indicated. The one exception may be the rare tumor that is larger than 2 cm. Because carcinoids can be multifocal, however, children with carcinoids of the appendix should be investigated to rule out other primaries.

CARCINOMA

Carcinoma of the large bowel is relatively rare in the pediatric age group. Less than 300 cases have been reported in the literature. The Third National Cancer Survey (Cutler, 1975) indicates an annual incidence of about 0.17 cases per 100,000 population in the 5- to 19-year age group. Caldwell and associates (1981) reported that the incidence of carcinoma at the St. Judes Children's Research Hospital was five times the expected rate. Pratt and associates (1977) reviewed 13 children with colorectal carcinoma during a 26 month period at this same institution. These 13 patients accounted for 2.2 percent of the total oncology admissions and represented 4.1 percent of the group of patients with malignant solid tumors during the time period studied. In our experience the incidence of carcinoma of the large bowel in this age group has been similar to that expected by the National Cancer Survey, with only 2 cases out of 212 malignant tumors during the past 10 years.

In general, children with carcinoma of the large bowel can be divided into two groups: those with known predisposing conditions, such as ulcerative colitis or polyposis syndromes, and sporadic cases.

It has been well established that both adults and children with ulcerative colitis are at increased risk for the development of carcinoma of the large intestine. The risk increases with the duration of illness. Devroede and co-workers (1971) found that approximately 3 percent of children with ulcerative colitis will develop colonic carcinoma within the first 10 years after the onset of disease. The probability of development of carcinoma then gradually increases with each decade of duration (to reach an estimated 43 percent 35 years after the onset of ulcerative colitis). Males and females appear to be equally affected. Ulcerative colitis rarely develops during the first decade of life. When it does, those patients need careful follow-up and may be candidates for prophylactic surgery.

Children and adolescents with a polyposis syndrome are also predisposed to the development of colonic carcinoma. As mentioned previously, patients with multiple familial polyposis and Gardner's syndrome have a definite increased risk for the development of large bowel cancer. Those children with multiple juvenile polyposis and Peutz-Jegher syndrome may also be at risk but at a significantly lower rate than those with the previously mentioned syndromes. Fortunately, these carcinomas rarely develop before puberty and the post pubertal growth spurt. Therefore, these children can be managed conservatively during a crucial period of growth and development.

Although ulcerative colitis and some of the polyposis syndromes predispose children to the development of a colonic carcinoma, most cases of large bowel carcinoma in children occur sporadically without obvious predisposing factors. There have been a number of epidemiologic studies concerning colorectal carcinoma in adults but very little research concerning this problem in children and adolescents has been carried out (Chablko and Fraumeni, 1975). Pratt and associates specifically reviewed epidemiologic factors in 13 patients at their institution. They found an equal distribution of colorectal carcinoma between males and females and Blacks and Caucasians. Geographically, the patients were concentrated in the tri-state area of Tennessee, Arkansas, and Mississippi, since the institution serves as a regional childhood cancer referral center for this area. Epidemiologic factors examined included population characteristics, water supply, and exposure to chemical agents. Nine of the 13 children were considered to have had significant exposure to chemicals. Unfortunately, neither a control group of children with other malignancies nor a group of children with nonmalignant conditions was reported for comparison. A retrospective examination of serum pesticide levels of 10 patients from the same institution was performed. Children from the Northwestern Mississippi Rheumatic Fever Clinic served as the controls (Caldwell et al., 1981). This study failed to reveal any significant difference in serum pesticide levels between patients and control groups, although two patients did have exceptionally high levels of DDT. Nevertheless, the authors stated that chemical exposure should not be totally discounted as a potential factor, since serum pesticide residue levels may not reflect environmental levels, route of exposure, or colonic pesticide contact.

There have been several large series and literature reviews of children and adolescents with carcinoma of the colon and rectum. These reports have revealed significant differences in the natural history of this disease in the pediatric age group compared with that occurring in the adult population. The most common presenting symptom in children is abdominal pain. This symptom was seen in 90 percent of 71 patients reviewed by Middlekamp and Hoffner (1963) and 23 of 24 patients reviewed by Odone and associates, 1982. Vomiting, changes in stool pattern, and rectal bleeding were much less common, occurring in 20 to 40 percent of children with colonic carcinoma. Hoerner and Middlekamp and Hoffner pointed out that presenting symptoms will vary somewhat based on whether the carcinoma occurs on the right side of the colon or on the left. Rectal bleeding, for instance, was seen in 22.6 percent of patients with left-sided lesions and in only 13.2 percent with right-sided lesions. An abdominal mass was the presenting symptom in 10.3 percent of children with right-sided lesions. It was not seen in any patients with carcinoma involving the left colon.

Primary tumors do not appear to have the marked predilection for the rectal sigmoid region, the location commonly associated with large bowel carcinomas in adults. The lesions presented in the series of Odone and associates (1982) were evenly distributed throughout the large bowel. In the series of Middlekamp and Hoffner (1963), only 23 percent of the 69 patients had lesions in the rectosigmoid area. Hoerner's series varies significantly in that he found 189 cases of carcinoma of the rectum and only 73 cases of carcinoma of the colon in the literature. However, he states that many cases of rectal carcinoma may have been included twice, owing to inability to determine overlap in previously reported series.

Perhaps most disturbing of all is that between 50 and 70 percent of children and adolescents with carcinoma of the colon have a poorly differentiated mucin-producing histologic type of adenocarcinoma (Fig. 16–5). This is in distinct contrast to the adult population in which this histologic variant accounted for only 5 to 15 percent of cases in two large series. Unfortunately, mucin-producing adenocarcinoma is an aggressive cancer with a very poor prognosis. The fact that this histologic type predominates in the pediatric age group has been well recognized, but no one thus far has been able to explain it.

Prognosis for children with carcinoma of the large bowel regardless of location has been dismal, with less than 5 percent surviving 5 years. This is related perhaps to several factors. First, the most common presenting complaint is abdominal pain. Unfortunately, this complaint is often vague and is very common in pediatrics. It is well known that abdominal pain in childhood, unless accompanied by weight loss or anemia, is seldom caused by significant disease (Stickler and Marly, 1979; Lebenthal, 1980). Because of this, the complaint is often not aggressively pursued and, therefore, there is frequently a delay in diagnosis. Several series include patients who had been initially operated on for presumed appendicitis and later reoperated on for the carcinoma. Also, since more than 50 percent of these patients have the mucin-producing, signet ring type of carcinoma, survival is decreased. Because of the combination of delayed diagnosis and aggressive histologic type of carcinoma, the majority of patients present with an advanced stage of disease, which is the single most important prognostic factor.

Once the presence of a mass has been determined by physical examination or x-ray contrast study, the diagnostic work-up of the patient is the same as that of an adult. It is significant that a metastatic work-up in a child must include a bone survey in addition to the bone scan because the metaphyseal growth areas will increase radionucleotide uptake.

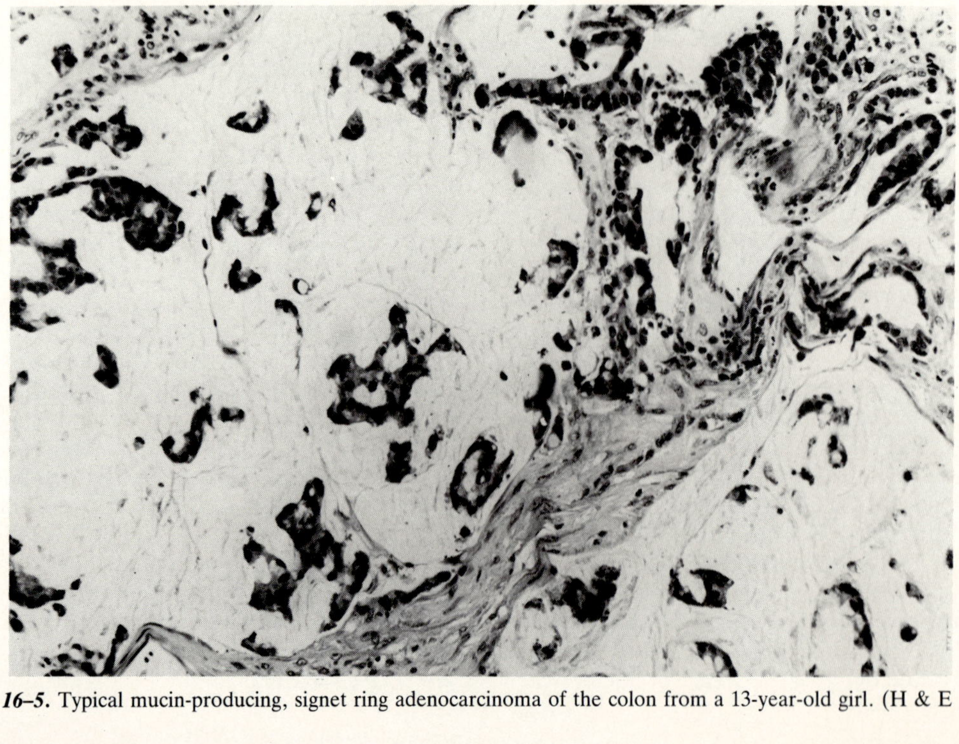

Figure 16–5. Typical mucin-producing, signet ring adenocarcinoma of the colon from a 13-year-old girl. (H & E ×250)

Both surgical and medical management of the carcinoma should proceed along the same lines as in the adult. No organized protocol management of these patients has been defined among the children's cancer study groups. Carcinoembryonic antigen as a tumor marker has proved to be of value in the detection of recurrent disease (Go and Zamcheck, 1982). Unfortunately, chemotherapy, primarily in the form of 5-fluorouracil has been of only limited value in treatment (Davis, 1982).

Acknowledgements

The authors thank Andrea Spalding for typing the manuscript.

References

Alexander RH, Beckwith JB, Morgan A, et al: Juvenile polyps of the colon and their relationship to allergy. Am J Surg 120:222–225, 1970.

Anderson A, Bergdahl L: Carcinoma of the colon in children—a report of six new cases and a review of the literature. J Pediatr Surg 11:967–971, 1976.

Bates HR Jr: Carcinoid tumors of the rectum. Dis Colon Rectum 5:270, 1982.

Bussey HJR: Familial polyposis coli: family studies, histopathology, differential diagnosis, and results of treatment. Baltimore, The Johns Hopkins University Press, 1975.

Caldarola VT, Jackman RJ, Moertel CG, et al: Carcinoid tumors of the rectum. Am J Surg 107:844–849, 1964.

Caldwell GG, Cannon SB, Pratt CB, Arthur RD: Serum pesticide levels in patients with childhood colorectal carcinoma. Cancer 48:774–778, 1981.

Chablko JJ, Fraumeni JF: Colorectal cancer in children—epidemiologic aspects. Dis Colon Rectum 10:1–3, 1975.

Chow EW, Sudha S, Campbell PE, Carter RF: Malignant carcinoid tumors in children. Cancer 48:802–811, 1982.

Cochet B, Carrel J, Desbaillets L, Widgren S: Peutz-Jeghers syndrome associated with gastrointestinal carcinoma: Report of two cases in a family. Gut 20:169–175, 1979.

Cutler SS, Young JL, Jr.: Third national cancer survey. incidence data. National Cancer Institute Monograph, 1975, p. 41.

Davis HL: Chemotherapy of large bowel cancer. Cancer 50:2638–2646, 1982.

DeCosse JJ, Adam MB, Condon RE: Familial polyposis. Cancer 39:267–273, 1977.

Devroede GJ, Taylor WF, Sauer WG, et al: Cancer risk and life expectancy of children with ulcerative colitis. New Engl J Med 285:17–21, 1971.

Donaldson MH, Taylor P, Rawitscher R, Sewell JB: Colon carcinoma in childhood. Pediatrics 48:307–312, 1971.

Erbe RW: Inherited gastrointestinal-polyposis syndromes. New Engl J Med 294:1101–1104, 1976.

Franklin R, McSwain B: Juvenile polyps in the colon and rectum. Ann Surg 175:887–891, 1972.

Gardner EJ: Follow-up study of a family group exhibiting dominant inheritance for a syndrome including intestinal polyps, osteomas, fibromas, and epidermal cysts. Am J Hum Genet 14:376–390, 1962.

Gardner EJ, Richards RC: Multiple cutaneous and subcutaneous lesions occurring simultaneously with hereditary polyposis and osteomatosis. Am J Hum Genet 5:139–147, 1953.

Gelb AM, Minkowitz S, Tresser M: Rectal and colonic polyps occuring in young people. NY State J Med 62:513, 1962.

Go VLW, Zamcheck N: The role of tumor markers in the management of colorectal cancer. Cancer 50:2618–2623, 1982.

Gold MS, Winslow PR, Litt IF: Carcinoid tumors of the rectum in children: a review of the literature and report of a case. Surgery 69:394–396, 1971.

Goodman ZD, Yardley JH, Milligan FD: Pathogenesis of colonic polyps in multiple juvenile polyposis: report of a case associated with gastric polyps and carcinoma of the rectum. Cancer 43:1906–1913, 1979.

Hoerner MT: Carcinoma of the colon and rectum in persons under twenty years of age. Am J Surg 96:47–53, 1958.

Holgersen LO, Miller RE, Zintal HA: Juvenile polyps in the colon. Surgery 69:288–293, 1971.

Horilens EG, Echert C, Ackerman LV: Polyps of the rectum and colon in children. Cancer 10:1210, 1957.

Howell J, Pringle K, Kirschner B, Burrington JD: Peutz-Jeghers polyps causing colocolic intussusception in infancy. J Pediatr Surg 16:82–84, 1981.

Jeghers H, McKusick VA, Katz KH: Generalized intestinal polyposis and melanin spots of the oral mucosa, lips, and digits. New Engl J Med 241:993–1005, 1031–1036, 1949.

Kottmeier PK, Clatworthy HW: Intestinal polyps and associated carcinoma in childhood. Am J Surg 110:709–716, 1965.

Lebenthal E: Recurrent abdominal pain in childhood. Am J Dis Child 134:347–348, 1980.

Linos DA, Dozois RR, Dahlin DC, Bartholomew LG: Does Peutz-Jeghers syndrome predispose to gastrointestinal malignancy? Arch Surg 116:1182–1184, 1981.

Lipper S, Kahn LB, Sandler RS, Varma V: Multiple juvenile polyposis. A study of the pathogenesis of juvenile polyps and their relationship to colonic adenomas. Hum Pathol 12:804–813, 1981.

MacDonald RA: A study of 356 carcinoids of the gastrointestinal tract. Am J Med 21:867–878, 1956.

Matuchansky C, Babin P, Coutrot S, et al: Peutz-Jeghers syndrome with metastasizing carcinoma arising from a jejunal hemartoma. Gastroenterology 77:1311–1315, 1979.

Mayo CW, Pagtalunan RJG: Malignancy of colon and rectum in patients under 30 years of age. Surgery 53:711–718, 1963.

Middlekamp JN and Hoffner H: Carcinoma of the colon in children. Pediatrics 32:558–571, 1963.

Moertel CG, Dockerty MB, Judd ES: Carcinoid tumors of the vermiform appendix. Cancer 21:270–278, 1968.

Morson BC: Some peculiarities of interestinal polyps. Dis Colon Rectum 5:237, 1982.

Naylor EW, Lebenthal E: Early detection of adenomatous polyposis coli in Gardner's syndrome. Pediatrics 63:222–227, 1979.

O'Brien SE: Carcinoma of the colon in childhood and adolescence. Can Med Assoc J 96:1217–1219, 1967.

Odone V, Chang L, Caces J, et al: The national history of colorectal carcinoma in adolescents. Cancer 49:1716–1720, 1982.

Ohman U: Colorectal carcinoma in patients less than 40 years of age. Dis Colon Rectum 25:209–214, 1982.

Pearce AGE: Histochemistry, Theoretical and Applied. London, Churchill Livingstone, 1954.

Pratt CB, Rivera G, Shanks E, et al: Colorectal carcinoma

in adolescents. Implications regarding etiology. Cancer 40:2464–2472, 1977.

Restrepo C, Moreno J, Duque E, et al: Juvenile colonic polyposis in Columbia. Dis Colon Rectum 21:600–612, 1978.

Romer H, Cotle C, Essenfeld-Yahr E: Behavior of the rectal juvenile polyp in vitro. Gut 12:194, 1971.

Root GT, Leddy W, MacDonald JL: Carcinoid tumors of the rectum. Am J Surg 98:243–247, 1959.

Roth S, Helwig EB; Juvenile polpys of the colon and rectum. Cancer 16:468, 1963.

Rubin SZ, Mancer JF, Stephens CA: Carcinoid in a rectal duplication: a unique pediatric surgical problem. Can J Surg 24:351–352, 1981.

Ryden SE, Drake RM, Franciosi RA: Carcinoid tumors of the appendix in children. Cancer 36:1528–1542, 1975.

Ryo UY, Roh SK, Balkin RB, et al: Extensive metastasis in Peutz-Jeghers syndrome. JAMA 239:2268–2269, 1978.

Sessions RT, Riddle DH, Kaplan HJ, Foster JH: Carcinoma of the colon in the first two decades of life. Ann Surg 162:279–284, 1965.

Shermeta DW, Morgan WW, Eggleston J, et al: Juvenile retention polyps. J Pediatr Surg 4:211–215, 1969.

Soper RT, Kent TH: Fetal juvenile polyposis in infancy. Surgery 69:692–698, 1971.

Stemper TJ, Kent TH, Summers RW: Juvenile polyposis and gastrointestinal carcinoma: A study of a kindred. Ann Intern Med 83:639–646, 1975.

Stickler G, Marly DB: Recurrent abdominal pain. Am J Dis Child 133:486–489, 1979.

Veale AMO, McCall I, Bussey HJR, et al: Juvenile polyposis coli. J Med Genet 3:5–16, 1966.

Watne AL, Lai HY, Carrier J, et al: The diagnosis and surgical treatment of patients with Gardner's syndrome. Surgery 82:327–333, 1977.

SEVENTEEN

Chemosensitivity of Human Colon Cancer Cells in Culture

M. T. Tseng, Ph.D.
G. Larson, M.D.

In the past few decades, despite extensive research, little progress has been made in the chemotherapeutic management of colonic cancer. Over half of patients with large bowel cancer develop disseminated and ultimately fatal disease. To date, no curative agent is available; therapy is essentially palliative and has only marginal impact on patient survival. Since its introduction in 1967, 5-fluorouracil (5-FU) (Heidelberger, 1967) has remained the single standard agent for chemotherapy of colonic cancer. Overall, in several studies only about one fifth of patients have been found to respond to 5-FU (Moertel et al., 1969; Wasserman et al., 1975). Results achieved with other cytotoxic agents, such as mitomycin C, BCNU, CCNU, cyclophosphamide, methotrexate, melphalan, actinomycin D, and Adriamycin, have been no more satisfactory (Moertel et al., 1969; Comis and Carter, 1974; Moertel, 1975). For combination chemotherapy, the most favorable results have been reported by Falkson and colleagues (Falkson et al., 1974). In these trials, 5-FU, BCNU, vincristine sulfate, and DTIC were randomized against 5-FU treatment alone. Other investigators, however, have failed to duplicate the 43 percent response rate with combination therapy (Macdonald et al., 1976). Clearly, chemotherapy in its present state is not the ultimate modality for colon cancer treatment.

The inadequate response of these tumors to chemotherapy may accurately reflect their biologic properties; however, it may also stem from suboptimal drug delivery at the tumor site. Factors such as absorption, metabolism, and clearance make it difficult for investigators to determine the "effective" drug concentration at any given location in the body. By administering a precisely measured amount of chemotherapeutic agent to tumor cells in culture, one can obtain an indication of the potential biologic response of a given tumor. Like clinical microbiologists who use cell culture to select appropriate antibiotics for a given patient, investigators who conduct chemosensitivity testing on the cultured tumor cells do so with the hope of screening multiple chemotherapeutic agents before committing the patient to any course of treatment. The results can be used to guide one in the selection of appropriate agents. In this chapter, a method that is used routinely in our laboratory for chemosensitivity testing is described, and the results regarding the drug sensitivity of several human colon tumor cell lines, two fibroblast cell lines, and 12 primary cultures of human colon cancer cells are presented and discussed.

PRIMARY CELL CULTURE AND MAINTENANCE OF ESTABLISHED CELL LINES

Commercial availability of synthetic cell culture media since the 1950s has made it possible for many researchers to develop in-vitro screening procedures for the prediction of the response of an individual patient's tumor to specific anticancer drugs. These anticancer agents are often tested on cells grown in monolayer (anchorage-dependent) cultures, and results are assessed according to (1) morphologic criteria (Wright et al., 1957; Lickiss et

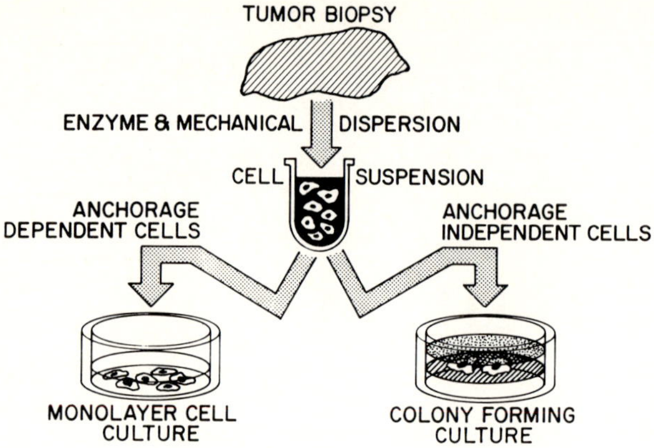

Figure 17–1. Diagrammatic comparison of two commonly used cell culture techniques for chemosensitivity tests.

al., 1974; Holmes and Little, 1974); (2) the degree of metabolic inhibition (DiPaolo and Dowd, 1961; Laszlo et al., 1958; Roper and Drewinko, 1976); or (3) inhibition of incorporation of radiolabeled precursors into DNA, RNA, and proteins (Volm et al., 1979; Bech-Hanset et al., 1977; Livingston et al., 1980). Although the anchorage-dependent culture technique permits the growth of the heterogeneous cell population making up a solid tumor, the inability to discriminate those cells possessing unlimited capacity to divide versus those that are terminally differentiated has led to increasing interest in the culturing of clones of cells in soft agar (Agrez et al., 1982; Albert et al., 1982). In 1961, Till and McCulloch showed that a subpopulation comprising less than 1 percent of the spleen cells of normal mice can repopulate the hemopoietic tissues of lethally irradiated syngeneic recipients. In 1971, Pike and Robinson reported the formation of cell colonies when cells were maintained in a two-layer soft agar system. This anchorage-independent cell growth technique was subsequently introduced into the in-vitro chemosensitivity test system by Salmon and colleagues in 1978. The principal difference between this type of chemosensitivity test and others in the method of cell maintenance is illustrated in Figure 17–1.

Although clonogenic assay permits the determination of the reproductive potential of selected cell subpopulations within a given tumor, it is a laborious technique and is plagued with extremely low plating efficiencies as well as a relatively long incubation period. In contrast, the anchorage-dependent cell cultures proliferate rapidly, preserve greater cellular heterogeneity of the tumors, and permit rapid and accurate quantification of results. Hence, in our laboratory the anchorage-dependent cell culture technique was chosen as the standard method, with the soft-agar clonogenic assay being employed only when specimen size permitted the maintenance of parallel cultures. For experimentation, four established colon cancer cell lines (SK-Co-1, SW-480, Colo-205, HT-29) and two human fibroblast cell lines (CCD-112-Co and CCD-18) were obtained from the American Tissue Type Culture Collection. These along with several human colon biopsy specimens were maintained in supplemented media. Four of the cell lines were maintained in supplemented Eagle's minimum essential medium (MEM) (CCD-112-Co, CCD-18, SK-Co-1, SW-480), one cell line was maintained in supplemented RPMI-1640 (Colo-205), and another was maintained in supplemented McCoy's 5A (HT-29). All were incubated at 37 degrees C in a humidified 95 percent air/5 percent CO_2 atmosphere. All supplemented cultures contained the following: 10 percent fetal calf serum, 10,000 units per ml penicillin, 10,000 μg per ml streptomycin, 25 μg per ml fungizone, 1 μg per ml insulin, 2 μg per ml corticosterone, and 1 μg per ml prolactin.

CHEMOSENSITIVITY TEST PROCEDURE

Our standard procedure measures the cell survival after 24 hours of continuous drug exposure. In one test, cells were plated in 24-well culture plates at a seeding density of 5×10^5 cells per well. Two to 3 days later, when the cells exhibited log phase growth, drug-containing media were introduced. As in the experiments of other investigators (Fink and Tseng, 1981; Safa and Tseng, 1983), a single drug concentration (10^{-5} M) was selected, and triplicate wells were assigned to a given drug. A randomized table was used, and nontreated controls received fresh media only. Twenty-

Table 17–1. IN-VITRO CHEMOSENSITIVITY* OF HUMAN COLON CELL LINES

Drug†	SK-Co-1	SW-480	Colo-205	HT-29	Mean Response
5-Fluorouracil	99.7	105.7	61.5	93.2	90.0 ± 19.7
BCNU	106.4	76.3	108.3	64.4	88.9 ± 21.9
Mitomycin C	97.2	102.6	12.3	46.8	64.7 ± 43.1
Melphalan	95.1	86.9	110.4	94.9	96.8 ± 9.8
Vinblastine	49.3	66.9	41.4	73.4	57.8 ± 14.9
cis-Platinum	94.7	120.8	141.1	144.4	125.3 ± 22.9

*Chemosensitivity is defined as percent survival after 24 hours of continuous exposure to drug.
†All drugs were given at 10^{-5} M final concentration.

four hours later, the medium was removed and the cultures were washed twice with MEM to remove any dead cells or cellular debris. Surviving cells were removed with the use of a trypsin-Versene mixture* and enumerated by employment of a Coulter counter. The percentage survival was normalized against the nontreated controls and formed the basis for ranking drugs in order of cytotoxicity. The results were further analyzed by the Wilcoxon Rank Sum test so that the statistical significance of differences could be determined. We have designated a tumor as a responder to a drug if the drug shows a cytotoxic advantage at a P value of 0.05 or less.

CHEMOSENSITIVITY OF ESTABLISHED COLON TUMOR CELL LINES, FIBROBLAST CELL LINES, AND COLON TUMOR CELLS IN PRIMARY CULTURE

The responses of the colon tumor cell lines to the drugs used in the test panel (Table 17–1) varied widely. In general, *cis*-platinum appeared to be mildly stimulatory to cell growth, whereas vinblastine sulfate and mitomycin C were seen to be the most cytotoxic of the agents tested. The responses of individual cell lines were also very diverse. For example, Colo-205 was extremely sensitive to mitomycin C (12.3 percent survival); however, it was resistant to BCNU, melphalan, and *cis*-platinum. Similarly, the most toxic agent for SK-Co-1 was vinblastine sulfate, whereas the same cells were entirely unaffected by 24 hours of continuous exposure to 5-FU, BCNU, mitomycin C, melphan, or *cis*-platinum. The mean responses obtained by averaging cell survival from these cell lines suggest that vinblastine sulfate is the most effective of the tested agents, followed by mitomycin C, BCNU, 5-fluorouracil, melphalan, and *cis*-platinum. Three points should be emphasized with regard to these data: (1) 5-fluorouracil is clearly not the most effective single agent; (2) the different biologic properties of tumor cell lines are reflected in differences in chemosensitivity; and (3) except for mitomycin C, which proved significantly cytotoxic in Colo-205 colon tumor cells, no other agent was found to be very effective against the cell lines tested. The presence of fibroblasts in primary cultures of human biopsy specimens can compromise results of chemosensitivity tests. Their luxuriant growth impedes the proliferation of tumor cells. Moreover, the contribution of fibroblast to the overall cytotoxicity response of the culture is largely unknown. Working with the relatively generous amount of tissue usually available from biopsies of colorectal carcinomas, we have found that if the suspended cells are seeded at a relatively high density, epithelial cells will anchor early, and thus cultures are rarely overwhelmed by fibroblastic growth.

The biologic response of normal colonic fibroblasts to therapeutic agents is not known, however. Two fibroblast cell lines derived from

*M. A. Bioproducts.

Table 17–2. IN-VITRO CHEMOSENSITIVITY* OF FIBROBLAST CELL LINES

Drug†	CCD-112-Co	CCD-18	Mean Response
5-Fluorouracil	92.8	105.1	98.9 ± 8.7
BCNU	107.0	113.1	110.1 ± 4.3
Mitomycin C	95.8	107.3	101.6 ± 8.1
Melphalan	92.7	141.7	117.2 ± 34.7
Vinblastine	121.8	124.6	123.2 ± 1.9
cis-Platinum	97.1	111.3	104.2 ± 10.0

*Chemosensitivity is defined as percent survival after 24 hours of continuous exposure to drug.
†All drugs were given at 10^{-5} M final concentration.

Table 17–3. **CHEMOSENSITIVITY* OF HUMAN COLON CANCER IN PRIMARY CULTURE**

Drug†	Initials of Patient								Mean Response
	J.J.	*L.T.*	*C.L.*	*R.C.*	*A.C.*	*H.H.*	*C.G.*	*W.M.*	
5-Fluorouracil	79.4	NT‡	85.3	101.0	90.3	48.4	111.0	52.6	81.1 ± 23.4
BCNU	90.8	56.6	84.8	NT	NT	NT	106.0	59.4	79.5 ± 21.1
Mitomycin C	90.8	NT	NT	61.2§	66.6	56.2	87.0	44.4	67.7 ± 18.0
Melphalan	98.5	NT	NT	NT	NT	NT	87.0	65.4	83.6 ± 16.8
Vinblastine	91.6	76.2	NT	69.4	76.1	81.5	83.0	58.9	76.7 ± 10,5
cis-Platinum	88.5	48.8	54.9	70.4	67.9	NT	68.0	73.9	67.5 ± 12.9

*Chemosensitivity is defined as percent survival after 24 hours of continuous exposure to drug.
†All drugs were given at 10^{-5} M final concentration.
‡NT, not tested.
§Chemosensitivity is significant at $P \leq 0.05$, Wilcoxon Rank Sum test.

the human colon were exposed to the same drug panel, and their responses were studied. The responses of CCD-112-Co and CCD-18 cells are presented in Table 17–2; clearly, neither line was markedly affected. The uniform resistance to the tested drugs is striking. Additional studies are under way to determine the basis for this apparent drug resistance. Should it prove to be a common property of colonic fibroblasts, it should be possible for investigators to discount the presence of small numbers of fibroblasts in primary cultures and to attribute the observed cytotoxic effects entirely to epithelial response.

Biopsy specimens from 12 randomly selected patients with colon and rectal cancer were included in our initial studies on the chemosensitivity of human colon cancer. Four cultures were overwhelmed by microbial contamination and were discarded. The remaining eight cultures were tested against three to six drugs, depending on the number of wells available. The results are summarized in Table 17–3. Of the eight tumors sampled, only one exhibited a statistically significant response ($P = 0.05$, patient R.C., to mitomycin C). Several other tumors showed varying degrees of growth inhibition to vinblastine sulfate, *cis*-platinum, or 5-fluorouracil. The mean response of these tumors suggests a low level of drug sensitivity in general. The finding of one potential responder in eight samples is consistent with the established clinical response rate of colorectal cancer patients to chemotherapy (Ausfield et al., 1977; Lavin et al., 1980; Davis, 1982). Results from other laboratories also indicate that few tumors of this type display in-vitro chemosensitivity (Ahmann et al., 1982; Schlag and Schreml, 1982). Large-bowel cancer appears to be intrinsically resistant to currently available therapeutic agents, and thus radically new chemotherapeutic agents appear to be needed for the treatment of colon and rectal cancer. Meanwhile, in-vitro chemosensitivity tests offer the potential of eliminating ineffective agents and a means of predicting the therapeutic efficacy of the few remaining agents.

TISSUE-SPECIFIC DRUG DELIVERY AND ENHANCED THERAPEUTIC EFFICACY

The idea of selective delivery of therapeutic agents by tissue-specific carriers was proposed in 1906 by Paul Ehrlich. The selectivity of anticancer agents can be enhanced by binding of the drug to carrier molecules. One recent development in the selective enhancement of drug uptake is the use of liposomes, which are closed multilamellar phospholipid spheres. They are internalized by endocytosis, and their contents are released by lysosomal action (Gregoriadis, 1978; Mayhow et al., 1978). This approach, however, does not yet qualify as a tumor-specific drug-delivery method. Although the existence of actual tumor-specific antigens remains an open question, the introduction of cell hybridization techniques for the production of monoclonal antibodies has stimulated a worldwide search for antibodies with specificity for cancer cells. In 1979, Herlyn and co-workers reported two monoclonal antibodies against human colorectal carcinoma, and in 1982 Atkinson and associates reported on their use of monoclonal antibodies generated by inoculating mice with colon cancer cell line SW-1116 to detect cancer in fixed, paraffin-embedded tissues by immunoperoxidase methods. The availability of a tumor-specific monoclonal antibody would open a new era in the immunochemotherapy of cancer, a field in which investigators have already reported enhanced cytotoxicity by covalently linking antibodies to toxins (Moolten et al., 1982; Ruben and Dulbecco, 1974), Adriamycin (Kitao and Hattori, 1977), melanotropin (Varga et al., 1977) to achieve the desirable local concentration and biologic response.

SUMMARY

We have used established colon tumor cell lines, colon-derived fibroblast cell lines, and primary cultures of 12 human colon cancers to assess their response to six clinically used chemotherapeutic agents. We have found that, as a rule, both the established cell lines and the primary cultures exhibit a high degree of drug resistance. Nevertheless, we advocate in-vitro chemosensitivity screening. We believe that until more effective drugs become available, it would be of benefit to incorporate the chemosensitivity test as a part of the management strategy for patients with colon cancer. Hybridoma technology may make it possible to generate quantities of antibodies that specifically recognize colorectal cancer tumors. If so, covalently linking drugs and antibodies offers a way to optimize drug delivery in recurrent cancer. However, the selection of the drug that will most effectively link to a specific carrier antibody will still require the use of some type of in-vitro chemosensitivity screening.

References

Agrez MV, Kovach, JS, Beart RW, et al: Human colorectal carcinoma: patterns of sensitivity to chemotherapeutic agents in the human tumor stem cell assay. J Surg Oncol 20:187, 1982.

Ahmann FR, Meyskens FL, Moon TE, et al: In vitro chemosensitivities of human tumor stem cells to the phase II drug 4-(9-acridinyl amino)methanesulfone-m-anisidide and prospective in vivo correlations. Cancer Res 42:4495, 1982.

Alberts DS, Mackel C, Pocelinko R, Salmon SE: Phase I clinical investigation of 9,10-anthracenedicarboxaldehyde bis [(4,5-dihydro-1H-imidazol-2-yl)hydrazone] dihydrochloride with correlative in vitro human clonogenic assay. Cancer Res 42:1170, 1982.

Atkinson BF, Ernst CS, Herlyn M, et al: Gastrointestinal cancer–associated antigen in immunoperoxidase assay. Cancer Res 42:4820, 1982.

Ausfield F, Klotz J, Nealon T, et al: A phase III study comparing the clinical utility of four regimens of 5-fluorouracil. Cancer 39:34, 1977.

Bech-Hansen NT, Sarangi F, Sutherland DJ, Ling V: Rapid assays for evaluating drug sensitivity of tumor cells. J Natl Cancer Inst 59:21, 1977.

Comis RL, Carter SK: A review of chemotherapy in gastric cancer. Cancer 34:1576, 1974.

Davis H: Chemotherapy of large bowel cancer. Cancer 50:2638, 1982.

DiPaolo JA, Dowd JE: Evaluation of inhibition of human tumor tissue by cancer chemotherapeutic drugs with an in vitro test. J Natl Cancer Inst 27:807, 1961.

Ehrlich P: Collected Studies on Immunity. Vol. II. New York, John Wiley and Sons, 1906, pp. 442–497.

Falkson G, Van Eden EG, Faulkson HC: Fluorouracil, imidazole carboximide dimethyltriazeno, vincristine and *bis*-chloroethylnitrosourea in colon cancer. Cancer 33:1207, 1974.

Fink S, Tseng MT: Effects of thiotepa on primary cultures of DMBA-induced mammary tumors of rats: kinetics and ultrastructure. Br J Cancer 44:762, 1981.

Gregoriadis G: Liposomes in therapeutic and preventive medicine: the development of the drug carrier concept. Ann NY Acad Sci 308:343, 1978.

Heidelberger C: Fluorinated pyrimidines, a new class of tumor inhibitory compound. Nature 179:663, 1967.

Herlyn M, Steplewski Z, Herlyn D, Koprowski H: Colorectal carcinoma–specific antigen: detection by means of monoclonal antibodies. Proc Natl Acad Sci (USA) 76:1438, 1979.

Holmes JL, Little JM: Tissue culture microtest for predicting response of human cancer to chemotherapy. Lancet 2:985, 1974.

Kitao T, Hattori K: Concanavalin A as a carrier of daunomycin. Nature 265:81, 1977.

Laszlo J, Stengle J, Wight K, Burk D: Effects of chemotherapeutic agents on metabolism of human acute leukemia cell in vitro. Proc Soc Exp Biol Med 97:127, 1958.

Lavin P, Mittelman A, Douglass H Jr, et al: Survival and response to chemotherapy for advanced colorectal adenocarcinoma: an Eastern Cooperative Oncology Group report. Cancer 46:1536, 1980.

Lickiss JN, Cane KA, Barkie AG: In vitro selection in antineoplastic chemotherapy. Eur J Cancer 10:809, 1974.

Livingston RB, Titus GA, Heilbrum IK: In vitro effects of DNA synthesis as a predictor of biological effect from chemotherapy. Cancer 40:2209, 1980.

Macdonald JS, Kisner DF, Smythe T, et al: 5-Fluorouracil (5-FU), methyl-CCNU and vincristine in the treatment of advanced colorectal cancer: phase II study utilizing weekly 5-FU. Cancer Treat Rep 60:1597, 1976.

Mayhow E, Papahadjaopoulos D, Rustam TM, Dave C: Use of liposomes for the enhancement of the cytotoxic effect of cytosine-arabinoside. Ann NY Acad Sci 308:371, 1978.

Moertel CG: Clinical management of advanced gastrointestinal cancer. Cancer 36:675, 1975.

Moertel CG, Reitemeier RJ, Hahn RG: Therapy with the fluorinated pyrimidines. *In* Moertel CG, Reitemeier RJ (eds): Advanced Gastrointestinal Cancer. New York, Hoeber-Harper, 1969, pp. 86–107.

Moolten FL, Schreiber BM, Zajdel SH: Antibodies conjugated to potent cytotoxins as specific antitumor agents. Immunol Rev 62:47, 1982.

Pike BL, Robinson WA: Human bone marrow colony growth in agar gel. J Cell Physiol 76:77, 1971.

Roper P, Drewinko B: Comparison of in vitro methods to determine drug-induced cell lethality. Cancer Res 36:2182, 1976.

Ruben RC, Dulbecco R: Augmentation of cytotoxic drug action by antibodies directed at cell surface. Nature 248:81, 1974.

Safa AR, Tseng MT: Doxorubicin-induced ultrastructural and growth changes in primary cultures of 7,12-dimethylbenz[a]anthracene–induced mammary tumors. J Natl Cancer Inst 70:535, 1983.

Salmon SE, Hamburger AW, Soehnlen BJ, et al: Quantitation of differential sensitivity of human tumor stem cells to anticancer drugs. N Engl J Med 298:1321, 1978.

Schlag P, Schreml W: Heterogeneity in growth pattern and drug sensitivity of primary tumor and metastases in the human tumor colony-forming assay. Cancer Res 42:4086, 1982.

Till JE, McCulloch EA: A direct measurement of the radiation sensitivity of normal mouse bone marrow cells. Radiat Res 14:213, 1961.

Varga JM, Asato N, Lande S, Lerner AB: Melanotropin-daunomycin conjugate shows receptor-mediated cytotoxicity in cultured murine melanoma cells. Nature 267:56, 1977.

Volm M, Wayss K, Kaufmann M, Mattern J: Pretherapeutic detection of tumor resistance and the results of tumor chemotherapy. Eur J Cancer 15:983, 1979.

Wasserman TH, Comis RL, Goldsmith M, et al: Tabular analysis of the clinical chemotherapy of solid tumors. Cancer Treat Rep 6:399, 1975.

Wright JC, Plummer-Cobb J, Gumport S, et al: Investigation of the relationship between clinical and tissue culture response to chemotherapeutic agents on human cancer. N Engl J Med 257:1207, 1957.

EIGHTEEN

Chemotherapy of Colorectal Cancer

N. Wolmark, M.D.
D. Haller, M.D.
J. Allegra, M.D.

Cancer of the colon and rectum is an extremely common disease in the United States. More than 110,000 new cases were diagnosed during 1982, and over 50,000 of these patients will die of advanced disease. The outlook for patients not cured by surgery is dismal and reflects our lack of effective drugs in the treatment of advanced disease and our inability to attain increased survival when drugs with even modest efficacy are used in the adjuvant setting.

In this chapter, we will provide information concerning the current status of advanced disease therapy and will attempt to summarize the results of completed and ongoing adjuvant trials.

CHEMOTHERAPY OF ADVANCED COLORECTAL CANCER

The necessity of developing chemotherapeutic strategies for managing the patient with advanced colorectal cancer is obvious upon inspection of data describing the incidence of this disease and the mortality associated with it (CA-A Cancer Journal for Clinicians, 1980). Surgical and radiotherapeutic techniques utilized in patients with recurrent disease have, except in uncommon instances, been only palliative. Therefore, large numbers of patients each year are eligible to receive some form of systemic therapy administered with the intent of alleviating symptoms or improving survival. Unfortunately, the literature fails to demonstrate that the treatment of this tumor has paralleled the development of chemotherapeutic strategies in other, more sensitive malignancies. The development of aggressive combination therapy regimens, the therapy of early disease, and none of the combinations of drugs with radiotherapy or immunotherapy have proved superior to single-agent chemotherapy or supportive care alone. In fact, although a controlled trial of chemotherapy versus supportive care alone has not been reported, retrospective data from the Mayo Clinic suggest no survival advantage associated with the most commonly employed single agent, 5-fluorouracil, when compared with matched, untreated controls (Moertel and Reitemeier, 1969).

Early data in the literature concerning the response rates achievable with common chemotherapeutic regimens are difficult to evaluate because of a lack of uniformity with regard to patient selection criteria, therapeutic response evaluation, and data analysis. Since survival, although easily measurable, has not been changed by the use of any therapy, response rates have been utilized as the chief means of comparing the various methods used to treat this malignancy; thus, recent data have shown somewhat less optimistic and more reproducible results (Moertel, 1982). Unfortunately, even though response criteria may be strictly observed in a particular trial, analysis of response in small numbers of patients may lead to large standard errors, and, consequently, false-positive studies. Larger studies often fail to confirm activity data from pilot studies, but they may provide insight into patient characteristics that might substantially affect response and survival. An analysis of

1314 patients treated with various drug regimens studied by the Eastern Cooperative Oncology Group suggested a number of factors that may have had more impact on patient survival than the specific chemotherapeutic treatment utilized (Lavin et al., 1980). Favorable response and survival statistics were more often seen in patients who had received no previous chemotherapy, no history of weight loss, an ECOG performance status of 0–1, or no liver or lung involvement. In these studies, patients who responded to therapy had a much longer interval from initial diagnosis to study entry (93 weeks) than those who failed to respond (52 weeks). The authors suggest that any survival advantage claimed for a responding population may actually be the result of a population or natural history variable rather than an indication of a treatment-related beneficial effect. It is important for the reader to recall these observations on the difficulty of adequately reporting response and survival data when evaluating reports of new treatments in the literature.

Single-Agent Chemotherapy

Nowhere is the effect of the variability of data-reporting more obvious than in the reports on the most commonly used drug in colorectal cancer, 5-fluorouracil (5-FU). In 1976, Carter reviewed collected series of over 2000 patients treated with this medication and calculated the response rate to be approximately 21 percent. However, in 1973 Moertel reported individual series with response rates varying from 8 to 85 percent.

Numerous studies have been performed to determine the optimal dose, schedule, and route of administration of 5-FU. Although this drug was originally administered intravenously, other routes (e.g., oral, intraluminal, and intra-arterial) have been utilized.

Oral 5-FU has been tested in a number of clinical settings. Although the drug is well tolerated by this route, in none of these studies were response or survival rates equivalent to, or better than, those provided by intravenously administered drug (Hahn et al., 1975; Amsfield et al., 1977).

Continuous infusion of 5-FU also has been tested and compared with bolus intravenous injection of the drug. In 1975, Seifert and coworkers reported a randomized series of 70 patients treated either with 30 mg per kg continuously infused over 24 hours for 5 days or with 12 mg per kg via bolus injection for 5 consecutive days. Stomatitis was dose-limiting in the prolonged infusion group, whereas myelosuppression was dose-limiting in the bolus group. These differences made it difficult to establish comparably toxic drug doses. Objective remissions were seen in eight of 36 (22 percent) patients treated via bolus injection and in 15 of 34 (44 percent) treated via infusion therapy. The median duration of response between the two groups was not different, and the average survivals in both were identical. The differences in response rates must be questioned because of the lack of patient stratification. Interestingly, all patients with hepatic metastases alone were excluded, since they were treated separately via hepatic artery infusion.

In order to delineate the role of hepatic artery infusions in the management of patients with hepatic metastases, the Central Oncology Group performed a randomized study comparing intrahepatic arterial 5-FU with systemically administered 5-FU (Grage et al., 1979). Seventy-four patients were treated with either (1) intrahepatic arterial infusion of 5-FU, 20 mg per kg per day for 14 days followed by 10 mg per kg per day for 7 days; or (2) systemic therapy consisting of bolus injection of 5-FU, 12 mg per kg per day for 4 days followed by 6 mg per kg per day every other day for 4 days. Both groups then received weekly maintenance doses of 5-FU. The response rate was 23 percent in the bolus therapy group and 34 percent in the infusion group; these results were not significantly different. The median survivals in these two groups were 15.4 months and 13.5 months, respectively.

The Central Oncology group also conducted one of the largest studies comparing various methods of administering 5-FU (Amsfield et al., 1977). In this clinical trial, 462 patients with colon, rectum, and breast cancer were randomized among the following four dosage regimens of 5-FU:

1. *Intravenous loading:* 12 mg per kg per day over 5 days followed by 11 half-doses on alternate days until toxicity was observed, followed by weekly maintenance doses of 15 mg per kg.
2. *Weekly intravenous:* bolus injection of 15 mg per kg per week over 4 days, with an increase to 20 mg per kg if no toxicity was observed.
3. *Nontoxic intravenous:* 500 mg per day over 4 days, followed by 500 mg per week.
4. *Oral:* 15 mg per kg per day over 6 days, followed by 15 mg per kg per week.

All drug regimens were continued until disease progression was documented. Of 198 patients with colorectal cancer, 36 (18 percent) demonstrated objective remission. Responses among the regimens were as follows: Regimen 1, 16 of 48 patients (33 percent); regimen 2, 7 of 52 patients (13 percent); regimen 3, 7 of 50 patients (14 percent); regimen 4, 6 of 48 patients (13 percent). Not surprisingly, regimen 1 was the most toxic. Although the duration of response was significantly longer with the intravenous loading regimen, the survival advantage was not significantly better for patients receiving that therapy. This study confirmed the lack of efficacy of 5-FU in nontoxic and oral regimens.

Moertel's data from the Mayo Clinic support the concept that moderate toxicity may be required to achieve the greatest number of objective responses but that excessive toxicity may militate against regressions (Moertel, 1982). In an analysis of 391 patients receiving either 5-FU or FUDR (the deoxyriboside of FU), the response rate seen in patients who suffered no leukopenia was 9.7 percent. In contrast, the response rates for patients with nadir white blood counts in the 1500 to 4500 per mm^3 range was 22.7 percent ($P > .01$). The response rate in patients who had white blood counts less than 1500 per mm^3 was 15 percent (statistically not significantly different from the 22.7 percent rate observed in the second group).

Numerous other single-agent chemotherapy regimens have been tested in advanced colorectal cancer. The nitrosoureas have received a great deal of attention both in patients with advanced disease and in those receiving adjuvant therapy. These drugs (BCNU, CCNU, MeCCNU, and chlorozotocin) have all produced responses in the 10 to 20 percent range (Moertel, 1973; Hoth et al., 1978). The response duration has generally been less than 6 months with these agents, and, as with 5-FU, survival advantages have not been demonstrated. Response rates of up to 16 percent have been achieved with mitomycin C in combined series, with response durations short compared with those associated with the nitrosoureas (Wasserman et al., 1975; Moertel, 1978).

In summary, the role of single-agent chemotherapy in advanced colorectal cancer is quite limited. Although survival is prolonged in patients who respond to treatment, the beneficial effect of therapy on overall survival has been impossible to demonstrate. In spite of a lack of survival benefit, chemotherapy may provide some patients with effective palliation of symptoms (e.g., relief of pain from malignant hepatomegaly). The intravenous loading regimen of 5-FU appears to have the best effect on tumor regression and toxicity; it is also relatively easily administered by an experienced chemotherapist. Whether or not patients have received 5-FU therapy, they should be encouraged to enter research protocols designed to evaluate activity of new drugs and other new modalities in advanced colorectal cancer.

Combination Chemotherapy

The concept of combination chemotherapy in the treatment of colorectal cancer was prompted by the early successes observed when these techniques were applied to other malignancies (e.g., leukemia, Hodgkin's disease, and breast cancer). In these diseases, improvements were seen not only in overall response rates but also in complete response rates, including the durations of response and of survival. With the hope of confirming this success in colorectal cancer, investigators in the mid 1970s initiated numerous combination chemotherapy trials.

One of the first reports of combination therapy in this disease was published in 1974 by Falkson and colleagues, who administered 5-FU, BCNU, vincristine, and DTIC together and compared the results with those obtained with 5-FU alone. The response rates in the two arms of this relatively small study were 43 percent and 25 percent, respectively, representing an insignificant difference. In 1975, Moertel reported a similar response rate of 43.5 percent, utilizing a combination of 5-FU, methyl CCNU, and vincristine. Soon, a number of researchers reported combinations identical with that used by Moertel's group as well as variations of their regimen. Although initial reports were consistent with Falkson's and Moertel's optimistic findings, later reports indicated the response rate with these combinations to be as low as 4 percent (Engstrom et al., 1978; Kemeny et al., 1977; Lokich et al., 1977).

In 1982, the Mayo Clinic updated their observations on the role of 5-FU and MeCCNU in advanced colorectal cancer (Schutt et al., 1982). In a comparative trial of 5-FU, MeCCNU, and triazinate; 5-FU, MeCCNU, and ICRF 159; and 5-FU, MeCCNU, and vincristine, an attempt was made to improve the response rate of 5-FU and MeCCNU through substitution of two agents with known response rates of 10 percent in place of vincristine, an inactive agent. In 163 patients whose responses could be evaluated, objective regressions were seen in five of 44 (11 percent) receiving the triazinate combination, in eight of 59 (14 percent) receiving the ICRF combination, and in ten of 60 (17 percent) receiving the vincristine combination. These response rates are not significantly different from those observed in previously quoted trials in which the effects of 5-FU alone were examined. In addition, the durations of response are not greater with these regimens, nor are median survivals significantly prolonged.

Other combinations have been extensively studied, including 5-FU and hydroxyurea (response rate, 21 percent); 5-FU, MeCCNU, vincristine, and streptozocin (27 percent); and 5-FU, Adriamycin, and mitomycin C (17 percent) (Engstrom et al., 1978; Kemeny et al., 1978; Haller et al., 1978). This last combination previously demonstrated response rates of 40 percent in upper gastrointestinal malignancies. Responses were particularly high in stomach cancer (Panettiere and Heilbron, 1979). No regimen to date has shown convincing benefits, in either response or survival, when compared with 5-FU alone.

Future Directions

Clearly, the future of chemotherapy of advanced colorectal cancer does not rest on currently available single agents or on combinations of those same relatively inactive drugs. A number of new approaches may inspire some interest and offer promise in the therapy of this disease. New drugs must continue to be screened for phase II activity as they become available following toxicity trials. The utilization of the tumor stem-cell cloning assay may assist investigators in two ways. First, the ability to test new drugs in vitro may shorten the testing period for each drug and may spare patients from being exposed to potentially toxic, inactive compounds. Second, the ability to test each individual's tumor may give the clinician a means of limiting drug treatment only to those patients whose tumors are known to be sensitive to particular drugs.

Investigators are also addressing issues relative to the enhancement of individual drug activities, based on biochemical modulations. With these techniques, the activities of individual drugs are metabolically improved by combination with other compounds. Examples of these modulations include combinations of 5-FU plus thymidine and 5-FU plus methotrexate. The proper sequencing of these drugs may significantly improve the activity of 5-FU.

Finally, investigators must continue to develop other modalities, including radiotherapy, hyperthermia, and immunotherapy, with the intent of combining these modalities with conventional chemotherapy techniques.

ADJUVANT CHEMOTHERAPY OF OPERABLE COLORECTAL CANCER

The degree of enthusiasm surrounding studies in adjuvant therapy for malignancy is invariably dictated by the natural history of the disease under consideration. Analysis of survival data for colorectal cancer indicates that a complacent attitude regarding primary operative therapy is unjustified. Results from various tumor registries suggest that the natural history of colorectal cancer has not been appreciably altered in the last 30 years, despite improved and more aggressive operative techniques. Indeed, the estimate that 50 percent of patients with colorectal cancer harbor disseminated disease at the time of diagnosis and the anticipated dismal survival rates in patients with Dukes' B and C tumors serve as constant reminders of the inadequacy of operative therapy (Astler and Coller, 1954; Dukes and Bussey, 1958; Bussey et al., 1960; McSherry et al., 1969; Kuehner et al., 1970; Franklin and McSwain, 1970). The assumption that the majority of failures in the treatment of colorectal cancer are due to disseminated micrometastatic foci that are present at the time of the initial operation provides the rationale for current efforts in assessing systemic therapy as an adjunct to operative resection. It is logical to postulate that gains in the treatment of colon cancer in which micrometastases are present will be made only with the use of a therapeutic modality that functions on a systemic level. The issues concerning the utility of systemic adjuvant therapy have been clouded by contentions that the results obtained with operation alone are highly variable and give rise to differences that make the accurate assessment of adjuvant therapy difficult.

More specifically, it has been argued that the operative technique employed is critical in determining ultimate survival, and it has been suggested that the routine employment of wide anatomic resection and radical lymphadenectomy (including hypogastric node dissection in rectal cancer) will significantly improve the national success rate (Enker et al., 1979). This thesis has been developed to imply that data from protocols evaluating adjuvant therapy, particularly from large cooperative groups, cannot be assessed because of the lack of uniformity in the operative technique and the failure to apply radical resection universally. This pessimistic view is counterproductive. The 30 percent 5-year survival rate among patients with Dukes' C tumors reported in the American College of Surgeons Cancer Survey and that of the Surveillance Epidemiology and End Results Report (SEER) provide the most compelling evidence of the value of adjuvant therapy protocols. Such an endorsement does not mean that optimal operative techniques that mandate wide anatomic dissection and high ligation of the blood supply should be abandoned. In short, the two goals are not mutually exclusive, and one should not be pursued at the expense of the other.

A high recurrence rate is not in itself a sufficient justification for the initiation of adjuvant therapy protocols. Under ideal circumstances, a solid theoretical basis should be available along with a suitable animal tumor model in which the relevant hypotheses may be tested. In addition, the agent or agents being considered for use in the adjuvant setting should demonstrate activity in advanced disease. The rationale for the use of adjuvant chemotherapy in the treatment of micrometastases and minimal residual disease, particularly with multiple agents, has been well established and need not be belabored. The encouraging results obtained from postoperative chemotherapy in other human solid tumors indicate that the principles of adjuvant therapy may be practically applied. Numerous examples of the efficacy of adjuvant therapy in animal tumor models are available. In 1977, Corbett and colleagues demonstrated synergism between fluorinated pyrimidines and nitrosoureas in chemically induced murine colonic adenocarcinoma, thus providing the rationale for the use of these combinations in the current generation of adjuvant therapy protocols. Perhaps the most significant drawback related to the use of adjuvant chemotherapy in colorectal cancer is the failure to identify agents with impressive activity in the advanced disease setting. The suggestive evidence from animal models nothwithstanding, colorectal cancer has proved particularly resistant to various chemotherapeutic manipulations, single or otherwise. The early promise of success in advanced disease with combinations such as MeCCNU, 5-FU, and vincristine (VCR) reported by Moertel and the Falksons (Moertel et al., 1975; Falkson and Falkson, 1976) was placed in a more somber perspective by the subsequent demonstration that these combinations may have no advantage over 5-FU alone. Nevertheless, despite the attenuated enthusiasm concerning the current group of agents utilized in advanced disease, the rationale is clearly available for the initiation of clinical trials in the adjuvant setting.

This review is not intended to serve as a comprehensive compilation of the current clinical trials in adjuvant therapy for colorectal cancer but rather to focus on selected examples in order to provide an overview of the present state of the art. This discussion in most instances will be limited to those studies conducted in a randomized prospective fashion in which a suitable concomitant control has been utilized.

Adjuvant Clinical Trials Utilizing Systemic Single Agents in Colorectal Cancer

The question regarding the efficacy of single agents in adjuvant trials in colorectal cancer may be focused on the utility of 5-FU. After considerable effort and the randomization of thousands of patients, the controversy surrounding 5-FU remains unresolved. The question is not only whether 5-FU is effective but also, more signifcantly, whether the natural history and the biology of colorectal cancer may be altered utilizing adjuvant therapy. It may be appropriate at this point to consider previous efforts with single agents in order to place the current controversy about 5-FU into perspective. Interest in adjuvant therapy is not a recent phenomenon; its origins may be traced to the late 1950s, when considerable excitement was generated by the National Cancer Institute in the evaluation of chemotherapeutic agents following the operative resection of visceral tumors and breast cancer. The initial adjuvant studies all utilized single agents that were administered intraoperatively or perioperatively in a single dose with the intent of eliminating circulating tumors dislodged by the surgical manipulation of the tumor. By 1959, the results of a randomized study assessing the efficacy of a single dose of intraoperative nitrogen mustard had become available (Mrazek et al., 1959). Several years later, multiple reports of clinical trials employing perioperative thiotepa and 5-FUDR were published (Higgins et al., 1962; Dwight et al., 1973). Despite the uniformly negative results obtained and the erroneous premise upon which these studies were based, they are historically significant in that they represent attempts to alter the natural history of a noeplastic process with systemic therapy. For a comprehensive analysis of the early adjuvant studies as well as some of the more recent protocols, the reader is referred to the 1978 review by Davis and Kisner.

VASOG. The possible beneficial effect of adjuvant chemotherapy was first suggested by two studies conducted by the Veterans Administration Surgical Oncology Group (VASOG), in which 5-FU was employed postoperatively with a concomitant untreated control (Table 18–1) (Higgins et al., 1971, 1976, 1978, 1981). In the initial study, carried out between 1965 and 1969, patient eligibility was restricted to males with colon cancer (lesions not accessible to the sigmoidoscope). Patients were classified into three separate groups on the basis of intraoperative evaluation of the extent of disease: (1) patients undergoing curative resection with neither residual metastasis nor tumor at lines of resection, (2) patients with histologically confirmed residual disease or tumor present at margins of resection, and (3) patients with histologically unconfirmed but clinically evident residual disease. Only the first group represents a test of adjuvant chemotherapy in that treatment followed "curative" resection. Patients in this first group were treated with two courses of 5-FU, with a 7-day interval in which 12 mg per kg were administered I.V. push for 5 consecutive days. The 5-year data from 338 patients indicated a survival rate of 58.2 percent among the patients treated with 5-FU, compared with 48 percent for those treated with operation only. This difference was not statistically important.

Table 18–1. ADJUVANT 5-FU TRIALS IN PATIENTS UNDERGOING CURATIVE RESECTION FOR COLORECTAL CANCER

Trial (Accrual Interval)	Number of Patients	Percent Survial (Follow-up Time)	
		Treated	*Control*
VASOG (1965–1969)	338	58.2	48.0
		(5 years)	
VASOG PIT (1969–1973)	518	49.1	44.7
		(5 years)	
COG (1971–1976)	233	68.0	62.0
		(2½ years)	

VASOG PIT. The second VASOG study, conducted between 1969 and 1973, was significantly different from the initial study with regard to both patient eligibility criteria and treatment regimen. Five-day cycles of 5-FU were commenced within 2 weeks postoperatively and administered at 6- to 8-week intervals for 18 months at a dose of 12 mg per kg. This study marked the first use of prolonged adjuvant chemotherapy and, consequently, has been designated as the "VASOG prolonged intermittent therapy trial" (VASOG PIT). Admission was restricted to those patients with high risk for recurrence, as indicated by histologically positive regional nodes, full-thickness tumor penetration, blood vessel and lymphatic invasion, and contiguous involvement of adjacent organs. Although excluded from the first study, patients with carcinoma of the rectum were included in the second one, and only two distinct groups were identified on the basis of intraoperative findings: (1) patients with "curative" resection and no residual disease, and (2) patients with palliative resections in whom residual disease or tumor at the line of resection was histologically confirmed. Again, only the first group is relevant to the surgical adjuvant setting, and the 5-year data obtained from 518 patients demonstrated a 49.1 percent survival rate for the group treated with 5-FU, compared with 44.7 percent for the untreated control group. This difference was not statistically significant. Although neither trial disclosed major differences, pooling the data from these two very distinct protocols yielded a p value of 0.05, obtained from a combined total of 856 patients. It is evident that such an exercise is inappropriate.

COG. The final study utilizing adjuvant 5-FU that warrants further discussion is that of the Central Oncology Group (COG) (Grage et al.,1979; Grage and Moss, 1981). In this study, nearly 400 patients were accrued between 1971 and 1976. As in the VASOG studies, eligible patients were divided into a curative and a palliative group. The curative group consisted of those patients with an "unfavorable prognosis" whose tumors were characterized by full-thickness penetration, involvement of adjacent organs by contiguity, and the presence of positive mesenteric nodes with no evidence of residual disease. In the palliative group, patients were characterized by histologically confirmed residual disease. In the curative group, the patients were randomized to an untreated control or to a regimen of 12 mg per kg of 5-FU, administered daily for 4 consecutive days, followed by 6 mg per kg on alternate days for five additional doses or until toxicity developed. In the treated group, weekly maintenance therapy was then commenced at a dose of 12 mg per kg for a period of 1 year. It was stipulated that therapy be instituted within 30 days of the operation. As of mid 1980, 233 patients in the curative group were available for analysis, with a median follow-up of 29 months. In the treated group, the disease-free survival rate was 62 percent, and the overall survival rate was 68 percent. Corresponding rates in the untreated group were 54 percent and 62 percent. The differences between the two groups were not statistically significant. When the data were analyzed according to subsets, however, it became apparent that those patients with Dukes' C lesions and those with rectal tumors had a significant advantage regarding disease-free survival when treated with 5-FU. It should be noted that drug-related life-threatening toxicity occurred in seven patients, wtih approximately half of all treated patients experiencing leukopenia, nausea, vomiting, and stomatitis.

Results. The interpretation of the data from the experience with 5-FR has been distorted by the introduction of confounding issues. In their fervent effort to demonstrate an effect from 5-FU, investigators have combined and analyzed the information from several 5-FU trials by every conceivable statistical measure. The issue is clearly not whether the differences obtained with 5-FU have statistical significance but whether there is any utility associated with the magnitude of the differences. It is not an unreasonable assumption that 5-FU in the adjuvant setting results in a small decrease in treatment failure. The magnitude of these putative differences and the risk associated with the treatment make the use of 5-FU in the adjuvant setting completely inappropriate. Although the results attributed to 5-FU cannot be regarded as a therapeutic breakthrough, they do not warrant an abrupt dismissal. Indeed, if any effect, no matter how small, is evident with 5-FU, it should be regarded as a conceptual advance that justifies the pursuit of adjuvant trials utilizing combinations that may have greater activity. Moreover, the initial trials with 5-FU provided an important framework upon which the current generation of adjuvant trials is based. The pioneering efforts of the VASOG in the area of colorectal cancer can only be lauded.

Adjuvant Clinical Trials Utilizing Systemic Multiple Agents in Colorectal Cancer

The initial findings concerning combination chemotherapy in advanced disease have been prematurely translated into the adjuvant setting. Consequently, current randomized prospective adjuvant trials involve a combination of fluorinated pyrimidines and nitrosourea analogues. The preceding discussion of the treatment on advanced disease emphasized that the initial optimism associated with these combinations was mitigated by an accumulating data base, suggesting no superiority of these combinations when compared with 5-FU alone. Although this information may seemingly make the validity of current trials questionable, it neither attenuates the biologic principles upon which these studies are based nor justifies premature condemnation of the efforts involved.

Representative adjuvant combination therapy trials that have been completed or that are currently in progress are depicted in Table 18–2. The stress placed on the assessment of BCG and BCG products is immediately apparent. Viewed in retrospect, this issue may seem to have been overemphasized, particularly in

Table 18–2. **ADJUVANT TRIALS IN COLORECTAL CANCER**

Trial (Accrual Interval)	Regimen	Number of Patients
VASOG 27A (1973–1979)	1. 5-FU + MeCCNU 2. Untreated	653
GITSG 6175 (1975–1979)	1. 5-FU + MeCCNU 2. MER 3. 5-FU + MeCCNU + MER 4. Untreated	621
SWOG 7510* (1975–1980)	1. 5-FU + MeCCNU + MER 2. 5-FU + MeCCNU + oral BCG	626
ECOG EST 2276 (1976–1978)	1. 5-FU 2. 5-FU + MeCCNU	866
NSABP C-01 (1977–)	1. 5-FU + MeCCNU + VCR 2. BCG 3. Untreated	1100
NCCTG 4852 (1978–)	1. Levamisole 2. Levamisole + 5-FU 3. Untreated	300

*Untreated control arm added in mid 1977.

view of the paucity of preliminary information that had been available concerning the efficacy of BCG in colorectal cancer. Indeed, the current pervasive view regarding BCG specifically and nonspecific immune stimulants in general is extremely pessimistic. The compelling results obtained with BCG from animal tumor systems, particularly the guinea pig hepatoma, provided the rationale for subsequent studies in human tumors. The preliminary studies in human colorectal cancer that have had a marked influence on the current series of adjuvant protocols were conducted in the M. D. Anderson Hospital and reported by Mavligit and colleagues in 1977 and 1978. The results of this study suggested a beneficial effect of BCG; however, the study unfortunately suffered because of the small sample sizes and, more importantly, because the untreated control consisted of an historical group of patients. Nevertheless, the impetus for the analysis of BCG was generated, and in spite of the drawbacks and current pessimism, these studies will enable an objective analysis of nonspecific immune stimulants in colon cancer.

An additional comment may be made with respect to the use of levamisole. This antihelminthic drug has been sporadically utilized as an immunotherapeutic agent in a wide range of malignancies. Results have been inconsistent, and at present there are no rigidly controlled trials in any tumor system that attest to its efficacy. Levamisole has demonstrated some intriguing properties in animal models, and this, coupled with the ease of administration and the lack of toxicity in humans, has made its consideration attractive (Amery et al., 1977).

NCCTG 4852. Currently, the North Central Cancer Treatment Group (NCCTG) is conducting a trial in which patients with carcinoma of the colon and rectum are randomized into three treatment arms following curative resection: (1) untreated controls; (2) patients receiving 50 mg of levamisole orally every 8 hours on days 1 to 3, with the course repeated every 14 days; and (3) patients receiving 450 mg per M^2 of levamisole plus 5-FU over days 1 to 5 of every month for 1 year. Approximately 300 patients of an estimated 400-patient sample have been randomized. The treatment groups have been coded, and the study should prove decisive in defining the role of levamisole in the adjuvant treatment of colorectal cancer.

It would serve little purpose to review here each study in detail, particularly since sufficient follow-up is unavilable to enable the formulation of definitive conclusions. It is particularly unfortunate that some of the studies did not include a concurrent untreated control, thus eliminating both the opportunity to analyze the data adequately and the ability to assess the natural history of the disease in the controlled-trial setting. In order to provide general insights into the current status of adjuvant therapy trials in colon cancer, we will review the studies of three cooperative groups: the VASOG, the Gastrointestinal Study Group (GITSG), and the National Surgical Adjuvant Project for Breast and Bowel Cancer (NSABP)

VASOG 27A. This trial, in which patients were accrued between 1973 and 1979, deserves special mention because it provides the longest follow-up period of any study employing combination therapy, with over half the patients having reached the 5-year mark (Higgins et al., 1981). Eligibility criteria were similar to those of the previously described VASOG PIT study. Patients randomized to receive chemotherapy were given intravenous 5-FU for 5 successive days at a dose of 9 mg per kg per day along with a single oral administration of MeCCNU, 120 mg per M^2 on day 1 only. Cycles were repeated every 7 weeks for 12 months. Of the eligible patients, 653 were evaluable, and no therapeutic benefit was observed from combination chemotherapy. No differences regarding survival were apparent; however, a small effect may be apparent with respect to disease-free survival, although the difference does not have statistical significance.

GITSG 6175. This study was initiated in 1975 and completed in 1979 after 621 patients had been randomized. It was a four-arm study evaluating combination chemotherapy (MeCCNU and 5-FU) and immunotherapy (MER-BCG). Eligible patients included only those having carcinoma of colon (more than 12 cm from the anal verge) with full-thickness tumor penetration and positive nodes (Dukes' B and C). Patients were classified according to the number of positive nodes, with a lesion being labeled "C"$_1$ if it had fewer than five histologically positive nodes and "C"$_2$ if it had five or more nodes. The schema and drug dosages appear in Table 18–3. Duration of treatment was 70 weeks. Preliminary results for a median follow-up period of 46 months were published by Lessner and coworkers in 1982. Recurrence rates were not significantly different for any of the treatment arms, although analysis of data according to subsets disclosed a prolonged time for recurrence in the group receiving chemoimmunotherapy among those patients with C_1 tumors. Actual recurrence rates were 29 per-

Table 18–3. GITSG 6175 COLORECTAL PROTOCOL: SCHEMA OF RANDOMIZED TREATMENTS

1. Control
2. Chemotherapy
   (a) MeCCNU: 130 mg/M² P.O. day 1, q 10 wks.
   (b) 5-FU: 325 mg/M² I.V. daily, days 1–5, q 10 wks.
3. Immunotherapy
   (a) MER: 1 mg in 5 sites (0.2 mg/site) injected intradermally on day 1 and at 1 wk.
   (b) MER: 0.5 mg in 5 sites (0.1 mg/site) injected intradermally at 5, 10, 15, 20, 25, 40, 55, and 70 wks if tolerated.
4. Immunotherapy + Chemotherapy
   (a) Immunotherapy as in item 3 above.
   (b) Chemotherapy as in item 2 above.

cent for the untreated controls, 28 percent for those receiving chemotherapy, 35 percent for those receiving immunotherapy, and 28 percent for those receiving chemoimmunotherapy. A critically important aspect of this study was the demonstration that 29 percent of the patients receiving chemotherapy developed grade II or worse hematologic toxicity, and five patients were diagnosed as having presumed drug-related leukemia or preleukemia. This information stresses the necessity of assessing any putative benefits in light of potential risks.

NSABP C-01. The final study to be described is that of the NSABP. This protocol was initiated in 1977, and as of mid 1983 over 1100 patients with B and C tumors have been accrued, the largest number in the current series of clinical trials. Patients are randomized into three arms: (1) untreated controls, (2) those receiving chemotherapy, and (3) those receiving BCG (Fig. 18–1). Eligibility is limited to patients with classic Dukes' B lesions (Kirklin B_2) and those patients with Dukes' C tumors. Patients with A and D lesions are registered but not randomized to treatment arms. An additional 300 patients with A and D tumors have thus far been registered. A colon tumor is defined by the protocol as any lesion that does not require opening of the pelvic peritoneum to determine the distal margin. The chemotherapy differs from that used in the other cooperative groups in that three drugs are utilized: 5-FU, MeCCNU, and vincristine (VCR). The dose schedule and cycle of 5-FU and MeCCNU are identical with those described for GITSG 6175, except that intravenous VCR is added at a dose of 1 mg per M² on days 1 and 36. The 70-day cycle is unchanged, and a total of eight cycles are administered. The patients randomized to BCG received 6×10^8 viable organisms (Pasteur) by scarification weekly for 12 weeks, followed by alternate weekly administration for a total of 45 doses.

It is anticipated that this study will provide essential information regarding propriety of

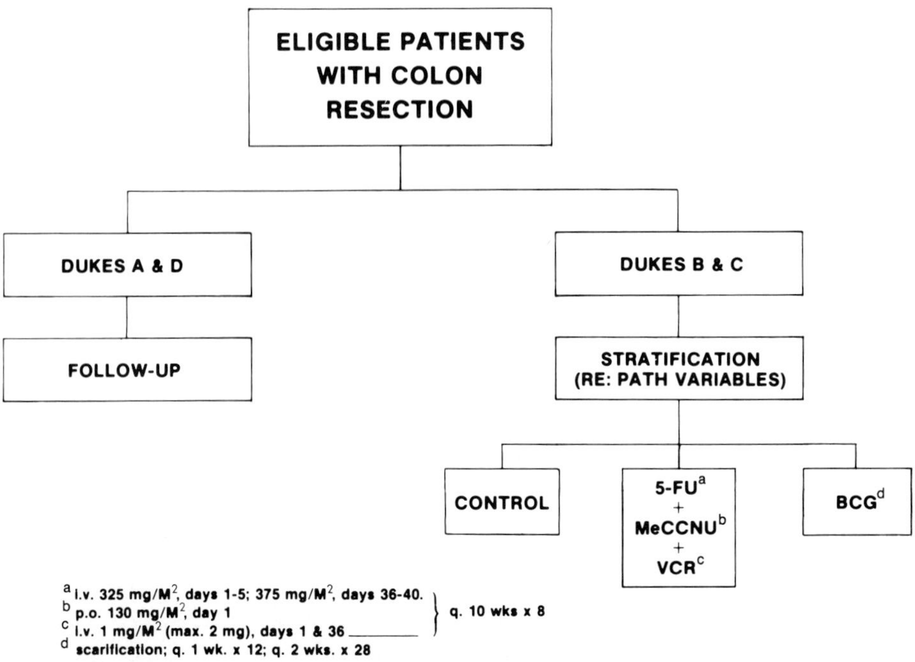

Figure 18–1. Schema of National Surgical Adjuvant Breast and Bowel Project (NSABP) Protocol C-01.

adjuvant therapy. However, with 28 months' mean follow-up time, conclusions concerning the therapeutic efficacy are impossible. The inclusion of an untreated control has made the subsequent analysis of the treatment arms possible and has provided a repository of natural history data that is crucial to the understanding of the biology of colon cancer.

Adjuvant Clinical Trials Utilizing Local and Regional Therapy in Colorectal Cancer

The use of adjuvant therapeutic strategies that are directed locally and regionally has been of long-standing interest to clinical investigators. The rationale for this kind of treatment is contingent on the basic assumption that adjuvant therapy that is successful in altering the disease on a local or regional level will result in prolonged disease-free survival and overall survival. This rationale was the basis for trials in which intraoperative 5-FU was instilled intraluminally with the intent of decreasing the incidence of anastomotic recurrence. The inherent supposition in this approach is that the successful control of local disease will result in increased survival rates and will not simply alter the pattern of first recurrences from a local site to a distant or systemic one. The initial reports by Grossi, updating a nonrandomized trial of Rousselot, demonstrated a suggestive but not statistically significant benefit associated with intraluminal 5-FU, particularly for Dukes' C and rectal lesions (Grossi et al., 1975). However, performing a similar study in a randomized prospective manner, Lawrence was unable to demonstrate any significant advantage resulting from intraluminal 5-FU (30 mg per kg) followed by five oral courses of 5-FU repeated every 2 months (Lawrence et al., 1975).

Before we discount regionally oriented studies, we must point out that the study that has to date provided the most intriguing preliminary results is based on precisely such a theme. In 1975, Taylor initiated an adjuvant trial in which the portal vein was infused with 5-FU following resection of the primary tumor (Taylor, 1981; Taylor et al., 1977, 1979). The rationale for this study is based on the contention that a significant proportion of patients with colorectal cancer will develop metastases in the liver as the first and only site of recurrence. The exact incidence of hepatic metastasis is difficult to establish, but it has been argued that a therapeutic regimen that could effectively decrease hepatic metastasis would alter the natural history of the disease and result in improved survival rates. Although most evidence suggests that established hepatic metastases are supplied predominantly by the hepatic artery, it has been suggested that the portal vein plays an important role, particularly in supplying smaller tumors (Taylor, 1981). As a consequence, a trial was undertaken in which patients were randomized to receive portal vein infusion via the umbilical vein or no further treatment. The treatment consisted of 1000 mg per day of 5-FU initiated postoperatively and administered over 7 successive days. In addition to the 5-FU, heparin was administered. Infusion was effected in 1 liter of fluid, and gravity drip was utilized. Between 1975 and 1981, 212 patients were randomized; 97 patients in the control group and 90 in the perfusion group were evaluable. In addition, 17 untreated patients developed hepatic metastases compared with five treated patients; however, the incidence of local and regional recurrences appeared unchanged. The patients who seemed to gain the greatest benefit from therapy had Dukes' B tumors, and those experiencing minimal effect had Dukes' C lesions. These results were achieved with very little toxicity.

A number of criticisms have been made concerning the design of the study and patient randomization. It has been noted that the 5-FU dose was constant and not determined by the patient's surface area. In addition, the effect of adding heparin to the infusate has not been controlled, and it is not inconceivable that heparin itself may have had a tumor-inhibiting effect. The patient-eligibility criteria were such that some patients with Dukes' D tumors were entered, making the data interpretation more difficult. Despite these criticisms, the study remains one that has provided preliminary results that warrant optimism. This treatment regimen is at least worthy of being tested within the context of the cooperative group setting involving large numbers of patients. The Mayo Clinic is currently accruing patients in a similar study of portal vein infusion and the Australia and New Zealand Bowel Cancer Trials Group has initiated a colon protocol designed to compare the portal-vein infusion of 600 mg per M^2 of 5-FU for 7 days with the identical regimen administered intravenously. An untreated control group completes the study regimen. Both these studies are now in progress, and the data will provide necessary information concerning the utility of portal vein perfusion.

The concept of regional hepatic therapy in the adjuvant setting has been pursued via other therapeutic methods. In 1979, the GITSG initiated a study involving whole-liver radiation. A total dose of 2100 rads was employed with adjuvant 5-FU (GITSG 6179). Patients treated with this regimen are compared with those in an untreated control group. Thus far, 130 patients have been entered. Severe toxicity has been a major problem with this regimen, necessitating dose modifications. Results from this study are at present unavailable.

Summary

Interpretations of the results concerning adjuvant therapy in colon cancer have often been divergent. The issues have in many cases been complicated by the lack of rigid definition of the characteristics of the various groups under study. Often, the results obtained in patients with tumors not resected for cure have not been differentiated from those undergoing curative resection, resulting in misleading impressions. The technique of pooling results from several studies in which different eligibility characteristics and drug dosages were employed has produced further uncertainty. It is, however, safe to conclude that single-agent intravenous 5-FU has no place in the current management of Dukes' B and C colon tumors. The results obtained with combination chemotherapy are preliminary, and no definitive conclusions can as yet be drawn. It is clear, however, that no striking benefit will be forthcoming, although improvement in specific subsets may yet become evident. Sufficient time has not elapsed to allow adequate assessment of the very real risks of adjuvant therapy, including the increased incidence of leukemias. It should be emphatically stated at this point that adjuvant therapy in colon cancer of any variety should not be utilized outside the context of a controlled clinical trial. The necessity of continuing the clinical trial process, particularly as related to promising leads such as portal vein infusion, must be underscored.

Adjuvant Clinical Trials in Rectal Cancer

There has been a general tendency not to differentiate between carcinoma of the colon and carcinoma of the rectum and to interpret the results with respect to adjuvant therapy in an indiscriminant fashion. It is critical that this distinction be made, particularly in light of the preliminary data from one cooperative group in which there is a putative advantage associated with the use of adjuvant therapy in carcinoma of the rectum. These results have been enthusiastically received and have had a considerable impact on the adjuvant therapy of carcinoma of the rectum in general clinical practice. It is therefore essential that the data available on adjuvant therapy for rectal cancer be critically reviewed, particularly in light of the not insignificant potential risks of the treatment.

The same biologic considerations that are relevant to carcinoma of the colon are, in general, applicable to carcinoma of the rectum. Consequently, similar therapeutic regimens have been applied to both tumors. The major difference regarding therapeutic strategy is that adjuvant radiotherapy is used for rectal tumors. The rationale for adjuvant radiotherapy is provided by an analysis of the location of recurrences following resection for Dukes' B and C rectal lesions. It is commonly believed that there will be local recurrence in a large proportion of patients following rectal operations either as the only apparent treatment failure or together with recurrent disease at other sites. Data supporting this contention are less than ideal, and documentation of location of treatment failure is not a straightforward matter. The information provided by Gunderson and Sosen in 1974 is unique in that the inaccuracies contingent on clinical and autopsy assessment of failure locations are avoided. In this study, patients with lesions up to 16 cm from the pectinate line in whom positive nodes were found at the initial curative resection were subjected to a planned "second-look" operation at 6 to 12 months following the first procedure. Of 74 evaluable patients, 52 were noted to have evidence of recurrent or residual tumor. In 25 of the 52 patients (48 per cent), local or regional tumor was the only site of recurrence, whereas in 48 of the 52 (92 percent) local or regional disease represented only part of the recurrence. Although other investigators (Cass et al., 1980; Olson et al., 1980) have reported a smaller percentage of patients with local or regional tumor as the only site of recurrence (8 to 25 percent), it is evident that local or regional recurrence is a formidable problem in carcinoma of the rectum. This predilection of carcinoma of the rectum to recur locally or regionally has led to the evaluation of radiotherapy in which the anatomic regions of the recurrence sites are encompassed. One must keep in mind when evaluating radiotherapy that the question is not simply whether local recurrence can be reduced but whether this reduction can be translated into a survival advantage. The possibility that must be entertained is that radiotherapy may simply alter the pattern of recurrence from one with a local or regional propensity to one in which distant disease will predominate.

Preoperative Radiotherapy

Initial emphasis was placed on preoperative radiotherapy, largely because it was believed that tumor seeding at the time of operation could be decreased and a precedent was available in which it was demonstrated that tumors could be rendered resectable with preoperative radiotherapy that otherwise could not have been removed. Following the 1959 retrospective analysis by Sterans, which indicated that preoperative radiotherapy provided an advantage, numerous attempts have been made to confirm this finding via randomized prospective trials. It is not unfair to state that despite these efforts, the suitability of preoperative radiotherapy remains unconfirmed. Stearns, in an effort to corroborate his initial conclusions, conducted a randomized prospective preoperative radiotherapy trial in which 376 patients received 2000 rad in eight fractions. No survival differences were evident; however, there appeared to be a decrease in local recurrences for Dukes' C tumors (Stearns et al., 1974). From 1964 to 1969, the VASOG conducted a similar study in which 700 patients were randomized to receive either 2000 to 2500 rad preoperatively in ten fractions or no further therapy (Higgins et al., 1981; Higgins, 1979). In the treated group, the 5-year survival was 35 percent; the corresponding survival in the untreated group was 29 percent. The overall differences were not statistically significant. When only those patients who underwent subsequent abdominoperineal resection were analyzed at 5 years, the survival rates were 40 percent in the treated group and 32 percent in the untreated group (P = .07). No survival differences were apparent at 12 years.

The second VASOG preoperative radiotherapy trial was conducted between 1973 and 1980, during which time 357 patients were randomized to receive either 3150 rad in 18 fractions preoperatively or no further treatment. Unlike the first study, the second trial disclosed at 5 years no survival differences either in the group as a whole or in that subgroup of patients undergoing resection. A number of other preoperative radiotherapy studies have been reported in which a bewildering variety of conclusions have been made. It is sufficient to say that the benefits of preoperative radiotherapy are elusive, and there is little justification for its use as an adjuvant in tumors that are technically resectable.

Postoperative Radiotherapy

The emphasis has shifted from preoperative radiotherapy to postoperative radiotherapy. Proponents of postoperative radiotherapy have emphasized that the strategy has a number of potential advantages as compared with preoperative radiotherapy. Postoperative radiotherapy does not interfere with tumor staging, and the "downstaging" attributed to preoperative therapy (particularly in cases of regional nodes) is avoided. Patients undergoing postoperative radiotherapy may be selected on the basis of the extent of disease found at operation. For exmaple, patients with Dukes' A tumors would be spared from receiving radiotherapy, and those with disease beyond the radiation field would similarly not be treated because both groups would be unlikely to benefit from such treatment. Contrariwise, preoperative radiotherapy is delivered to all patients when the tumor stage and extent of disease are not known at the time of treatment. Finally, it has been argued that with postoperative radiotherapy the surgeon may perform technically taxing procedures (e.g., sphincter-preserving operations) requiring low anastomoses without the added risk of an irradiated field.

Despite the increasing popularity of postoperative radiotherapy, there are insufficient data from prospective clinical trials to justify the current endorsement of the strategy. Even the ancedotal retrospective analyses that have been published are based on small sample sizes and heterogeneous patient characteristics. The studies of Withers (Withers and Romsdahl, 1977; Withers et al., 1979) performed at M. D. Anderson Hospital warrant further emphasis not for the beneficial effects of postoperative radiotherapy demonstrated in those studies but for the potential complications. In this historically controlled retrospective study, patients were treated with 5000 rads in 6 weeks. The alarmingly high incidence of small bowel obstruction emphasizes that postoperative radiation is not a benign therapeutic mode.

The role of postoperative radiotherapy in the management of patients with rectal cancer is illustrated in current randomized prospective

Table 18–4. **ADJUVANT TRIALS IN RECTAL CANCER**

Trial (Accrual Interval)	Regimen	Number of Patients
GITSG 7175 (1975–1980)	1. 5-FU + MeCCNU 2. Postoperative radiotherapy 3. 5-FU + MeCCNU + radiotherapy 4. Untreated	194
ECOG EST 4276 (1976–)	1. 5-FU + MeCCNU 2. Postoperative radiotherapy 3. 5-FU + MeCCNU + radiotherapy	279
NSABP R-01 (1977–)	1. 5-FU + MeCCNU + VCR 2. Postoperative radiotherapy 3. Untreated	400

trials. In many of the protocols that have been undertaken for rectal cancer, there has been an inadequate number of patients, necessitating that study be discontinued in many cases. There are three cooperative group studies of rectal cancer in which chemotherapy and postoperative radiotherapy have been evaluated and in which over 150 patients have been accrued. These studies are outlined in Table 18–4.

Representative Trials

GITSG 7175. The first study is that of the GITSG, in which a beneficial effect has been claimed for adjuvant therapy. Because of the important potential and actual influences of these findings, it is essential to review the data in some detail. This study was initiated in 1975 and terminated in September of 1980 after 245 patients (of whom 194 were evaluable) had been randomized. The study defines a rectal cancer as being within 12 cm of the pectinate line. Patients were randomized into four arms (Table 18–5): (1) an untreated control group; (2) patients receiving chemotherapy consisting of MeCCNU and 5-FU; (3) patients receiving postoperative radiotherapy consisting of 4000 to 4800 rad delivered in 4½ to 5½ weeks; and (4) patients receiving a combination of radiotherapy and chemotherapy. The chemotherapy schema and dosages are identical with those described in the GITSG 6175 colon protocol. According to initial projected sample-size estimates, 520 evaluable patients were required for detection of a 50 percent increase in median survival time for 2 to 3 years.

In February of 1980, it was noted that one of the randomized arms was inferior to the other three, and therefore the group was unblinded. The inferior arm proved to be the untreated control group, and randomization into this arm was discontinued. Following this event, there was an insufficient number of patients entered, and the study was discontinued 6 months later, far from having achieved the original sample-size estimates. Consequently, the number of patients in each group is at best perilously small. Of the 194 evaluable patients, 58 were untreated, 48 received chemotherapy, 49 received radiotherapy, and 39 were treated with a combination of chemotherapy and radiotherapy.

Preliminary 2-year results of this study, which have been widely quoted, indicated that 52 percent of the control group experienced recurrence, compared with 39 percent of those receiving chemotherapy alone; 36 percent of those receiving radiotherapy; and 21 percent of those receiving a combination of radiotherapy and chemotherapy (Sugarbaker et al., 1982; Enker et al., 1981). Later analyses have disclosed no major changes in the results. The overall differences in the treatment groups concerning disease-free survival are not statistically significant. The only significant difference was noted when the untreated control patients were compared with those receiving a combination of radiotherapy and chemotherapy. The strongest therapeutic benefits were evident in patients with C_1 tumors (fewer than 5 nodes), in whom significant differences were evident among the treatment arms. Information concerning recurrence site suggested that patients receiving combined treatment had a clear advantage. Survival data disclosed no significant advantage associated with any of

Table 18–5. **GITSG 7175 RECTAL PROTOCOL: SCHEMA OF RANDOMIZED TREATMENTS**

1. Control
2. Chemotherapy
   (a) 5-FU: 235 mg/M² I.V. days 1–5, 375 mg/M² I.V. days 36–40.
   (b) MeCCNU: 130 mg/M² P.O. day 1. Repeat therapy every 10 wks for 18 months.
3. Radiotherapy: 4000 or 4800 rad in 4½ to 5½ wks with 5 treatments/wk. Institutional preference.
4. Radiotherapy + chemotherapy
   (a) Radiotherapy: 4000–4400 rad.
   (b) 5-FU: 500 mg/M² I.V. days 1–3 and on last 3 days of radiotherapy. At wk 10, therapy as described in item 2 above begins and continues for total of 18 months.

the three treatment strategies compared with operation alone.

Often neglected in the wave of enthusiasm in which these data have been received is the very real incidence of treatment toxicity. Over one half of the patients receiving a combination of radiotherapy and chemotherapy have had a severe toxic reaction, compared with 29 per cent of those receiving only chemotherapy and 16 percent of those receiving radiotherapy alone. There have been two treatment-associated patient deaths in the combined treatment arm attributed to radiation enteritis. The long-term incidence of radiation enterocolitis has yet to be determined. The design of the GITSG 7180 trial, the replacement for the GITSG 7175 trial, perhaps offers the strongest evidence of the toxicity of the combined regimen. In essence, this study represents a retreat from GITSG 7175 in that the identical combined radiotherapy and chemotherapy arm is compared with one in which the MeCCNU has been eliminated altogether and replaced by 5-FU alone.

The information obtained from GITSG 7175 must be regarded as a major conceptual advance and viewed as an important initial indicator for the value of adjuvant therapy in patients with Dukes' B and C rectal cancers. However, with only 39 patients available for analysis in the group demonstrating the greatest benefit and with the magnitude of major toxicity encountered, it is premature and inappropriate for investigators to extrapolate these results for treatment of patients outside the context of clinical trials. In short, the GITSG results must await confirmation from trials in progress in which adequate sample sizes are available.

ECOG EST 4276. The second study in which there has been significant accrual of patients is being conducted by ECOG. This study was activated in 1976, and as of November 1981, 279 patients have been entered, with patient accrual continuing as of mid 1982. Patients with B (full-thickness penetration) and C lesions are randomized into three treatment arms that are very similar to the three groups receiving therapy in GITSG 7175: patients receiving chemotherapy, patients receiving radiotherapy, and patients receiving a combination of radiotherapy and chemotherapy. An important difference is that the ECOG study does not include a concomitant untreated control. Consequently, it is not possible to compare the results of any of the treatment arms with an appropriate control. This omission significantly compromises analysis of data and makes confirmation of preliminary GITSG results impossible. All things considered, preliminary analysis of the groups discloses no differences to date.

NSABP R-01. The final study that merits review is being conducted by the NSABP. This study was initiated in 1977, and to date over 350 patients with B and C rectal lesions have been randomized into three treatment arms. An additional 120 patients with A and D tumors have been registered but not randomized to treatment. The schema for this study includes an untreated control group; a group receiving chemotherapy consisting of 5-FU, MeCCNU, and VCR in the regimen outlined for NSABP C-01; and a group receiving postoperative radiotherapy. Postoperative radiotherapy was delivered in an average dose of 3200 to 4000 rad in 18 to 22 fractions. A rectal tumor is defined by this study as one that requires the intraoperative opening of the pelvic peritoneum in order to distinguish the distal margin of the lesion. This study, in which to date the most patients have been accrued, is the only one that currently allows comparison of patients receiving adjuvant chemotherapy and radiotherapy with those in a concomitant untreated control group. Consequently, the results of this study are of pivotal significance. As of late 1982, the average study time has been 36 months, and conclusions concerning the efficacy of the treatment modalities cannot be formulated. Until the results of this study become available. adjuvant therapy in the form of chemotherapy and radiotherapy must be regarded as experimental.

Other Strategies

Other methods that are being considered for the adjuvant treatment of rectal cancer include "sandwich" radiotherapy, in which a low-dose preoperative course is followed by postoperative radiotherapy, intraoperative radiotherapy, interstitial radiotherapy, radiotherapy with hyperthermia, and the use of radiation sensitizers and protectors. Whether these innovative methods will provide an advantage over radiotherapy as currently employed remains conjectural.

Summary

Current efforts in adjuvant therapy in rectal cancer have provided encouraging preliminary results. The information obtained from GITSG 7175, which suggests that the combination of radiotherapy and chemotherapy is

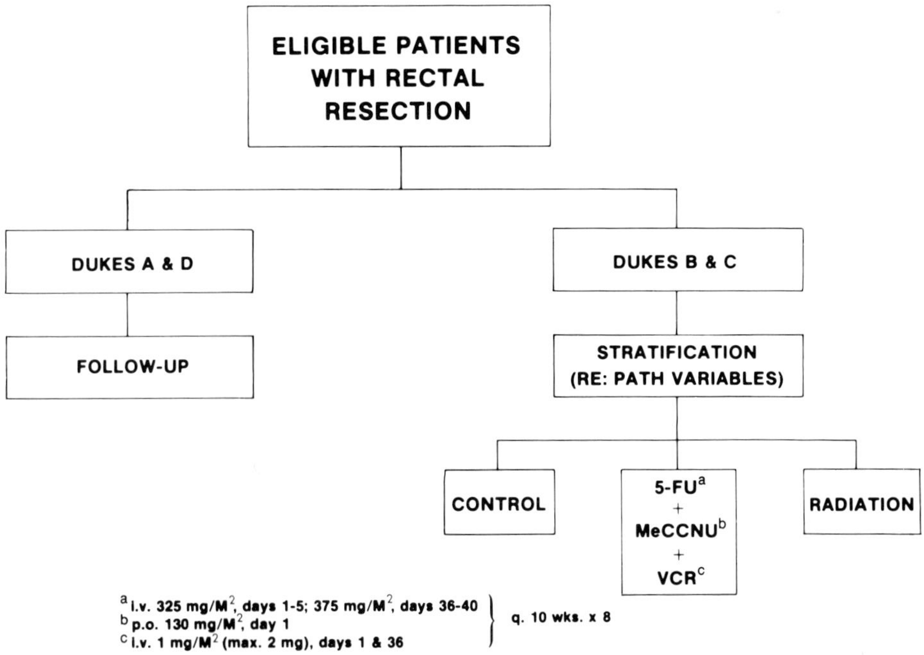

Figure 18–2. Schema of National Surgical Adjuvant Breast Project (NSABP) Protocol R-01.

beneficial, should be regarded as a promising preliminary lead. It must be emphasized that the small sample size in this study and the formidable toxicity of the combined regimen necessitate a cautious interpretation of the data. Until these findings can be confirmed from current randomized prospective trials, adjuvant therapy for rectal carcinoma must be regarded as experimental. Consequently, patients with Dukes' B and C rectal cancer should not be treated in the adjuvant setting outside the context of a clinical trial.

References

Amery WK, et al: Adjuvant treatment with levamisole in cancer. A review of experimental and clinical data. Cancer Treat Rev 4:167–194, 1977.

Ansfield R, Klotz J, Nealon T, et al: A phase III study comparing the clinical utility of four regimens of 5-fluorouracil. Cancer 39:34–40, 1977.

Astler VB, Coller FA: The prognostic significance of direct extension of carcinoma of the colon and rectum. Ann Surg 139:846–852, 1954.

Bussey, et al: Results of the surgical treatment of rectal cancer. *In* CE Dukes (ed): Cancer of the Rectum. London, E & S Livingstone, Ltd., 1960, pp. 267–280.

CA: Cancer Statistics, 1980. A Cancer Journal for Clinicians. Vol 30, No 1. January/February 1980, pp. 23–38.

Carter SK: Editorial: Large-bowel cancer—the current status of treatment. J Natl Cancer Inst 56:3–10, 1976.

Cass AW, et al: Patterns of recurrence following surgery alone for adenocarcinoma of the colon and rectum. Cancer 37:2861–2865, 1976.

Corbett TH, et al: Evaluation of single agents and combinations of chemotherapeutic agents in mouse colon carcinomas. Cancer 40:2660–2680, 1977.

Davis HL, Kisner DL: Analysis of adjuvant therapy in large bowel cancer. Cancer Clin Trials 1:273, 1978.

Dukes CE, Bussey HJR: The spread of rectal cancer and its effect on prognosis. Br J Cancer 12:309–320, 1958.

Dwight RW, et al: FUDR as an adjuvant to surgery in cancer of the large bowel. J Surg Oncol 5:243–249, 1973.

Engstrom P, MacIntyre J, Douglass H Jr et al: Combination chemotherapy of advanced bowel cancer. Proc AACR-ASCO 19:384, 1978.

Enker WE, et al: Enhanced survival of patients with colon and rectal cancer is based upon wide anatomic resection. Ann Surg 190:350–360, 1979.

Enker WE, et al: Defining the needs for adjuvant therapy of rectal and colonic cancer. Surg Clin North Am 61:1295–1310, 1981.

Falkson G, Falkson HC: Fluorouracil, methyl CCNU, and vincristine in cancer of the colon. Cancer 38:1468–1470, 1976.

Falkson G, Van Eden EG, Falkson HC: Fluorouracil, imidazole carboxamide dimethyl triazeno, vincristine and bis-chloroethyl nitrosourea in colon cancer. Cancer 33:1207–1208, 1974.

Franklin F, McSwain B: Carcinoma of the colon, rectum and anus. Ann Surg 171:811, 1970.

Grage TB, Moss SE: Adjuvant chemotherapy in cancer of the colon and rectum: Demonstration of effectiveness of prolonged 5-FU chemotherapy in a prospectively controlled, randomized trial. Surg Clin North Am 61:1321–1329, 1981.

Grage TB, Vasilopoulos PP, Shingleton WW, et al: Results of a prospective randomized study of hepatic artery infusion with 5-fluorouracil versus intravenous 5-fluorouracil in patients with hepatic metastases from colorectal cancer: A Central Oncology Group Study. Surgery 86:550–555, 1979.

Grage TB, et al: Adjuvant chemotherapy in large bowel

cancer. (Update analysis of single agent chemotherapy.) *In* Jones SE, Salmons SE (eds): Adjuvant Therapy of Cancer II. New York, Grune and Stratton, 1979.

Grossi CE, et al: Intraluminal and intravenous 5-FU chemotherapy adjuvant to surgery for resectable colorectal cancer: a clinical cooperative multi-hospital trial. Chir Gastroenterol 9:61–68, 1975.

Gunderson LL, Sosin H: Areas of failure found at reoperative (second or symptomatic look) following "curative surgery" for adenocarcinoma of the rectum. Clinicopathologic correlation and implications for adjuvant therapy. Cancer 34:1278–1292, 1974.

Hahn RG, Moertel CG, Schutt AJ, et al: A double-blind comparison of intensive course of 5-FU by oral vs intravenous route in the treatment of colorectal carcinoma. Cancer 35:1031–1035, 1975.

Haller DG, Woolley PV, MacDonald JS: Phase II trial of 5-fluorouracil, adriamycin and mitomycin C in advanced colorectal cancer. Cancer Treat Rep 62 563–565, 1978.

Higgins GA: Adjuvant radiation therapy in colon cancer. Int Adv Surg Oncol 2:1, 1979.

Higgins GA, et al: The Veterans Administration Surgical Adjuvant Group interim report. Cancer Chemother Rep 16:141–148, 1962.

Higgins GA, et al: Fluorouracil as an adjuvant to surgery in carcinoma of the colon. Arch Surg 102:339–343, 1971.

Higgins GA, et al: Adjuvant chemotherapy in the surgical treatment of large bowel cancer. Cancer 38:1461–1967, 1976.

Higgins GA, et al: The case for adjuvant 5-fluorouracil in colorectal cancer. Cancer Clin Trials 1:35–41, 1978.

Higgins GA, et al: Adjuvant therapy for large bowel cancer: update of Veterans Administration Surgical Oncology Group Trials. Surg Clin North Am 61:1311–1320, 1981.

Holden WD, et al: The use of triethylenethiophosphoramide–adjuvant to the surgical treatment of colorectal carcinoma. Ann Surg 165:481–503, 1967.

Hoth D, Butler T, Winolur S, et al: Phase II study of chlorozotocin. Proc AACR-ASCO 19:381, 1978.

Kemeny N, Yagoda A, Golbey R: Randomized study of 2 different schedules of methyl CCNU, 5-fluorouracil and vincristine for metastatic colorectal carcinoma. Proc AACR-ASCO 18:336, 1977.

Kemeny N, Yagoda A, Golbey R: Methyl CCNU, 5-fluorouracil, vincristine and streptozotocin for metastatic colorectal cancer. Proc AACR-ASCO 19:354, 1978.

Kuehner CR, et al: Comparison of surgical techniques in the treatment of carcinoma of the colon. Surg Gynecol Obstet 131:63–64, 1970.

Lavin P, Mittleman JA, Douglass H: Survival and response to chemotherapy for advanced colorectal adenocarcinoma: an Eastern Cooperative Oncology Group report. Cancer 46:1536–1543, 1980.

Lawrence W Jr, et al: Chemotherapy as an adjuvant to surgery for colorectal cancer. Ann Surg 181:616–623, 1975.

Lessner HE, et al: Adjuvant therapy of colon cancer—A prospective randomized trial. Proc Am Soc Clin Oncol 1:351, 1982.

Lokich J, Skarin A, Mayer R, et al: Lack of effectiveness of combined 5-FU and methyl CCNU therapy in advanced colorectal cancer. Cancer 49:2792–2796, 1977.

Mavligit GM, et al: Clinical immunotherapy as adjuvant therapy for colon and rectal cancer. *In* Enker WE (ed): Carcinoma of the Colon and Rectum. Chicago, Year Book Medical Publishers Inc, 1978, pp. 133–171.

Mavligit GM, et al: Adjuvant immunotherapy and chemoimmunotherapy in colorectal cancer. (Dukes Class C). Cancer 40:2726–2730, 1977.

McSherry CK, et al: Carcinoma of the colon and rectum. Ann Surg 169:502–509, 1969.

Moertel CG: Large bowel. *In* Holland JF, Frei E (eds): Cancer Medicine. Philadelphia, Lea & Febiger, 1973, pp. 1597–1626.

Moertel CG: Therapy of advanced gastrointestinal cancer with the nitrosoureas. Cancer Comother Rep 4:27, 1973.

Moertel CG: Chemotherapy of gastrointestinal cancer. New Engl J Med 299:1049–1052, 1978.

Moertel CG: Large Bowel. *In* Holland JF, Frei E (eds): Cancer Medicine. Philadelphia. Lea & Febiger, 1982, pp. 1830–1858.

Moertel CG, Reitemeier RJ: Advanced Gastrointestinal Cancer. Clinical Management and Chemotherapy. New York, Harper & Row, 1969.

Moertel CG, Shutt AJ, Hahn RG, et al: Therapy of advanced colorectal cancer with a combination of 5-fluorouracil, methyl-1, 3-*cis*(2-chloroethyl)-1-nitrosourea and vincristine. J Natl Cancer Inst 54:69–71, 1975.

Mrazek R, et al: Prophylactic and adjuvant use of nitrogen mustard in the surgical treatment of cancer. Ann Surg 150:745–755, 1959.

Olson RM, et al: Patterns of recurrence following curative resection of adenocarcinoma of the colon and rectum. Cancer 45:2969–2974, 1980.

Panettiere FJ, Heilbron L: Experiences with two treatment schedules in the combination chemotherapy of advanced gastric carcinoma. *In* Carter SK (ed.): Mitomycin-C. New York, Academic Press, 1979, pp. 145–157.

Schutt AJ, Scott M, Moertel C: Combination chemotherapy in advanced colorectal cancer. Proc ASCO 1:101, 1982.

Seifert P, Baker LH, Reed ML, Vaitkevicius VK: Comparison of continuously infused 5-fluorouracil with bolus injection in treatment of patients with colorectal adenocarcinoma. Cancer 36:123–128, 1975.

Stearns MW Jr, Deddish MR, Quan SH: Preoperative roentgen therapy for cancer of the rectum. Surg Gynecol Obstet 109:225–229, 1959.

Stearns MW Jr, Deddish MR, Quan SH, et al: Preoperative roentgen therapy for cancer of the rectum and rectosigmoid. Surg Gynecol Obstet 138:584–586, 1974.

Sugerbaker PH, et al: Colorectal cancer. *In* Devita FT, Hellman S, Rosenberg SA (eds): Cancer, Principles and Practice of Oncology. Philadelphia, JB Lippincott, 1982, pp. 643–723.

Taylor I: Studies on the treatment and prevention of colorectal liver metastases. Ann R Coll Surg Engl 63:270–276, 1981.

Taylor I, et al: Adjuvant liver perfusion in colorectal cancer. Br Med J 2:1320–1322, 1977.

Taylor I, et al: Adjuvant cytotoxic liver perfusion for colorectal cancer. Br J Surg 66:833, 1979.

Wasserman TH, Comis RL, Goldsmith M, et al: Tabular analysis of clinical chemotherapy of solid tumors. Cancer Chemother Rep 36:399–419, 1975.

Withers HR, Romsdahl MM: Post-operative radiotherapy for adenocarcinoma of the rectum and rectosigmoid. Int J Radiat Oncol Biol Phys 2:1069–1074, 1977.

Withers HR, et al: Postoperative radiotherapy for rectal cancer. *In* Jones SE, Salmon SE (eds): Adjuvant Therapy for Cancer II. New York, Grune and Stratton, 1979, pp. 621–628.

NINETEEN

Place of Radiotherapy in the Management of Cancer of the Rectum and the Anal Canal

J. Papillon, M.D.

MANAGEMENT OF RECTAL CANCER

Since the early 1960s there has been a growing recognition of the need for a multidisciplinary approach in the management of rectal cancer. Previously, radiotherapy was only used for palliation in patients with inoperable or recurrent rectal tumors. In recent years, there has been a revival of interest in the possible role of radiotherapy in the treatment of cancer of the rectum. There are several reasons for this: (1) There is greater knowledge of the natural history of the disease; (2) there is a growing awareness of the limitations of rectal surgery; and (3) there has been technical progress with the advent of supervoltage external beam radiotherapy and the development of intracavitary methods of irradiation.

Radiotherapy in the management of rectal cancer can be adjuvant, in a combined radiosurgical approach; definitive, as a conservative procedure; and palliative.

Adjuvant Radiotherapy

Irradiation combined with surgery may be carried out to (1) improve surgical results, (2) increase resectability, and (3) enlarge the field of conservative and sphincter-preserving treatments. The first purpose is the most commonly known, the second is usually given little consideration, and the third is new and rarely discussed.

Improvement of Surgical Results

After curative surgery, the average 5-year survival rate is 50 percent. This means that one in two patients will die from cancer or intercurrent disease within 5 years after surgery. This figure has been static for many years.

Local recurrence is one of the principal causes of treatment failure following surgery. After abdominoperineal resection, most recurrences occur in the perineum or pelvic region. After anterior resection, the cancer recurs around the suture line or in the pelvis. These recurrences are due to the presence of viable neoplastic cells beyond the surgical field or to the spillage or dissemination of cancer cells during manipulation at the time of operation.

The average rate of local recurrence of rectal cancer is 20 percent. It is significantly higher (more than 30 percent) when the lesions have a high histologic grade, when there is gross involvement of the perirectal fat, or when there is lymphatic metastasis (Dukes' B or C tumor). Morson (1966) has shown that although patients with Dukes' B or C tumors of the middle or lower third of the rectum account for less than 60 percent of patients coming to resection, they make up over 85 percent of those likely to develop recurrence and thus form an "at risk" group suitable for adjuvant therapy.

Local recurrence is a problem that adjuvant therapy is designed to solve. Of the possible treatment modalities available, chemotherapy alone has proved unrewarding in rectal adenocarcinoma. By contrast, several trials have indicated that radiotherapy given before or after radical surgery may be valuable as an adjuvant to surgery.

Preoperative Irradiation

The rationale of preoperative irradiation is to try to reduce viability of tumor cells at operation by destroying the cancer cells already present in lymph nodes or perirectal tissues or rendering them incapable of further growth. In this way incidence of recurrences due to seeding of malignant cells is reduced.

Various protocols of irradiation have been suggested. They differ markedly in terms of target-volume, tumor-dose, dose-time factor, and optimum time between radiotherapy and surgery.

In 1969, an important randomized trial was conducted by Higgins and Roswit (1981) of the Veterans' Administration Oncology Group, based on treatment of 700 male patients presenting with operable rectal carcinoma. Radiotherapy was administered in a dosage of 2000 rad through two opposed anteroposterior (AP)-posteroanterior (PA) fields over a 2-week period, with 500 rad boosters for those whose tumor was within 8 cm of the anal verge. Resection was carried out as soon as feasible. The most significant results were obtained in the group of 305 patients with low-lying lesion who underwent abdominoperineal resection after radiotherapy (Table 19–1).

In 1976, a second preoperative radiotherapy trial was conducted by Higgins and Roswit (1981). Radiotherapy was administered only to tumors suitable for abdominoperineal resection. The radiotherapy dosage was 3150 rad in 18 fractions over 24 days. Preliminary results showed improved 5-year survival in the combined therapy groups.

A nonrandomized study conducted by Stevens and associates (1976) at the University of Oregon was based on treatment of 58 patients with resectable tumors. A dosage of 5000 rad over 5 to 8 weeks was delivered to the area of the tumor. Surgical excision was carried out 4 to 7 weeks following the completion of irradiation. In the group of patients with resectable tumors, there was no local recurrence of cancer in the pelvis, and in 5 cases, no tumor could be found in the specimen. The 5-year survival rate of the group treated preoperatively with radiotherapy compared with the group treated surgically showed an improvement of 17 percent (55 percent versus 38 percent). Kligerman (1977), Simbertseva and associates (1975), Gary Bobo and co-workers (1979), and Rider (1975) reported series that stressed the efficacy of preoperative irradiation. Boulis-Wassif (1982), Buroker and associates (1976), and Sischy (1982) reported favorable results using a combination of irradiation and chemotherapy (5-flurouracil [5-FU], with or without mitomycin C) preoperatively. In 1982, Sischy reported a series of 48 patients treated by preoperative radiation and chemotherapy in which there was a regression of tumor volume of more than 50 percent in all cases and six tumor-free specimens.

At the present time, sufficient data have been accumulated to define the effects of preoperative irradiation. They may be summarized as follows:

1. Regression of bulky lesions and reduction in adherence to adjacent structures.
2. Decrease in the expected rate of lymphatic involvement.
3. Decrease in the rate of local recurrence.
4. Increase in survival rate.

Preoperative irradiation is especially advisable in patients not older than 75 years of age, who have extensive but resectable tumors of the lower two thirds of the rectum, and who are most likely to develop local recurrence after abdominoperineal resection. These patients have tumors that are larger than 5 cm in diameter, ulcerative, and infiltrating, with fair or impaired mobility. These tumors do not cause symptoms of bowel obstruction and do not show signs of dissemination.

Large tumors of the upper third of the

Table 19–1. **RESULTS OF THE VETERANS' ADMINISTRATION SURGICAL ADJUVANT GROUP STUDY OF PATIENTS WITH LOW-LYING TUMORS**

	Surgery Group (%)	Preoperative Radiotherapy + Surgery Group (%)
Rate of patients with positive lymph nodes	44	26
Rate of local recurrences	40	29
5-year survival rate	34	47

rectum that are suitable for anterior resection may be treated by the same procedure (Stevens et al., 1976; Bugat et al., 1981), and it has been demonstrated that surgical anastomosis is not a problem after carefully planned preoperative irradiation.

As to the technique of irradiation, several protocols are used. In most institutions a dosage of 3000 to 4000 rad over a 2 to 4 week period is delivered through two opposed AP-PA fields to a target-volume that is either large and encompasses the entire pelvis (sometimes extending to the lumbar region up to L2) or limited to the perirectal area and main lymphatic drainage areas. Radical excision is usually carried out very soon after completion of irradiation. However, if one wants to take advantage of the optimum radiologic effect, a delay of 5 to 7 weeks is advisable. Most protocols are represented in Table 19–2.

One of the main criticisms of preoperative irradiation concerns the alleged inability of clinicians to adequately assess the extent of the disease, resulting in the possible use of unnecessary irradiation in a number of patients who could have been cured by surgery alone or who have distant metastasis and are not suitable for curative treatment. Other criticisms of preoperative irradiation are that it causes an increase in postoperative morbidity and delayed wound healing.

In fact, it is not true that the extent of the disease can only be assessed by surgery. Nicholls and associates (1982) have compared clinical with pathologic findings in a series of 70 patients and demonstrated that clinical staging is more accurate than it is usually thought to be. One can easily distinguish tumors confined to the bowel wall or tumors with slight extrarectal spread from tumors with moderate or extensive extrarectal spread. Pretreatment evaluation enables the clinician to define, with a rather good approximation, the extent of the tumor and especially the degree of infiltration of the rectal wall, as long as the work-up includes careful rectal palpation, endoscopy, and systematic search for pararectal metastatic lymph nodes in cases of low-lying tumor. Computed tomography is useful only in cases of extensive transmural penetration (Nicholls et al., 1982). Double contrast barium enema study, level of plasma carcinoembryonic antigen (CEA), and abdominal and liver CT scans are used in order to exclude from preoperative irradiation tumors that have a high probability of having extrapelvic or distant metastases or multicentric cancers.

When the protocol of irradiation is carefully

Table 19–2. **METHODS OF PREOPERATIVE IRRADIATION OF RECTAL CANCER**

Dosage in Rads	No. of Fractions	No. of Days	Target-Volume	Time of Surgery (days)	Institutions
Low					
500	1	1	pelvis	next day	Princess Margaret Hospital (Toronto) Medical Research Council (MRC) (England)
Moderate					
2,000	8	10	pelvis	0–10	Memorial Sloan Kettering Cancer Center (N.Y.) MRC (England)
2,000–2,500	10	12	pelvis	0–10	Vasag
2,400	3	3	pelvis	10–15	Cleveland Clinic
3,000	10	12	tumor area	50	Centre Léon Bérard (Lyon)
3,150	18	24	pelvis	21	Vasag
3,450	15	18	pelvis → L2	15	Radiotherapeutisch Institut (Rotterdam)
3,450	15	19	pelvis → L2	21	European Organization on Research and Treatment of Cancer
3,600	15	18	pelvis	15	Toulouse (France)
4,000	18	21	pelvis	0–10	Montpellier (France)
High					
4,500	23–25	31–33	pelvis	28	Yale University Massachusetts General Hospital
5,500	25–30	33–40	tumor area	28–50	Oregon University

planned, with close collaboration between surgeon and radiotherapist, there should be no problems at the time of surgery and no increase in postoperative morbidity. The following protocols are used at the Centre Léon Bérard (Lyon).

Protocol of Preoperative Irradiation

The technique of irradiation varies according to the site of the cancer. When the tumor is more than 5 cm from the anal verge, irradiation is directed to the posterior part of the pelvis from the supra-anal area to L5. A tumor-dosage of 3000 rad, calculated at 8-cm depth, is delivered in 10 fractions within 12 days by cobalt-60 (^{60}Co) 120 degree arctherapy through a posterior field measuring 10 by 14 cm. The patient is in the prone position (Fig. 19–1).

When the tumor is less than 5 cm from the anal verge, the target-volume encompasses the posterior part of the pelvis and the perineal area. A tumor-dosage of 3000 rad is delivered in 10 fractions over 12 days. Two fixed fields are used: Through a perineal field, a dose of 1500 rad calculated at 6-cm depth is delivered, and through a sacral field with a 45-degree wedge filter, a dose of 1500 rad, calculated at 8-cm depth, is given. The dose at the surface of the perineum does not exceed 2200 rad.

Surgery takes place 7 to 8 weeks after completion of irradiation, and there is no delay in perineal wound healing attributable to radiotherapy. In our own series of 40 cases, not yet published, there was no regrowth of the tumor during the 2 months following such irradiation.

Postoperative Irradiation

Advantages of postoperative irradiation over preoperative irradiation are that (1) it is easier to select cases suitable for combined treatment; (2) pathologic study and grading of the tumor is facilitated; (3) there is better definition of treatment volumes.

Usually a depth dosage of 4500 rad is delivered to the posterior part of the pelvis and to the perineum over 5 to 7 weeks, utilizing posterior and lateral fields or two parallel opposed AP-PA fields. A booster dose of up to 5500 rad can be given to areas suspected of having residual disease. Gunderson and associates (1976), Romsdahl and Withers (1978), Zucali and co-workers (1980), and Turner and associates (1977) have reported preliminary results of trials showing a decrease of recurrence rates at 2 or 3 years in series of patients

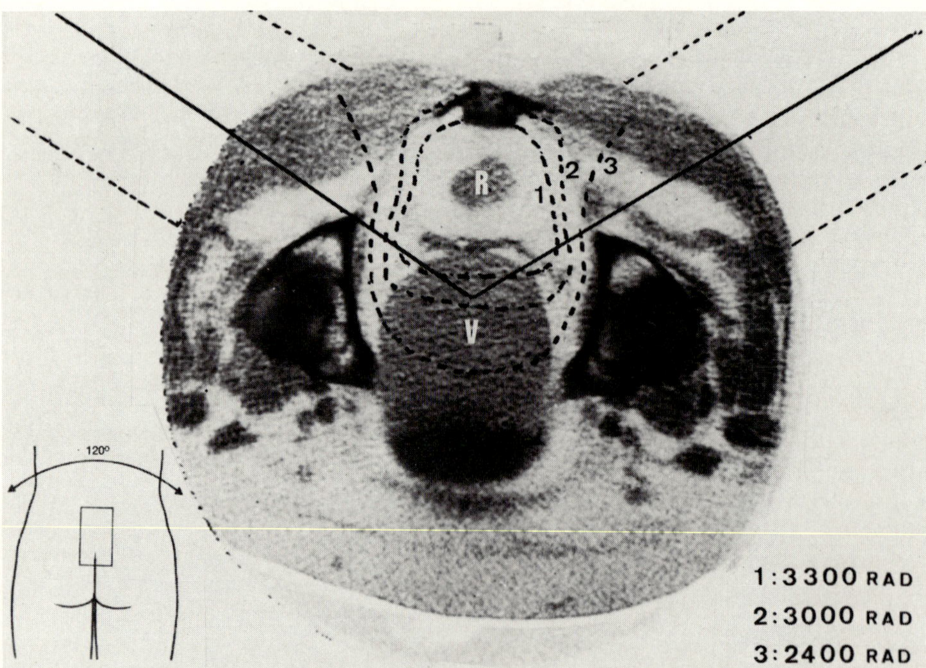

Figure 19–1. Isodose distribution of preoperative irradiation using cobalt-60 (^{60}Co) for cancer of the middle third of the rectum. The lower end of the tumor is more than 5 cm above the anal verge and the patient is in the prone position. Radiation is delivered through a 10 x 14 cm sacral field using ^{60}Co arc therapy 120 degrees. The axis of rotation is 10 cm depth. A dose of 3000 rad calculated at a 8-cm depth is delivered in ten fractions over 12 days. The 80 percent isodose curve encompasses the periorectal area and most lymphatic drainage areas.

treated with radiation postoperatively as compared with series of patients treated by surgery alone.

One of the most interesting randomized trials was conducted by the Gastro-Intestinal Tumor Study Group (GITSG) (Thomas et al., 1982). This trial started in August 1975. It compared the effects of postoperative radiotherapy with and without adjuvant chemotherapy (5-FU and MeCCNu) with the effects of adjuvant postoperative chemotherapy (5-FU and MeCCNu) alone, and with the effects of surgery alone. Two-year results of this trial showed a decrease in recurrence rates for those treated with a combination of modalities compared with those treated by surgery alone. With median follow-up of 11.8 months, the difference in recurrence rates between the surgery-only group and the other treatment groups was statistically significant (p = 0.05). The difference was highly significant between the surgery-only group and the radiotherapy-chemotherapy group (p = 0.001)—a 19 per cent versus a 3 per cent local recurrence rate. The improvement shown by those treated with adjuvant therapy was so striking that GITSG terminated patient entry into the surgery-only arm in February 1980.

The conclusion that radiation used adjuvantly has a positive effect on patient outcome has been drawn from studies by the Radiation Therapy Oncology Group (RTOG) (Davis, 1982) and by Mohiuddin and associates (1981). Both groups used the *"sandwich technique,"* with or without cytotoxic drugs. In this technique, a single exposure of 500 rad is given preoperatively followed by surgery within 24 hours and postoperative irradiation (4500 rad in 5 weeks) for Dukes' B and C tumors. However, a longer follow-up is needed to determine if the improvement due to postoperative irradiation will hold up and if the efficacy of postoperative irradiation is comparable to that of preoperative irradiation. The following protocol of postoperative irradiation is used at the Centre Léon Bérard (Lyon).

Protocol of Postoperative Irradiation

For patients who have undergone an abdominoperineal resection, the irradiation therapy should be conducted as follows:

The aim is to deliver a dosage of 3500 rad in 15 fractions over 19 days to a target-volume encompassing the perineal area and the posterior part of the pelvis, with satisfactory protection of small bowel and urinary bladder. Two fields are used: Through a perineal field, a "given dose" of 3600 rad (at the surface) is delivered in nine fractions; the cobalt beam is inclined 10 degrees downwards on the horizontal line. Through a sacral field with a 45-degree wedge filter, a dose of 2000 rad is delivered in six fractions. The isodose curve (Papillon, 1982) shows that a homogeneous dose is delivered to the whole target-volume and only a small dose to the small bowel in the pelvis. The tolerance to the radiation by the patient is quite good.

Preoperative versus Postoperative Irradiation

At the moment, some physicians favor preoperative irradiation as an additive therapy to surgery for rectal cancer, whereas others favor postoperative irradiation. Both have advantages and disadvantages. Gunderson et al. (1976) stressed that "theoretical considerations favoring preoperative therapy are that there would be less likelihood of dissemination of viable tumor at the time of surgery and that tumor cells are more likely to be better vascularized than in the postoperative state and, therefore, would require less dosage for similar results. Postoperative therapy offers greater flexibility for the type of operation and the extent of disease established by the surgeon and pathologist."

I have emphasized that careful pretreatment evaluation can define rather accurately the indications for preoperative irradiation. This method has demonstrated its efficacy by a decrease of local recurrences. Study of operative specimens after preoperative irradiation and delayed surgery gives an interesting idea of the differences of responsiveness of the tumor to radiotherapy, which can hardly be foreseen.

In the case of postoperative irradiation, small bowel complications may occur if the bowel is fixed with adhesions in the pelvis. At times, owing to the late healing of the perineal wound or the late recovery of the patient, irradiation is started only 2 months after surgery. So far, an increase in the 5-year survival rate after postoperative irradiation has not been widely demonstrated, and randomized trials comparing the results of preoperative irradiation with those of postoperative irradiation would be informative.

For all these reasons and because of its three purposes, I favor the use of preoperative irradiation. However, it requires teamwork, with close collaboration between surgeon and radiotherapist, whereas for postoperative irradiation, the decision to refer the patient to the radiotherapist is made by the surgeon alone after surgery and pathologic study of the specimen.

Improvement of Resectability

It has been demonstrated that radiation therapy applied to clinically inoperable or borderline resectable tumors may render some of them suitable for resection and, in some instances, permit cure in a previously incurable situation.

Stevens and co-workers (1976) reported on 17 of 46 patients with initially unresectable tumor who underwent resection of the tumor within 10 weeks of completion of irradiation at a tumor-dose of 5000 rad. Two of the patients were alive and well at 5 and 10 years. Two died without tumor at 14 and 19 months.

Kligerman (1977) reported on a series of 43 patients with inoperable tumor. Thirteen were suitable for exploration after irradiation. Nine patients underwent resection, although four of them had undergone exploration previously and were found to have unresectable tumor. Three patients were alive free of disease from 2 to 7 years.

Other cases of tumors that were considered unresectable but that could be resected after irradiation have been reported by Emani and associates (26 out of 44) in 1979 and by Overgaard and associates (three out of 15) in 1982. The main criticism that can be made of these series is that there was a lack of consistency concerning the clinical definition of unresectability.

However, these data show that radiotherapy may convert unresectable cases into resectable cases, and some patients with very advanced local disease in the pelvis may respond so favorably to radiation that they have a chance of cure after further intensive irradiation. In such cases, a combination of radiotherapy and chemotherapy (5-FU and MeCCNu) may be used to reinforce the efficacy of treatment (Boulis-Wassif, 1982).

Enlargement of the Field of Conservative and Sphincter-Saving Treatments

In the determination of the efficacy of preoperative irradiation, two points, not commonly stressed, must be emphasized:

1. In several series (Stevens et al., 1976; Kligerman, 1977; Roe et al., 1982), the occurrence of Dukes' A tumors is significantly greater after preoperative irradiation (27 to 45 percent) than after surgery (15 to 25 percent). This indicates that some tumors that had involved the perirectal fat, shrunk in such a manner that they became confined to the rectal wall.

2. Some tumors may be controlled by external beam irradiation alone. It has been reported that, after preoperative irradiation, when the operation has not taken place "too early," some operative specimens are free of tumor cells, the lesion being totally sterilized (Williams and Horwitz, 1956; Wang and Schultz, 1962; Stevens et al., 1976; Bugat et al., 1981; Roe et al., 1982; Boulis-Wassif, 1982; Sischy, 1982). In our own series, which is not yet published, in eight cases out of 40, the operative specimen was tumor-free and theoretically the abdominoperineal resection could have been avoided.

Such examples may indicate that major surgery can be prevented in some instances or that a restorative operation should sometimes be performed instead of a radical excision. This problem is a new advance in the framework of preoperative irradiation.

At the time of diagnosis, most patients present with large, infiltrating, well- or moderately differentiated adenocarcinoma with impaired mobility. Clinical examination indicates that these tumors have moderate or extensive extrarectal spread (Nicholls et al., 1982). The incidence of metastatic lymph nodes is high and patients with these tumors should have major surgery, preferably with adjuvant irradiation. On the other hand, some patients (10 to 15 percent) present with small tumors, less than 4.5 cm in diameter, that are freely mobile and considered to be confined to the bowel wall. These tumors are suitable for conservative treatment.

Between both these groups are tumors 4 to 6 cm in diameter that are mobile, and too large and too thick to be suitable for conservative treatment but whose clinical staging indicates that they have slight extrarectal spread or are still confined to the bowel wall. In such cases, the probability of lymphatic spread is less than 20 percent. After carefully planned external beam irradiation (3000 rad in 12 days concentrated to the tumor area), the shrinkage that is apparent 7 weeks later may be so significant that the prospect of abdominoperineal resection is abandoned in favor of a conservative procedure (interstitial curietherapy or electrocoagulation in elderly patients unfit for surgery and a low anterior resection in younger patients if the tumor is located in the middle rectum). At the Centre Léon Bérard (1979 to 1982) 27 patients with well-differentiated adenocarcinoma that was not deeply infiltrating were studied. The tumor became amenable to a conservative treatment in 25 of these poor-risk patients (median age 77 years), and in two cases it was treated using a sphincter-saving operation.

In these cases, external beam irradiation was used to convert tumors initially suitable only for major surgery into lesions suitable for a conservative procedure. The preliminary results of such policy are encouraging. They warrant this new approach, which supports a plea in favor of preoperative irradiation, whose range is larger than usually thought acceptable and whose technique should be adapted for this purpose.

Definitive Irradiation as a Conservative Procedure

Substantial progress has been made in the detection of rectal cancer at an early stage, and it is now admitted that small tumors can be treated without radical surgery. When conservative treatment is considered, two conditions must be met: There must be proper selection and there must be good follow-up.

Selection

Local treatment involves the rectal tumor and a limited margin of surrounding tissues but does not concern the lymphatic chains. The principal objection made to local treatment concerns the supposed inability to clinically determine the presence or absence of metastatic nodes. Accordingly, conservative treatment should only be applied to tumors that are thought to have no lymphatic spread. Concerning the probability of lymph node involvement, three criteria must be considered:

Histologic Grading. Only well- and moderately well-differentiated adenocarcinomas should be accepted for conservative treatment. Anaplastic and colloid carcinomas must be excluded because of their high rate of lymphatic dissemination.

Local Spread. Morson (1966) has shown that there is a close relationship between local spread and lymphatic spread, with tumors confined to the bowel wall, which have low probability of lymph node involvement (6 to 12 percent) in the first category and tumors with extrarectal spread, which have a 50 percent chance of lymphatic spread in the latter (Fig. 19–2). Only tumors confined to the rectal wall may be treated conservatively. Configuration, consistency, and mobility of the tumor are reliable means of assessing the degree of infiltration of the tumor in the rectal wall.

The ability to stage rectal cancer clinically has long been questioned. Nicholls and associates (1982) compared clinical and pathologic findings and demonstrated that growths confined to the bowel wall are correctly identified by the clinician in 80 percent of cases.

Radiation response can help the radiotherapist to define with great accuracy the degree of infiltration of the rectal wall. The "third-week test" consists of comparing the appearance of the ulcerative lesions on the first day with their appearance on the 21st day after two applications of contact x-ray therapy (on days 1 and 8). On the 21st day it is easy to distinguish tumors that remain hard and deeply ulcerative from tumors that have shrunk significantly. The former have a transmural pen-

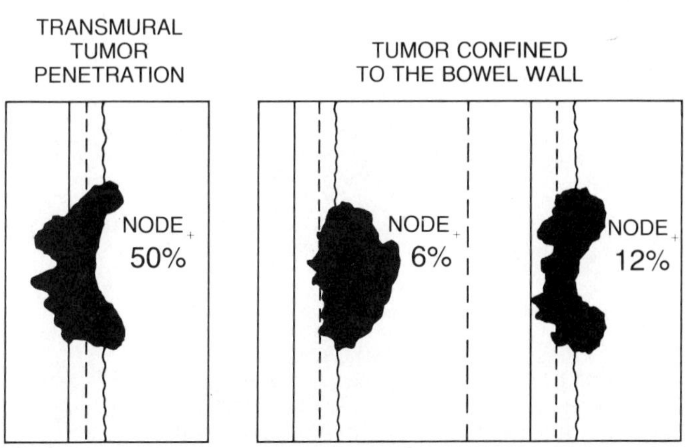

Figure 19–2. The probability of lymphatic spread is related to the local spread of rectal cancer. Tumors that have spread beyond the rectal wall have a high rate of lymph node involvement (50 percent), whereas well-differentiated adenocarcinomas confined to the rectal wall have a much lower risk of lymphatic spread (6 percent in cases of polypoid tumor, 12 percent in cases of ulcerative tumor).

etration and must be treated by major surgery. The latter are surely confined to the bowel wall and are suitable for conservative treatment.

Absence of Palpable Metastatic Nodes in the Mesorectum. In the case of tumor located in the lower rectum, systematic search for metastatic nodules in the rectal wall above the primary tumor is a very important way of approaching the problem of lymphatic dissemination. In a series of 154 patients with low-lying tumor seen since 1965, in 17 cases, hard nodules were discovered. In all these cases, the operative specimen confirmed the metastatic nature of the nodes (Fig. 19–3).

In the selection of patients, the most suitable for local treatment are elderly, frail or poor-risk patients; however, middle-aged and even young patients may also be treated in this way.

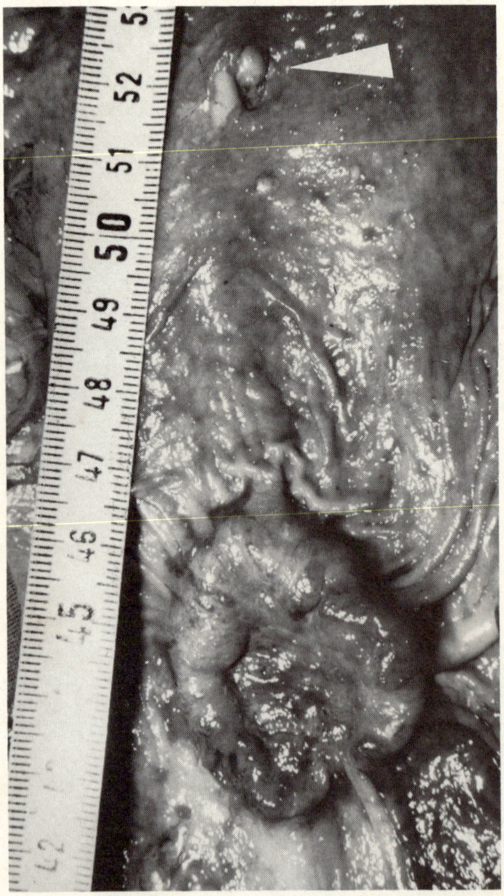

Figure 19–3. Operative specimen of a 50-year-old female patient referred for intracavitary irradiation of this limited, ulcerative, well-differentiated adenocarcinoma (2.8 cm in diameter). Rectal digital examination showed a small nodule in the mesorectum. The patient was not irradiated and underwent an anteroposterior resection. The arrowhead shows the metastatic node discovered by palpation (after incision of the mucosa).

Follow-Up

Conservative treatment requires regular follow-up after control of the rectal tumor to detect local and nodal treatment failures. Besides general and clinical examinations, cytologic examination of scrape smears taken from the treated area as well as digital examination for the search for pararectal metastatic nodes in the case of low-lying tumor may be helpful.

Although most patients treated conservatively are elderly, some are middle aged and robust. In such cases, a laparotomy with *inferior mesenteric and perirectal lymphadenectomy* may be considered and carried out 2 months after completion of conservative treatment. This operation, developed by Mayer and associates (1982), may be compared with neck dissection for carcinoma of the tongue or pelvic lymphadenectomy for carcinoma of the uterine cervix. It is an answer to the criticism made of local treatment, which itself does not involve the lymphatic drainage areas.

Surgical Technique

Through a midline incision, the liver is examined and the paraortic and common external iliac nodes are palpated to check that the tumor has not spread throughout the abdomen. Then the sigmoid colon is freed from its congenital adhesions to the peritoneum in the left iliac fossa. Left and right ureters are identified at the level of the iliac arteries. The posterior parietal peritoneum is incised above and below the origin of the inferior mesenteric artery. The incision follows the right side of the rectum and crosses in front of the rectum, entering the pouch of Douglas before continuing along the left side of the rectum up to the origins of the sigmoid arteries. Inferior mesenteric nodes are resected after the artery is isolated at its origin. The dissection is extended along the artery up to the trunk of the sigmoid artery. Sigmoid nodes are excised, and if there is any suspicion about their nature, they are sent for a frozen section examination. The dissection of the mesorectum is then undertaken. The operator enters the retrorectal space with his right hand. The posterior surface of the rectum is freed from the sacrum down to the levator ani muscles. The lateral ligaments of the rectum are stretched and the superior hemorrhoidal pedicle is isolated at its origin and held in a ligature.

With his left hand, the operator pulls the pedicle above and to the left while the assistant, with his right hand, pushes the rectosigmoid colon anteriorly and to the left. A good exposure of the mesorectum is obtained. The bifurcation of the superior hemorrhoidal artery is identified, and the principal nodes are excised and sent for a frozen section examination. The dissection is continued along the right branch of the left superior hemorrhoidal artery up to its entry into the muscular layer of the rectal wall, and any lymphatic tissue is excised. This dissection, which exposes the posterior and lateral sides of the rectum, with minimal blood loss, permits excision of the (Gerota) anorectal lymph nodes. Ligation of one of the branches of the superior hemorrhoidal artery may be necessary if its termination is surrounded by fibrotic tissue. At times, the nodes may be adherent to the rectal wall, which is repaired with silk thread. Then the middle hemorrhoidal pedicles are sectioned near their points of origin, and tissues bearing lymph nodes are excised up to the rectal wall. The next stage of the operation is the excision of the posterior obturator lymph nodes situated at the bifurcation of the primitive iliac artery. A suction drain is put in the posterior rectal space and brought out through the left and right iliac fossae. The pelvic and parietal peritoneum is sutured, and the abdomen is closed.

After surgery, recovery is rapid and in a series of 30 patients, who underwent this operation at the Centre Léon Bérard since 1970, no complications were recorded.

If pathologic study of the specimen does not show any metastatic nodes, the patient is followed as usual. If one or several nodes are found involved, radical surgery should be carried out, since it represents the most reliable procedure.

Intracavitary Irradiation

In the control of limited rectal cancers, external beam irradiation is much less efficient than intracavitary irradiation, which comprises two modalities: contact x-ray therapy and interstitial curietherapy.

Contact X-Ray Therapy

Contact x-ray therapy is the principal method that uses the Philips RT 50 unit. The x-ray tube is light and easily held in the right hand of the operator. The tip of the x-ray tube is inserted in a special rectoscope held by the left hand. The characteristics of the tube are as follows: low voltage (50 kV), short focal distance (4 cm), high-dose rate (2000 rad per min in air, with a filter of 0.5 mm Al), and substantial absorption of the x-ray beam (90 percent) in the first 2 cm. The field of irradiation is circular and is 3 cm in diameter. Two overlapping fields can be used, one upper and one lower for tumors larger than 3 cm. A small number (4 to 5) of short applications (2 to 4 min) are given over a period of 6 weeks. The treatment is carried out in the out-patient department and is compatible with normal active life. It is easily applicable to elderly, frail, or handicapped patients (Fig. 19–4).

The high exposure dose given at every application (2500 to 4000 rad) produces rapid shrinkage of the exophytic part of the lesion. Hence, at the second (eighth day) and third applications (21st day), the tumor has a greatly

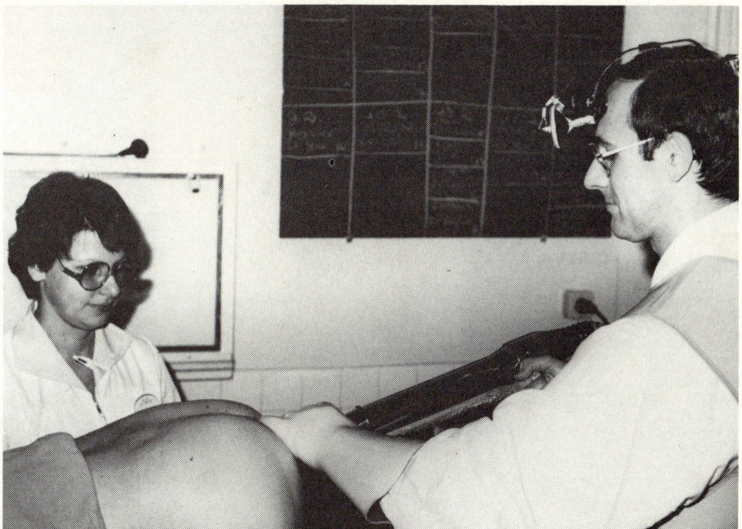

Figure 19–4. Application of contact x-ray therapy with the Philips RT 50 machine. During treatment the operator wears a forehead lamp, a leaded rubber apron, and a leaded rubber glove on the left hand. The x-ray tube held by the right hand is fitted in the treatment applicator, which is firmly held by the left hand.

reduced size. The dose per application, the size of the field, and the intervals between each application are calculated according to the speed of shrinkage of the tumor. The total exposure dose is between 10000 and 14000 rad.

Interstitial Curietherapy

Interstitial curietherapy is used only as a supplementary method to give a booster dose of radiation to the bed of the tumor when the cancer is ulcerative or slightly infiltrating. The patient undergoes this therapy 4 to 6 weeks after completion of contact x-ray therapy. The material used is a rigid steel fork, with two straight hollow prongs preloaded with two iridium wires 4 cm long. For the insertion of the radioactive implant, the unanesthetized patient is placed in the knee-chest position. The implant should deliver a dose of 2000 to 4000 rad. The implant should not remain in place longer than 36 hours. The iridium-192 (^{192}Ir) implant increases the chance of local control of the cancer and is used in 40 percent of cases (Fig. 19–5).

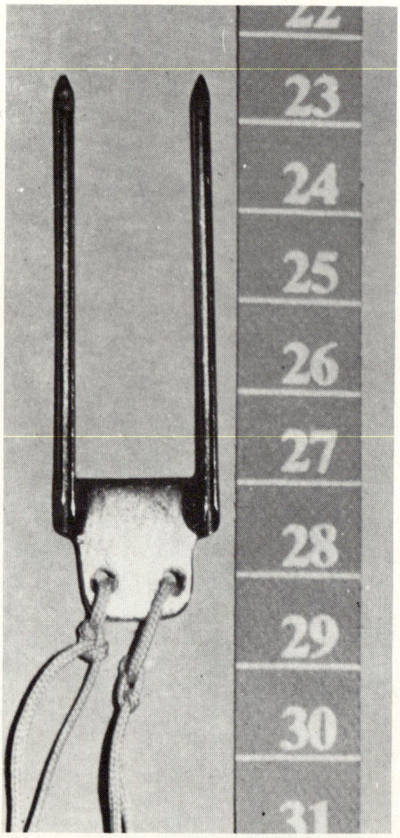

Figure 19–5. Steel fork with two hollow prongs 16 mm apart used for iridium-192 (^{192}Ir) implant of a slightly infiltrating rectal adenocarcinoma. Each prong is preloaded with an iridium wire 4 cm long. The insertion of the fork in the rectal wall is carried out 1.5 months after completion of contact x-ray therapy.

Results

Both these methods of treatment are simple and easily carried out. As long as the technique is correct, there is almost no morbidity except for the occurrence of mild rectitis a few weeks after the last treatment (Fig. 19–6).

Three hundred and ten patients were treated by intracavitary irradiation at the Centre Léon Bérard; 231 were followed more than 5 years; 177 were followed more than 10 years. The results of the treatment are reported in Tables 19–3 to 19–5.

All patients treated had invasive, well-dif-

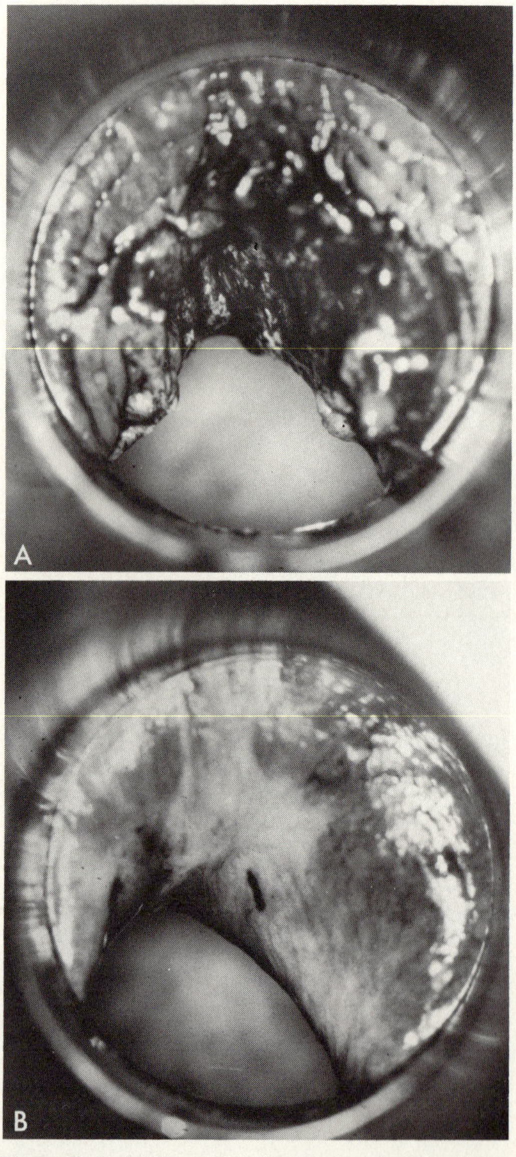

Figure 19–6. *A,* Ulcerative adenocarcinoma of the rectum, 3 cm in diameter, before treatment. *B,* The same case after four applications of contact x-ray therapy (total exposure 11,000 rad). The patient is alive and well 11 years after treatment.

Table 19–3. **RESULTS AT 5 YEARS FOLLOWING INTRACAVITARY IRRADIATION FOR RECTAL CARCINOMA, 1951–1977**

No. of Cases	Alive and Well	Intercurrent Disease	Death Rate Postoperative	Cancer
231	171* (74%)	14%	2%	10%

*Ten after surgery (seven abdominoperineal resections, one anterior resection, two lymphadenectomies).

Table 19–4. **FAILURES FOLLOWING INTRACAVITARY IRRADIATION OF RECTAL CANCER**

	No. of Cases*	Alive and Well
Local failures	12 (5.2%)	3
Nodal failures	12 (5.2%)	3†

*231 cases followed more than 5 years.
†One after abdominoperineal resection; two after lymphadenectomy (without colostomy).

ferentiated or moderately well-differentiated adenocarcinoma. Excluded from this therapy were patients with carcinomas in situ, degenerated villous tumors, and cancers in polyps. There were no patients lost to follow-up. The rate of death from cancer was 10 percent at 5 and 10 years follow-up. Among the group of 171 patients alive and well at 5 year follow-up, ten underwent life-saving surgery (seven abdominoperineal resections, one anterior resection, two lymphadenectomies). The results obtained in trials by Sischy (Rochester, N.Y.) (1982) and Jelden (Cleveland) (1981) were similar.

Indications

Intracavitary irradiation has proved its ability to control most limited, well-differentiated rectal adenocarcinomas that are not greater than 4.5 cm in length and 3 cm in width and that are accessible. Polypoid carcinomas located up to 12 cm above the anal verge can be treated, whereas ulcerative carcinomas should be palpable, i.e., located in the distal 9 cm above the anal verge (Fig. 19–7).

When comparing surgical procedures (excision, electrocoagulation) with intracavitary irradiation for the treatment of limited rectal cancers, certain advantages of irradiation become apparent:

1. Treatment is ambulatory.
2. There is no danger of rectovaginal fistula.
3. There is a lower rate of local failure.
4. It is well tolerated even by the senile and other poor-risk patients.

It has been emphasized that intracavitary irradiation as well as other methods of local treatment are only applicable to strictly selected cases, representing 10 to 15 percent of all patients with rectal cancer.

For example, elderly and frail patients with tumor primarily considered to be unsuitable for local treatment or a borderline indication for local treatment might be able to undergo conservative treatment after external beam irradiation. This new approach combining external beam and intracavitary irradiation in order to increase the field of conservative treatment deserves special attention (Fig. 19–8).

To summarize, intracavitary irradiation must be conceived as a modality requiring teamwork between radiotherapist and surgeon. The radiotherapist must be fully aware of the responsibility he is taking in starting the treatment and must keep in mind that patients who undergo a local treatment could have been cured by radical surgery.

Palliative Treatment

Radiotherapy of Inoperable Rectal Cancers

Patients who are considered inoperable have tumors that are bulky, deeply infiltrating, and fixed to the pelvic wall or pelvic structures, with or without distant metastasis. These pa-

Table 19–5. **RESULTS AT 10 YEARS FOLLOWING INTRACAVITARY IRRADIATION FOR RECTAL CANCER, 1951–1972**

No. of Cases	Alive and Well	Intercurrent Disease	Death Rate Postoperative	Cancer
177	101 (57%)	30%	2.2%	10%

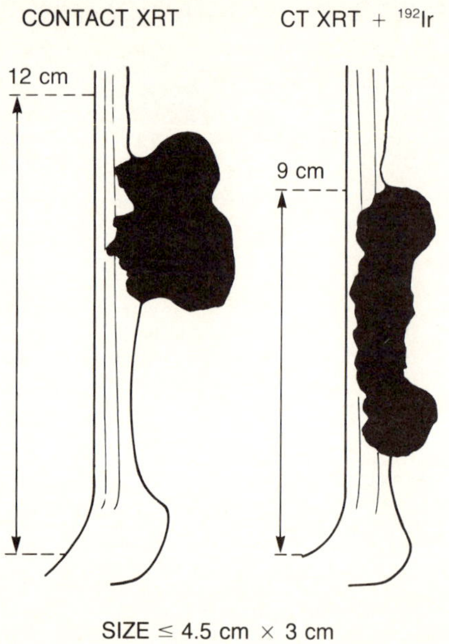

Figure 19–7. Well-differentiated polypoid adenocarcinomas up to 12 cm from the anal verge are suitable for contact x-ray therapy. Ulcerative carcinomas of the lower two thirds of the rectum are suitable for conservative treatment by contact x-ray therapy and ^{192}Ir implant, so long as they are confined to the bowel wall (third-week test) and the size of the tumor does not exceed 4.5 × 3 cm.

tients may be in good or poor condition. They are not considered suitable for surgery with curative intent.

The principal role of irradiation is to relieve the most distressing symptoms, such as bleeding, discharge, tenesmus, troubles of defecation, pain, and pressure symptoms (hydronephrosis). An other objective of irradiation is to delay or avoid colostomy.

The radiation dosage commonly used is 4500 to 5000 rad in 4.5 to 5 weeks, delivered to a target-volume that encompasses the tumor and a large part of the posterior pelvic cavity, but not systematically the entire pelvic area. An equivalent dosage (3000 rad in 12 days) may also be given with the same chance of effectiveness. For incurable patients, this latter dosage has a psychologic advantage in that overall treatment time is shorter.

The protocol of irradiation must be adapted to the extent of the disease and to the general condition of the patient. It is recommended that intensive radiation be administered to patients who have inoperable tumor because of disease localized to the true pelvis and that in such cases a protocol similar to that given in preoperative irradiation be used. Lower radiation dosage is used for patients with distant metastasis or poor general condition who have a short life expectancy.

Williams and Horwitz (1956) reported a series of 189 inoperable patients treated by supervoltage irradiation (6000 rad over 6 to 8 weeks). Relief of symptoms was obtained in 76 percent of those with rectal bleeding, 48 percent of those with pain, and 47 percent of those with mucous discharge. Because of this treatment many patients were able to avoid colostomy.

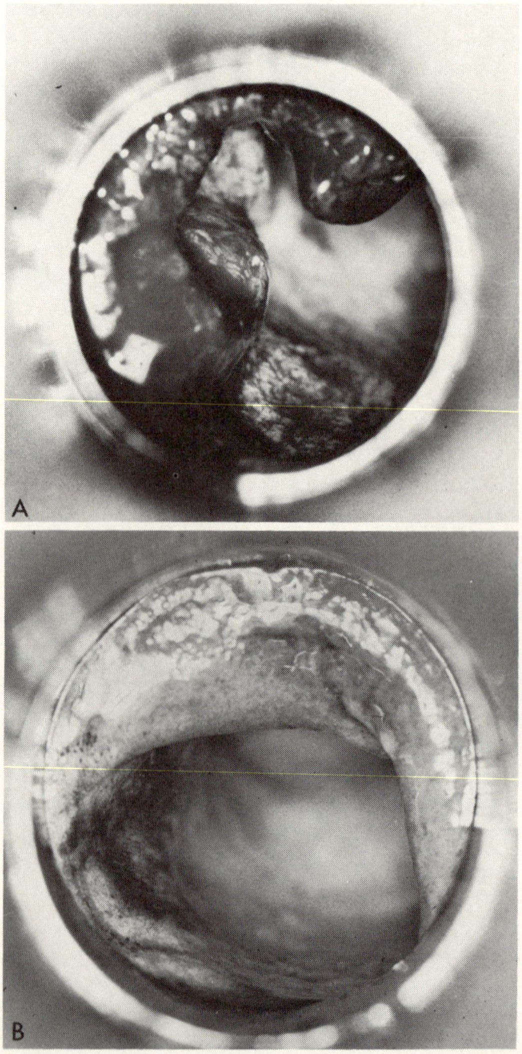

Figure 19–8. *A*, Female patients, age 73 years, with an ulcerative, vegetating rectal adenocarcinoma invading more than half the circumference of the rectal wall. Before treatment, the adenocarcinoma was 5 cm long, too large to be treated by intracavity irradiation. *B*, The same patient after treatment using external beam irradiation by ^{60}Co arc therapy (3000 rad in 10 fractions over 12 days) and a ^{192}Ir implant with template (6 wires 5 cm long); the dose was 3000 rad. The implantation was carried out 2 months after the use of ^{60}Co. The patient is alive and well 2 years after treatment.

Urdaneta-Lafee and associates (1972) reported a series of 43 patients with nonresectable tumor who were irradiated with a dose of 4000 rad. Symptomatic relief was obtained in 80 percent of the patients. Colostomy was avoided in 71 percent.

Irradiation of big, very hard, stony masses reveals that these tumors are slightly radiosensitive because of the large amount of anoxic tumor cells. The size of the mass may often not be significantly reduced, but pressure symptoms are relieved. The duration of survival is not substantially increased, but the quality of life is almost always improved.

Radiotherapy of Recurrent Rectal Cancer

The value of radiotherapy in the management of locally recurrent rectal cancer has been substantiated by a number of authors. Treatment failures after abdominoperineal resection are often localized to the pelvis. In female patients, tumor masses are easily palpated, whereas in male patients, pain and pressure symptoms are the only indicators of pelvic recurrence. Pain may be caused by invasion of presacral nerves or branches of the lumbosacral plexus or by involvement of the prostate or pelvic soft tissues. Complete and lasting relief of pain is obtained in one third of patients after radiotherapy. The others have incomplete or transient relief. Irradiation does not alter the duration of survival. The palliative effect shows no definite relationship to the radiation dose, and in all cases, the importance of preventing late radiation complications must be stressed.

Large tumor recurrence in the perineal region may be associated with pelvic treatment failure. A dose of 4500 to 5000 rad should be applied to a target-volume encompassing pelvic and perineal areas. Sometimes, however, the recurrent cancer is made up of only limited tumor and is easily accessible to palpation, especially in female patients. If there is no sign of dissemination, such a lesion may be suitable for intensive irradiation, using either a combination of external beam radiotherapy (perineal field) and interstitial curietherapy or electron beam therapy (5000 to 6000 rad). The irradiation is concentrated to the perineal area and aimed at controlling the disease. Some cases of long-term control of perineal treatment failures have been reported.

Treatment failures after anterior resection are often localized to the suture line. They may present as small exophytic lesions involving a limited portion of the anastomotic area. It would be an error to consider such lesions suitable for treatment with conservative procedure because they are always more infiltrating than they may seem. The part of the lesion that is visible in the rectal lumen is only a small portion of the tumor, which extends into the pelvis.

External beam irradiation has usually a purely palliative purpose, except in those rare cases in which an abdominoperineal resection is scheduled and can be associated with preoperative radiotherapy. Radiotherapy is also indicated to relieve pain from hepatic involvement or metastasis to the spine. Priestman (1977) recommended that a dosage of 2500 rad in 2.5 weeks be applied to the liver when manifestations of liver involvement are not controlled by chemotherapy. High-dose irradiation may be of some value in cases of brain or bone metastasis.

Summary

Radiation therapy has gained an important place in the management of rectal cancer, especially as a definitive and adjuvant treatment, and the radiotherapist must be aware of the role he has to play in conjunction with the surgeon.

MANAGEMENT OF EPIDERMOID CARCINOMA OF THE ANAL CANAL

Squamous cell carcinoma of the anal canal has long been overshadowed by cancer of the rectum and treated as a poor relative in the family of tumors of the distal part of the bowel. In many institutions in the United States and in England, squamous cell carcinomas of the anal canal and adenocarcinomas of the lower rectum are still treated by radical surgery, i.e., abdominoperineal resection. In some radiotherapy centers, such as Institute Curie and Institut Gustave Roussy in France, squamous cell carcinomas of the anal canal are still treated by external beam irradiation alone in the same manner as epidermoid carcinomas of the pharyngolarynx: 6000 rad in 6 weeks. The results of such policies are reported in Table 19–6.

In Table 19–6 the striking difference in the 5-year survival rates obtained at the Mayo Clinic and at the Memorial Sloan Kettering Cancer Center (S.K.C.C.) during the period

Table 19–6. EPIDERMOID CARCINOMA OF THE ANAL CANAL: RESULTS OF TRADITIONAL METHODS

Radical Surgery	No. of Cases	5-yr Survival Rate (%)
St Mark's Hospital, London, (1968)	92	48
Mayo Clinic, Rochester (1976)	80	60.7
Memorial SKCC, New York (1944–1963)	109	57
(1963–1970)	65	33
External Beam Irradiation (^{60}Co)		
Institut Curie, Paris, (1979)	128	48
Tumor ≤ 4 cm	57	68
Tumor > 4 cm	71	32
Institut G. Roussy, Villejuif (1979)	109	42
Tumor ≤ 4 cm		62
Tumor > 4 cm		26

from 1963 to 1970 is explained by a larger number of advanced cases in the series of the latter institution. The results of treatment using external beam irradiation have proved to be unsatisfactory for tumors larger than 4 cm, and the rate of radionecrosis, around 20 percent, indicates that this method cannot be considered reliable for the treatment of large tumors.

Both treatment modalities shown in Table 19–6 do not take into consideration the true nature of squamous cell carcinoma of the anal canal, which is a peculiar disease and deserves a specific approach. The most important characteristics of this disease are as follows:

1. It is possible to assess the extent of the primary tumor and of the lymphatic spread in the pelvis with great accuracy, since most metastatic nodes are palpable as long as rectal digital examination is performed carefully and methodically, with the patient in the knee-chest position. This accessibility also makes the use of interstitial curietherapy possible.

2. Carcinomas of the anal canal are more radiosensitive than is generally realized. This quality is true not only of the primary tumor but also of the metastatic nodes. The pace of shrinkage, however, is particularly slow, and optimum effect of irradiation is not obtained until 2 months after the last application.

3. Radionecrosis is one of the well-known complications of irradiation of tumors of the anal area, and there is a narrow margin between local treatment failures due to underdosage and severe radionecroses due to overdosage.

4. Pelvic metastatic lymph nodes located either in the pararectal area (visceral route) or along the pelvic wall (parietal route) are common even at an early stage of the disease, and this must be taken into account in all treatment planning. No local procedure, such as local excision or irradiation of the anal area alone, should be attempted.

During the past 10 years, two new therapeutic approaches have been defined. Both give a prominent place to radiotherapy and aim at increasing the chance of control of the disease for patients with large tumor and avoiding the necessity of a permanent colostomy. These two treatments are as follows: (1) preoperative irradiation with or without chemotherapy, which has been initiated in the United States and in France, and (2) split-course irradiation, which has been especially developed in Lyon.

Preoperative Irradiation with or without Chemotherapy

In 1973, Nigro and associates (1974) published the cases of three patients with primary operable epidermoid carcinoma of the anal canal who were treated by a presurgical approach consisting of external irradiation by ^{60}Co (3000 rad in 3 weeks) and a short course of chemotherapy (5-FU during the first 5 days and mitomycin C during the first day of irradiation). Abdominoperineal resection was performed 6 weeks later in two of the three patients. No tumor was found in the operative specimen. The third patient refused operation and was well some years later.

Using the same protocol Nigro and associates (1981), Newman and Quan (1976), Wanebo and associates (1981), and Bruckner and co-workers (1979) reported a series of patients with significant shrinkage or disappearance of the primary tumor. As a result some of these patients underwent local surgery or no surgery and were therefore spared radical operation.

Loygue and associates (1981) and Parks (1981) suggested that radical surgery alone be abandoned in patients with large tumors in favor of irradiation at a dosage of 4000 rad in 4 weeks. After a delay of 1 to 3 months, the decision was made to perform radical excision in patients with substantial residual tumor or, alternatively, to continue irradiation, up to 6500 rad, in patients in whom there was substantial shrinkage of the lesion. Loygue reported a 50 percent 3-year survival rate for patients with large tumors treated by radiotherapy and surgery and an overall 3-year survival rate of 67 percent.

Experience with Irradiation as a First Approach at the Centre Léon Bérard: Material and Methods

Since 1971, 253 patients have been treated by irradiation as a first approach at the Centre Léon Bérard; 156 have been followed for more than 3 years, 104 for more than 5 years.

The presentation of patients with squamous cell carcinoma of the anal canal differs markedly according to the stage of the disease, the presence or absence of lymphatic spread, and the condition of the patient. It is illogical to deal with so many variables using a single approach—either surgery or external beam irradiation.

Pretreatment Evaluation

To evaluate the limits of the tumor in the circumference of the anus and its upper and lower ends, rectal digital examination must be carried out methodically, with the patient in the lithotomy position and in the knee-chest position. The operator uses the right index finger as well as the left, depending on the site of the lesion. Vaginal digital examination is of great help in defining the upper limit of the tumor and the degree of infiltration of the rectovaginal wall by tumors located in the anterior part of the canal. The lymphatic spread must be assessed not only by palpation of the inguinal areas but also by systematic search for pelvic metastatic nodes in the mesorectum and along the pelvic wall by digital examination. Grossly involved nodes are always indurated and situated a few centimeters above the primary tumor. For this assessment, all patients should be re-examined under general anaesthesia. Lymphangiography is only justified in cases of obvious involvement of inguinal nodes to visualize the external iliac chains. Liver scan and intravenous pyelography are not part of the usual investigation except for advanced cases.

At the Centre Léon Bérard, the following clinical staging has been adopted.

- T1: Tumors less than 2 cm in diameter.
- T2: Tumors between 2 and 4 cm in diameter.
- T3: Tumors larger than 4 cm that are mobile, and that are not infiltrating either the vaginal mucosa or more than two-thirds of the circumference of the anus.
- T4a: Tumors invading the vaginal mucosa or more than two thirds of the circumference.
- T4b: Tumors with extension to neighboring structures other than the skin, rectum, and vaginal mucosa, or tumors fixed to the pelvic wall.

Treatment Policy

Carcinoma of the anal canal can be classified into three groups according to the resectability of the tumor and the possibility of preservation of anal function. Each requires a particular approach. Three protocols have been designed that take into consideration the substantial progress that has been made in the field of irradiation of carcinoma of the anal canal and especially the radiation response of this tumor and the tolerance of perianal structures to radiation. In no case was surgery alone used. Histologic type, i.e., squamous cell or cloacogenic carcinoma, does not affect treatment policy.

Combination of External Irradiation and Iridium Implant in a Split-Course Regimen

The first group is composed of patients with T1, T2, or T3 tumor, whether they are operable or not. Irradiation alone should be suitable treatment for the tumor and should provide the patients with a good chance of controlling the disease, with preservation of anal function. This group represents 75 to 80 percent of cases. This protocol is also applied to patients who have undergone a local excision (Fig. 19–9).

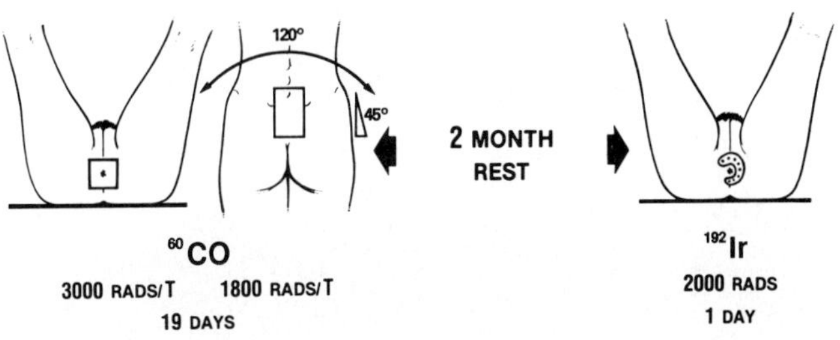

Figure 19–9. Protocol for irradiation for carcinoma of the anal canal suitable for curative and conservative treatment. Split-course irradiation with ^{60}Co and ^{192}Ir with a free interval of two months is adapted to the slow regression rate of this tumor. The moderate dosage of radiation is designed to reduce the incidence of radionecrosis.

The protocol consists of two stages, separated by an interval of 2 months. Cobalt therapy aims to deliver a minimum tumor dosage of 3000 rad in 19 days to a target-volume that encompasses the anal area and main pelvic lymphatic drainage areas, i.e., the most important parts of the presacral and posterior pelvic region. Two fields are used. A dosage of 3000 rad, calculated at 5 cm depth, is delivered through a direct 8 by 8 cm perineal field in 10 fractions over 16 days. The given dose under the skin of the perineum is 4200 rad. This irradiation is performed with the patient in the lithotomy position; the buttocks are taped apart so that the perineum presents as flat as possible. Presacral irradiation with ^{60}Co is applied using arctherapy (120 degrees with a 45-degree wedge filter) through a field 7 by 12 cm, directed to the sacral area, with the patient in the prone position. The lower limit of the field is situated 7 cm above the anal verge. This irradiation gives a depth dose of 1800 rad at 8 cm in six fractions. The overall treatment time is 19 days.

After this first sequence of treatment, there is a two-month rest before insertion of the iridium implant. This long interval is adapted to the slow pace of regression after irradiation of epidermoid carcinoma of the anal canal. The purpose of ^{60}Co is to reduce the size of the tumor to a volume suitable for interstitial curietherapy.

In the second stage, the ^{192}Ir single plane implant delivers a booster dose of 2000 rad to a limited target-volume in that part of the circumference of the anal canal that was involved by tumor before cobalt therapy was started. With the patient under general anesthesia, five to seven wires, usually 5 cm long, are introduced in steel needles inserted through a crescent-shaped plastic template containing a series of holes 1 cm apart. The template is sutured to the perineal skin by four stitches and placed in the quadrants of the anus originally involved by the tumor. The dose is calculated according to the "Paris system" at 85 percent of the basal dose. The implant remains in place from 18 to 28 hours (Figs. 19–10 to 19–12).

The immediate and late tolerance of patients to this schedule is quite good, with a low rate of necrosis; there is no fibrosis of the perianal area and there are no problems if subsequent surgery is required.

Preoperative Irradiation and Chemotherapy (5-FU and Mitomycin C) Followed by Radical Surgery

Operable patients with T4a tumor or with large T3 tumor associated with large perirectal metastatic nodes are not suitable for curative irradiation with potential preservation of the anal sphincter. They can be treated by abdominoperineal resection but, as it has been demonstrated, the chances of control of the disease

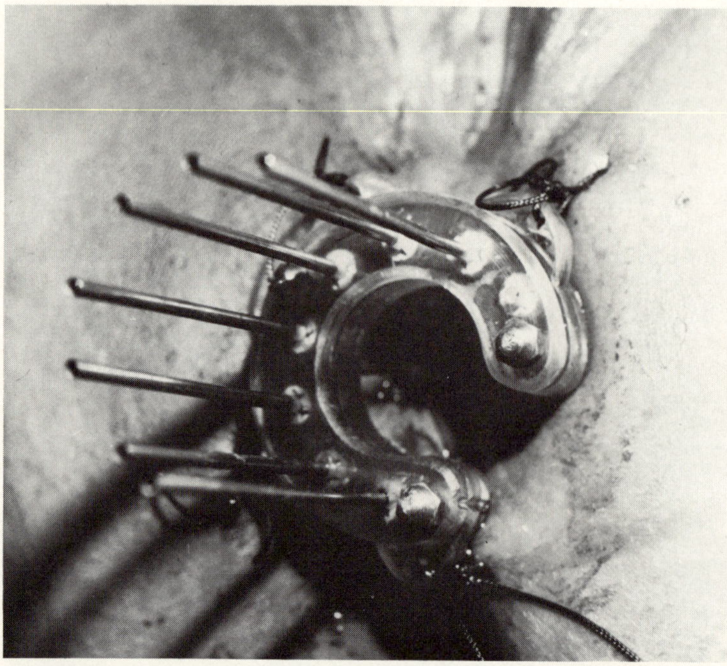

Figure 19–10. One-plane ^{192}Ir implant is carried out 2 months after completion of Cobalt therapy. A plastic template with a series of holes 1 cm apart is sutured to the perianal skin. Steel needles (5 to 7) that will receive the 5-cm long iridium wires are inserted. The dose delivered is 2000 rad.

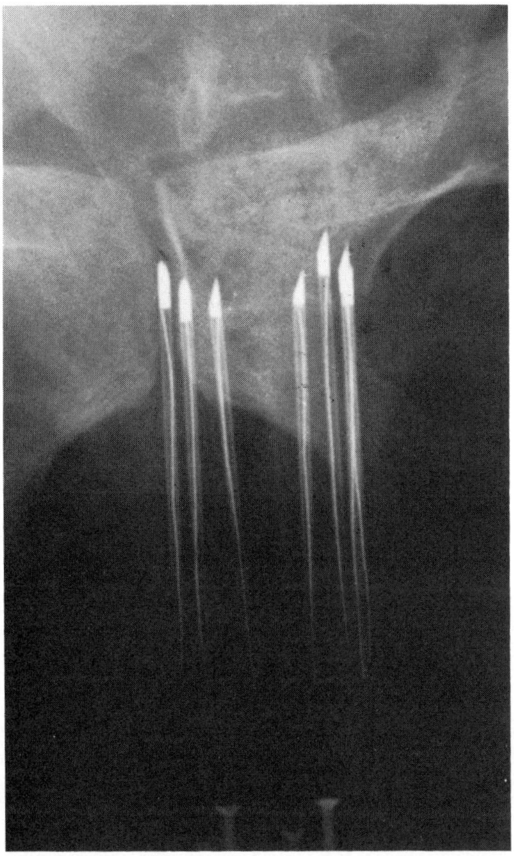

Figure 19–11. X-ray film of a ^{192}Ir implant. Notice the good parallelism of the seven radioactive wires.

are increased by preliminary irradiation with ^{60}Co or 18 MeV x-rays combined with 5-FU and mitomycin C. This group represents approximately 10 percent of cases.

The aim of irradiation is to deliver a dosage of 3000 rad through two portals in ten fractions over 12 days to the anal and presacral areas: (1) a direct perineal field 8 by 8 cm through which a tumor dose of 1500 rad is delivered at a 5 cm depth in five fractions and (2) a direct sacral fixed field, 8 by 14 cm, with a 45-degree wedge filter. A dosage of 1500 rad calculated at an 8 cm depth is given in five fractions. The lower end of this field is 3 cm above the anal verge. Both fields are used alternatively.

The operation must not be carried out before 8 weeks have passed because the best radiobiologic effect is obtained at that time. After surgery, there is no problem in the healing of the perineal wound and there are no complications related to radiotherapy.

To reinforce the efficacy of radiotherapy, a short course of chemotherapy is given during the first 5 days of irradiation (5-FU, 900 mg as a continuous 24-hour infusion for 5 days; and mitomycin C, 18 mg as a single bolus injection on the first day). *The same regimen of chemotherapy may be combined with the first protocol in cases of T3* tumor, when there are no contraindications.

Large-Field Pelvic and Anal Irradiation for Unresectable Tumors

At the time of diagnosis, 15 percent of patients present with very advanced and unresectable tumor. There are lesions that are infiltrating the surrounding structures deeply and are hardly movable or are fixed to the pelvic wall. In most cases, there is large inguinal lymph node involvement as well as pelvic node metastases. Generally, the irradiation has a purely palliative effect. However, high-dose radiation properly applied to well defined target-volumes may result in some long-term survival in spite of the extent of the disease.

Irradiation is carried out with high energy 18 MeV x-rays rather than cobalt. Utilizing

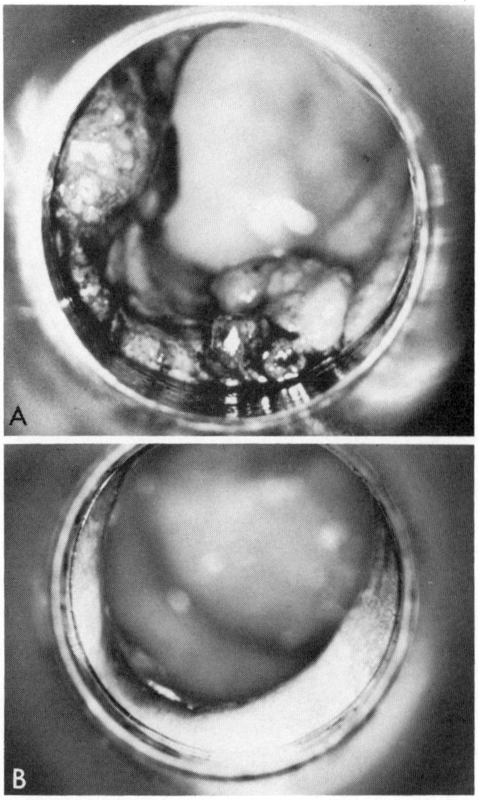

Figure 19–12. Female patient, aged 63 years. *A,* Ulcerative epidermoid carcinoma deeply infiltrating the anorectal junction, before split-course irradiation. *B,* After treatment, anal function is entirely normal. Note the white color of the anal mucosa in the treated area. There is no fibrosis. The patient is alive and well more than 5 years after treatment.

Table 19–7. **EPIDERMOID CARCINOMA OF THE ANAL CANAL***

	At 5 Years Follow-Up		At 3 Years Follow-Up	
	No. of Cases	*5-Year Survival Rate (%)*	*No. of Cases*	*3-Year Survival Rate (%)*
Resectable Tumors	88	62	132	70
Unresectable tumors	16	18	24	17.5

*Data from the Centre Léon Bérard.

two opposed fields, a dose of 4000 rad at the midline is delivered in 4 weeks to the whole pelvis. The anterior field encompasses the inguinal areas. The posterior field encompasses the anal area. This irradiation can also be performed utilizing three fields, one posterior and two lateral, in order to protect the bladder and small bowel and to concentrate the beams on the posterior part of the pelvis. In the latter protocol, inguinal areas are irradiated by electrons, without interference with the pelvic irradiation. Booster doses of up to 5500 rad are given to limited target-volumes such as the anal area (by x-rays or iridium implant) or pelvic mass (by x-rays) or inguinal nodes (by electrons). The overall treatment time is 6 to 7 weeks, with a break after the dose of 4000 rad has been distributed.

A short course of chemotherapy (5-FU and mitomycin C) is usually performed during the first 5 days if the general condition of the patient warrants it.

Results

Since 1971, at the Centre Léon Bérard, 223 patients have been treated with curvative intent either by irradiation alone (first protocol—200 patients), or by preoperative irradiation (second protocol—23 patients), and 30 patients had unresectable tumor and were treated according to the third protocol.

In the group of patients treated with curative intent, the 5-year and 3-year survival rates were 62 percent and 70 percent, respectively (Table 19–7), and the death rate from cancer was 17.5 and 18 percent at 3 and 5 years follow-up. Almost all treatment failures were observed during the first few months following the treatment and before 2-year follow-up. Of the patients alive and well at 3 years, three out of four had normal anal function; one out of four had had a colostomy.

In the group of patients with large, unresectable tumor, four out of 24 were alive and well at 3 years and three out of 16 were tumor-free at 5 years.

These results demonstrate that properly planned irradiation (combined with chemotherapy for large tumors), with or without subsequent surgery, gives the patient a better chance for control of the disease than do either traditional surgical or radiotherapeutic methods and spares many of them a permanent colostomy.

The management of epidermoid carcinoma of the anal canal can be summarized in Figure 19–13 using data from the Centre Léon Bérard.

Management of Lymph Node Metastasis

Treatment of inguinal node metastasis is presented in Figure 19–14.

Presentation		**Modality of Treatment**
Tumors invading less than two thirds of the circumference of the anal canal; mobile; involving neither the vaginal mucosa nor surrounding structures (excluding rectum and skin)	⟶	Irradiation by photons and ^{192}Ir implant in a split-course regimen (with or without 5-FU and mitomycin C)
Tumors invading more than two thirds of the circumference of the anal canal or the vaginal mucosa; or large tumors (one half the circumference), with large but mobile pararectal metastatic nodes in operable cases	⟶	Preoperative radiochemotherapy (5FU and mitomycin C) followed by abdominoperineal resection 8 weeks later
Tumors, invading surrounding structures or with significant metastatic lymph nodes; tumors fixed to the pelvic wall; or disseminated tumors	⟶	External beam irradiation associated with 5FU and mitomycin C

Figure 19–13. Management of epidermoid carcinoma of the anal canal.

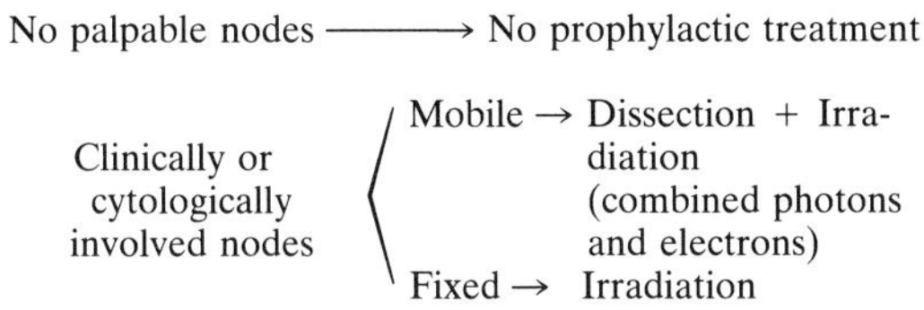

Figure 19–14. Treatment of inguinal node metastasis.

Prophylactic dissection has been generally abandoned, except for patients who cannot be followed regularly (Stearns and Quan, 1970; Wolfe, 1968; Beahrs, 1979). The role of irradiation used postoperatively (4500 rad in 4.5 weeks) or exclusively in fixed nodes (5500 rad) should not be underestimated. In case of operable inguinal involvement, the performance of superficial groin dissection combined with postoperative irradiation is the routine policy. In the statistics of the Centre Léon Bérard, out of 223 patients treated with curative intent, 34 developed either synchronous (19) or metachronous (15) inguinal metastases. Twelve patients (35 percent) died of cancer. Contrary to what is generally believed, the date of appearance of the groin metastasis does not seriously influence prognosis.

Pelvic Lymph Nodes

Pelvic node metastases located either in the pararectal area or along the pelvic wall are common even at an early stage and must be sought by a careful digital examination. They are more radiosensitive than expected and in many cases can be controlled by properly planned irradiation (Fig. 19–15).

In the experience at the Centre Léon Bérard, pelvic nodes considered metastatic were discovered in 66 patients (26 percent of cases); 52 of these patients were treated curatively, and 14 were treated palliatively.

In the group of patients treated with curative intent, and followed more than 2 years, 13 (25 percent) died of cancer, 33 are alive and well (30 without colostomy), three died from intercurrent disease before 5 years, and two died postoperatively.

It is now admitted that pelvic metastatic lymph nodes may be controlled by carefully planned irradiation and that prophylactic treatment of the pelvic lymphatic chains is needed in all cases—even in small early carcinoma of the anal canal without palpable nodes in the pelvis (Fig. 19–16).

Summary

Carcinoma of the anal canal should not be irradiated according to the same guidelines as those applied to most pelvic tumors, such as uterine cervix or bladder cancers (i.e., the use of two opposed AP-PA fields and calculation of the dose at the midline of the pelvis). New protocols of radiotherapy better adapted to the natural history of anal canal cancer are required that are based on the use of specific techniques of radiotherapy. The main characteristics of these protocols are as follows: perineal and sacral fields, split-course regimen, moderate dosage, great care in positioning the patient at each application, and appropriate use of ^{192}Ir implant as a boost to limited target-volumes. The radiotherapist in charge of such a treatment must be fully aware that it is a demanding approach, which requires a perfect definition of target-volumes, dose, and frac-

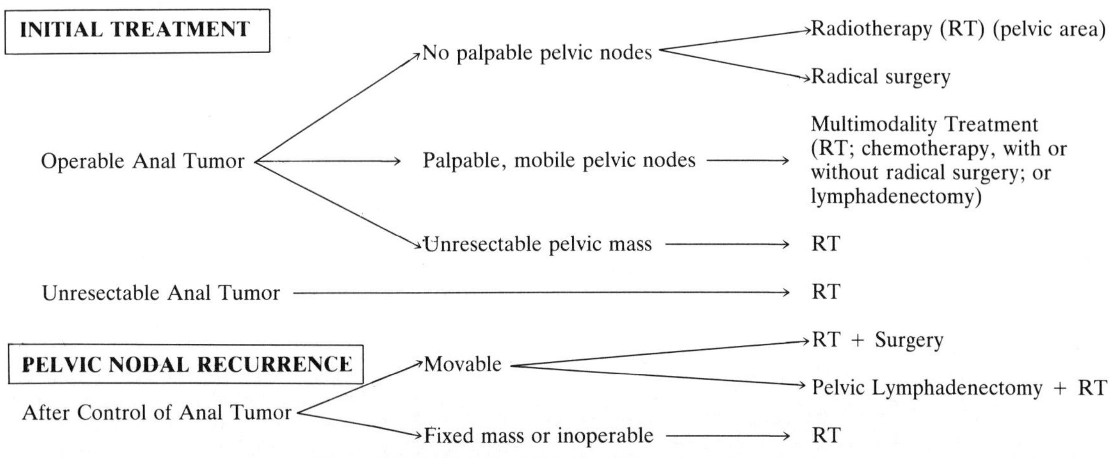

Figure 19–15. Management of pelvic metastatic nodes.

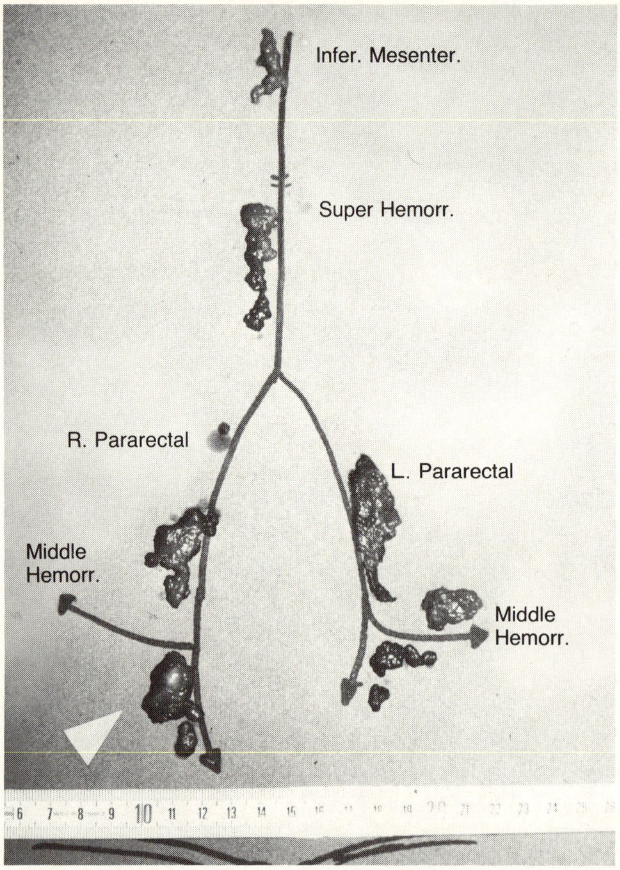

Figure 19–16. Operative specimen of a mesenteric and perirectal lymphadenectomy from a patient treated by split-course irradiation for a carcinoma of the anal canal that was locally controlled. This patient developed a pararectal metastatic node, which was discovered at follow-up examination. The metastatic lymph node is indicated by the arrowhead on the right side. Histopathological examinations of all other lymph nodes removed were negative for cancer. The patient is alive and disease-free 4 years after treatment.

tionation and regular follow-up. Faulty techniques often lead to failure or necrosis. Treatment given along these lines controls resectable tumors in two out of three patients, and 75 percent of those cured do not need a permanent colostomy. Subsequent surgery, if needed, can be carried out without a substantial increase in postoperative morbidity.

Radiation therapy deserves a prominent place in the management of squamous cell carcinoma of the anal canal. Its application requires close collaboration between surgeon and radiotherapist.

References

Beahrs OH: Management of cancer of the anus. AJR 133:791–795, 1979.

Boulis-Wassif S: The role of pre-operative adjuvant therapy in the management of borderline operability rectal cancer. Clin Radiol 33:353–358, 1982.

Bruckner HW, Spigelman MK, Mandel E, et al: Carcinoma of the anus treated with a combination of radiotherapy and chemotherapy. Cancer Treat Rep 63:395–398, 1979.

Bugat R, Nguyen TD, El Safadi N, et al: L'irradiation pré-opératoire des cancers du rectum. A propos d'une série de 96 cas. Bull Cancer (Paris) 68:363, 1981.

Buroker J, Nigro N, Correa J, et al: Combination preoperative irradiation and chemotherapy in adenocarcinoma of the rectum. A preliminary report. Dis Colon Rectum 19:660–663, 1976.

Davies L: personal communication, 1982.

Dukes CE: Cancer of the rectum. Livingstone, Edinburgh, London, 1960.

Emani B, Willet C, Pile Prich M, Miller H: Preoperative radiotherapy of unresectable colorectal carcinoma. Int J Radiat Oncol Biol Phys (Suppl) 6:39, 1979.

Eschwege F, Breteau N, Chavy A, et al: Complications de la radiothérapie trans-cutanée des épithéliomas du canal anal. Gastroentérol Clin Biol (Paris) 3:183–186, 1979.

Gary Bobo J, Pujol J, Solassol C, et al: L'irradiation pré-opératoire du cancer rectal. Résultat à 5 ans de 116 cas. Bull Cancer (Paris) 66:491–496, 1979.

Gunderson L, Sosin H: Areas of failure found at reoperation (second or symptomatic look) following "curative surgery" for adenocarcinoma of the rectum. Cancer 34:1278–1292, 1974.

Gunderson L, Votava C, Brown RC, Plenk HP: Combined treatment with surgery and postoperative irradiation. LDS Hospital experience (Abstr). Int J Radiat Biol (Suppl) 1:64, 1976.

Hardcastle JD, Bussey JR: Results of surgical treatment of squamous cell carcinoma of anal canal and anal margin seen at St. Mark's Hospital. Proc Roy Soc Med 61:629–630, 1968.

Higgins GA, Roswit B: The role of radiotherapy in the surgical treatment of large bowel cancer. Prog Clin Cancer 7:71–81, 1981.

Jelden G, Dhalival R, Lavery I, et al: Definitive treatment of rectal carcinoma with intracavitary irradiation therapy. Int J Radiat Oncol Biol 7:1207, 1981.

Kligerman MM: Radiotherapy and rectal cancer. Cancer 39:896–900, 1977.

Loygue J, Laugier A, Parc R, Weisgerber G: Carcinome épidermoïde de l'anus à propos de 149 observations. Chirurgie 109:710–711, 1981.

Mayer M, Papillon J, Bobin JY, Ardiet JM: La lymphadénectomie mésentérique inférieure et périrectale dans le traitement conservateur des cancers de la partie inférieure de l'ampoule rectale. Chirurgie 108:479–483, 1982.

Mohiuddin M, Dobelbower RR, Kramer S, Marks G: Adjuvant radiotherapy with selective sandwich technique in treatment of rectal cancer. Results of continuing study. Dis Colon Rectum 24:76–79, 1981.

Morson BC: Factors influencing the prognosis of early cancer of the rectum. Proc Roy Soc Med 59:607–608, 1966.

Newman HK, Quan SH: Multimodality therapy for epidermoid carcinoma of the anus. Cancer 37:12–19, 1976.

Nicholls RJ, Mason A, Morson BC, et al: The clinical staging of rectal cancer. Br J Surg 69:404–409, 1982.

Nigro MD, Vaitkevicius VK, Buroker T, et al: Combined therapy for cancer of the anal canal. Dis Colon Rectum 24:73–75, 1981.

Nigro MD, Vaitkevicius VK, Considine BJ: Combined therapy for cancer of the anal canal. A preliminary report. Dis Colon Rectum 17:354–356, 1974.

Overgaard M, Overgaard J, Sell A: Radiation therapy of recurrent or inoperable carcinoma of the rectum. Proc Cong Europ Soc Ther Rad Onc (London) 1982, p. 36.

Papillon J: Rectal and anal cancers. Conservative treatment by irradiation. An alternative to radical surgery. New York, Springer Verlag, 1982.

Parks A: Squamous carcinoma of the anal canal. Ann Gastroenterol Hepatol 17:103–107, 1981.

Priestman TJ: The place of radiotherapy in the management of rectal adenocarcinoma. Cancer Treat Rev 4:1–12, 1977.

Quan SHQ: Squamous cancer of the anorectum. Int J Radiat Oncol Biol 5:63, 1979.

Rider WD: Is the Miles operation really necessary for the treatment of rectal cancer? J Can Assoc Radiol 26:167–175, 1975.

Roe JP, Kodner IJ, Walz B, Fry RD: Preoperative radiation therapy for rectal carcinoma. Dis Colon Rectum 25:471–473, 1982.

Romsdahl M, Withers HR: Radiotherapy combined with curative surgery. Its use as therapy for carcinoma of the sigmoid colon and rectum. Arch Surg 113:446–453, 1978.

Rousseau J, Mathieu G, Fenton J: Resultats et complications de la radiothérapie des épithéliomas du canal anal. Etude de 128 cas traités de 1956 à 1970. Gastroenterol Clin Biol (Paris) 3:207–208, 1979.

Simbertseva LP, Sneshko LI, Smirnov NM: Results of intensive combined therapy for carcinoma of the rectum. Vopr Onkol 21:7–9, 1975.

Sischy B: The place of radiotherapy in the management of rectal adenocarcinoma. Cancer 50:2631–2637, 1982.

Sischy B, Remington JH, Sobel SH: Treatment of rectal carcinomas by means of endocavitary irradiation. Cancer 42:1073–1076, 1978.

Stearns MW, Quan SHQ: Epidermoid carcinoma of the anorectum. Surg Gynecol Obstet 131:953–957, 1970.

Stevens K, Allen C, Fletcher WS: Preoperative radiotherapy for adenocarcinoma of the rectosigmoid. Cancer 37:2866–2874, 1976.

Thomas PRM, Ellenberg SS, Knowlton AM, et al: Adjuvant therapy following apparently complete excision of adenocarcinoma of the rectum. Results of a multi-institutional trial. Int J Radiat Oncol Biol Phys 8:119, 1982.

Turner SS, Vieira EP, Gaer PI, et al: Elective postoperative radiotherapy for locally advanced colorectal cancers. Cancer 40:105–108, 1977.

Urdaneta-Lafee N, Kligerman MM, Knowlton AH: Evaluation of palliation in rectal carcinoma. Radiology 104:673–677, 1972.

Wanebo HJ, Futrell JW, Constable WC, Rosenoff S: Multimodality approach to the surgical management of locally advanced epidermoid carcinoma of the anorectum. Cancer 47:2817–2829, 1981.

Wang CL, Schulz MD: The role of radiation therapy in the management of carcinoma of the sigmoid, rectosigmoid and rectum. Radiology 79:1–5, 1962.

Williams JG, Horwitz H: The primary treatment of adenocarcinoma of the rectum by high voltage roentgenrays (1000 kV). AJR 76:919–928, 1956.

Wolfe HRI: The management of metastastic inguinal adenitis in epidermoid cancer of the anus. Proc Roy Soc Med 61:626–628, 1968.

Zucali R, Gardani G, Volterani F: Adjuvant postoperative radiotherapy in locally advanced rectal and rectosigmoid cancer. Tumori 66:595–600, 1980.

TWENTY

Stomas and Their Care

P. J. Martin, B.S.N., E.T.
J. S. Spratt, M.D.

The stoma is defined as the portion of the intestinal tract or urinary system brought to the skin's surface. A stoma can be temporary or permanent. Planned surgical procedures known as *ostomies* date back to the 1700s. For over two centuries systematic thought was concentrated on the management skills needed to maximize the quality of life after survival from the surgery. Since the early 1960s, formal programs designed to plan systematically for ostomies and to educate the new ostomate have been evolving. Our purpose here is not to present an exhaustive review of surgical techniques because others have done this so well, such as Shackelford and Zuidema (1982). Rather, we wish to stress the importance of preoperative and postoperative programs.

Under Turnbull's leadership, the role for ostomy specialists was first defined. The first training program was established in 1961. All the first students were ostomates. The initial education was rudimentary and was offered on a one-to-one basis, with most instructions being given at the bedside. Enterostomal therapists are now available in most hospitals that perform a significant number of ostomies.

An enterostomal therapy hospital program promotes organized care of ostomy patients. The primary role is planned rehabilitation of individuals with stomas. The enterostomal therapist provides direct care or serves as a health team member with surgeons, staff nurses, dietitians, social workers, and others. Physically and psychologically, rehabilitation is the responsibility of all members of the health team. People with stomas must have access to an effective ostomy program. Both the disease requiring the stoma and the stoma itself may impose totally disabling limitations on patients. These limitations may necessitate special approaches to daily living. Planned and responsive support should also be directed toward psychologic needs, as an individual requires a strong self-image in order to make the necessary adjustments to an ostomy.

The ostomate needs basic knowledge of gastrointestinal physiology, making it easier to understand the malfunctions and effects of stomas. Urostomy patients also require an understanding of genitourinary physiology.

The maintenance of skin integrity is an ongoing process for the person with a stoma. The ostomy patient is more susceptible to skin irritations because of fecal and urinary drainage, adhesive material from appliances, occasional skin allergies, and bacterial or fungal infections. Perspiration rash under the pouches can be troublesome.

There are many surgical procedures that produce both gastrointestinal and genitourinary stomas. These procedures are thoroughly reviewed by Shackelford and Zuidema (1982). A temporary stoma is performed with the intention of closing it in the future. Some stomas originally intended to be temporary may end up permanent. Permanent stomas are

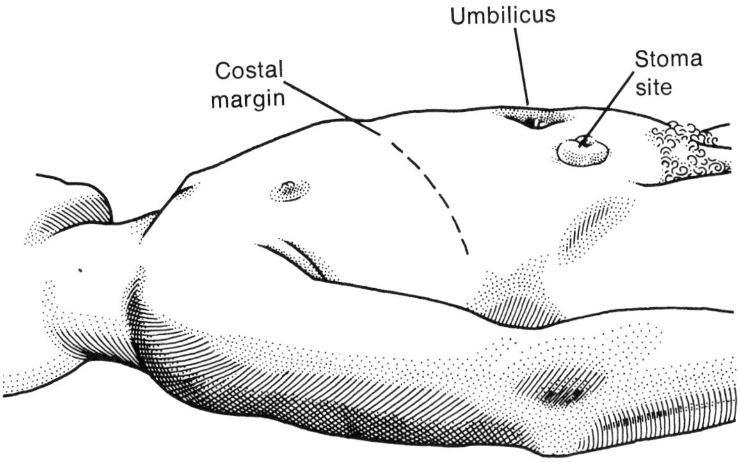

Figure 20–1. Lower quadrant abdominal stoma site of a supine adult of normal weight. (From Watt RC: Stoma placement. *In* Broadwell DC, Jackson BS (eds): Principles of Ostomy Care. St Louis, CV Mosby Co, 1982.)

those created with no plan or option for future closure (e.g., when the distal portion of bowel or urinary tract has been removed, leaving no anastomotic possibilities available) (Broadwell and Jackson, 1982). Typical stomas are shown in Figures 20–1 to 20–3.

PREOPERATIVE TEACHING AND PLANNING

"Preoperative teaching can benefit the patient by reducing anxiety, shortening hospital stays, reducing analgesic needs postoperatively, increasing trust in hospital personnel, and promoting patient compliance." (Shrankel, 1978). Ideally, a stomal therapy program will provide for careful preoperative assessment, stomal location planning, and patient and support group education. This involves the development of a care plan. The patient's mental and physical conditions will influence the degree of preparation that can be expected preoperatively.

The fear of ostomy surgery is interrelated with past experiences. Preoperative education

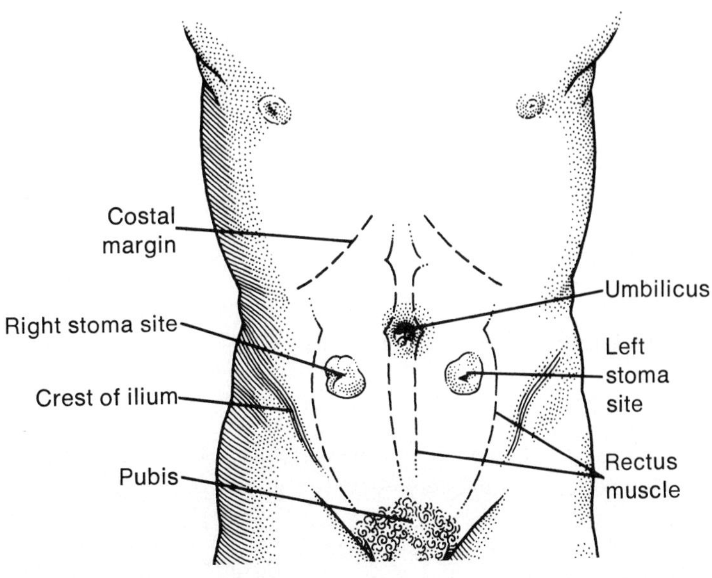

Figure 20–2. Right and left lower quadrant abdominal stoma sites of an ambulatory adult of normal weight. (From Watt RC: Stoma placement. *In* Broadwell DC, Jackson BS (eds): Principles of Ostomy Care. St Louis, CV Mosby Co, 1982.)

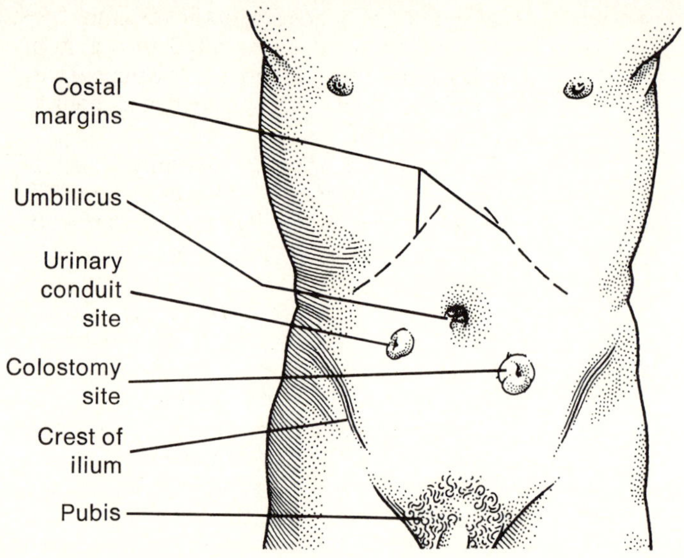

Figure 20–3. Two abdominal stomas (urinary diversion, right lower quadrant site, and fecal diversion, left lower quadrant site) of an adult patient. (From Watt RC: Stoma placement. *In* Broadwell DC, Jackson BS (eds): Principles of Ostomy Care. St Louis, CV Mosby Co, 1982.)

should emphasize improvements in ostomy equipment. A complete ostomy program with a trained staff present provides reassurance and relieves anxiety and uncertainty. Teaching patient and family self-help skills aids greatly in lowering anxiety levels.

All principles that affect the teaching-learning situation apply to ostomy education. The amount and type of education given preoperatively may depend on the diagnosis. Retention of information during this time may be limited. Explanations should be clear and brief, and time should be allowed for questions. Preoperative teaching should be initiated gradually, with evaluation of the patient's response. The patient will rarely ask for more information than he is ready to assimilate. Teaching should be paced according to each individual's rate of assimilation.

Stoma Site Selection

Abdominal assessment and determination of the best stoma site are critical preoperative procedures. A poorly situated stoma has a negative influence on a patient's adjustment to an ostomy. The patient's diagnosis and disease process should be well understood before the site is marked.

Ideally, the stoma site is away from skin folds, scars, previous radiation therapy skin ports, the patient's normal beltline, and bony prominences.

In avoiding areas of past or future radiation therapy at the stoma site, accurate definition of these treatment ports is essential. The radiation therapist should be consulted to be sure that stomas will not be in these ports (Spratt and Sala, 1962; Spratt, 1974). Wrinkles and folds not obvious when the patient is lying flat can be identified by having him sit, bend, and stand. Once the site has been identified, it is marked with an intradermal injection of a sterile solution of methylene blue.

Careful preoperative assessment of the aforementioned factors has a favorable influence on postoperative rehabilitation, allowing the patient to return more quickly to normal physical and social activities. Stoma site consideration and placement are illustrated in Figures 20–1 to 20–3.

POSTOPERATIVE CARE

In the recovery room or operating room, a drainable, odor-resistant, disposable pouch is applied. The pouch is clear so that the stoma can be observed frequently. Important postoperative aspects are stoma viability and peristomal skin integrity. The type of stoma and its discharge usually dictate the approach to stomal management.

Ideally, a hospital-based enterostomal therapist is not assigned to a single nursing unit and can provide continuity of support for the ostomate as he progresses through convalescence and is transferred through a sequence of graded-care nursing units.

ILEOSTOMIES

Discharge from an ileostomy generally appears 12 to 36 hours after surgery. A clear, drainable, disposable appliance with a skin barrier (Stomahesive or HolliHesive) is applied immediately in the operating room or the recovery room to catch this effluent. The peristomal skin must be protected from the irritating enzymes and bile salts that are present in the ileostomy discharge. Ideally, the ileostomy stoma is nippled and protrudes ½ to 1 inch to facilitate drainage into the pouch (Fig. 20–4) (Spratt et al., 1973). Symptoms such as burning and itching or signs of leakage require that the appliance be changed immediately.

During the first 6 to 8 weeks, the edematous stoma decreases in size. With this normally subsiding edema and contracture, the appliance opening may need periodic resizing. Most reusable equipment is not fitted to the stoma opening until 2 to 3 months following surgery, when most edema has subsided and contracture has become stable.

The effluent from the ileostomy is usually dark green, watery, and odorless when functioning begins. Gradually, the discharge becomes thicker and yellowish-brown. The effluent is normally pasty in consistency unless the ostomate is having diarrhea secondary to gastroenteritis or a problem with eating or drinking.

In the postoperative period, the output from the ileostomy should be accurately measured. When the patient's physical strength returns, he will undertake the first step in self-care, emptying the pouch. When feasible, self-care practices should be performed in the bathroom for convenience and privacy. The frequency of pouch emptying usually depends on oral intake. With the introduction of solid foods, habits will develop and the pouch can be emptied after meals and before sleep. Hill advised "slow introduction of solid food postoperatively because too rapid introduction in the first postoperative week can be associated

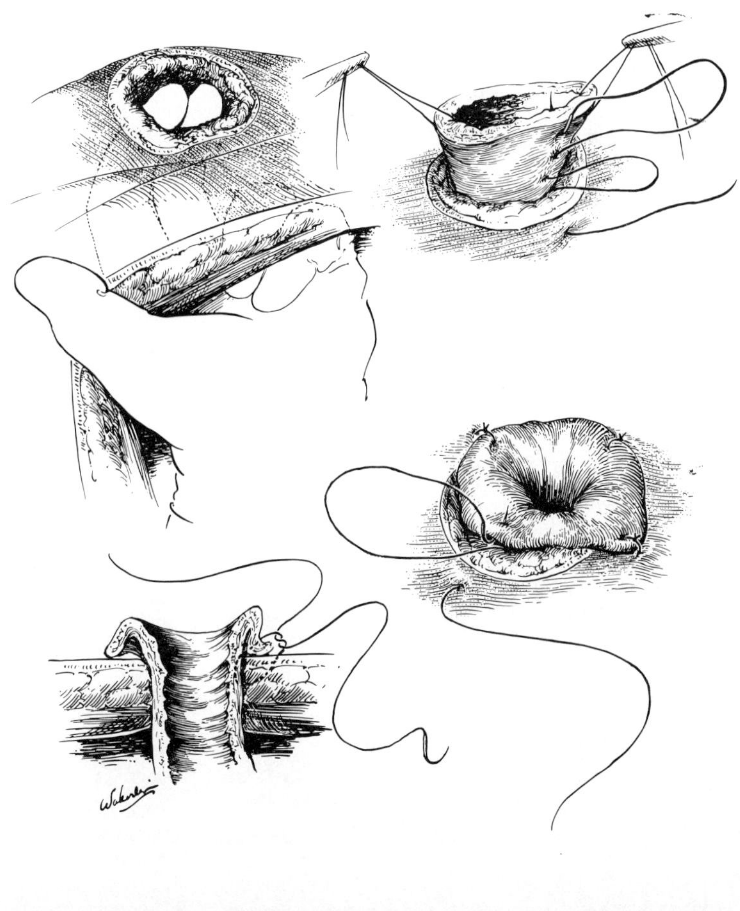

Figure 20–4. The ends of either the ileum or the colon are approximated to the skin in the same manner. Either interrupted fine silk or fine catgut sutures are placed by traversing skin and the seromuscular layer of the intestine about 1 cm proximal to the end and full thickness at the cut end of the intestine. (From Spratt JS Jr, Butcher H, Bricker ER: Exenterative Surgery of the Pelvis. Philadelphia, W. B. Saunders, 1973.)

with cramps and nausea, even when ileostomy is functioning normally." He suggested that intravenous fluid supplementation continue "until adequate oral intake is tolerated" (Hill, 1976).

Controversy concerning dietary limitations persists. Regardless of the diet prescribed, the ostomate should be taught to chew food thoroughly to prevent food blockage. Foods should be added to the diet one at a time so that the way in which individual foods affect the ileostomy can be determined. Foods higher in fiber and cellulose may cause mechanical blockage of an ileostomy. High-roughage foods should be eaten slowly and chewed thoroughly.

The large-bowel function of absorbing sodium and water is lost with the resection of the colon. Increased intake of fluid and electrolytes is important until adaptation occurs. "The process of thickening of ileostomy fluid with lessening of daily volume during the weeks and months after surgery for an ileostomy (a process known as ileostomy adaptation) is a physiologic response of the small intestine to body salt and water depletion" (Hill, 1976). The well-functioning ileal stoma excretes about 60 mEq of sodium and 500 ml of water daily. Sodium and water losses may exceed daily intake if ileostomy volume is abnormally high.

Associated Odors and Flatus

The presence of an ostomy often enhances awareness of bowel gas and its odors.

Flatus is composed predominantly of three gases: hydrogen, methane, and carbon dioxide. Hydrogen and methane are not normal metabolic products and are produced by the endogenous gastrointestinal bacterial flora. The amount often varies with the quanity and type of substrate and variations in endogenous flora. Carbon dioxide is a product of both bacterial metabolism and intraluminal interaction of bicarbonate and hydrogen ions. Swallowed air, carbon dioxide, methane, and hydrogen are all odorless. Knowledge of the numerous sources of fecal odor are incomplete.

The bacteria that produce hydrogen and methane are located in the colon. Production requires that fermentable carbohydrate reach the colon. Breath hydrogen can actually be monitored to assay the amount of carbohydrate reaching the colon (Haines et al., 1977).

Certain foods (e.g., baked beans) contain oligopolysaccharides that reach the colon undigested, where they are fermented. Methane production is extremely variable. Patients with carcinoma of the colon have been reported to have a higher prevalence of methane production.

Most ostomy appliances are odor-proof or odor-resistant, but other methods of odor control may be desired. Internal and external deodorizers are available. Many deodorants and cleaning agents are available for pouches. The patient will find that he can best control odor by keeping the pouch empty and clean and by changing the appliance on a regular basis. Certain foods (e.g., onions, cabbage, spicy foods, and fish) as well as antibiotics and vitamin preparations can produce an odorous effluent. Ingestion of yogurt, buttermilk, and parsley may help with odor control.

Voluntary control of the passage of flatus is not possible because the stoma has no sphincter. Many ostomates can anticipate the passage of flatus, and they can muffle the sound by folding their arms and pressing against their abdomen or stoma. Excessive flatus can be caused by air swallowing, eating rapidly, talking while eating, gum-chewing, drinking carbonated beverages, or using drinking straws.

Flatulence may be reduced by restricting the quantity of carbohydrate ingested. A diet low in lactose, legumes, and wheat is often helpful (Levitt, 1981).

Changing the Appliance

When possible, the patient should select a time during which the stoma is inactive to change the appliance. Prior to meals, before bedtime, and 2½ to 4 hours after eating, the stoma is usually quiet. Changing an appliance too frequently or scrubbing or scratching the area excessively can cause skin irritation. The use of oily soaps or bath oils is discouraged because the residue left by them decreases the effectiveness of adhesives. Simple washing with nonoily soap and warm water is more than adequate.

The first step a patient takes in learning to accept the stoma is to observe and touch it. Touching the stoma reassures the new ostomate that it is not fragile and can withstand physical contact and pressure. Cleaning the peristomal skin and stoma will frequently precipitate slight stomal bleeding that is due to the local vascularity. Stoma movement is also normal owing to the peristaltic wave of the intestine. The new ostomate must be taught to expect an unplanned discharge occasionally and to cope with the occurrence.

The choice of appliance takes into consideration the patient's dexterity, his life style, his personality, and the type and location of the stoma. The appliance should be properly fitted and odor-proof or odor-resistant, and it should be successfully managed by the ostomate to prevent stoma injury or skin irritation before the patient is discharged from the hospital.

Ileostomy Complications

There are various complications related to all ostomies, but one unique to ileostomy is food blockage. This problem can be caused by inadequately digested food or a stenosed stoma. Some foods likely to cause food blockage are those of high fiber and cellulose content. Foods most often causing food blockage are popcorn, peanuts, coconut, chinese vegetables, string beans, and olives. "Food blockage is mainly caused by two factors: inadequately digested food and stenosed stoma" (Broadwell and Jackson, 1982).

When symptoms of food blockage occur, the appliance must be removed immediately to reduce the risk of stomal edema and injury. Lying down or sitting in a knee-chest position will sometimes move the food out of the stoma. Massaging the abdomen may also help the blockage. A digital examination may relieve the blockage. When all else fails, an experienced person can perform an ileostomy lavage using 30 to 50 ml of warm saline, slowly allowing the solution to return each time before adding more. Several hours may be required to relieve a blockage. If excessive vomiting occurs, intravenous fluid replacement may be indicated. Although it is not desirable for the patient to lavage the ileostomy, knowledge of the proper procedure is necessary. If all conservative measures fail to give relief, the surgeon may have to remove the obstruction by operation. Many of the principles of care for ileostomy apply to colostomies of the transverse and right colon, where liquid effluents are common.

LOOP COLOSTOMIES

Loop colostomies are usually temporary and are more often performed in emergencies, as for intestinal obstruction. Preoperative preparation is often minimal and inadequate. The stomal site may be located in an area in which there is difficulty attaching a pouch. The stoma may be extremely large and edematous with a support device that makes it difficult to secure a leak-proof appliance. Although these operations are emergency in nature, time should be taken to select and mark a proper stomal site if feasible.

A variety of support devices can be used with the loop colostomy: a rubber catheter, a glass rod with rubber tubing connected, the Hollister bridge, the Loop-Loc by Bard, or the T-rod by Marlen. The support device is usually left in place for at least 6 to 10 days postoperatively. Patient and family education in stoma care should be deferred until surgical steps are completed and the support device has been removed (Broadwell and Jackson, 1982) Typical support devices for loop colostomies are shown in Figure 20–5.

The authors have found that when performing loop colostomies for distal loop colonic obstructions, a technique of great value is the insertion of a large Pezzer catheter into the loop secured by a purse-string suture. The Pezzer is attached to a closed drainage system for as many days as are necessary to allow colonic decompression, uncontaminated wound healing, and thickening of the stool. Then the colostomy can be opened and sutured to the skin. Most sutures should be on the proximal side, constructing a very large-mouthed stoma proximally and a very small-mouthed stoma distally. This reduces spillage of fecal content into the distal loop. Placing a row of staples across the distal loop is also helpful in assuring that feces do not enter the distal bowel.

DOUBLE-BARREL COLOSTOMIES

A double-barrel colostomy has a functioning and nonfunctioning stoma. The proximal (functioning) stoma is covered with a clear, drainable, odor-proof pouch. The distal (usually nonfunctioning) stoma may have a pouch or a nonadherent absorbent dressing. Rectal discharge and sensations that accompany a conventional bowel movement may be expected periodically from a retained rectum.

Although a double-barrel colostomy is usually temporary, it becomes permanent in a variety of clinical situations. Stomas located on the transverse colon generally cannot be regulated by irrigation, diet, or medications. Care of those stomas are similar to that employed for ileal stomas.

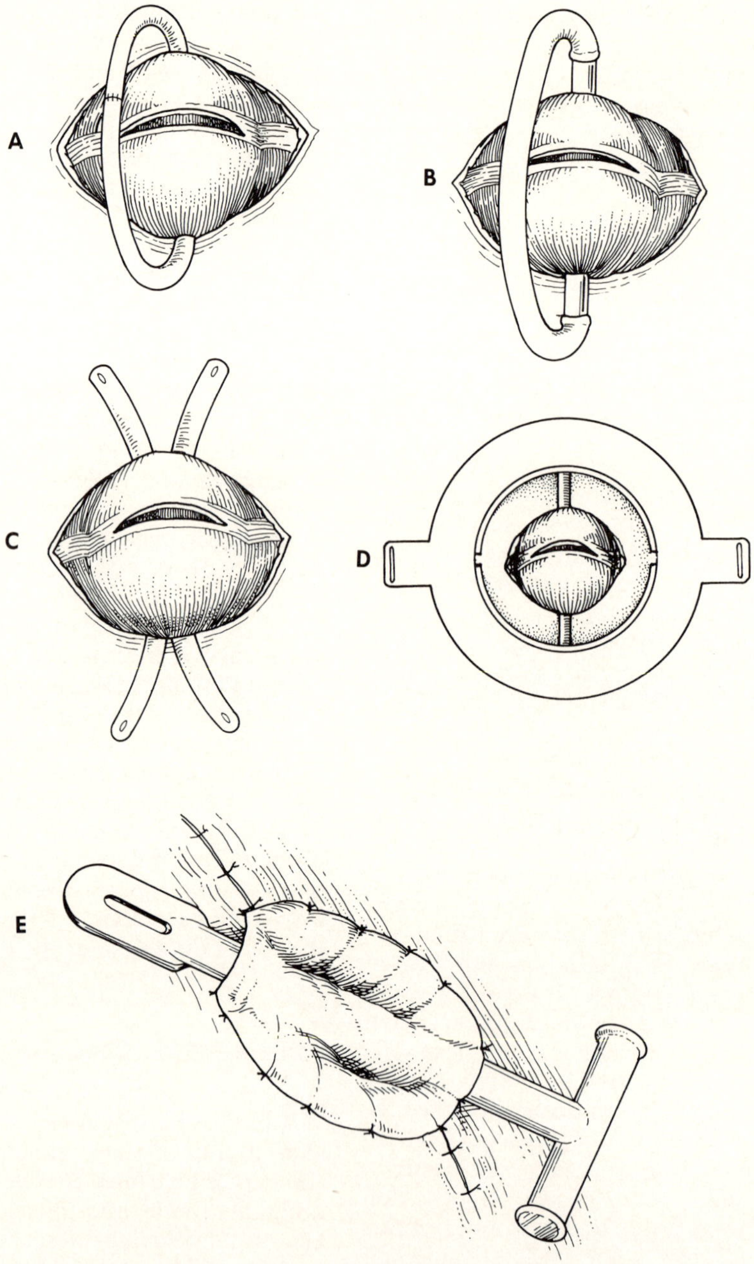

Figure 20–5. *A,* A no. 26 red rubber catheter is placed under the bowel to provide support. This is contraindicated in obese patients and in those with a short mesentery. This is a very flexible system and is easy for staff and patients to manage. *B,* A glass rod is used to support the bowel. A piece of rubber tubing is connected to each end of the rod to prevent it from slipping. The rod may be carefully slipped vertically so that a skin barrier and pouch may be applied. *C,* A Hollister bridge is usually sutured to the skin. A skin barrier and pouching system is available that fits over this. *D,* Loop-Loc set (Bard). A skin barrier is applied under the plastic ring up to the base of the stoma; a disposable pouch is attached to the gasket. *E,* A Marlen T-rod may be used when the stoma is matured at the time of surgery. (From Dudas S: Postoperative considerations. *In* Broadwell DC, Jackson BS (eds): Principles of Ostomy Care. St Louis, CV Mosby Co, 1982.)

SIGMOID COLOSTOMIES

Sigmoid colostomies and end colostomies of the left colon are most commonly performed when permanent fecal diversion is indicated. Abdominoperineal resection and pelvic exenterations as well as unresectable anorectal cancers necessitate a permanent colostomy.

The initial effluent from this type of stoma is liquid to pasty in consistency. As the patient begins to eat solid foods, the stool gradually becomes formed. Management options for the sigmoid colostomate are colostomy irrigation, dietary planning, and natural evacuation.

Colostomy irrigation remains a controversial procedure. When the patient and a selected assistant are taught to irrigate with safe, appropriate equipment, no complications will occur. Colostomy irrigation is successful when there is no stool spillage from one irrigation to the next. Irrigation can be done daily or every other day, according to the needs of each person. The procedure should always be performed at about the same time, planned according to the individual's life style. After each irrigation, the patient should cover the stoma with a small protective dressing. The patient should be aware that the intestine could become disturbed unexpectedly by gastroenteritis or by problem foods or drink, resulting in diarrhea. Ostomates are advised to carry a disposable, drainable pouch in case such an emergency arises.

Not all sigmoid stomas will be successfully managed with irrigation. Many patients have limited physical dexterity, deficits in learning ability, and irregular bowel activity prior to surgery. These individuals may simply choose to learn only about the necessary procedures for pouch care.

When radiation therapy or chemotherapy is being administered, it is wise to wait until after treatments are completed before daily colostomy irrigation. These treatments often cause diarrhea, and the use of an odor-proof, drainable pouch with a skin barrier is often necessary to collect the stool and protect the peristomal skin.

When appropriate, the new ostomate is taught the procedure for irrigation and given the opportunity to practice before going home. "The life style, personal goals and aspirations, and abilities of the individual person should be considered before the patient decides whether or not to irrigate" (Mahoney, 1976). Colostomy irrigation, when successful, can give the ostomate a sense of security and better control over his daily schedule.

The colostomy irrigation procedure may be performed with the equipment of various manufacturers, but the principles of irrigation will remain the same. The general guidelines to the patient regarding irrigation are as follows:

1. Select a time when the bathroom will not have to be shared. In the beginning, plan for at least 1 hour. As the procedure becomes familiar, less time is usually required. Irrigate at about the same time daily until regularity is established. After this is achieved, irrigation time is not as critical. (One hour one way or another should not upset your schedule.)
2. Do not rush! In a rushed atmosphere, evacuation may be incomplete, resulting in a discharge later.
3. The easiest method of irrigation is to sit on the toilet in the normal fashion with the long plastic drain (sleeve) between the legs and into the bowl. Colostomates who have had a surgical procedure that has left a wound in the perineum may find it more comfortable to sit on a chair (with a pillow) in front of the toilet.
4. It is not necessary to sit the entire time. Once the initial rush of water has passed (15 to 20 minutes), the plastic sleeve can be folded and clamped shut. Proceed with other activity. Usually after another 30 to 40 minutes, no more stool or water returns.
5. Do not be concerned if water does not return. The two most common reasons are failure to use enough water or failure to allow enough time for return. Be patient! Don't let an occasional failure of irrigant to return discourage you. Try again. If difficulties occur during 3 to 4 consecutive days, notify the surgeon.
6. Lubricate the irrigation cone tip or catheter with water or some other substance. If there is difficulty introducing the device there might be hardened stool. Relax. Keep the water flowing and gently insert the tip. *Never force it!* There are no sensory nerves in the colon. It can be injured, even pierced, without any pain or warning sensation. If difficulty persists after several efforts, call the surgeon or wait until the next time for irrigation. If abdominal pain, bleeding, or fever develops, consult the surgeon.
7. Air in tubing can cause cramps. Let the air run out of the tubing before inserting the irrigator tip into the stoma. Irrigation solution should be close to body temperature. Cold water causes cramping. If cramping occurs with warm water, the water may be going in too rapidly. Clamp the tubing closed and keep the cone (or device being used) in the stoma until

cramping subsides. When cramps subside or become tolerable, continue with irrigation.

8. *Never* connect irrigating equipment to a faucet.

The person who prefers the natural method of evacuation for the colostomy can wear an odor-proof, drainable pouch. With this approach, it is important that problem foods be tried one at a time so that the effects of each can be determined. Also, too frequent changes of appliance can precipitate peristomal irritation.

UROSTOMIES

Immediately following a urostomy (e.g., ureterocutaneous stoma or ileoneocystostomy), a disposable transparent pouch is applied. A urine meter attached to a bedside collection device is connected to the pouch, and the urinary output is closely monitored in the early postoperative period. Initially, the urine may be tinged with blood, but its color generally clears to light amber in the first postoperative week.

At the surgeon's option, ureteral catheters, which are called stents, are used to traverse the ureters through the conduit stoma. The stents prevent stricture of the ureteroileal anastomoses and sometimes simplify a difficult ureteroileal anastomosis. The surgeon may secure these catheters in a variety of ways. With each pouch change, these ureteral stents are carefully threaded into the pouch, and gravity drainage is employed until the appropriate time for removal. Removal of the stents can be done when urine flow is well established, with no leakage. If there is doubt about leakage, a radiologic ileogram can be performed through the stoma, using absorbable contrast medium.

The urostomy pouch has a valve that allows convenient emptying. The valve also can be connected to the bedside drainage collector. Once the patient resumes walking, he should be taught how to disconnect the urostomy pouch from the bedside collector for freedom of ambulation. A night drain collector is useful even after discharge so that sleep is not disturbed with the need to empty the bag during the sleep cycle.

Urostomies (ileal or colonic conduit) are not reservoirs or storage units for urine. The conduit is a passageway from the urinary tract to the skin and does not regulate the urine flow. The amount of urine depends on fluid intake. Any sudden change of urinary output not related to fluid intake should be reported to the surgeon.

Foul-smelling urine may be a symptom of a urinary tract infection. Maintaining an acid urine may help prevent or reduce the chance of infection, crystal formation in the urine, skin irritation secondary to alkaline urine, and odor. "Methods of internal acidification are by oral administration of ascorbic acid and a diet high in acid-ash foods including cranberry juice intake" (Chezem, 1976).

The new urostomate needs to evaluate the frequency of appliance change to suit his own life style. There is no set time at which the appliance must be changed. The length of time for which the appliance may adhere will vary; the average duration is from 2 to 14 days. It is best to change the appliance in the morning before eating because urine output is reduced at that time. The appliance is gently eased from the skin. The peristomal skin is washed with warm water and dried thoroughly. The patient can apply rolled gauze, tampons, or dental wicks over the stoma to absorb the urine while preparing the skin for the clean appliance. A skin barrier is recommended to all urostomates to protect the peristomal skin from urine.

Before being discharged from the hospital, the new ostomate is given information about local suppliers of ostomy equipment. Selection of equipment is an individual choice that is based on the type of stoma and life style of the ostomate. Wait 6 to 8 weeks before sizing reusable equipment to permit stomal edema to subside. Proper sizing of reusable equipment allows ⅛ inch so that the stoma can move normally. When reusable equipment is chosen, it is recommended that the patient keep two complete sets so that one set is ready at all times. Urine crystal buildup may occur on reusable equipment. The patient manages this problem by soaking the equipment in one part water and one part vinegar for 20 to 30 minutes.

Routine urinary function tests of culture and sensitivity and intravenous pyelogram are usually done every 6 to 12 months or as indicated. A sterile urine specimen should be taken directly from the urinary stoma (conduit stoma). Using a sterile technique, insert a catheter 1 to 2 inches into the stoma and collect the specimen in a sterile container.

In addition to the ileal conduit, there are other urinary diversions such as ureterostomy, ureterosigmoidostomies, or other ureterocolostomies. Ureterostomy stomas generally are tiny and flush with the skin, making pouching a problem. A vesicostomy is also performed for a neurogenic bladder. This type of diversion can be managed with an intermittent catheter or with a Foley catheter that is left in place to drain the bladder.

SURGICAL MANAGEMENT OF TOTAL PELVIC EXENTERATION

The patient who has a total pelvic exenteration with two ostomies will require special management. The operation includes a colostomy and a urinary diversion, with complete removal of all pelvic viscera. The time required for complete healing of the large pelvic defect varies. The patient will have to adjust to many physiologic and psychologic changes. The female patient is unable to have sexual intercourse unless vaginal reconstruction can be accomplished successfully. If reconstruction is feasible, it may be done at the time of the exenteration or at a later date.

The ostomies are managed as discussed earlier. The surgeon generally locates the colostomy lower than the conduit in case a belt is worn with the urostomy appliance. Wound healing may be slow in patients who have previously had radiation therapy. Such patients are particularly prone to intestinal obstruction and fistula formation. Care of these patients can present the most difficult problems in stomal management (Spratt et al., 1973).

COMPLICATIONS AFTER OSTOMIES

Complications following ostomy surgery are the same as those that can occur after any surgery. The patient having an ostomy is particularly vulnerable to intestinal obstruction, fistula formation, and complications related to the stoma itself, including stomal perforation, necrosis, stenosis, retraction, and prolapse as well as peristomal skin irritations and peristomal hernia. The stomas may also be the site of metastatic or implanted cancer.

Wound infection is a common complication of colon surgery. An optimal plan for stomal care ensures that stool and urine are contained in a secure pouching system that prevents the output from contaminating the incision and greatly reduces continuing contamination if open wound management is required. Aside from indicated surgical management of the wound, skilled stomal management is mandatory in this situation.

Postoperative intestinal obstruction in the presence of stomas must take into consideration the possibility of internal or parastomal hernia incarceration, stricture, adhesion, or recurrent cancer (Shackelford and Zuidema, 1982).

Stomal complications can occur from surgical trauma, edema, or compromised mesenteric circulation, which causes ischemia in the stoma. If the stoma becomes dusky, light gray, or blue, the stoma may be ischemic, with progression to infarction. A surgical reconstruction with viable bowel may be required. "Stomal edema can be caused from too tight a pouch opening, stomal prolapse or stomal stenosis. Dilatation of the stoma is recommended by some surgeons to keep the stoma from stenosing. This procedure is controversial. More stenosis may actually occur from this dilatation since the fibrous ring surrounding the stoma is torn and even more scar tissue forms. If stenosis is causing symptoms of obstruction, a surgical revision of the stoma is indicated" (Hill, 1976). Attentive nursing care is critical in these situations, and surgical correction is often required.

Stomal prolapse is seen frequently with loop ostomies. Retraction of the stoma results from scar tissue formation around the stoma, with a shrinkage of the fascial structures causing the stoma to be pulled inward.

Following conduit surgery, ureteral obstruction can occur. Early, this can be caused by a mucus plug in the stoma. Swelling at the ureterointestinal anastomosis can cause oliguria in the early postoperative period. Urine leakage from the anastomotic site into the pelvis or peritoneal cavity may cause irritation and perineal drainage. The frequency and management of complications, both early and late, associated with ileoneocystostomy was reviewed previously and is not further discussed here, since only an occasional advanced but still localized anorectal cancer will require replacement of the urinary bladder (Spratt et al., 1973).

POSTOPERATIVE CARE OF PERISTOMAL SKIN

The most important layer of peristomal skin is the epidermis. The keratin layer of the epidermis is a shield against the tissue-destructive effect of moisture. The integrity of the epidermis can be compromised by the type of stomal drainage, consistency of the drainage, some medications (particular fat solvents), surgical construction and location of the stoma, improper nursing care of the stoma, the patient's skill and interest in self-care, and choice of equipment.

Skin allergies to ostomy equipment can occur, but a true allergic reaction is rare. Symptoms that may be indicative of a skin allergy include itching, stinging, and burning. The first step in treatment involves the identification and discontinuance of the offending product. Occasionally, a dermatologist may need to be consulted. Minor skin problems may be treated as follows:

Treatment for Erythematous Skin

1. *Gently* remove appliance every 24 to 36 hours.
2. Clean skin with warm water and air dry.
3. Treat irritated skin with room air, the light of a 60-watt bulb (12 to 14 inches from the irritated area), or moderate heat from a hair dryer.
4. Cover irritated skin with a skin barrier (Stomahesive or HolliHesive). Cut an opening in the skin barrier to fit very snugly around the stoma. If a reusable face plate is used, it must be ⅛ inch larger than the stoma.

Treatment for Broken Blistered Skin

1. *Gently* remove the appliance every 24 to 36 hours.
2. Clean skin area with warm water and air dry.
3. Apply warm water soaks for 15 to 20 minutes (this cleans and soothes the area and stimulates blood flow).
4. Expose the irritated area to light, air, and heat as in step 3 for treatment of reddened skin.
5. Cover with skin barrier as in step 4 for reddened skin treatment.
6. Finish application of device as usual.

Residual soap, detergents, or solvents may also cause irritation. When using any of these items, always make sure to rinse and dry peristomal skin thoroughly before equipment is applied.

Urine also causes skin problems when the appliance has not been fitted properly. Urine constantly bathing the skin, especially alkaline urine, causes erythema, maceration, and epidermal hyperplasia. The recommended treatment for these symptoms is application of soaks of one part vinegar and one part water to the irritated area for 15 to 20 minutes with each appliance change. This is followed with the light, heat, and air regimen used to treat reddened and excoriated skin.

Improper sizing and fitting is one of the main reasons for peristomal skin irritations. Skin problem complaints indicate the need for reassessment of equipment currently in use. If equipment has not been fitted to within ⅛ inch of the stoma, new sizing and equipment may be indicated. Urine crystal buildup may be seen on face plates of equipment. This crystallization can be a problem, acting as both a chemical and mechanical irritant. It can cause bleeding from the gritty salts rubbing against the stoma. More frequent cleaning and increased fluid intake may be required (Broadwell and Jackson, 1982).

The peristomal skin is an important area of ostomy care. Prevention of skin irritation is much easier than its treatment. Meticulous skin care is essential in stomal management.

PATIENT EDUCATION AND DISCHARGE PLANNING

As the patient's physical status improves, the focus of education turns to the physical changes and the informational needs of the ostomate after his discharge from the hospital. "Patient educators must apply the principles of the learning theory in both the creation and presentation of educational materials. Effective patient education should incorporate information about what any patient 'ought to know' with what the patient thinks he needs to know" (Newby et al., 1978). Patient education should begin on the day of admission. Some patients, overwhelmed by a cancer diagnosis, may not immediately be able to assimilate stomal care information. Therefore, information should be presented in small increments and reinforced by practice.

The nursing staff may initially handle all aspects of stomal care, but when the patient is more comfortable and alert, he will probably be curious about how to manage it himself. One of the first steps in acceptance of an ostomy is viewing the stoma. The gradual progression from simple to complex tasks gives the patient time to accept and apply this new information to learning self-care skills. The patient must be an active learner. Each new ostomate needs time and sufficient opportunities to practice techniques of ostomy care. The patient's self-esteem and confidence will be reinforced when he can successfully care for himself.

There is no "right" time to teach patients self-care skills. Assessment of individual patient needs and comfort levels is important in finding the optimal time for effective teaching.

An unhurried and private environment creates a better climate for learning new skills. The ostomate's health and physical limitations are considered when a teaching plan is being established. Management skills, any physical changes that affect daily living, any dietary limitations, sexual implications, and signs or symptoms that may require a physician's attention are taught to the new ostomate and to the family members or friends selected by him.

PSYCHOSOCIAL EFFECTS OF OSTOMIES

Education of a new ostomate usually involves one other person. This person can be the spouse, a relative, or a friend of the patient's choice. This person will learn ostomy care with the patient, ensuring adequate support at home.

Physical limitations, including arthritic disability, poor vision, and paralysis, may hamper the patient's ability to care for himself. Mental limitations may also inhibit learning and require a more studied approach. The stoma usually alters the ostomate's self-image, and therefore a period of psychologic adjustment is needed. Acceptance of an ostomy is greatly influenced by the way a person feels about himself and the support systems available.

The patient with an ostomy may require support in the physical environment and psychosocial areas. The ostomate's coping abilities and his support systems (both personal and professional) influence his acceptance of an altered body image and adaptation to the ostomy. Each patient as an individual brings factors that affect the psychologic reaction to ostomy surgery. These factors are age, personality, intelligence, independence, and prognosis. Open preoperative relationships with others will have a significant impact on the patient and family after surgery. Normally private experiences of bowel and bladder control are now shared with medical personnel and family. Initially, new ostomates are overwhelmed by the stress of major physiologic and psychologic changes.

Responsibilities of ostomy care should be introduced gradually to reduce anxiety and facilitate learning. Many new ostomates view discussion of bodily functions as an invasion of privacy. At the same time, loss of these functions may cause depression and doubts about the ability to manage bodily changes. This makes the ostomate dependent on others for relearning the most intimate types of personal care.

As the new ostomate starts to show interest in his bodily changes, it is appropriate to establish the goal of self-care and encourage the patient toward independence. Fears of social rejection and social relationships are normal following ostomy surgery. The ostomy patient requires psychologic support from persons who are sensitive, patient, sympathetic, and knowledgeable about all aspects of postoperative care.

Bowel and bladder control have many symbolic social and cultural meanings that must be resolved before some ostomates can adjust to the bodily function alterations. There seems to be no correct way of defining proper or improper behavior as the patient adjusts to an ostomy. There is no established schedule that the patient must follow to master self-care skills. The appropriate time is determined by the individual patient's readiness to participate in his care. Temporary dependence is permitted, but prolonged dependence is not. If the patient cannot accept altered bodily function, his recovery and rehabilitation will be prolonged. The patient may need psychiatric counseling to facilitate the recovery and rehabilitation process.

Sexual intercourse may vary in its importance to a person at different points in life. Health professionals need to be thorough in explaining the sexual dysfunctions associated with ostomies and any related surgical resections.

The creation of a stoma will not increase or decrease a person's sex drive. The type of physical sexual activity may need to be modified or changed. There are many ways to give and receive sexual pleasure. The individual's values and preferences directly affect the acceptance of these modifications and changes made in sexual expression. Sexual counseling is often helpful to patients and their mates.

Males may experience sexual dysfunction resulting from nerve damage after surgical dissection of the rectum or bladder or both. Females may experience sexual dysfunction, dyspareunia, and loss of pelvic sensation. "The high incidence of dyspareunia can be secondary to the formation of fistulae or abscesses in the perineal region or within the vagina itself as complications of virulent inflammatory bowel disease and in part because of vaginal scarring" (Koloday et al., 1979).

Complications resulting from resumation of sexual activity before physical strength has returned may suggest organic disease when none is present. Return of sexual function will depend on the type of surgery, any underlying disorders, other chronic diseases, and the individual's recuperative powers.

By observing personal hygiene, avoiding problem foods, and ensuring that the pouch is clean and odor-free prior to sexual activity, the ostomate will increase the satisfaction that he derives from the experience.

SELF-HELP ORGANIZATIONS

Self-help groups support patients and families following ostomies and other operations requiring special postoperative care. Talking with one who has been through a similar experience can be invaluable. The national organization for ostomates, The United Ostomy Association (2001 W. Beverly Boulevard, Los Angeles, CA 90057), has information on all local chapters.

References

Broadwell DC, Jackson BS: Principles of Ostomy Care. St. Louis, CV Mosby Co., 1982.

Chezem JL: Urinary diversion: select aspects of nursing management. Nurs Clin North Am 11:445–456, 1976.

Haines A, Metz G, Dilwasi J, et al: Breath-methane in patients with cancer of the large bowel. Lancet 2:481–483, 1977.

Hill GL: Ileostomy. Surgery Physiology and Management, New York, Greene and Strollen, Inc., 1976.

Koloday RC, Masters WH, Johnson VE, Biggs MA: Textbook of Human Sexuality for Nurses. Boston, Little, Brown & Co., 1979.

Levitt M: Intestinal gas production—recent advances in flatology. N. Engl. J. Med. 302:1474–1475, 1981.

Mahoney JM: Guide to Ostomy Nursing Care. Boston, Little, Brown & Co., 1976.

Newby L, Spratt JS Jr, Alfieri Z: A conceptual model for evaluation of patient education for cancer. J. Graham Brown Cancer Center, University of Louisville. Presented at American Educational Research Association, Toronto, March, 1978.

Rizzo M: Here's to progress: the IAET comes of age. ETJ 4:1, 1977.

Shackelford RT, Zuidema GD: Surgery of the Alimentary Tract. Vol. 3. 2nd ed. Philadelphia, W.B. Saunders Co., 1982, pp. 198–242.

Shrankel DP: Pre-operative teaching. Supervisor Nurse 9:82–90, 1978.

Spratt JS: Surgery and radiobiological changes. *In* Lee YTN, Spratt JS: Malignant Lymphoma: Nodal and Extranodal Diseases. New York, Grune & Stratton, 1974.

Spratt JS Jr. Butcher H, Bricker ER: Exenterative Surgery of the Pelvis. Philadelphia, W. B. Saunders Co., 1973.

Spratt JS, Sala JM: The healing of wounds within irradiated tissue. Mo. Med 59:409–411, 1962.

TWENTY-ONE

Special Problems Associated with Colorectal and Anal Cancers

J. S. Spratt, M. D.

This chapter reviews a series of studies dealing with special problems unique to cancers of the colon, rectum, and anus. The implications of these situations, when they occur, must be understood so that the most appropriate actions can be taken for the patient's well being.

URINARY RETENTION AND INFECTION AFTER ABDOMINOPERINEAL RESECTION

Urinary retention after abdominoperineal resection can be a major cause of postoperative morbidity in men (Cook et al., 1963). The operation is usually performed in an age group that has a significant incidence of prostatic hypertrophy and symptoms of bladder neck obstruction. The surgical interruption of pelvic nerves (McCrea and Kimmel, 1953) and extensive dissection immediately adjacent to the lower urinary tract (Campbell and Gislason, 1950) are associated with at least temporary inability to void in most patients recovering from abdominoperineal resection (Cunningham and Young, 1962). The necessity of an indwelling catheter is associated with a high incidence of urinary tract infection, which may result in prolonged morbidity and occasionally in earlier death years later.

Some authors have proposed that perineal prostatectomy be performed at the same time as abdominoperineal resection in selected patients to avoid some of these problems (Leadbetter and Leadbetter, 1958), whereas others believe that the necessity for prostatectomy cannot be determined until several months after operation.

To study this problem Glass and Spratt (1968) reviewed 147 abdominoperineal resections performed on men at the Ellis Fischel State Cancer Hospital. The purpose of the study was to determine the natural history of urinary tract problems in these patients and to develop a rational approach to their management.

The median age of patients requiring prostatectomy was 67 years, and of patients not requiring prostatectomy, 68 years. Patients were followed for a median period of 27 months, over a range of from 2 to 258 months. Only 2 percent of patients were lost to follow-up. Eight patients followed fewer than 6 months were voiding well when last seen.

The indwelling catheter routinely inserted at operation was usually removed on the seventh postoperative day. Twenty-four of the 147 patients (16 percent) had urinary retention after removal of the Foley catheter and required recatheterization during the first postoperative month (Table 21–1). Fourteen of these patients ultimately voided well without prostatic surgery. Most patients who had urinary retention in the early postoperative period regained satisfactory bladder function within 6 weeks of abdominoperineal resections without prostatectomy; a few spontaneously regained normal function as late as 6 months postoperatively.

In 1953, McCrea and Kimmel demonstrated by careful anatomic dissection two routes of vesical innervation with overlapping functions.

Table 21–1. PERSISTENT URINARY RETENTION IN THE FIRST MONTH AFTER ABDOMINOPERINEAL RESECTION*

Total no. of patients	24
Required prostatectomy	10 (42%)†
Ultimately voided well without prostatectomy	14 (58%)

*Adapted from Glass RL, Spratt JS: Urinary complications after abdominoperineal resection of the rectum in men. Am Surg 34:238–241, 1968.

†Three prostatectomies performed in first postoperative month.

The pelvic plexus courses around the rectum and is resected with the wide resection indicated for rectal cancer. The second route is along the lateral (hypogastric) vessels. These nerves are not destroyed by the standard rectosigmoidectomy but probably are temporarily disturbed by stretching and edema. However, after lateral dissection including the perivascular structures of the hypogastric vessels, the contents of the obturator fossae, and the internal genitalia of the female (the so-called "posterior" pelvic exenteration) satisfactory bladder function may still occur (Table 21–2).

Campbell and Gislason (1950) believe that traumatic pericystitis with edema and resultant immobility of the detrusor is a major factor in urinary retention after abdominoperineal resection. Marshall and associates (1964), in reviewing 600 abdominoperineal resections, found a 19.66 percent incidence of "severe" urinary difficulties in the immediate postoperative period, but by 3 months prostatectomies were necessary in only 2.83 percent of the cases. On the basis of these data, he advised conservative management for 3 months.

The results of prostatectomies performed during the first postoperative month suggested that several might have been unnecessary had several weeks been allowed for further return of neuromuscular function of the bladder (Cunningham and Young, 1962).

In 1963, Cook and associates found a 24.1 percent incidence of urinary retention after operations on the bowel in 29 men who had previously had prostatectomy and a 28.5 percent incidence in 414 with no previous prostatic surgery; the difference was not significant.

Table 21–2. VOIDING PATTERNS AFTER POSTERIOR EXENTERATION*

Total no. of patients	5
Voided well (2–8 weeks postoperatively)	3
Never voided (neurogenic bladder)	2

*Adapted from Glass RL, Spratt JS: Urinary complications after abdominoperineal resection of the rectum in men. Am Surg 34:238–241, 1968.

Among patients who had prostatectomies more than a month after abdominoperineal resection, 11 developed symptoms of bladder neck obstruction after a variable period of satisfactory voiding. Two patients never voided satisfactorily after surgery and had prostatectomies in the second and third month after abdominoperineal resection. Five patients developed obstructive urinary symptoms coincident with pelvic recurrence of cancer and did not benefit from prostatectomy. Of these five, the symptoms of obstructive uropathy were the first signs of recurrent cancer. In three of these five, recurrent cancer could not be detected at the time of prostatectomy but became apparent 1 to 2 months later.

An attempt was made to select on the basis of preoperative symptoms those patients most likely to develop major urinary tract complications postoperatively (Table 21–3). The patients classified as having minimal urinary symptoms either had no symptoms preoperatively or had nocturia only once or twice. Those with nocturia three or more times or other symptoms such as retention, dribbling, dysuria, and hesitancy were classified in the second group of patients considered to have major preoperative urinary symptoms. No significant difference in the number of prostatectomies after abdominoperineal resection was noted between these two groups. A subgroup of those with major preoperative urinary symptoms were patients who clearly dated the onset of urinary symptoms coincident with the onset of rectal symptoms. Several of these patients had remarkably benign postoperative courses in spite of severe urinary symptoms in the period before abdominoperineal resection. Resection of rectal cancer relieved their urinary symptoms.

Table 21–4 depicts the course of those patients who never developed obstructive urinary symptoms. In addition to the four with persistent evidence of infection in this nonobstructed group, two had recurrent urinary infection after prostatectomy and two eventually died from causes directly related to infection.

The necessity of an indwelling catheter after abdominoperineal resection is not questioned. However, as Beeson (1958) and Levin (1964) pointed out, pyuria follows 48 hours of catheterization in essentially 100 percent of patients and may persist if untreated. It can ultimately contribute to death.

Table 21–3. **ASSOCIATION OF PREOPERATIVE SYMPTOMS WITH POSTOPERATIVE COMPLICATIONS***

	Patients with Minimal Preoperative Symptoms†	Patients with Major Preoperative Urinary Symptoms‡
No prostatectomy	72	51
Prostatectomy		
Preoperatively	5	2
1st month postoperatively	3	1
2–3 months postoperatively	3	1
	(8%)	(10%)
3rd month postoperatively‡	4	5
Total	87	60

*Adapted from Glass RL, Spratt JS: Urinary complications after abdominoperineal resection of the rectum in men. Am Surg 34:238–241, 1968.

†0–2 × nocturia without other urinary symptoms.

‡3 × nocturia and/or other urinary symptoms.

Glass and Spratt (1968) concluded that urinary retention after abdominoperineal resection in men was related to temporary neural dysfunction and local edema. Spontaneous return of bladder function after abdominoperineal resection may not occur for 3 months postsurgery. In general, prostatectomy was not required sooner. The late development of symptoms of bladder neck obstruction after abdominoperineal resection was often the first sign of recurrence of cancer. These patients did poorly after prostatectomy. As a general rule, continued difficulty in urination after an abdominoperineal resection in men proved to be a symptom that required evaluation for persistent pelvic cancer.

On the basis of preoperative symptoms, prediction of patients who would require prostatectomy postoperatively was not possible. Were it possible, these cases might benefit from a prostatectomy at the time of abdominoperineal resection. In some cases, major urinary symptoms associated with symptoms of rectal cancer were relieved by abdominoperineal resection.

Table 21–4. **URINARY TRACT INFECTIONS IN PATIENTS WITHOUT POSTOPERATIVE OBSTRUCTIVE URINARY SYMPTOMS***

Occurrence of Postoperative Infection	No. of Patients
1st month	17
2nd to 6th month	4
6th month to 3 years	4
3 years +	4†
No occurrence (no signs of infection)	106
Total	123

*Adapted Glass RL, Spratt JS: Urinary complications after abdominoperineal resection of the rectum in men. Am Surg 34:238–241, 1968.

†Two of these patients died as a result of urinary infections.

Urinary tract infections uniformly followed the use of an indwelling catheter and were difficult to eradicate. When return of function is prolonged, consideration should be given to managing these cases as neurogenic bladders are managed, i.e., with intermittent catheterization. Patients with urinary tract infection persisting after abdominoperineal resection should be completely examined and treated aggressively and persistently. Long-term management of these patients must include evaluation for asymptomatic pyuria to help reduce the problems of chronic urinary tract infections in an aging population.

The preoperative and intraoperative evaluations of the entire urinary tract are integral parts of colorectal and anal cancer management. Contiguous involvement of the urinary tract by these cancers is commonplace, and the surgeon must be prepared to resect, reconstruct, and rehabilitate as the nature of the problem dictates. Operations occasionally required include en bloc nephrectomies, segmental ureterectomies, partial to total cystectomies, prostatectomies, urethrectomies and combinations thereof. Reconstructive operations vary according to the type of resection performed, from the simplest procedures to the most complex, e.g., ileoneocystostomies. The preparative evaluation of the urinary tract should include biochemical assays of urinary tract function, diagnosis and treatment of urinary tract infections, intravenous pyelograms and, when indicated, transurethral cystoscopy, assessment of bladder function, and cystograms. Particular attention to the size and consistency of the prostate is always required. Prostatic cancers can present in the rectum, mimicking rectal cancers, and primary rectal cancers can invade the prostate and bladder.

OBSTRUCTING COLORECTAL CARCINOMA

The colorectal cancers that present with obstruction create unique problems in management and have grave implications for prognosis (Ragland et al., 1971). Colorectal cancer is the most common cause of obstruction of the large intestine (Hickey and Hyde, 1965; Ulin and Ehrlich, 1962). The prognosis of patients with obstructing colorectal carcinoma is worse than for patients with nonobstructing lesions. This is true even after the patients have survived resection of the obstructing carcinoma (Hickey and Hyde, 1965; Ulin and Ehrlich, 1962; Chang and Burnett, 1962; Floyd and Cohn, 1967; Loefler and Hafner, 1964; Minster, 1964; Nickell and Dockerty, 1948; Thompson and Mark, 1968; Wilder et al., 1961). A study by Ragland and associates (1971) was undertaken in an effort to define cancer-host-treatment factors associated with poor prognosis.

Among the colorectal carcinomas reported in detail (Spratt and Spjut, 1967), 227 (20 percent) were obstructing lesions. This group was further subdivided according to the degree of obstruction. The patient was considered partially obstructed if he was still passing stool or flatus or had gas distal to the area of obstruction on the roentgenogram. Roentgenographic observation of fecal stasis, bowel distention, or failure to canalize the tumor site on barium contrast study was not considered adequate evidence of complete obstruction. One hundred sixteen patients (10.2 percent) were considered partially obstructed and the remaining 111 (9.8 percent) were considered completely obstructed. However, of this 111, 38 patients had complete obstruction diagnosed at another hospital, and the bowel had been decompressed by various means before the patient was transferred. The study focused on the 73 patients who had complete obstruction and whose entire course of therapy was carried out at the same hospital. Clinical reports of these patients were reviewed, and a 100 percent follow-up evaluation was obtained.

In this series, 59 percent of the patients were males. The peak age at the time of obstruction was in the eighth decade, with 75 percent of the patients being older than 60 years of age. Twelve percent were below the age of 50. Thus, these cancers occurred primarily in an elderly population. Segments of the colon most frequently involved were the rectum and sigmoid, with the cecum being the third most frequent site.

The most frequent symptom was pain, followed by constipation, weight loss, and mild bleeding. Only one patient in the group had obstruction as the first symptom. The average duration of symptoms was 7 months. However, 37 percent had symptoms of less than 6 months' duration, and 20 percent had symptoms for more than 20 months prior to obstruction.

Surgery was performed with the intent to palliate in 36 patients (49.4 percent) and with the intent to cure in 35 patients (47.8 percent). Two patients died before surgery could be performed. Twenty-eight patients had colostomy alone, and 28 had an initial decompressive colostomy followed by subsequent resection. Fourteen patients had primary resection (Table 21–5). One patient received only celiotomy and biopsy. Sixty-one of the 73 patients with total obstruction required emergency surgery for decompression, whereas 11 patients were decompressed nonoperatively with a long intestinal tube. One patient died prior to any treatment.

The complication rate in the small number of patients who were decompressed by nonoperative means and subsequently underwent

Table 21–5. **RESULTS OF PRIMARY RESECTION FOR TREATMENT OF COMPLETE OBSTRUCTION***

Procedure	No. of Patients	Anastomotic Complication	Other Complication
Right colectomy	4	1	1
Transverse colectomy	1	0	1
Abdominoperineal resection	4	0	2
Hartmann's procedure	2	0	0
Mikulicz or obstructive resection	2	0	0
Other	1	0	0
Total	14	1	4

*Adapted from Ragland JJ, Londe AM, Spratt JS Jr: Correlation of the prognosis of obstructing colorectal carcinoma with clinical and pathologic variables. Am J Surg 12:552–556, 1971.

surgery was approximately equal (41 percent) to that of patients requiring emergency surgery for decompression (45.5 percent). Nearly one half the patients (48 percent) had obstruction for 3 days or less, and 90 percent had obstruction less than 10 days before treatment. The surgical complication rate was 34.3 percent in those with obstruction for 3 days or less as compared with 50 percent in those in whom the duration of obstruction was greater than 3 days. The complication rate produced in those patients who had primary resection was not significantly different from that produced in those who had colostomy followed by resection. The largest number of complications occurred in those patients who had colostomy only. The resection of a second organ did not increase the complication rate significantly. The rate was 44.4 percent in those who had a second organ resected and 42.8 percent in those who had no additional organ resected.

Complications were related to the extent of the tumor as correlated by the feasibility of a palliative resection only or colostomy. Complications could also be related to age. There were 39 patients under 70 years of age and 34 patients over 70. In the group over 70 years of age, the complication rate was 47 percent, whereas in the group under 70, the complication rate was 38.4 percent. Fatal complications were highest in those patients with angina pectoris, previous myocardial infarction, hypertension, cardiac decompensation, and pulmonary disease.

Operative mortality, meaning death from any cause within 30 days after operation, was highest in the group of patients who had colostomy only (28.6 percent). Operative mortality was 14.3 percent in those who had a colostomy followed later by resection, and 7.1 percent in the group that had primary resection.

Each group consisted of selected cases in which the condition of the patient and the extent of the tumor dictated the treatment. The patients who had only a colostomy had the most extensive disease or were in the poorest condition. Those who had colostomy followed by resection had less extensive disease. Primary resection was performed in those patients who were in satisfactory condition and whose bowel was not dilated to the point of vascular compromise.

The overall 5-year survival rate in this series was 15.1 percent. There was a 34.4 percent 5-year survival rate in those who had a resection thought to leave no gross residual cancer. None of those undergoing a palliative operation survived more than 3 years, and 31 of 35 died in the first year.

The incidence of obstruction in this series in all cases of cancer of the colon was 20 percent. This is nearly the same as that of other large series (Chang and Burnett, 1962; Floyd and Cohn, 1967; Loefler and Hafner, 1964; Minster, 1964; Fletcher et al., 1963).

Pain, constipation, weight loss, and bleeding were common symptoms in reported series of patients with obstructing or nonobstructing tumors of the colon, although the place of each in the order of frequency varied from series to series (Chang and Burnett, 1962; Floyd and Cohn, 1967; Minster, 1964; Fletcher et al., 1963; Botsford et al., 1965). The series of Ragland and associates (1971) of patients with totally obstructing tumors also had a sex ratio and age distribution that were similar to those found in series that contained patients with both obstructing and nonobstructing tumors (Spratt and Spjut, 1967; Fletcher et al., 1963). Likewise, in cases of totally obstructing tumors, the location of the tumors in the large bowel and the incidence of symptoms were similar to those in cases of nonobstructing tumors.

Ragland and associates (1971) included only patients with complete obstruction of the large bowel in their series. With this criterion for selection, it was found that the overall 5-year survival rate was only 15.5 percent. This compared well with an 11 percent 5-year survival rate reported by Loefler and Hafner (1964), who used a similar criterion. In 1962, Chang and Burnett reported a 19 percent 5-year survival rate in a series of patients with completely obstructing tumors of the colon. The 5-year survival rate in a group of patients with nonobstructed tumors was reported by Minster (1964) to be 53 percent. Others have noted this poorer prognosis in patients with obstructing carcinomas (Hickey and Hyde, 1965; Ulin and Ehrlich, 1962; Floyd and Cohn, 1967; Loefler and Hafner, 1964; Nickell and Dockerty, 1948; Thompson and Mark, 1968; Wilder et al., 1961).

Effect of Obstruction and Other Tumor Characteristics on Prognosis

In this study (Ragland et al., 1971), several characteristics were associated with a poor prognosis. These included a low rate of resectability, presence of lymph node metastasis, extension of tumor into an adjacent organ, unfavorable marginal characteristics, and a brief duration of symptoms.

The resectability of these obstructing carcinomas was only 57.5 percent, whereas in a previous review of all colorectal carcinomas at the same hospital, the resectability for the entire series was 73.3 percent (Spratt and Spjut, 1967).

The 5-year survival also was affected by the number of positive lymph nodes. Of 32 patients who had resection, 15 had lymph node metastasis (47 percent). This percentage of lymph node involvement is nearly the same as that reported in the total series of colorectal carcinomas (Spratt and Spjut, 1967). However, the involvement of lymph nodes as well as the presence of an obstructive cancer was an ominous sign. When all lymph nodes were negative, the 5-year survival rate was 58.8 percent in resected cases. With one to five positive nodes, the 5-year survival rate dropped to 16.7 percent. No patients with obstructing cancers and six or more lymph nodes containing metastases survived for 5 years. In the total series with five or fewer nodes involved, the survival rate was 24.1 percent, and with six to ten nodes involved, 8.6 percent. Only when 16 or more nodes were involved did all patients die. This suggests that tumors with proven ability for metastasizing that have the additional characteristic of being obstructive are very lethal.

When tumor was shown microscopically to extend into an adjacent organ, there were no 5-year survivors in the group of patients with completely obstructing colorectal carcinomas. In the absence of complete obstruction with proven tumor invasion, a 5-year survival of 20 percent was obtained by resecting adjacent organs en bloc (Spratt and Spjut, 1967). Inflammatory adhesion does not carry the same poor prognosis as actual tumor invasion; this was demonstrated by several patients in the series. Since tumor invasion and inflammatory adhesion frequently cannot be differentiated clinically, en bloc resection of tissues and organs adherent to tumor is still desirable.

Surgical pathologists at the institution where the study was conducted customarily recorded certain tumor characteristics that were correlated with prognosis (Spratt and Spjut, 1967). When the entire margin of the lesion appeared to be infiltrating normal tissue, the prognosis was significantly worse than when there was a well-circumscribed, "pushing" margin or mixed margin. Of the resected cases in the series of Ragland and associates (1971) in which marginal characteristics were determinable, 78.3 percent were infiltrating, 13.5 percent were mixed infiltrating and pushing, and 8.2 percent were pushing. This compared with 64 percent infiltrating, 19.1 percent mixed, and 12.7 percent pushing in the previously reported total series of colorectal carcinomas (Spratt and Spjut, 1967). Among the 5-year survivors having obstructing cancers that were resected, 72.7 percent had infiltrating tumor margins, 18.3 percent had mixed infiltrating and pushing margins, and 9.1 percent had pushing margins. There was a 27.6 percent 5-year survival rate for patients with obstructing cancers with infiltrating margins compared with a 40 percent 5-year survival rate for those with cancer with mixed pushing and infiltrating margins; there was a 33.3 percent survival rate for those with cancer with pushing margins only.

The duration of symptoms before complete obstruction and celiotomy had some prognostic significance. Thirty-seven percent had symptoms of less than 6 months' duration. In the group with a shorter interval of symptoms, only 11.1 percent survived 5 years compared with a 25 percent 5-year survival rate in the group of patients who had symptoms for more than 20 months before obstruction. In a large series of patients with colon cancers reported from Massachusetts General Hospital in 1962 (Welch and Burke, 1962), those who entered the hospital after a brief period of symptoms also had a poorer prognosis. This paradoxical, but consistent, observation is discussed in greater detail in Chapters Two and Ten.

The low percentage of resectability, in the presence of a high percentage of cases with a brief duration of symptoms, suggests that obstructing colorectal carcinomas are among the more virulent or malignant variants of colon and rectal carcinomas. This is further substantiated by the fact that a large percentage of these cases have unfavorable marginal characteristics. These, plus the observation that obstruction may be associated with widespread dissemination, may account for the poorer prognosis associated with obstructing colorectal carcinoma.

In those completely obstructing tumors available for pathologic study, in all cases, the margin of the tumor extended into the outer layer of muscle of the bowel wall. The importance of the outer (longitudinal) layer for normal intestinal transit was emphasized by Schiller and associates (1967) in experiments in which the other layer was stripped away. They found that with the outer layer removed, a sphincter was produced, and the outer layer was identified as the "opening component." In light of these studies, invasion of the outer layer of muscle by carcinoma with subsequent loss of the "opening component" might be important in the development of complete obstruction.

Primary Resection of Obstructing Lesions

Primary resections of obstructing lesions of the colon are fraught with danger. The morbidity and mortality of primary resection should decrease with the availability of better preoperative and supportive measures; improved techniques in anesthesia; the avoidance of procedures that include a primary anastomosis; and the judicious use of proper fluids, antibiotics, the long intestinal tube, aseptic anastomosis, and delayed wound closure. This was the experience of Ragland and associates (1971) in the few patients in whom primary resection was performed. This experience in no way confirms primary resection to be the procedure of choice, only that it be considered more often in carefully selected cases.

Patients with obstructing colorectal carcinomas have a poor prognosis, which may be due to the fact that the more malignant variants of colorectal carcinoma lead to obstruction. Extension of neoplasm into the outer layer of intestinal musculature is postulated to be important in the development of complete obstruction. In carefully selected cases, primary resection was shown to be a worthwhile procedure and to have no adverse effects on morbidity or mortality.

In the presence of an obstructing cancer, the passing of a long tube past the pylorus to decompress an obstructed small intestine can be expedited by attaching it to a flexible duodenoscope. It can then be delivered directly to the jejunum. With the tube in the jejunum, safe decompression without contamination can be obtained before operation. Although this will not ensure decompression of the proximal colon in the presence of a competent ileocecal valve, it has numerous other benefits, such as easier exposure and wound closure, reduced risk of intraoperative perforation, enhanced blood flow to a distended bowel, reduced risk of aspiration, and continued postoperative decompression.

ADENOCARCINOMA OF THE LARGE INTESTINE AND RECTUM WITH PERFORATION OR INTERNAL FISTULAS

Until the early 1960s, a spontaneously perforated adenocarcinoma of the large intestine was generally regarded as ensuring an ominous prognosis. This attitude was based almost entirely on the infrequent occurrence of this complication in the individual surgeon's experience. Detailed reports in the literature of groups of such cases were infrequent. To ascertain the validity of this pessimistic attitude, a review was made of all patients with perforated carcinoma of the large intestine and rectum admitted to Ellis Fischel State Cancer Hospital over a 21-year period (Sperling et al., 1963).

Fourteen cancers that had perforated into the free peritoneal cavity and four rectal cancers that had perforated into the perirectal fat with abscess formation were studied. Cancers invading adjacent organs without producing peritoneal soilage or abscess formation were excluded. Review of the histopathology of all included cases confirmed the gross impression of perforation with extravasation of luminal contents into the free peritoneal cavity or perirectal fat. The 18 perforated cancers occurred among 1137 consecutive cancers of the large intestine and rectum treated at the Ellis Fischel State Cancer Hospital between 1940 and 1961, providing an incidence of 1.6 percent. The follow-up after treatment was 100 percent. The age and sex of the patient, anatomic distribution, and pathologic characteristics of the cancer, diagnostic and surgical procedures, operative mortality, and host survival data were reported on these 18 cases. No significant peculiarities of these perforating cancers were evident in the distributions according to age and sex of host or the anatomic segment of colon that contained the cancer.

Some pathologic characteristics were distributed differently from those recorded for the parent series. Higher grade carcinomas with infiltrating margins were the predominant variant (Table 21–6). The infiltrating cancers tended to penetrate all layers of the intestinal wall while the primary cancers were small (Spratt and Ackerman, 1962). Their ulcerodestructive characteristics were associated with the presence of perforation.

A surprising characteristic was the tendency of these cancers to be localized, with neither regional lymph node nor distant metastases being present. This favorable observation was reflected in the equally favorable host survival rates following resection (Table 21–7).

All 18 patients presented with the signs and symptoms of sepsis. In the preoperative evaluation, 14 patients were examined by barium enema study. In each case, the radiologist filled the colon under fluoroscopic control only to the lower margin of the cancer. As a result of

Table 21–6. **PATHOLOGIC CHARACTERISTICS OF PERFORATED CARCINOMAS OF THE LARGE INTESTINE AND RECTUM***

Tumor Grade	No. of Tumors
Well differentiated (grade 1)	1
Poorly differentiated (grade 2)	14
Undifferentiated (grade 3)	1
Mucinous	1
Not determinable	1
Total	18
Tumor Margin	**No. of Tumors**
Infiltrating margin	15
Circumscribed or pushing margin	1
Marginal characteristics indeterminable	2
Total	18
Gross Characteristics	
Entire circumference of the intestine involved with cancer	11 of 18 (61%)
Mean tumor length	5 cm.
Secondary external fistula formation	4 of 18 (22%)
Mesenteric Lymph Node Metastases	**No. of Cases**
Metastases present	5
Metastases absent	11
Status of lymph node metastases not determined	2
Total	18
Distant Metastases	**No. of Cases**
None discovered	15
Presence confirmed	2
Indeterminable	2
Total	19

*Adapted from Sperling D, Spratt JS Jr, Carnes VM: Adenocarcinoma of the large intestine with perforation. Mo Med 60:1104–1107, 1963.

this conservative approach, barium was not extravasated into the free peritoneal cavity in any of these cases. Barium extravasation was not seen on any of the roentgenograms.

A few barium particles were observed microscopically in the perforations and meat and vegetable fibers were also present extraluminally. Consequently, in the presence of perforation from a colonic cancer, filling of the colon with barium contrast medium under cautious fluoroscopic control may be employed, when needed, to locate the diseased segment without creating a source of morbidity from barium soilage of an infected peritoneal cavity.

The surgical therapy for these carcinomas was variable (Table 21–8). Nine perforations were treated primarily by some form of diverting colostomy proximal to the perforation. Four of these patients were never in condition for a subsequent surgical procedure and died within 30 days following the diverting procedure. Four patients had subsequent resections, and two of these were alive and apparently free of cancer 36 and 130 months after the original resection. The ninth patient died of cancer 5 months after the diversion.

In the operative notes of two of the 18 cases, the surgeon stated positively that he had performed a "conservative" surgical procedure because he believed that no patient having a perforation of a colonic cancer was ever cured of cancer by surgical resection. Both of these patients died of their cancer. The belief that perforation of a colon cancer produced an incurable situation was the prevalent clinical opinion before Donaldson's report of 1958, although earlier reports from the Ellis Fischel State Cancer Hospital had shown the efficacy of en bloc resection of fistulas arising from colonic cancers (Sugarbaker, 1946; Sugarbaker and Wiley, 1950). The survival data in Table 21–7 following the resection of perforated cancers shows the importance of the definitive resection of the perforated cancer as soon as the patient's condition permitted. When a preliminary diversion was required, complete diversion of the colon was required. A proximal colostomy totally diverting the fecal stream was essential. Without complete diversion, continued peritoneal soilage through the perforation occurred. The only certain method of stopping peritoneal soilage at once was to resect or exteriorize the perforated cancer.

The survival data on the case material showed that patient survival after perforation through a colonic or rectal cancer was no worse than the gross 32 percent 5-year survival rate for all patients with colonic cancers and the 66 percent survival rate for all patients with resectable colonic cancers reported by Gilbertsen (1959). A 76.9 percent (40 of 52) hospital mortality rate occurred in Goliger and Smiddy's (1957) series when suture closure of perforations and colostomy were employed. The hospital mortality rate was 23.8 percent (five deaths among 21 patients) when primary resection was employed. Madden and Tan (1961) also showed the importance of definitive resection in the treatment of perforated colon cancers and paraphrased the old philosophy, "the patient was too ill to withstand other than the minimum emergency surgical procedures," to read "the patient was too ill to withstand other than a primary resection." As previously stated, the report by Donaldson (1958) supported the point of view that the presence of perforation was no more ominous than the

Table 21–7. **SURVIVAL OF PATIENTS WITH PERFORATED CARCINOMAS OF THE LARGE INTESTINE AND RECTUM***

Follow-up Interval (Years)	*Patients at Risk*	*Dead*	*Withdrawn From Follow-up Alive*	*Annual Survival*	*Accumulative Survival Rate*
All Patients Regardless of Therapy					
0–1	18	5	0	72.2	72.2
1–2	13	0	0	100.0	72.2
2–3	13	2	2	77.7	61.1
3–4	9	2	2	77.7	47.5
4–5	5	0	0	100.0	47.5
All Patients Undergoing a Primary or Staged Resection of the Perforated Cancer					
Follow-up Interval (Years)	*Patients at Risk*	*Dead*	*Withdrawn From Follow-up Alive*	*Annual Survival*	*Accumulative Survival Rate*
0–1	13	0	0	100.0	100.0
1–2	13	0	0	100.0	100.0
2–3	13	2	2	84.6	84.6
3–4	9	2	2	77.7	65.7
4–5	5	0	0	100.0	65.7

*Adapted from Sperling D, Spratt JS Jr, Carnes VM: Adenocarcinoma of the large intestine with perforation. Mo Med 60:1104–1107, 1963.

presence of the cancer alone, providing that definitive resective therapy was carried out as soon as possible.

Possibly the failure of extensive peritoneal and implantation metastases to develop after the perforation of colonic and rectal cancers was attributable to the presence of infection. Both Vink (1954) and Cohn and Atik (1960) showed in rabbits that "there is an increased danger in implanting tumor in a 'sterilized' bowel as compared to an unclean one." The presence of greater numbers of bacteria within the colons of rabbits that had received no preoperative antimicrobial drugs was associated with a significant reduction in the number of successful implants of Brown-Pearce carcinomas in lines of intestinal anastomosis compared with rabbits that had received these drugs. The cancer implant in the rabbit colon seemed less likely to survive and grow in a dirty wound than in a clean one, and the same generalization might conceivably apply to perforated cancers of the human colon and rectum. Certainly, in this study, the mechanical dissemination of cancer upon the peritoneal surface occurred with the perforations, and the seeds for the development of metastatic implants were therefore available.

The conclusion was that on the basis of the relationships between survival, pathologic characteristics, and therapeutic approach, tumor removal, performed at the earliest time that the patient could tolerate resective surgery, was necessary for optimal results with perforated cancers. Frequently resectability was limited by the patient's ability to survive

Table 21–8. **MORTALITY OF PATIENT WITH PERFORATED CARCINOMA ACCORDING TO SURGICAL PROCEDURE***

Surgical Procedure	**No. of Patients**	**Death Within 30 Days of Surgical Operation**
Diversion only	4	4
Diversion and resection (staged)	4	0
Resection and primary anastomosis	3	0
Diversion and closure perforation	1	0
Abdominoperineal resection	4	0
Hartmann's procedure	1	0
Modified pelvic exenteration	1	0
Total	18	4

*Adapted from Sperling D, Spratt JS Jr, Carnes VM: Adenocarcinoma of the large intestine with perforation. Mo Med 60:1104–1107, 1963.
†Death occurring within 30 days of operation.

the sepsis of the perforation, colostomy, and drainage, but this should not deter the surgeon from completing standard therapy whenever possible. Unwarranted pessimism regarding perforated cancers of the large intestine and rectum does not justify compromised surgical therapy.

In other reviews of the management of free intraperitoneal perforations, Muller (1969) concurred that primary resection was the treatment of choice.

PERFORATIONS OF CANCERS INTO PARACOLONIC SPACES

Perforations may also occur from all segments of the colon into adjacent tissues without entering the free peritoneum. Contiguous abscesses in various paracolonic spaces occur. As a consequence, the existence of a perforated colorectal cancer must always be considered in the differential diagnosis when evaluating patients with unusual abscesses. As a general rule, these are best managed, as is cancer perforating into the free peritoneal cavity, by resection of the cancer, and, when possible, its contiguous abscess. Freeman and associates (1979) provide a review with additional case reports reaffirming these surgical principles.

The cancers may also form a wide assortment of internal fistulas—gallbladder, stomach, small intestines, and urinary tract. No controlled data exist on these complicated surgical problems, but certain general principles do appear to be associated with better results. In general, if the area of involvement can be resected, resection should be done. Anastomoses frequently fail in the presence of sepsis, abscess formation, or obstruction with dilatation of bowel. In these situations, exteriorization of the ends of bowel, exteriorization of tenuous anastomoses, and proximal diversion (complete) may all be required in various circumstances. The second generalization is to recall that in comparing the results of single staged procedures with those of multiple staged procedures, the *accumulation* of morbidity and mortality of the multiple stages must be weighed against that of single staged procedures. Each stage imposes additional physiologic stress on the patient. Therefore, in between each stage of multistaged procedures, vigorous supportive care including hyperalimentation may be essential to get the patient in optimum condition for the next stage.

LOCALLY ADVANCED CANCERS OF THE RECTUM OR ANUS

An occasional cancer of the lower rectum or anal area and lower sacral chordomas present with posterior fixation to the lower sacrum, which requires modification of the posterior and perineal dissection in order to encompass the cancer. In 1981, Wanebo and Marcove reported on an approach to some of these cases, with or without adjuvant chemotherapy or radiation therapy. Computerized transaxial tomography has proved very helpful in delineating the extent of these neoplasms before surgery. The intra-abdominal part of the dissection is similar to that reported for a total or posterior pelvic exenteration (Spratt et al., 1973). The dissection must proceed posteriorly to below the S2 level. The abdomen is then closed and the patient is repositioned in the prone position. A midline incision is made that begins in the midsacrum and extends down to encircle the gluteal fold. Flaps are created that expose the gluteus maximus. The sciatic nerve is identified and looped with a Penrose drain, since the nerve passes between the ischial tuberosity and the femoral trochanter. The sacrotuberous and sacrospinous ligaments are next transected. The gluteal muscle is detached from the sacrum to above the point of transection of the sacrum. By placing a finger below the piriform muscle but over the sciatic nerve and through the sciatic notch (Fig. 21–1), one can break through the facia and feel the tumor margin adherent to the sacrum. This examination determines the level at which the sacrum should be transected. A laminectomy is done next at the level of sacral transection, protecting all possible nerve roots. The dural sac is ligated through the laminectomy. The sacrum is then divided and the entire specimen removed. Sliding pedicles then permit closure. Wanebo and Marcove (1981) have successfully carried out this approach for selected tumors, even those persistent after administration of as much as 9000 rad.

Rarely, advanced local cancers can invade the musculoskeletal pelvis in such a manner as to require en bloc hemopelvectomy. Techniques for this operation have been reported previously (Spratt et al., 1973).

COLONIC ADENOCARCINOMAS IN PATIENTS WITH URETEROSIGMOIDOSTOMIES

The time interval between the performance of ureterosigmoidostomies and the appearance

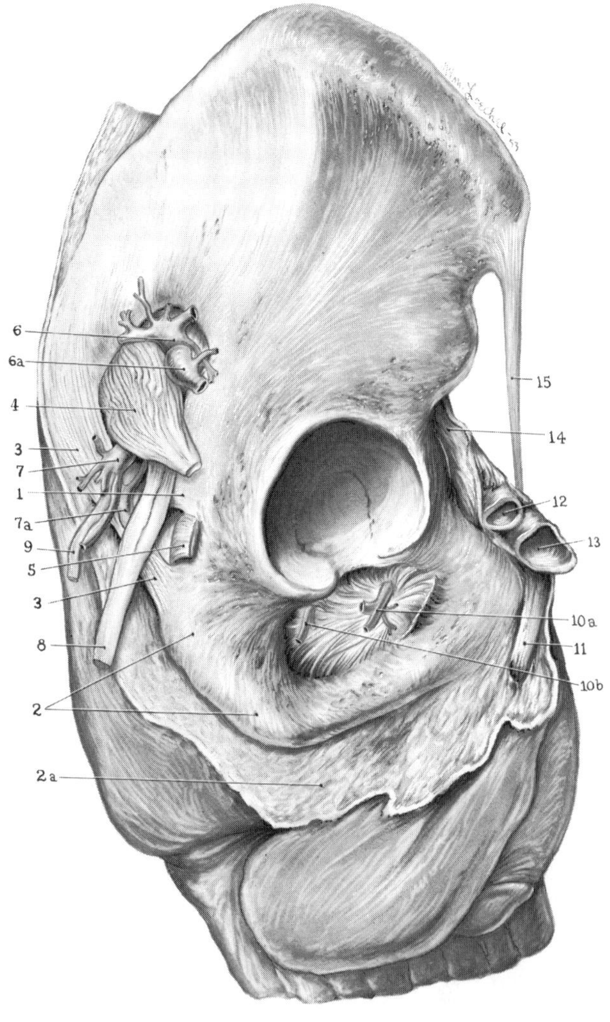

Figure 21–1. 1, Sacrospinous ligament; 2, superior ramus of ischium; 3, sacrotuberous ligament; 4, piriform muscle; 5, internal obturator muscle; 6, superior gluteal artery; 6a, superior gluteal vein; 7, inferior gluteal artery; 7a, inferior gluteal vein; 8, sciatic nerve; 9, posterior femoral cutaneous nerve; 10a, anterior ramus of obturator artery; 10b, posterior ramus of obturator artery; 11, spermatic cord; 12, femoral artery; 13, femoral vein; 14, pectineal ligament; 15, inguinal ligament. (From Spratt JS Jr, Butcher HR Jr, Bricker EM: Exenterative Surgery of the Pelvis. Philadelphia, WB Saunders Company, 1973.)

of cancers at the site of anastomoses is so great that these cancers are still appearing, even though the use of this operation is now infrequent. Urdaneta and associates (1966) estimated the lifetime risk for cancers of these anastomoses to be about 500-fold greater for patients who underwent ureterosigmoidostomies than for the normal population. In contrast, cancers have not been reported at ureteroileal anastomoses.

By 1979, Labow and associates reported the 31st and 32nd of colonic adenocarcinomas in patients with ureterosigmoidostomies. The cancer appeared 17 and 41 years, respectively, after the anastomoses were performed. Warren and associates (1980) reported an interval of 49 years between diversion and cancer.

Leadbetter and associates (1979) reviewed 45 cases from the literature and added two of their own. Time intervals between diversion and the appearance of cancer ranged from 6 to 50 years. When implants were performed after age 40, the mean lag time was 8.7 years. Before age 40, the lag time was 21.4 years. Actually, these gross figures provide limited insight into the true *rate* for the appearance of cancers. To calculate that, the age specific number of person-years of follow-up accumulating after diversion would have to be tabulated. Then the cancers could be placed in the numerator to calculate the age-specific incidence rate per person-year of postdiversion follow-up. An interval would probably exist beyond which the risk of cancer exceeded the risk of reoperation. At reoperation before cancer develops, both the most distal ureter and the contiguously involved colon must be excised.

In these cases, reported by Leadbetter and associates (1979), no reports of carcinogen in the urine could be found. However, a colonic mucosa contiguous with the anastomosis first exhibits hyperplasia then atrophy. As discussed under the etiology of colonic cancers, the "Two Hit Theory" is a plausible explanation of the cause of the adenocarcinomas. The first hit induces the cancerous changes in the target cells, and almost any factor can serve as a promoter that stimulates hyperplasia. The urine is probably the promoter. The uretero-ileal anastomosis plus urine might provide the "hit two" or promotional phase of carcinogenesis, promoting a second primary cancer from a colonic mucosa already affected by a "hit one" carcinogen.

TOTAL PARENTERAL NUTRITION

The survival value, feasibility cost, and perhaps even ethics of total parenteral nutrition of the patient with advanced colon cancer is an area that merits further study. In the presence of complications after treatment, total parenteral nutrition (TPN) is definitely justified, particularly when prognosis after cancer management might be favorable.

In the absence of a chemotherapeutic agent capable of providing a high probability of tumor response, justification of TPN to improve a patient's tolerance to chemotherapy is a considerably more difficult issue to address.

A useful study by Nixon and associates (1981) addresses the value of TPN in patients with advanced colon cancer. These investigators randomly selected 50 patients to receive either chemotherapy alone or the same drugs following TPN for 14 days before drug treatment and for variable periods thereafter. The overall survival rate was significantly *decreased* in the TPN patients ($p < 0.03$). The survival rate was significantly decreased in the TPN patients who had lost the *least* percentage of premorbid weight (0 to 6 percent) (66 vs. 398 days, $p < 0.02$). All males receiving TPN lived for shorter periods (61 vs. 209 days, $p < 0.03$). TPN did not increase survival in any subcategory. The authors concluded that not only did TPN not prolong median survival in any category, it may have shortened duration of survival in males and in patients who had not experienced a weight loss.

Controlled studies such as these help clarify a very complicated issue. The real possibility exists that the cancer may benefit preferentially over the host from TPN. The growth of cancers are slowed in the presence of starvation, and the belief that cancer cachexia is a host defense mechanism can be argued. For this reason, extensive review of the role TPN may have in colon cancer treatment has been withheld here. There may be other reasons for its use, but enhanced survival in the presence of advanced colorectal cancers has not yet been proved to be one of these reasons.

References

Beeson PB: The case against the catheter. Am J Med 24:1–3, 1958.

Botsford TW, Aliapoulios MA, Curtis LE: Results of treatment of colorectal cancer at the Peter Bent Brigham Hospital. Am J Surg 109:566–571, 1965.

Campbell EW, Gislason GJ: Urologic invalidism following abdominoperineal rectosigmoidectomy. Ann Surg 132:85–93, 1950.

Chang WY, Burnett WE : Complete colonic obstruction due to adenocarcinoma. Surg Gynecol Obstet 114:353–356, 1962.

Cohn I Jr, Atik M: The influence of antibiotics on the spread of tumors of the colon: an experimental study. Ann Surg 151:917–929, 1960.

Cook EN, Ten Cate HW, Potter WM: Urinary retention following operations on the bowel. J Urol 89:225–259, 1963.

Cunningham EF Jr, Young GA: Bladder dysfunction following abdominoperineal resection. Am Surg 28:56–58, 1962.

Donaldson GA: The management of perforated carcinoma of the colon. N Engl J Med 258:201–207, 1958.

Fletcher WS, Krippaehne WW, Harcwick CE, Dunphy JE: Carcinoma of the colon and rectum. Results of treatment in a county hospital population. Am J Surg 105:117–125, 1963.

Floyd CE, Cohn I Jr: Obstruction in cancer of the colon. Ann Surg 165:721–731, 1967.

Freeman HP, Oluwole SF, Granepola GAP: Unusual presentations of carcinoma of the right colon. Cancer 44:1533–1537, 1979.

Gilbertson VA: Adenocarcinoma of the large bowel. 1340 cases with 100 percent follow-up. Surgery 46:1027–1042, 1959.

Glass RL, Spratt JS: Urinary complications after abdominoperineal resection of the rectum in men. Am Surg 34:238–241, 1968.

Goliger JC, Smiddy FG: The treatment of acute obstruction or perforation with carcinoma of the colon and rectum. Br J Surg 45:270–274, 1957.

Hickey RC, Hyde HP: Neoplastic obstruction of the large bowel. Surg Clin North Am 45:1157–1163, 1965.

Johnson FW, Goodale RL, Leonard AS, Varco RL: Rapid long tube intubation of the jejunum by a new endoscopic device. Am J Surg 131:91–93, 1976.

Labow SB, Hoexter B, Walrath DC: Colon adenocarcinomas in patients with uterosigmoidostomies. Dis Colon Rectum 22:157–158, 1979.

Leadbetter GW Jr, Leadbetter WF: A new approach to the problem of urinary retention following abdominoperineal resection for carcinoma of the rectum. Surg Gynecol Obstet 107:333–338, 1958.

Leadbetter GW Jr, Zickerman P, Pierce E: Ureterosigmoidostomy and carcinoma of the colon. J Urol 121:732–735, 1979.

Levin J: The incidence and prevention of infection after urethral catheterization. Ann Intern Med 60:914–922, 1964.

Loefler I, Hafner CD: Survival rate in obstructing carcinoma of colon. Arch Surg 89:716–718, 1964.

McCrea LE, Kimmel DL: New concept of vesical innervation to bladder management following abdominoperineal proctosigmoidectomy. Arch Surg 66:84–93, 1953.

Madden JL, Tan PY: Primary resection and anastomosis in the treatment of perforated lesions of the colon, with abscess or diffusing peritonitis. Surg Gynecol Obstet 113:646–650, 1961.

Marshall VF, Pollack RS, Miller C: Observations on urinary dysfunction after excision of rectum. J Urol 55:409–416,1946.

Minster JJ: Comparison of obstructing and nonobstructing carcinoma of the colon. Cancer 17:242–247, 1964.

Muller CA: A plea for primary hemicolectomy in perforated cancer of the right colon. Int Surg 52:234–247, 1969.

Nickell DF, Dockerty MB: Five year survival rate in cases of completely obstructing annular carcinoma of descending colon and sigmoid; pathologic study. Surg Gynecol Obstet 87:519–524, 1948.

Nixon DW, Lawson DH, Kutner MH, et al: Effect of total parenteral nutrition on survival in advanced colon cancer. Cancer Detect Prev 4:421–427, 1981.

Ragland JJ, Londe AM, Spratt JS Jr: Correlation of the prognosis of obstructing colorectal carcinoma with clinical and pathologic variables. Am J Surg 121:552–556, 1971.

Schiller WR, DiDio LJA, Anderson MC: Production of the large intestine with perforation. Mo Med 60:1104–1107, 1967.

Sperling D, Spratt JS Jr, Carnes VM: Adenocarcinoma of the large intestine with perforation. Mo Med 60:1104–1107, 1963.

Spratt JS Jr, Ackerman LV: Small primary adenocarcinomas of the colon and rectum. JAMA 179:337–346, 1962.

Spratt JS Jr, Butcher HR, Bricker EM: Exenterative surgery of the pelvis. Major Probl Clin Surg 12:1–171, 1973.

Spratt JS Jr, Spjut HJ: Prevalence and prognosis of individual clinical and pathologic variables associated with colorectal carcinoma. Cancer 20:1976–1985, 1967.

Sugarbaker ED: Coincident removal of additional structures in resections for carcinoma of colon and rectum. Ann Surg 123:1036–1046, 1946.

Sugarbaker ED, Wiley HM: Significance of fixation in operable carcinoma of the large bowel. Surgery 27:343–347, 1950.

Thompson RW, Mark JB: Obstructing adenocarcinoma of the right side of the colon. Arch Surg 96:100–103, 1968.

Ulin AW, Ehrlich EW: Current views related to management of large bowel obstruction caused by carcinoma of the colon. Am J Surg 104:463–467, 1962.

Urdaneta FF, Duffell D, Creevy CD, Aust JB: Late development of primary carcinoma of the colon following ureterosigmoidostomy: Report of three cases and literature review. Ann Surg 164:503–513, 1966.

Vink M: Local recurrence of cancer in large bowel: Role of implantation metastases and bowel disinfection. Br J Surg 41:431–433, 1954.

Wanebo HJ, Marcove RCC: Abdominal sacral resection of locally recurrent rectal cancer. Ann Surg 194:458–471, 1981.

Warren RB, Warner TF, Hafez GR: Late development of colonic adenocarcinoma 49 years after ureterosigmoidostomy for exstrophy of the bladder. J Urol 124:550–551, 1980.

Welch CE, Burke JF: Carcinoma of the colon and rectum. N Engl J Med 266:211–219, 1962.

Wilder TC, Dockerty MB, Waugh JM: A clinicopathologic study of obstructing carcinomas of the right portion of the colon. Surg Gynecol Obstet 113:353–359, 1961.

TWENTY-TWO

Recurrent Carcinoma of the Colon and Rectum

H. C. Polk, Jr., M.D.
D. J. Vandertoll, M.D.

Carcinoma of the colon and rectum continues to be a significant health problem in the United States in spite of ever-increasing levels of medical surveillance and care. Over 110,000 new cases of carcinoma of the colon occur each year and more than 50,000 deaths occur as a result of this malignancy (Malcolm et al., 1981). Survival rates do not exceed 40 to 50 percent, in spite of alleged better methods of detection and treatment (Olson et al., 1980). A significant number of patients dying from this carcinoma are those who have undergone surgical resection for cure and who, therefore, represent failures in treatment. As with any malignant tumor, recurrent or metastatic disease, or both, can occur anywhere; however, the most common sites of recurrence are liver, lung, and incision, and in cases of local recurrences, in and about the primary tumor site.

CLASSIFICATION OF RISK OF RECURRENCE

The impact of various clinical, pathologic, and therapeutic variables on host survivorship is reviewed in Chapter Ten. The data from a major study reviewed in that chapter (Spratt and Spjut, 1967) were further analyzed, not for the purpose of determining survival rates per se, but for predicting, detecting, and treating recurrent cancer (Polk and Spratt, 1971).

The study by Polk and Spratt (1971) was confined to 386 patients from the Spratt and Spjut (1967) study in whom according to the operating surgeon all gross cancer had been removed and a resection had been done for cure. The annual recurrence rate is shown in Figure 22–1. The significant factors associated with recurrence were a mixed or infiltrating cancer margin, nodal metastases, and the inclusion of only a limited number (< 6) of lymph nodes in the resected mesentery. However, not one of the subsets was strong enough as a predictor to use alone in the planning of a follow-up strategy. The actual plan of follow-up is discussed in Chapter Four.

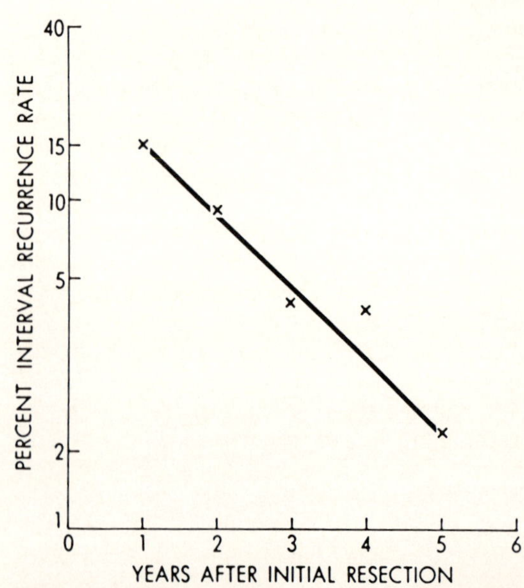

Figure 22–1. Interval recurrence rate on an annual basis for the first five years of follow-up examinations after resection intended for cure of carcinoma of the colon and rectum. (From Polk HC Jr, Spratt JS Jr: Recurrent colorectal carcinoma: Detection, treatment, and other considerations. Surgery 69:9–23, 1971.)

PREVENTION OF RECURRENCE

Ancillary precautionary measures that are believed to be important and that are instituted by most surgeons at curative operation to reduce the risk of recurrent tumor are as follows:

Soon after the peritoneal cavity is entered and prior to exploration, the edges of the incision should be draped, preferably with impermeable pads. This not only affords some protection from bacterial contamination, but minimizes the chance of implantation by malignant cells. The pad should be dry and maintained in position throughout the operation. If these pads become soaked with blood, they should be changed. Smith and associates (1958, 1963) reported that they found malignant cells in the washings from the wounds in 26 percent of patients undergoing operations for all types of cancer. Also, the tumor itself should be covered at the onset of surgery, if possible, and this covering should be maintained for the entire operation. The use of impervious material to cover the tumor has been recommended. This is particularly important for lesions that have penetrated the bowel wall (Pomeranz and Garlock, 1955). Gloves, instruments, and drapes should be changed if there is the slightest chance that contamination with malignant cells has occurred.

In the preliminary exploration, the surgeon should attempt to minimize the manipulation of the tumor when determining resectability, to minimize the spread of malignant cells intravascularly and by desquamation within the bowel and within the peritoneal cavity if the tumor has extended through the serosa.

Early ligation of the vascular supply (arterial and venous) is widely recommended to prevent tumor emboli (Cole et al., 1954). Preliminary ligation of the bowel above and below the tumor is advocated to prevent viable cells from being desquamated from the tumor and implanting at the suture line or from being desquamated into the free peritoneal cavity. This, along with irrigation of the exposed bowel lumen, may be important in reducing the possibility of postoperative recurrences at the anastomosis (Cole, 1952; Southwick and Cole, 1955).

Several studies (DiVincenti and Cohn, 1965; Gubareff and Suntzeff, 1962) have shown that iodized suture has an inhibitory effect on the growth of experimental cancer cells. Local recurrence rates apparently are reduced at the anastomosis when iodized sutures are used.

There is a relatively high incidence of local recurrence in and about the suture line in patients who had colon resection followed by end-to-end anastomosis, particularly when the cancer involved the rectosigmoid and rectum. The reported incidence of suture line recurrence varies but averages between 10 and 15 percent (Vandertoll and Beahrs, 1965). McGrew and associates (1954) examined the contents of the bowel in patients undergoing surgery for carcinoma of the colon and found viable-appearing malignant cells as far as 21 cm from the tumor in two thirds of the cases. These desquamated malignant cells are believed to be responsible for the recurrent malignant disease. Although it is unlikely that these free cells can implant in normal mucosa, it has been shown experimentally that they can implant in open wound or ulcerated areas and grow. Because of the large number of cancers in the rectosigmoid and rectum, the surgical manipulation that is necessary to free the extraperitoneal colon precludes adherence to some of the principles stated previously, e.g., early ligation of the bowel proximal and distal to the lesion.

In spite of improving surgical techniques and postoperative care, survival and recurrence rates have not changed appreciably for patients with cancer of the colon and rectum. Overall, there is a high degree of pessimism in regard to recidivated cancer of the colon, and a review of the literature indicates that colorectal adenocarcinoma recurrence is highly lethal. An overall recurrence rate of 27 percent was reported by Malcolm (1981) in his retrospective analysis of 285 patients undergoing curative resections for all areas of the colon and rectum. Lesions involving the sigmoid and rectum classified as Dukes' B2 or greater in this study had a recurrence rate of 50 percent or more.

Radiation therapy administered preoperatively and/or postoperatively has been advocated as adjuvant therapy, particularly for malignancies of the rectum and rectosigmoid area. In two series (Dwight et al., 1972; Quan et al., 1960) of patients treated with both radiation and surgery, survival rates remained in the 30 to 44 percent range. Statistically improved survival rates did occur in one series (Dwight et al., 1972) of patients who underwent abdominoperineal resection and who also received x-ray therapy. Many surgeons prefer postoperative radiation for a number of reasons: (1) The tumor can be staged adequately if the surgery is carried out initially; therefore, a number of patients who have cancers associated with a low probability of recurrence might avoid receiving radiation therapy. (2) The patients are not detained or delayed in undergoing surgical therapy. (3) A patient who has not been given preoperative radiation tends to heal better postoperatively and, therefore, significant postoperative morbidity for the patient might be avoided. In theory, the purpose of postoperative x-ray therapy is to alter the lymphatic bed and the malignant desquamated tumor cells so that the viability of the tumor cells and their ability to grow in the tissues are impaired.

Tumors with unfavorable pathologic characteristics usually have a distinct propensity for local recurrence. The frequency of recurrence varies directly, according to the presence of high-grade malignancy, local spread, size of tumor, and bowel wall penetration with lymph node metastasis (Malcolm et al., 1981; Morson et al., 1963). Certainly, patients with tumors with unfavorable pathologic characteristics, such as high grade malignancy, lymph node metastasis, and extensive local spread should be watched very closely for postoperative recurrence. Additionally, patients who have undergone low anterior resection seem to have a propensity for recurrence.

DETECTION

Gerster (1885) first suggested that there was the possibility that cancer could be spread by massaging the area involved. Lack (1896) first stressed the danger of tumor implantation in gastrointestinal cancer. Current recognition of the problem of tumor implantation at the time of surgery of the gastrointestinal tract malignancy is of more recent origin (Cole, 1951, 1952; Goligher, 1952; Lloyd-Davis, 1948). In an attempt to deal with the propensity of colon malignancies to recur locally and to metastasize to distinctive sites and not further disseminate for an extended period of time, Wangensteen (1951) proposed the so-called second-look procedure. This procedure was to be done within the first postoperative year to see if early recurrence could be found and resected. The procedure was never widely accepted because there were often negative results at laparotomy and because of the morbidity and mortality associated with surgery. In view of this, only symptomatic second-look procedures have been utilized at the University of Minnesota since 1964. More recently, carcinoembryonic antigen (CEA) selective second-look procedures have been advocated (Martin et al., 1976, 1977, 1979; Meeker, 1978; Wanebo et al., 1978). Martin and associates (1979) reported on 40 patients with elevated CEA levels; 36 (90 percent) were found to have an intra-abdominal recurrence at laparotomy. Ideally, CEA follow-up, as advocated by these authors, was monthly for 2 years, every 2 months for 3 years, semi-annually for 2 additional years, and annually after the seventh year. Whether this will alter the outcome of retreatment for attempted cure remains to be seen.

The important role of roentgenographic studies and the technique of their utilization in detecting recurrent cancer is covered in Chapter Five.

Greater responsibility is advocated for the surgeon-endoscopist in the follow-up of patients to detect early recurrent disease. Whether this will truly influence ultimate survival is doubtful. Kiselow and associates (1967) treated certain patients with carcinomas of the sigmoid and rectum by pelvic exenteration and reported a 30 percent 5-year survival rate; however, the majority of their patients had advanced primary cancers. Bacon and Berkley (1959) reported on 79 patients with recurrent pelvic tumor, 32 of whom underwent reresection. More than 30 percent (11 patients) were alive beyond 5 years; 20 patients lived more than 2 years; 16 patients lived more than 3 years. It appears then that reresection is justified, not only for prolonging survival, but also for enhancing the quality of life. Long-term cure is seldom achieved in patients with reresected recurrent carcinomas of the colon and rectum when the primary operation has been a standard one; however, significant palliation can result in carefully selected cases.

Detection and treatment obviously are a function of location of recurrence. Symptoms of recurrent colorectal carcinoma are protean in nature, and unless the patient and physician have a high index of suspicion, delay in diagnosis is the rule (Long et al., 1950; Olsen et al., 1980; Polk and Spratt, 1971; Welch and Donaldson, 1978). Perineal discomfort aggravated by sitting is a sure harbinger of recurrence of cancer in patients who have undergone abdominoperineal resection. It antedated a palpable recurrence by 1 to 9 months in Polk and Spratt's series (1971). Failure of the perineum to heal completely or dull aching pain in the perineum warrants prompt investigation by the physician. Sinus tracts should be scraped for histopathologic or cytologic assessment and "blind" needle biopsy should be performed immediately. Wide excision with or without radiation therapy should be considered.

Rectal bleeding is a highly significant symptom in patients who have undergone resection and anastomosis for carcinoma of the bowel. In the Polk and Spratt series (1971), patients who developed recurrent carcinoma in or about the anastomosis had rectal bleeding. Visualization of the colon, particularly the anastomosis, should be obtained by barium enema study and colonoscopy.

Weight loss, abdominal pain, anorexia, or any deviation in postoperative well-being warrant a complete and thorough work-up to rule out recurrent malignancy. A palpable mass in the perineal scar, in the abdominal incision, or intra-abdominally may be the only sign of recurrent carcinoma and may antedate other systemic signs and symptoms of recurrent disease considerably. Discovery of any mass, regardless of size, justifies immediate biopsy.

Chest x-ray every 6 months during the first 48 postresection months should be an integral part of the patient's postoperative follow-up. Although carcinoma of the colon has a tendency to recur locally, it also has a propensity to metastasize to distant sites and not progress further for protracted periods of time. An isolated pulmonary metastasis with no further evidence of disease certainly warrants an aggressive approach. Reports of long-term cure after resection are not unusual (Habein, 1959).

Physical examination of patients who had curative resection of carcinoma of the colon or rectum or of both, is particularly important. Careful palpation of surgical scars in operative sites is mandatory. The clinician should conduct a careful abdominal examination, looking for masses and additional indications of hepatomegaly, and the anastomotic site should be directly visualized by endoscopy.

TREATMENT OF RECURRENT DISEASE

Given the propensity of the carcinoma to recur locally and early, what protocol should be followed in patients who have undergone curative resection for malignancy of the large bowel? Mayo (1942) reported that 7 percent of patients dying in the immediate postoperative period (30 days) who had undergone apparently curative resection did, in fact, have residual carcinoma. This probably accounts for the very early recurrence of carcinoma in patients during the first 6 months. In the series reported by Polk and Spratt (1971) (see Figure 22–1), 65 percent of the patients had recurrence by the end of the second year and 88 percent had recurrence by the end of the fourth year. To attempt to detect these recurrences early, follow-up examination should be performed every 2 months the first year, every 3 months the second year, and every 6 months the third and fourth years, and annually thereafter. This is an empiric schedule and whether it truly results in the discovery of more clinically occult and, therefore, truly treatable recurrent disease, has not been proved.

SUMMARY

Recurrences after curative resection should be studied very thoroughly. If recurrence appears to be localized without evidence of widespread metastasis, resection should be attempted, and in the case of abdominal wall recurrences, i.e., incisional or drain site recurrence, radical excision should be carried out, if possible. If an anastomotic recurrence has occurred after low anterior resection, abdominoperineal resection should be contemplated even if resection is not curative. This can result in excellent palliation. In the case of pulmonary metastases, a similar approach is advocated, as significant long-term cures have been reported after pulmonary resection for metastases from colorectal cancer. Roentgenographic therapy is especially good for reducing the pain from perineal recurrences in patients who are not candidates for reresection. It should be an integral part of the treatment of these patients with or without repeat surgery. Unfortunately, even early detection seldom results in cure for the patient, and patients with recurrent carcinoma of the colon and rectum have extremely high rates of mortality and morbidity.

References

Bacon HE, Berkley JL: The rationale of re-resection for recurrent cancer of the colon and rectum. Dis Colon Rectum 2:549, 1959.

Cole WH: Measures to combat the menace of cancer. Am Surg 17:660, 1951.

Cole WH: Recurrence in carcinoma of the colon and proximal rectum following resection for carcinoma. Arch Surg 65:264, 1952.

Cole WH, Packard D, Southwick HW: Carcinoma of the colon with special reference to prevention of recurrence. JAMA 155:1549, 1954.

DiVincenti FC, Cohn I Jr: The role of suture material on tumor implantation. JAMA 191:107, 1965.

Dwight RW, Higgins GA, Roswit B, et al: Preoperative radiation and surgery for cancer of the sigmoid colon and rectum. Am J Surg 123:93, 1972.

Gerster AG: The surgical dissemination of cancer. NY State Med J 41:233, 1885.

Goligher JC, Dukes CE, Busseys HJR: Local recurrences after sphincter-saving excisions for carcinoma of the rectum and rectosigmoid. Br J Surg 39:199, 1951.

Gubareff N, Suntzeff V: Preliminary report on application of iodine in prevention of surgical dissemination of viable malignant cells. J Surg Res 2:144, 1962.

Habein HC Jr, Clagett OT, McDonald JR: Pulmonary resection for metastatic tumors. Arch Surg 78:716, 1959.

Kiselow M, Butcher HR Jr, Bricker EM: Results of the radical surgical treatment of advanced pelvic cancer. Ann Surg 166:428, 1967.

Lack HL: A contribution to the operative treatment of malignancies of the larynx with special reference to the dangers of cancerous wound infection. Lancet 1:1638, 1896.

Lloyd-Davies OB: Discussion on radical excision of carcinoma of the rectum with conservation of the sphincter. Proc Roy Soc Med 41:822, 1948.

Long JW, Mayo CW, Dockerty MB, et al: Recurrent versus new and independent carcinoma of the colon and rectum. Mayo Clinic Proc 25:169, 1950.

McGrew EA, Laws JF, Cole WH: Free malignant cells in relation to recurrence of carcinoma of the colon. JAMA 154:1251, 1954.

Malcolm AW, Perencevich NP, Olson RM, et al: Analysis of recurrence patterns following curative resection for carcinoma of the colon and rectum. Surg Gynecol Obstet 152:131, 1981.

Martin EW Jr, Cooperman M, King G, et al: A retrospective and prospective study of serial CEA determinations in the early detection of recurrent colon cancer. Am J Surg 137:167, 1979.

Martin EW Jr, James KK, Hurtubise PE, et al: The use of CEA as an early indicator for gastrointestinal tumor recurrence and second look procedures. Cancer 39:440, 1977.

Martin EW Jr, Kibbey WE, Sampson R, et al: Carcinoembryonic antigen in colorectal practice. Dis Colon Rectum 19:99, 1976.

Mayo CW, Schlicke CP: Carcinoma of the colon and rectum: A study of metastasis and recurrences. Surg Gynecol Obstet 74:83, 1942.

Meeker WR Jr: Use and abuse of CEA test in clinical practice. Cancer 41:854, 1978.

Morson BC, Vaughan EG, Bussey HJR: Pelvic recurrence after excision of rectum for carcinoma. Br Med J 2:13, 1963.

Olson RM, Perencevich NP, Malcolm AW, et al: Patterns of recurrence following curative resection of adenocarcinoma of the colon and rectum. Cancer 45:2969, 1980.

Polk HC Jr, Spratt JS Jr: Recurrent colorectal carcinoma: Detection, treatment, and other considerations. Surgery 69:9, 1971.

Pomeranz AA, Garlock JH: Postoperative recurrence of cancer of colon due to desquamated malignant cells. JAMA 158:1434, 1955.

Quan SH, Deddish MR, Starns MW: Effect of preoperative roentgen therapy upon the 10 and 5 year results of the surgical treatment of cancer of the rectum. Surg Gynecol Obstet 111:507, 1960.

Smith RR, Ketcham AS, Malmgren RA, et al: Cancer cell wound contamination associated with surgical therapy of carcinoma of the cervix. Cancer 16:1100, 1963.

Smith RR, Thomas LB, Hilberg AW: Cancer cell contamination of operative wounds. Cancer 11:53, 1958.

Southwick HW, Cole WH: Prophylactic measures in local recurrence in venous metastases in carcinoma of the colon. Surg Clin North Am 35:1363, 1955.

Spratt JS, Spjut HJ: Prevalence and prognosis of individual clinical and pathological variables associated with colorectal carcinoma. Cancer 20:1976, 1967.

Vandertoll DJ, Beahrs OH: Carcinoma of rectum and low sigmoid: Evaluation of anterior resection of 1,766 favorable lesions. Arch Surg 90:793, 1965.

Waltzer AK, Altemeier WA: Studies on the mechanism and prevention of recurrence of carcinoma at the suture line. Ann Surg 172:273, 1970.

Wanebo HJ: Are carcinoembryonic antigen levels of value in the curative management of colorectal cancer? Surg 89:290, 1981.

Wanebo HJ, Rao B, Pinsky CM, et al: Preoperative carcinoembryonic antigen levels as a prognostic indicator in colorectal cancer. N Engl J Med 299:448, 1978.

Wangensteen OH, Lewis FJ, Tongen LA: The second look in cancer surgery. Lancet 71:303, 1951.

Welch JP, Donaldson GA: Detection and treatment of recurrent cancer of the colon and rectum. Am J Surg 135:505, 1978.

TWENTY-THREE

Misadventures with Sigmoidoscopes, Flexible Endoscopes, Barium Enemas, and Colorectal Surgery

J. S. Spratt, M.D.

The purposes of this chapter are to report on the occurrence and treatment of various misadventures associated with the use of diagnostic interventions and the prevention, management, and cost of these problems. Previously, we reviewed the misadventures resulting from barium enema and sigmoidoscopic examinations in patients treated at the Ellis Fischel State Cancer Hospital (EFSCH) from 1962 through 1967. A review of the literature was presented, and conclusions regarding management were drawn from the available data (Kiser et al., 1968). To this must now be added a consideration of perforations associated with the use of flexible endoscopes and an update of that earlier review. This review also considers the ramifications and costs of complications in general.

At EFSCH, 7000 proctoscopic examinations were performed between January 1962 and December 1967. Proctoscopic study of the mucosa of the anus, rectum, and lower sigmoid colon was used as a screening procedure on all new patients and on patients seen again 1 year or more after the last proctoscopic examination. All these examinations were performed in a well-equipped proctosigmoidoscopic examining room after a disposable Clyserol* enema had been given and expelled. During this same period, 2150 barium enemas were performed. For patients who had no symptoms of partial intestinal obstruction, preparation consisted of 30 ml of castor oil given on the evening before the examination and saline enemas administered until clear on the morning of the examination.

In this interval, 353 carcinomas of the colon and rectum were diagnosed. Of these, 239 (67.7 percent) involved the rectum and lower sigmoid. More than 300 benign polypoid tumors were removed through the sigmoidoscope. The majority of the benign lesions and four of the carcinomas were found as a result of proctoscopic examination of asymptomatic patients.

PERFORATIONS WITH THE SIGMOIDOSCOPE

Five rectal or colonic perforations occurred during the sigmoidoscopic examinations, with one occurring during a repeat examination to control bleeding from a biopsy site. Sigmoidoscopic findings were normal in the other four patients. In four of the cases, perforation occurred at the junction of the rectum and the sigmoid colon, where the bowel was sharply angulated. One woman developed incapacitating pain during the enema used to prepare her for sigmoidoscopy. This cleansing enema probably produced the perforation. In all but one

*Clyserol Laboratories, Oklahoma City, OK.

of the cases, perforation was suspected during the examination, and all were confirmed by the radiographic demonstration of intraperitoneal free air. Pain was absent in two cases (Table 23–1).

All five patients were given antibiotics immediately, and celiotomies were performed within 5 hours of the time of perforation. The sites of colonic perforation were identified and closed. The pelvic cavities were drained transabdominally in four cases. Colostomies were not performed for any perforations caused by the sigmoidoscope. Four of the patients (three with drainage and one without) were fully recovered and were discharged within 10 days. The fifth patient had a pelvic abscess drained on the eighteenth day and was discharged on the thirty-eighth day.

Perforation of the bowel can be caused by unskilled insertion of the sigmoidoscope, by an attempt to force the instrument past an organic stricture or persistent area of spasm (Seman and Wells, 1965), and by the sudden movement of a nervous patient during the examination.

In 1962, Thorbjarnarson reported five cases in which either sigmoidoscopic biopsy or removal of a polyp through the sigmoidoscope resulted in a perforation. He pointed out that one can perforate the bowel by taking too

Table 23–1. PERFORATIONS OCCURRING DURING SIGMOIDOSCOPIC EXAMINATIONS AND BARIUM ENEMAS*

Age (Years)	Primary Disease	Mode of Perforation	Site of Perforation	Procedure	Course
69	No colon disease, basal cell cancer of face	Sigmoidoscope	Free peritoneum, distal sigmoid	Closure and drainage	Uncomplicated
49	Anemia, no colon lesion	Sigmoidoscope	Free peritoneum, distal sigmoid	Closure and drainage	Patient discharged eighth postoperative day
49	Carcinoma thyroid, no colon disease	Enema before sigmoidoscopic examination	Free peritoneum, 10 cm of distal sigmoid	Closure	Patient discharged ninth postoperative day
87	Bleeding at site of sigmoid polyp biopsy	Sigmoidoscope	Free peritoneum, distal sigmoid	Closure and drainage	Pelvic abscess drained on eighteenth day, patient discharged well on thirty-eigth day
82	Carcinoma rectum, A-P resection 3 years before	Barium enema via colostomy (outside hospital)	Sigmoid adjacent to colostomy, local abscess	Local resection drained	Patient discharged fourteenth postoperative day
76	Carcinoma cecum	Barium enema perforation vagina	Vagina, free peritoneal cavity	Drained	Patient expired 24 hours postoperative
86	No colon disease	Barium enema	Sigmoid colon	Closure and colostomy	Colostomy closed 2 mos later, patient expired from unrelated cause 2 mos later
47	Carcinoma rectosigmoid, low anterior resection 3 years before	Sigmoidoscopy with biopsy	Sigmoid colon	Closure and drainage	Patient discharged eleventh postoperative day, demonstrated concomitant chronic granulocytic leukemia

*Adapted from Kiser, J. L., et al.: Colon perforations occurring during sigmoidoscopic examinations and barium enema. Mo. Med. 68:969–974, 1968.

deep a bite with biopsy forceps from a sessile lesion, by performing a biopsy of an ulcer that has caused thinning of the bowel wall, and by pulling a polyp too far down before removing it with a snare. Not only a pathologic bowel but also a normal one can be perforated by a deep biopsy (Seman and Wells, 1965). Whether the perforation due to a biopsy is intraperitoneal or extraperitoneal depends on the site from which the biopsy specimen is taken.

PERFORATIONS FROM BARIUM ENEMAS

Complications of barium enemas were treated three times at EFSCH during the same period. Only one perforation occurred among the 2150 patients receiving barium enemas performed in the hospital (0.05 percent). Two additional patients were referred with colonic perforations that had occurred in roentgen diagnostic facilities outside EFSCH and were included for the purpose of discussing the management of the complication.

One of the three patients developed a localized barium abscess adjacent to an old colostomy. This patient's enema had been performed through the colostomy. The abscess was treated by drainage and resection of the colostomy along with the perforation. A new colostomy was then constructed with the more proximal bowel. The patient was discharged after 14 days of an uncomplicated postoperative course.

Two patients with widespread barium peritonitis were treated. The first case was caused by perforation through the posterior fornix of the vagina. A Bardex* catheter, used for instilling barium, had been incorrectly placed in the vagina. This complication was recognized, and corrective surgery was performed within 8 hours. Shock persisted through surgery despite appropriate treatment. The patient died 24 hours later.

The second case of perforation occurred through a normal sigmoid colon into the free peritoneal cavity in an 86-year-old man. Figures 23–1 and 23–2 show the widespread barium in this case. Treatment 12 hours later consisted of oversewing the perforation and constructing a transverse colostomy. This man recovered fully; 2 months later the colostomy was closed.

In all, one death was attributed directly to perforation from barium enema performed during 2150 examinations. Two additional deaths occurred during or immediately after the examination from myocardial infarction and cerebral vascular accidents. No mortality attributable to intestinal preparation alone without performance of the examination occurred during the period studied, although morbidity and death can occur as a result of this preparatory effort. Such deaths are rarely included in mortality registers, since the patients dying never actually have the contemplated examinations. In elderly patients, cardiovascular accidents occasionally occur after intense intestinal preparation, and careful consideration should be given to the physiologic status of any elderly individual in whom a barium enema is contemplated. The mortality rate associated with the barium enema examination in the aforementioned study was 0.14 percent. No deaths resulted from proctosigmoidoscopic examinations, but celiotomies performed for management of perforations were required for five of 7000 patients receiving proctosigmoidoscopic examinations at the EFSCH.

IATROGENIC COMPLICATIONS IN COLORECTAL EXAMINATION: ADDITIONAL CONSIDERATIONS

Other studies show as many as one to three carcinomas discoverable per 1000 sigmoidoscopic examinations performed on asymptomatic patients. Several investigators found that polyps were present in from 3 to 5 percent of patients (Crumpacker et al., 1956; Wilson and Dale, 1955). This incidence increased with age (Helwig, 1947). In all screening studies, controlled clinical trials are desirable. At the very least, data must show that the complication and mortality rates associated with the examinations or the preparations for them do not exceed the prevalence rate of cancer at first examination or the annual incidence rate of cancers at annual re-examinations. Also, any mortality and morbidity attributable to the biopsy or treatment of benign, premalignant, or asymptomatic neoplasms discovered by these examinations must be considered when one is assaying the net worth of the screening examinations. A long lead-time bias is always associated with the removal of indolent tumors. More on the epidemiologic considerations on which these observations are based can be found in Chapter One.

Only a small number of iatrogenic colonic

*C. R. Bardex Company, Inc., Murray Hill, NJ

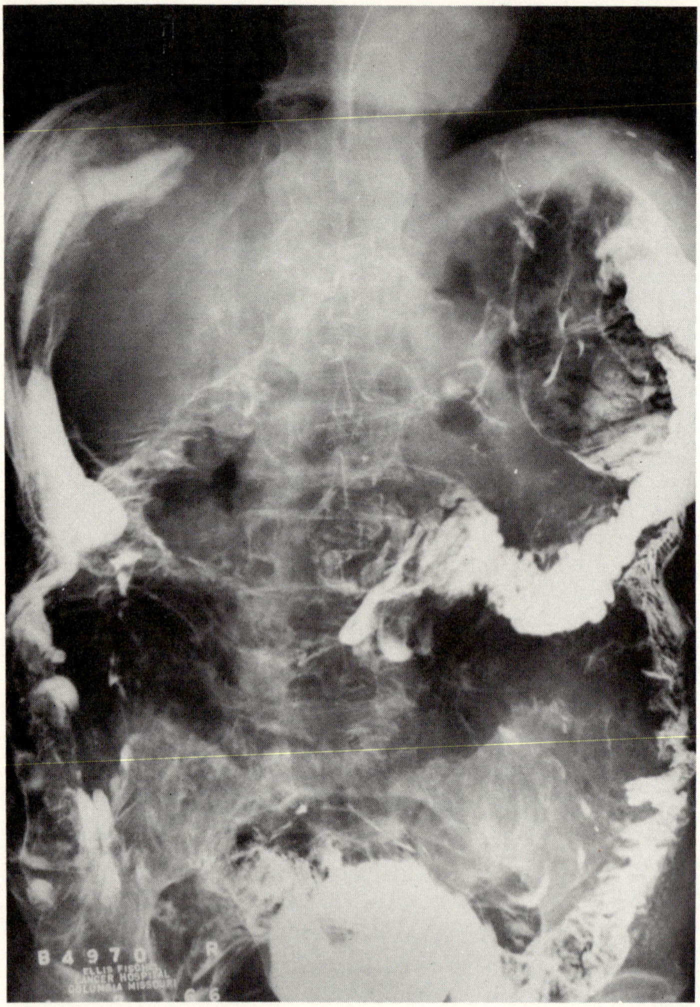

Figure 23–1. This is the roentgenographic appearance of the abdomen immediately after the rupture of the colon by a barium enema. (From Kiser JL, Spratt JS Jr, Johnson CA: Colon perforations occurring during sigmoidoscopic examinations and barium enemas. Mo Med 68:969–974, 1968.)

injuries have been reported in the literature. The earliest report was published by Schmidt in 1912. In 1947, Andresen reviewed 48 case reports of proctoscopic perforations from the literature and collected 47 case reports of perforations in response to a questionnaire submitted to 340 members of the American Gastroenterological Association and the American Proctologic Association (Andresen, 1947). Andresen indicated that mortality among patients who had been operated on was related to the length of time between perforation and surgery, and that prompt laparotomy and closure of the perforation are essential to achieving optimal survival rates. Of 12 patients operated on immediately, only one mortality occurred. In 22 cases, the patients were observed until signs of peritonitis developed and 11 (50 percent) of these patients died.

Other case reports of colonic perforations by a proctoscope have been published. Only one perforation was reported among 50,000 patients who had been examined at the Cancer Detection Center of Chicago between 1943 and 1955, indicating that a well-organized, properly staffed, and appropriately equipped clinic can keep the risk of perforation very low. Rapid recovery followed immediate surgical closure (Portes and Majarakis, 1957). At the University Clinic Frankfurt am Main, three perforations due to a sigmoidoscope and five due to barium enema occurred between 1944 and 1964. Over half of these patients died (Blaha, 1965).

In 1953, Klein and Scarborough reviewed reports of 50 perforations of the rectum and distal colon. They stated: "Characteristically, there are no prompt dramatic symptoms when

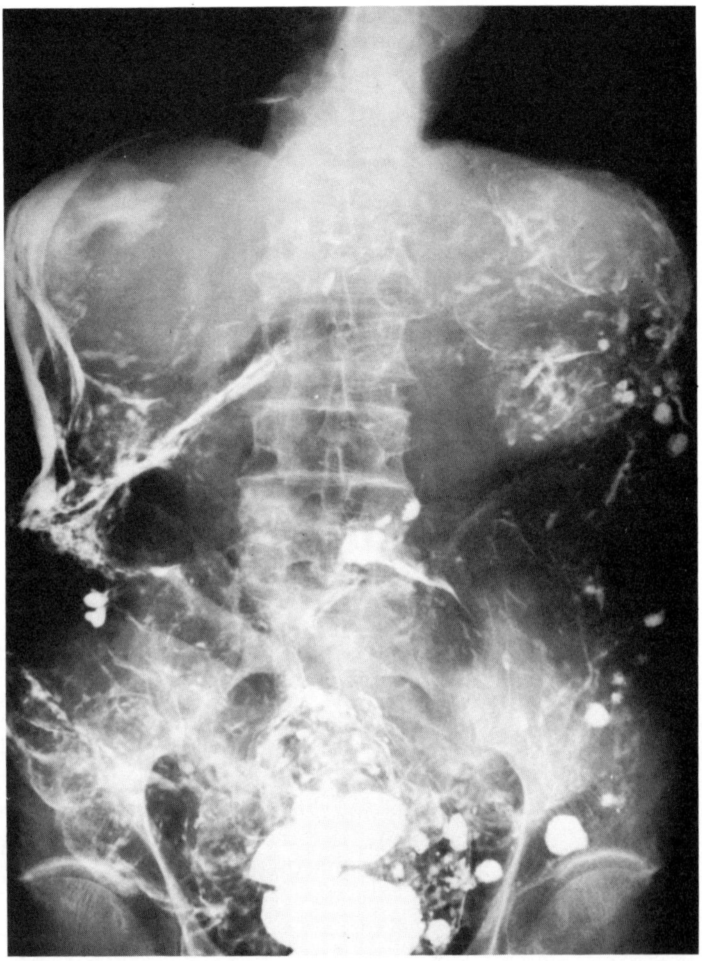

Figure 23–2. This is the roentgenographic appearance of the same abdomen shown in Figure 23–1 two months later, showing retained barium. (From Kiser JL, Spratt JS Jr, Johnson CA: Colon perforations occurring during sigmoidoscopic examinations and barium enemas. Mo Med 68:969–974, 1968.)

the rectum is perforated." Eleven of these perforations were attributable to proctosigmoidoscopic examinations. Of eight patients operated on immediately, one died. Of three patients operated on after 18 hours, two died. In intraperitoneal perforations, surgery must be performed before the development of signs and symptoms of peritonitis. Many of the cases reported in the literature as operative mortalities were managed expectantly until peritonitis was well established.

Klein and Scarborough reported 20 cases of perforation of the extraperitoneal rectum. Seventeen patients were treated with no surgical drainage, resulting in two mortalities. Almost all proctoscopic perforations occurred where the intestine was sharply angulated at the distal sigmoid.

Proctoscopic examination in newborn children has been found to be more hazardous than in older children and adults. In a 1965 report of ten iatrogenic perforations in newborn infants at the Columbus Children's Hospital, Fonkalsrud stated that there was much greater risk of perforation by sigmoidoscopy in this age group than in older children and adults. He recommended that barium enema be performed as the initial diagnostic procedure.

Perforation may occur after a cleansing enema and not be recognized until the sigmoidoscopic examination has been performed. This probably occurred in one of the EFSCH cases. Similarly, perforation due to sigmoidoscopic examinations may go unrecognized until a barium enema is performed (Issacs, 1952).

Most of the reported perforations due to barium enema have been through ulcers, tumors, diverticula, or other diseased areas (Portes and Majarakis, 1957; Hamit, 1955). In 1952, using a questionnaire, Zheutlin and colleagues collected 53 cases of perforations. Details regarding the type of operation were not recorded for the other 29 patients who underwent celiotomy, but the mortality rate was less in this group. Prompt celiotomy, closure, and drainage with antibiotic coverage have prevented death in several reported cases (Hamit, 1955; Greentree and Funske, 1962; Hartman and Kills, 1957). In the late follow-up, 30 percent of the survivors underwent laparotomy for adhesions. This was necessary in approximately the same percentage of the surgical and nonsurgical groups (Zheutlin et al., 1952).

Chemical additives to the enema and fecal contamination of the peritoneal surface have complicated the problem of perforation resulting from diagnostic enemas. Earlier, tannic acid was used as an adjuvant in approximately 25 percent of barium enemas to produce puckering of the mucosa, to stimulate peristalsis, and to precipitate mucin (Portin, 1963; Rambo et al., 1966). Tannic acid irritates the peritoneum. In addition, tannic acid may cause fatal liver necrosis when added to enemas. This observation was reported first in 1963 by McAlister and co-workers. Three children with hepatic necrosis died within 7 days after receiving enemas containing 0.75 percent tannic acid. Studies in animals have shown that barium alone is less toxic to the peritoneum than barium and feces, emphasizing further the importance of a thorough colon preparation before any elective examination and early laparotomy to reduce the chance of fecal soilage (Kleinsasser and Washaw, 1952). Tannic acid is rarely used anymore.

In their 1966 experimental evaluation of the treatment of barium peritonitis in animals, Westfall and associates concluded that the best treatment consisted of antibiotics and early closure of the perforation. Within an hour, clumps of barium are held to the peritoneum by a layer of fibrin. Copious irrigation of the peritoneal cavity with saline can wash much of the barium free early. Some barium must be left in order to prevent undue abrasion of the serosal surface.

Misadventures With Flexible Endoscopes

The flexible colonic endoscope has now become widely available. The basic considerations for its use are the same as those discussed for sigmoidoscopes and barium enemas—the risk of intervention to find asymptomatic disease must be less than the incidence of the disease. Actually, proving its value is much more complicated. The final proof lies in being able to test the hypothesis that a particular strategy for endoscopic examinations, as well as the other components of a screening program for colorectal cancers, reduces the chance of premature death or morbidity from the cancers. The principle of early recognition and prompt management of perforations remains unchanged.

The use of the flexible scope is associated with an array of unique problems, the most significant being high silent perforations and hemorrhage. A controlled clinical trial will ultimately be required to determine the optimal strategy for the flexible colonoscope. The author was consulted on the type of problem that could significantly reduce the public health value of the flexible colonoscope, were it to become very prevalent or remain unreported. A 46-year-old high-school coach had a checkup at which a 4-mm polyp at 15 cm was removed (pathology not available). A barium enema was performed that showed a 1.5-cm polyp in the sigmoid colon. The lesion was removed following colonoscopy and was designated a benign adenomatous polyp. A perforation went unrecognized, and the patient was discharged from the hospital. Over a period of days, and despite frequent contacts with physicians and hospitals, symptoms of the perforation progressed to massive gaseous gangrene, requiring life-saving debridement of bowel and abdominal wall. The patient survived, but with lifelong morbidity. Treatment, including transport to a hyperbaric oxygen center, was extremely expensive. Only an occasional case like this can negate the public health value of endoscopic removal of benign lesions in the name of cancer prevention. Such cases emphasize the importance of clear indications for and local quality control of the endoscopic examination of the asymptomatic, plus the need for controlled clinical trials to define the optimal strategy for its use.

Perforation During Cleansing Enema

The introduction into the rectum of a hard object such as the nozzle of a Higginson's syringe can injure the bowel. The rectal wall, even in the absence of disease, can be perforated by the tip of a rubber catheter introduced for the purpose of administering a simple cleansing enema. This may happen if a relatively inflexible catheter is introduced in such a way that its tip impinges heavily on the anterior wall of the rectum.

A large-bowel perforation that occurs during the administration of a simple enema can also occur at a site that precludes injury by the catheter as the cause. In that event, the perforation occurs at some point at which the bowel is diseased. The assumed cause is a rise in the intraluminal pressure, perhaps brought about by an active contraction of the bowel. We know of one such case in which the perforation occurred in the cecum, where there was an unusual lesion—a localized area of gangrene.

Precautions with Barium Enema

When a radiologist who is performing a barium enema examination sees evidence of leakage of barium out of the lumen of the bowel, he has several possibilities to consider. Barium may have entered an abscess cavity; it may have passed through a fistula into some other viscus; or it may have leaked through a recent perforation in the bowel wall. If the radiologist thinks it is likely that there is a recent perforation, he may have to consider whether this has been caused by a cleansing enema, an endoscopic examination, a biopsy, or the barium enema itself.

Assuming that there had been no preceding endoscopic examination and that the performance of the barium enema was responsible, one finds that damage to the bowel might have occurred in one of three possible ways. First, the bowel might have been injured by the catheter or tube used for giving the enema, in the same way as can happen when a cleansing enema is given. Second, if an inflatable balloon catheter has been used, injury might have been caused by overinflation of the balloon. Among thirteen patients reported in 1965 by Seaman and Wells with colonic rupture as a complication of a barium enema, there were six in whom overinflation of a balloon catheter was regarded as a possible cause, although only one was an adult in whom the injury could be attributed to the inflation of a balloon in the rectum. Of the remaining five patients, three were infants and two were patients to whom enemas were given through colostomies. In another report, the deaths of four elderly patients were attributed to the catheter (Ansell, 1968).

The third possibility is that the rupture was due to an excessive rise in intraluminal pressure. We have already referred to a case in which this appeared to be the cause of rupture during the administration of a cleansing enema, and there can be no doubt that a barium enema can produce the same complication.

Barium Enema After Biopsy

In 1963, Hemley and Kanick reported two cases of rectal perforation as a result of rectal biopsy followed by barium enema. Sigmoidoscopy and biopsy were performed in one of their patients on the same day as the enema, and in the other these procedures were done 2 days earlier. In both patients, the perforation was below the peritoneal reflection, and bar-

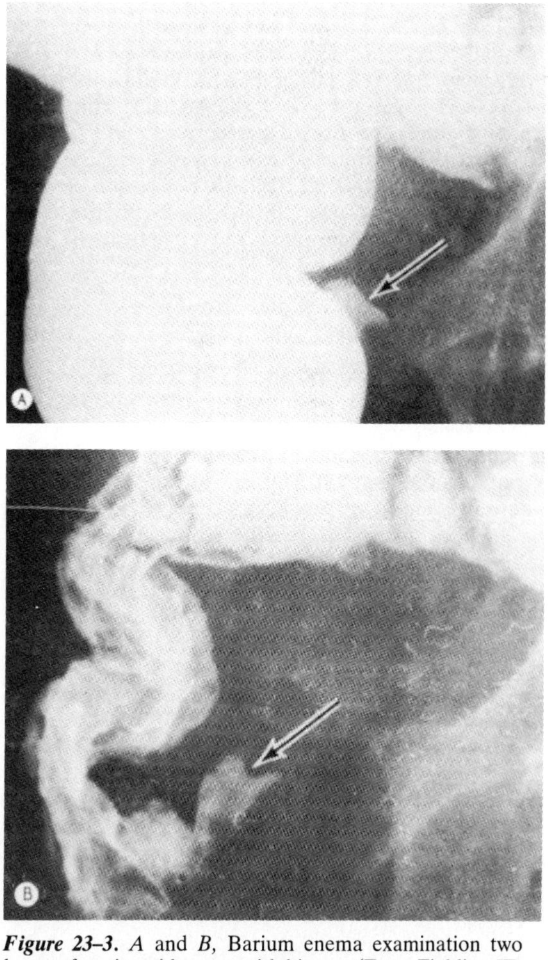

Figure 23–3. *A* and *B,* Barium enema examination two hours after sigmoidoscopy with biopsy. (From Fielding JF, Lumsden K: Large bowel perforations in patients undergoing sigmoidoscopy and barium enema. Br Med J 1:471–473, 1973.)

ium was extravasated into the perirectal tissues. Both were treated conservatively, and both died from peritonitis.

Other fine points in technique essential to obtaining high-quality barium contrast studies of the colon with minimal complications are discussed in Chapter Five.

Limitations Imposed by Misadventures or Incidence Rates of Neoplasms

In the continued absence of a controlled clinical trial on the optimal strategy for the use of the proctosigmoidoscope, flexible endoscope, and barium enema in asymptomatic people, the following generalizations can serve as a guide:

1. Proctosigmoidoscopic and flexible colonoscopic examinations and barium enema are important methods for examining *symptomatic* persons.

2. The small but measurable morbidity and mortality restrict the use of the examination in asymptomatic patients to those older than 45 years of age when the probability of finding disease becomes great enough to justify the effort and exceeds the small but measurable morbidity and mortality rate of the examination. The exception might be the person with a strong family history of colon neoplasia.

3. When used in asymptomatic persons who are older than 45 years of age and when the examinations were within normal limits, the rate of new growth was slow enough to reduce the need for re-examination to once every 2 to 3 years. Some more acute and rapidly growing cancers may still attain a size that will produce symptoms during this period.

4. Previous studies have shown that the *entire* population is increasingly at risk to develop colorectal carcinomas with advancing age, regardless of the presence or absence of various benign growths, making the identification of a group with a high cancer risk difficult (Koppel, 1962). The only significant exceptions are familial adenomatous polyposis and ulcerative colitis (Greentree and Funske, 1962). The major complication of both sigmoidoscopic examination and barium enema is perforation. When these perforations are intraperitoneal, the most effective treatment consists of prompt celiotomy and primary closure. Drainage and colostomy are rarely necessary. The stress of these examinations on elderly people can also precipitate lethal cardiovascular accidents, and in rare cases hemorrhage and sepsis from biopsy may occur.

In all, eight patients with iatrogenic colonic perforations were treated at the Ellis Fischel State Cancer Hospital during the period of the review, including two with barium peritonitis. Antibiotics and *prompt* closure of the perforation were essential to survival. Colostomy was generally unnecessary in acute perforations produced by the sigmoidoscope.

The one patient who died as a result of perforation was 76 years old and had a very large cecal carcinoma with extensive local invasion and numerous other chronic diseases identified at autopsy. At this age, without the cecal cancer, the patient probably would have survived approximately another 7.6 years (Kiser et al., 1968). With such a large cecal cancer, no more than one year of life was lost as a result of the complications associated with 9150 colonic and rectal examinations by proctosigmoidoscopic study and barium enema after treatment of the several complications. No deaths occurred among disease-free asymptomatic patients. However, among 100,000 persons being examined annually by these methods, as many as 11 deaths might occur if the observed rate were to remain constant. The incidence of colorectal cancer does not exceed 13 per 100,000 per year until age 45 years. The risk associated with repetitive examinations in asymptomatic patients must remain less than the known incidence. Any mortality associated with the treatment of still asymptomatic cancer must be counterbalanced by an actuarial gain in the balance of the examined and treated population. Use of proctosigmoidoscopic examination and barium enema as part of the routine physical examination in asymptomatic patients must be combined with an appreciation and avoidance of the potential complications and prompt management when complications occur. The detection of predisease states must similarly be succeeded by equally nondestructive treatment methods. Morbidity and mortality undoubtedly vary in different clinics; however, until the rates are zero, the methods cannot be considered "nondestructive," and frequent and indiscriminate use in asymptomatic patients has to be restricted to a strategy that will provide the greatest benefit.

A not generally appreciated effect of barium enemas is the fact that they produce a transient bacteremia in at least 11 percent of the examinations. In 1975, Le Frock and colleagues performed pour-plate blood cultures 5, 10, 15, and 30 minutes following barium enemas. Cultures remained positive for as long as 15 minutes but were usually negative by 30 minutes. Positive cultures were seen with all types of disorders. The authors suggested that recent barium enemas might be the cause of endocarditis and that the risk of bacteremia should be considered whenever a barium enema might be indicated in patients with known cardiac valvular disease.

Clearly, experience with sigmoidoscopic examination and barium enemas stresses that these procedures can be associated with serious complications that must be prevented when possible but managed appropriately when they do occur. The vital importance of prompt diagnosis, celiotomy, and closure of the perforations cannot be overemphasized. Other precautions relate to the general condition of the patient.

Holes in the Lower Bowel

The seriousness of small holes in the colon whose presence goes unrecognized for a while is periodically reaffirmed. In 1973, Fielding and Lumsden reviewed the perforations associated with cleansing enemas, sigmoidoscopic examinations, and barium enemas. The ideal is to prevent perforations; however, these complications continue to occur occasionally in all clinics, and, when they do occur, prompt recognition and laparotomy are life-saving necessities. Prompt closure and exteriorization should be performed when they are feasible; when they are not, a diverting proximal colostomy is required as soon as possible. Culture, drainage, antibiotics, and supportive care must be part of careful management aimed at preventing development of gaseous gangrene and multiorgan failure.

The Cost of Misadventures

In 1978, Couch and co-workers estimated the "cost of error" arising from failure to diagnose colonic leakage and failure to perform a safe colostomy associated with routine colon surgery. The mortality was increased by tenfold, the cost by sevenfold, and the length of hospitalization by fourfold.

Therapeutic accidents contribute to the increasing need for high-cost care. In some cases, elaborate and expensive hospital care is mandated because of misadventures in standard procedures. One group of investigators, using colonic surgery as a model (or example), analyzed a random series of 16 patients, all of whom required intensive care owing to misadventures in colonic surgery that seemed, in retrospect, to have been avoidable. Aspects of cost and analysis of adverse outcomes were described (Couch et al., 1978).

Through the years, important lessons in colonic surgery have been learned. Early experience with appendicitis showed that the peritoneum was able to cope with a single, small contamination by organisms of average virulence, although a persistent intestinal leak became lethal unless localized and drained. If the leak was from the colon, treatment had to include a proximal diversion to minimize soilage. If standard principles were neglected, peritonitis (often followed by sequential system failure) occurred. Support of such patients for longer intervals is now possible, and even survival can be achieved. The fatality rate remains high in the presence of established peritonitis because of pulmonary, renal, and hepatic failure and the cerebral consequences of sepsis or a prolonged low-flow state. With survival, the costs in money, in professional effort, and in suffering are becoming increasingly high.

In the 1978 study by Couch and colleagues, there were nine male and seven female patients, ranging in age from 14 to 80 years. Their primary diagnoses were adenocarcinoma (four patients), diverticulitis (seven patients), iatrogenic colonic perforation (three patients), and ulcerative colitis (two patients). Eleven of this group were referred from other hospitals for intensive care when very ill. Five patients suffered complications arising in the same hospital.

When the patients' clinical patterns of adverse outcome were classified according to primary episode of management failure, the following three groups were defined:

1. Group I included those patients characterized by unrecognized or undiagnosed peritoneal sepsis of colonic origin who, lacking any treatment, developed dangerous or lethal peritonitis.
2. Group II included those patients in whom no proximal colonic diversion was performed, either at the time of precarious anastomosis or at the time of colonic leakage.
3. Group III included those patients in whom colonic exteriorization was performed inadequately, resulting in retraction and local sepsis.

Although the operative approaches to the colon have been established and accepted for many decades, the authors were impressed by the unremitting abundance of related misadventures and the occasional requirement for extensive and costly intensive care after surgery of the colon. Colonic surgery always tests the surgeon's knowledge, judgment, skill, and rapport with his patient. The surgeon must explain when a temporary colostomy and staged operations will probably be needed. Determination of the total cost of complications would require a major surveillance program, with analysis of all morbidity and mortality. Some idea of the mortality rate associated with colon resections by competent surgeons can be found in the literature: approximately 5 percent for ulcerative colitis (Abrams, 1975; Aylett, 1971); 2 to 5 percent for adenocarcinoma (Mzabi et al., 1976; Wilson and Beahrs, 1976); and approximately 8 percent for diverticulitis (Botsford et al., 1971).

As surgical technology evolves, principles of safe surgical management are established. Once these principles become familiar, they frequently are overshadowed by new discoveries. Surgical teachers must emphasize commonplace principles and the penalties for ignoring them.

As applied to colonic surgery even for the seemingly simple polyp, the list of principles should include the following:

1. Preoperative preparation of the bowel as discussed in Chapter Seven, nasogastric tube or alternative upper gastrointestinal suction drainage.

2. Ensure adequate blood supply to all stomas or anastomoses with no tension.

3. Avoid fecal spillage and contamination by quarantining sheets, and discarding soiled instruments, gowns, and gloves after bowel is closed.

4. Perform proximal complete colonic diversion whenever (a) the colon has been perforated, (b) an anastomosis appears precarious or has leaked, (c) immunosuppression or immunologic disorders exist, or (d) there is any possibility that one or both ends of the anastomosed bowel may have received significant radiation. If in doubt, a frozen section examination of the ends of the intestines can sometimes lead to the discovery of significant radiation damage, particularly to small blood vessels.

5. When signs of peritoneal or systemic infection appear postoperatively, search diligently for the source (e.g., radionuclide and ultrasonic scanning and barium radiography). Exploration should be carried out without delay. Antibiotics can never substitute for drainage and colon exterioration.

6. Promptly discontinue ineffective antibiotics and avoid nephrotoxic antibiotics in critically ill patients.

7. Use only the most definitive surgical procedures for all patients including specifically high risk groups.

The teaching of such principles may compete with other curricula. In residency programs, the staff may become preoccupied with more interesting or "frontier" areas, and thus the teaching of the commonplace is overlooked. The time is at hand for surgeons to adapt more of the techniques of "risk management" from the managerial science field to reduce the probability that misadventures will occur.

Among the most common errors in colonic surgery were those that arose from unwarranted confidence in colonic anastomoses and misplaced optimism when postoperative sepsis occurred. Inattention to detail for such minor procedures as polyp removal can be catastrophic.

The 16 patients discussed in the review by Couch and associates in 1978 would ordinarily have required approximately 235 days of hospitalization had there been no complications. Because these patients were hospitalized at different times and at varying hospital charges over a 10-year period, the expenses were calculated for all on the basis of current charges. In January 1977, at the Peter Bent Brigham Hospital, the average daily total charge for a bed in the intensive care unit was approximately 680 dollars, whereas the average daily total charge for a standard bed was approximately 400 dollars, making a day in intensive care about 1.7 times as expensive as a day in the standard bed. Thus, the total hospital charge for all sixteen patients would have been about 94,000 dollars, had their courses not been complicated. In reality, they required 984 days of hospitalization (a fourfold increase), almost all in intensive care. Their total bill would have been about 670,000 dollars (a sevenfold increase). The "cost" in terms of physical and emotional suffering and death was not measured.

An important and often neglected step in cost-benefit analysis in medical care is the analysis of the origin and cost of errors. Various investigators, in an effort to gather reliable data on medical or surgical accidents, have suggested and tried several mechanisms to monitor all complaints, complications, and adverse outcomes (American Surgical Association, 1976). Such a general mechanism, although useful for investigating some adverse events (e.g., transfusion reactions, electronic hazards, and mechanical errors), would be ineffective in identifying and preventing poor results of more complex genesis that originate in nonmonitored hospitals and lead to patient transfers. Preventability and frequency need to be examined, along with any abnormally high rates of errors associated with particular hospitals or physicians.

Because of pervasive fears of malpractice litigation, it would be in the interest of all involved physicians to participate in the evaluation and prevention of misadventures and to develop effective corrective, continuing education programs. The current abundance of such lawsuits could cause physicians to conceal unfavorable outcomes, resulting in obstruction of medical progress. Unfortunately, openness is sometimes impeded by the principles of the common law, which hold that no one can be relieved of responsibility and liability of his own acts. The author (JSS) believes that economic motivation has a great impact on performance after education in the basics are provided. If all remuneration in medicine were based on patient outcome rather than on a "piecework-wage" system, the frequency of misadventures would dramatically decline (Spratt, 1975a, 1975b). Risk management techniques might also assist in reducing the incidence of misadventures.

SUMMARY

Perforation of the large bowel can occur as a complication of sigmoidoscopy, rectal or sigmoid biopsy, flexible endoscopy, barium enema, a simple cleansing enema, and various surgical procedures. If the perforation is extraperitoneal, there may be no early symptoms, and, consequently, there may be delay in diagnosis. The risk of perforation during these procedures is small, but it cannot be ignored. The performance of a barium enema shortly after a rectal or sigmoid biopsy may slightly increase the risk by converting a partial perforation into a complete one. Precautions can be taken to minimize the hazard.

Sigmoidoscopic, colonoscopic, and endoscopic biopsy as well as barium enema examinations are so widely used in the investigation of disease of the large bowel, and there have been so few reports of serious complications arising from their use, that these procedures are often considered virtually free from hazard. Each of them, however, can produce a perforation of the wall of the bowel, even when it is healthy, and we believe this risk should be widely understood and properly managed. The same principles apply to colonic surgery in general, as has been briefly considered in this chapter.

Since so many patients undergo sigmoidoscopy, rectal biopsy, barium enema examination, and colon surgery without developing complications, the chances of bowel perforation in these procedures, or of postoperative leaks, are certainly small. Nevertheless, perforations and leaks do occur often enough to warrant consideration of means to minimize the risks.

For sigmoidoscopy, the patient must be reassured and placed in the position of choice of the endoscopist. It is important that once the instrument has passed through the anal canal its further advancement should be in a posterior direction towards the patient's sacrum, since the long axis of the lower rectum is set approximately at a right angle to the direction of the anal canal. The instrument should be advanced only under direct vision, and insufflated air should be kept to a minimum. It is also necessary to avoid the use of undue force if the instrument encounters resistance, due either to spasm of the bowel or to organic disease (e.g., a stricture). If a biopsy specimen is taken, the site must be subsequently visualized to determine the depth of the tissue removed.

Various types of catheters have long been used for giving cleansing enemas, and although there is the possibility of even the healthy rectum being injured by these catheters, their use is essential. If any catheter meets with resistance when it is being inserted, it should be retracted a short distance (approximately 2 cm), rotated through an angle of 60 to 90 degrees, and then gently advanced again. If this simple maneuver is not immediately successful, it may be repeated. Alternatively, the person who is administering the enema may try the effect of running enema fluid through the catheter; this often causes enough rectal distention to allow the catheter to be introduced further into the rectum with ease.

For barium enemas, the bulbous tip of the rectal tube should be situated in the lower rectum, just above the anal canal, when the tube has been correctly inserted. The enema must be given slowly from a reservoir that is adjusted so that its contents can be delivered by gravity at a low pressure. A balloon catheter is rarely necessary.

When the anal sphincter is incompetent, the use of a balloon catheter may be required. Certain precautions must be taken (Margulis, 1967). For example, rectal disease should have been excluded by a sigmoidoscopy. Also, some barium should be run into the bowel before the balloon catheter is inflated; if the patient cannot retain the enema, the balloon should be inflated under fluoroscopic control. Also, the balloon should be in the lower rectum, with only the bulbous tip of the rectal tube projecting into the lumen beyond, and it should never be overinflated. The use of balloon catheters in infants is not only dangerous but also unnecessary; if this type of catheter is used for giving an enema through a colostomy, the inflated balloon should be *outside* the colon and held against the colostomy opening, preferably by the patient himself.

Some authors have recommended that after a rectal or sigmoid biopsy the performance of a barium enema should be delayed for at least 7 days (Margulis, 1967) or 14 days (Hemley and Kanick, 1963). The basis for such a recommendation is the belief that the rise in intraluminal pressure resulting from the enema may convert a partial perforation of the bowel into a complete one. At the same time, any difference in the risks between the two groups is a very small one.

If this view is correct, it follows that it is desirable (although not entirely necessary) that after the patient has had a biopsy of the rectum or sigmoid, there should be a lapse of 1 or 2 weeks before a barium enema is performed. It also follows that in those cases in which it is thought justifiable to perform a biopsy followed by a barium enema on the same day, the radiologist should be aware that the patient has had a biopsy and should know its site. In making his examination, the radiologist should pay special attention to the condition of the rectum and sigmoid before proceeding to study other parts of the bowel. He should also refrain from overdistension of the colon by either barium or air. A number of cases have been reported of retroperitoneal and interstitial emphysema as a complication of barium enema, and the most common cause is the performance of a double-contrast examination when there is rectal damage (Brunton, 1960).

If the decision is made to perform a barium enema on a patient who has recently undergone sigmoidoscopy, regardless of whether or not there has also been a biopsy, a plain radiograph of the abdomen may be taken to look for possible evidence of retroperitoneal gas before starting the enema. If such evidence is found, the enema should be deferred. In the absence of signs of air, the radiologist can proceed cautiously with the enema, using a flexible plastic tube with a bulbous tip, as already described. The bag containing the enema fluid should be suspended at a low enough level to ensure a very slow rate of delivery of the barium into the rectum

By paying attention to the precautions outlined, further reductions of the risks to patients undergoing sigmoidoscopic and barium enema examinations can be obtained, irrespective of the temporal relationship of these examinations (Fielding and Lumsden, 1973). If the least suspicion of perforation exists, the patient must be retained under close surveillance and undergo corrective surgery before peritonitis becomes well established.

In 1982, Adar and associates came to a similar conclusion in studying iatrogenic complications in general and vascular surgery. These complications tend to be infrequent and sporadic. However, reduction in frequency requires objective study, unencumbered by the intimidating impact of psychologic and medicolegal pressures.

The professional dialogue must remain open, accurate, analytical, and corrective. If complications occur too frequently, conventional approaches to the solutions of these problems may need to be replaced by more reliable ones.

References

Abrams JS: Surgical treatment of inflammatory bowel disease of the colon: Ulcerative colitis and granulomatous (Crohn's) colitis. Am J Surg 130:528–531, 1975.

Adar R, Bass A, Walden R: Iatrogenic complications in surgery. Ann Surg 166:725–729, 1982.

American Surgical Association Statement on Professional Liability, September, 1976. N Engl J Med 295:1292–1296, 1976.

Andresen AFR: Perforations from proctoscopy. Gastroenterology 9:32–43, 1947.

Ansell G: A national survey of radiological complications: interim report. Clin Radiol 19:175–191, 1968.

Aylett SO: Ileorectal anastomosis: review 1952–1968. Proc R Soc Med 64:967–971, 1971.

Blaha H: Dickdarm Perforations. Der Chirug 36:267–270, 1965.

Botsford TW, Zollinger RM Jr, Hicks R: Mortality of the surgical treatment of diverticulitis. Am J Surg 121:702–705, 1971.

Brunton FJ: Retroperitoneal emphysema as a complication of barium enema. Clin Radiol 11:197–199, 1960.

Couch NP, Tilney NL, Moore FD: The cost of misadventures in colonic surgery. A model for the analysis of adverse outcomes in standard procedures. Am J Surg 135:641–646, 1978.

Crumpacker EL, Baker JP, Ballou HC, Morhous EJ: Proctosigmoidoscopy in the general examination: an analysis of 5158 examinations. Arch Int Med 98:314–321, 1956.

Fielding JF, Lumsden K: Large bowel perforations in patients undergoing sigmoidoscopy and barium enema. Br Med J 24:471–473, 1973.

Fonkalsrud EW: Accidental perforation of colon and rectum in new born infants. N Engl J Med 272:1097–1100, 1965.

Greentree LN, Funske W: Perforation of normal colon by barium enema. Report of a case with uncomplicated survival. Ohio Med J 58:1150–1151, 1962.

Hamit HF: Perforation of the colon after barium enema and air contrast studies. Am Surgeon 21:1226–1234, 1955.

Hartman AW, Kills WJ: Rupture of colon in infants during barium enema. Ann Surg 145:712–717, 1957.

Helwig EB: The evolution of adenomas of the large intestine and their relation to carcinoma. Surg Gynecol Obstet 84:36–49, 1947.

Hemley SD, Kanick V: Perforation of the rectum: a complication of barium enema following rectal biopsy. Report of 2 cases. Am J Dig Dis 8:882–884, 1963.

Issacs I: Intraperitoneal escape of barium enema fluid; perforation of sigmoid colon. JAMA 150:645–646, 1952.

Kiser JL, Spratt JS Jr, Johnson CA: Colon perforations occurring during sigmoidoscopic examinations and barium enemas. Mo Med 65:969–974, 1968.

Klein RD, Scarborough RA: Traumatic perforations of the rectum and distal colon (50 cases). Am J Surg 86:515–522, 1953.

Kleinsasser LS, Washaw, H: Perforations of sigmoid during barium enema. Ann Surg 135:560–565, 1952.

Koppel M: Incidence of cancer in the colon and rectum among polyp-free patients. Dis Colon Rectum 5:349–355, 1962.

Le Frock J, Ellis CA, Klainer AS, Weinstein L: Transient bacteremia associated with barium enema. Arch Int Med 135:835–837, 1975.

Margulis AR: Alimentary tract radiology. *In* Margulis AR, Burhenne HJ (eds): Alimentary Tract Roentgenology. Vol 2. St Louis, CV Mosby, 1967.

McAlister WH, Anderson MS, Bloomberg GR, Margulis A: Lethal effects of tannic acid in barium enema. Report of three fatalities and experimental studies. Radiology 80:765–773, 1963.

Mzabi R, Himal HS, Demers S, McLean LD: A multiparametric computer analysis of carcinoma of the colon. Surg Gynecol Obstet 143:959–964, 1976.

Portes C, Majarakis JD: Proctosigmoidoscopy—incidence of polyps in 50,000 exams. JAMA 163:411–413, 1957.

Portin BA: Colon perforation during barium enema—case report. Dis Colon Rectum 6:308–310, 1963.

Rambo ON, Zboralske FF, Harris PA, et al.: Toxicity studies on tannic acid administered by enema. I. Effects of enema-administered tannic acid on the colon and liver of rats. Am J Roentgenol 96:488–497, 1966.

Schmidt A: Perforation of the rectum by proctoscopy. Munchen Med Wchnschr 59:154, 1912.

Seaman WB, Wells J: Complications of the barium enema. Gastroenterology 48:728–737, 1965.

Spratt JS Jr: The physician's role in minimizing the economic morbidity of cancer. Sem Oncol 2:411–417, 1975a.

Spratt JS Jr: The relation of human capital preservation to health costs. Am J Econ Sci 34:295–307, 1975b.

Thorbjarnarson B: Iatrogenic and related perforations of the large bowel. Arch Surg 84:608–614, 1962.

Westfall RH, Nelson RH, Musselman MM: Barium peritonitis. Am J Surg 152:760–763, 1966.

Wilson GS, Dale EH, Brines DA: An evaluation of polyps detected in 20,847 routine sigmoidoscopic examinations. Am J Surg 90:834–840, 1955.

Wilson SM, Beahrs OH: The curative treatment of carcinoma of the sigmoid, rectosigmoid, and rectum. Ann Surg 183:556–565, 1976.

Zheutlin N, Lassey EC, Rigler LG: Clinical studies on effect of barium in the peritoneal cavity following rupture of the colon. Surgery 32:967–979, 1952.

APPENDIX FOR PUBLIC EDUCATION

Good Health and the Avoidance of Cancer

J. S. Spratt, M.D.

The results of epidemiologic research strongly suggest that variations in exposure to environmental agents and in social practices are largely responsible for variations in the incidence of cancers among different groups of people. Therefore, if harmful environmental exposures and social practices could be identified and eliminated, many cancers in man might be prevented.

The prevention or avoidance of cancer by changing behavior and environmental and social practices is a very complicated process. Much detailed and time-consuming scientific detective work is needed to identify the causes and to eliminate the harmful factors and associated social practices. Prevention in an individual will never be possible without the practice of lifelong habits that will reduce the chances of developing cancer. This article identifies some individual behavioral practices that, if followed, should reduce an individual's chances of being exposed to factors known to increase the incidence of cancer. Simultaneously, these practices should enhance each individual's physical well being and general health.

Most cancers seem to require a "starter," most commonly a cancer-causing chemical, and growth promoters. The higher the exposure and the earlier in life that exposure and promotion begins, the greater is the lifetime risk. The cancer itself expresses and transmits to successive generations of daughter cells the basic molecular damage (Weinberg, 1983; Yunis, 1983).

CANCER AND DIET

A relationship between various forms of cancer and diet and personal habits is becoming increasingly well established. Organs involved are usually those in the digestive tract, but diet also has been associated with cancer in other parts of the body. Food may contribute to both the causation and prevention of cancer in several ways (Ames 1983).

For example, cancer-inducing chemicals, such as pesticides and by-products as a result of smoking meats and fish, are present in food itself. Chemical compounds called nitrosamines and polycyclic hydrocarbons also have been implicated as likely causative agents of many cancers. Nitrosamines are present in some foods, but may also be manufactured in man's own intestinal tract from compounds that are not carcinogenic (cancer producers), such as nitrates and secondary amines. Bacteria are involved in the conversions. One should reduce intake of foods and drugs likely to form nitrosamines in the intestines. Foods often containing nitrites include ham, corned beef, bacon, and most canned and smoked fish and meat. Most tranquilizers, antihistamines, antimalarials, appetite control agents, some hypoglycemic (low blood sugar) agents, and some antibiotics interact easily with nitrites to form nitrosamines. Other common potential sources of nitrosamines are beer, wine, and tobacco smoke.

Another class of agents implicated as cancer causing includes the so-called natural by-products or metabolites of molds and fungi. Aflatoxin, one of the most potent, causes liver cancer when included in the diet of test animals. Legumes (peanuts, soybeans), grains (corn, wheat), and aged meats (sausage, salami) are all prime candidates for aflatoxin contamination. In humans, a healthy liver may help protect the body from this compound by converting the aflatoxin into a harmless substance, which is subsequently excreted. In certain areas of the world, aflatoxin contamination has been implicated as a possible cause of liver cancer. A liver toxin capable of producing tumors also has been isolated from another common fungus, *Penicillium rubrum* (the antibiotic penicillin is not implicated), which has been found to contaminate rice in Japan. Several plants and plant components are known to cause cancer.

Consumption of coffee and sugar has recently been investigated in relation to cancer incidence. Consumption of each has been correlated with prostatic cancer. Excessive sugar intake also was found to be related to breast, ovarian, bladder, intestinal, and rectal malignancy. There is varying evidence that a high consumption of sugar is a contributory factor in several human diseases besides cancer—notably dental caries, obesity, coronary thrombosis, diabetes, and certain diseases of the skin, digestive tract, and the joints. Attention also has been focused on the caffeine in coffee, tea, and carbonated soft drinks as a possible carcinogen. In the United States, a high correlation between oral cancer and excessive alcohol consumption has been reported.

Diet as a whole, which possibly plays a more important role in the development of cancer than the occasional carcinogenic contamination in individual foods, is currently being evaluated in relation to the incidence of several types of cancer. There seems to be a relationship between the *quantity* of food eaten and cancer. People who overeat or who are overweight when past middle age are more likely to die of cancer than people who are average weight or less. However, people with protein, vitamin, or mineral deficiencies or general malnutrition are more susceptible to cancers of the liver, gallbladder, and upper alimentary tract.

Epidemiologic surveys have shown that the incidence of colon cancer is greater in Western Europe and the United States than in East Africa, Asia, and South America. Attempts have been made to relate these findings to dietary differences. People living in the industrialized Western countries tend to eat larger amounts of fat, animal protein, and refined carbohydrates, such as granulated sugar. In the developing areas, people eat largely vegetarian diets, with little fat or animal protein. The intestines of the people in the Western countries contain more bacteria capable of converting fats and steroids into cancer-causing compounds. It is thought that refined carbohydrates, such as sugar and white flour, play a major part in the origin of cancer of the bowel and colon. Geographic variations in the incidence of breast cancer have also been correlated with the fat content of diets.

Another notable difference between the diet of the Western World and that of developing countries is the proportion of unabsorbable fiber in the diet. The fiber content of diet affects the time food takes to travel through the intestines, the bulk and consistency of stools, and the bacterial population of the colon. The low-residue diet of Westerners increases the time that the food is retained in the colon and prolongs the opportunity for colon bacteria to convert dietary materials into cancer-causing compounds. Of the various types of fiber, wheat fiber seems to be most valuable in prevention. Studies thus far have provided convincing evidence that diet is important in many respects other than in meeting nutritional requirements. As research continues, we will probably become increasingly aware of the relationship between diet and disease, especially cancer.

Fratkin (1978) has observed that breast cancers occur largely among those people with "bovine" type of culture, which is associated with a lifetime exposure to a high intake of dairy products. Fratkin implicated beta estradiol in milk as being causative. However, radioimmunoassay for beta estradiol of milk and cheese products commercially available in Louisville revealed very low quantitites in these pasteurized products (Yussman and Rao, 1983). Minton (1983) considers that the tyramine present in ripe cheeses is a major culprit. Tyramine follows a metabolic degradation pathway similar to xanthines. Minton reports that both lead to an elevation of serum catecholamines. Tissues supersensitive to catecholamines will be stimulated to undergo a series of catecholamine-induced biochemical events. In breast tissue with increased intracellular levels of cyclic adenosine 3′, 5′-monophosphate (CAMP), this predisposes to chronic cystic mastopathy. Its effect could be similar on other tissues with an increased intracellular CAMP. Its effect on the colonic mucosa has not been reported.

Gaskill and associates (1979) expand on the relation of dairy products to breast cancer. There are parallels in the occurrence of colon and breast cancer in both animal and man. A diet useful in reducing dairy product intake is provided in Table 1.

Reduction of the Incidence of Cancer Through Diet

Diets associated with low incidences of various forms of cancer have several features in common. However, it should be remembered that none of these factors is absolute. Many nutrients, when present in sufficient amounts, enhance the body's defenses against disease but, when in short supply, decrease this defense. These nutrients, which are well dispersed in a variety of foods, include protein, vitamins, and minerals. The incidence of cancer could be reduced by developing the general eating habits that incorporate the nutrients described in the following paragraphs. Ames (1983) concludes that the ideal diet will be rich with anticarcinogens.

Be sure to eat a well-balanced selection of foods that are nutritionally adequate. Avoid prolonged cooking and excessive use of salt, pepper, condiments, and nutritionally empty foods such as sugar and alcohol. Since excessive use of refined sugar may replace other foods in your diet, it will reduce the intake of nutrients. Of all common foods, refined sugar uniquely supplies only calories with no protein, fats, vitamins or minerals.

The most nutritious foods containing protein are obtained largely from animal and some plant sources. One must be careful, however, to consume only small amounts of animal fats and fats from dairy products. To do this effectively and still receive adequate protein, keep consumption of processed meats, such as ham, lunch meat, and wieners to a minimum. Substitute, but eat in moderation, defatted animal protein, such as roast beef and skinned chicken, or fish. Excellent sources of animal protein besides meat, fish, and fowl are eggs. Include a high percentage

Table 1. **DIET TO REDUCE THE CHANCE OF CANCER***

Allowed	Prohibited†
Beverages: Water, fruit juices, noncaffeine drinks	Milk of any kind (when milk has to be consumed, use skimmed milk), caffeine beverages
Breads: Any kind;‡ whole grain breads preferred	Commercially prepared baked goods; commercially prepared mixes (hot cakes, waffles); soda crackers, cheese crackers, popovers
Cakes and Cookies: e.g., angel food cake, ladyfingers, Chinese Chews, Arrowroots, graham wafers	Check recipes; commercially prepared mixes
Candies: Gum drops, hard candies	Chocolates or creamed candies
Cereals: Dry cereals, cream of wheat, wheat, oatmeal, rolled oats, wheat germ, granola (from all sources, the diet should contain 25–30 gm of wheat fiber daily)	Check labels
Desserts: Gelatin, jellies, tapioca, rice, pies‡	All types made with milk, butter, i.e., ice cream, ice milk, sherbet, custard, pudding mixes
Cheeses	All kinds, including rarebit
Eggs: Any style except prohibited	Milk or fats added, i.e., fried, scrambled, omelet, soufflé
Fats and Oils: Some margarines;‡ corn, cottonseed, peanut, safflower, sesame, soy bean and olive oils	Butter, some margarines
Fish: Any kind	Fried in butter or batter
Fowl: Any kind	Fried in butter or batter
Fruits and Fruit Juices: Any kind, i.e., fresh, frozen, canned (but with no sugar added)	
Gravies and Sauces: Roux made with special margarines, flour, and water	Made with milk, butter, cheese, i.e., tartar sauce, butter sauce, hard sauce
Lentils: Split peas, dried beans	
Meat: Any kind; excess fat should be removed and the meat should not be cooked in fat	DES fed animals; some prepared meats, i.e., bologna, wieners, sausages, frozen beef patties, macaroni loaf, paté de foie gras, beef, chicken and pork spreads, meatballs in gravy
Nuts: Any kind	
Pastas: Spaghetti, noodles, macaroni	
Potatoes: Baked, steamed, boiled, sweet	French fries, mashed, scalloped, instant,‡ au gratin
Salad Dressings: French, homemade, mayonnaise (check recipe)	Boiled, commercially prepared‡
Soups: Any kind except prohibited	Cream or bisques, canned or packaged‡
Vegetables: Any kind, i.e., fresh, frozen, canned; mushrooms	Creamed or with butter sauce
Miscellaneous: Salt and pepper, pickles, spices, vinegar, herbs, condiments, jams, jellies, honey, marmalade	Popcorn, made with butter
Tobacco: Avoid in all forms	
Alcohol: Consume in moderation if at all	
Supplements: One adult multiple vitamin capsule daily. Add enough vitamin C or ascorbic acid, taken in divided doses throughout day, to total 3000 mg per day. For those with breast disease, add vitamin E, 200 IU twice daily. Elderly and those with stomach problems often need supplementary folic acid—about 1 mg daily.	

*Courtesy of Leonard B. Fratkin, M.D.

†Labels of food products should be checked for the addition of milk, lactose, and milk solids, particularly milk fats. When these are listed as ingredients, the food should be avoided. When the composition of the food is in doubt, an appropriate source should be consulted. One should realize that food prepared outside the home may contain prohibited substances. Total caloric intake balanced against daily exercise should keep body weight at or slightly below ideal for age and height (see Table 2).

‡Check label.

of bulk in your diet by eating whole grain cereals, salads, raw fruits, and vegetables with the peelings, unsweetened stewed fruits, and bran. When possible, total wheat fiber intake should approach 30 gm per day. Fiber content of various cereals is often stated on the package. Fresh, uncooked seasonal fruits and vegetables should be eaten daily. Unsweetened citrus fruit, in addition to juice, should definitely be included in the diet. Vegetables of the deep yellow and dark green varieties are excellent sources of fiber, vitamins, and betacarotene. A variety of these, occasionally including the potato and its peeling, should be eaten daily either cooked or raw. Eating a raw carrot a day is an excellent habit. Vegetables should never be fried or served with high-fat condiments, such as butter or sour cream. Be sure to wash the surface of all fresh fruits and vegetables carefully to reduce the intake of pesticides. However, soaking them and drying their surfaces after washing causes nutrient loss. In general, in order to get optimum nutrients from fruits and vegetables, you should eat them fresh. Many canned and stewed fruits are undesirable because of sweetening with refined sugar and loss of vitamins in cooking.

To reduce dairy product intake, check the labels on packages. Generally, most breads, sugarless cereals, eggs, corn and vegetable oils, fish, fowl, and nuts are satisfactory as are a variety of other foods.

I also suggest that you have an adequate daily fluid intake, consisting of fresh fruit juices (purchase only varieties to which sugar has not been added or prepare your own fresh fruit juice and drink without sweetening), tomato juice, and water, and that you take a daily multiple vitamin supplement. Keep consumption of coffee, tea, and alcohol to a minimum.

Appetite and flow of digestive juices can be greatly enhanced by preparing colorful and flavorful meals. Your dining environment may also be very important in that a relaxed, peaceful atmosphere with soft conversation promotes healthy digestion. Any disruptive influences, such as excessive noise, distracting television programs, or family arguments actually promote gastrointestinal disturbances. These points cannot be overemphasized, since no meal, no matter how nutritious, is of any value if not eaten or digested properly.

RECOMMENDATIONS FOR THE PREVENTION OF CANCER

Your entire behavioral pattern may affect the development of cancer. Many environmental factors are now recognized as cancer-causing. Each individual can make behavioral choices to avoid cancer or he can ignore the facts and possibly expose himself to potential cancer-causing factors. Diet has been discussed. Listed below are some other suggestions that could affect the development or nondevelopment of cancer in the individual:

1. To avoid excess body weight, adjust your daily caloric intake according to your work habits and body build (Table 2). (Correlations have been shown between obesity and cancer, as well as between obesity and heart disease.)
2. Get a good, sound, natural sleep every night.
3. Avoid use of tobacco in any form. The correlation between lung and oral cancers and tobacco has been strongly established, and tobacco has been implicated as causative of other cancers.
4. Practice good oral hygiene and have regular examinations by a dentist.
5. Avoid prolonged exposure to direct sunlight. If you work in the sun, wear protective clothing, including a hat with a brim and gloves. Prolonged exposure to direct sunlight has been directly linked to skin cancer. Do not use a sun lamp.

Table 2. **HEIGHT-WEIGHT SCREENING TABLES**

	Weight (lb)			
	Men		*Women*	
Height	*Minimum*	*Maximum*	*Minimum*	*Maximum*
4′ 10″	—	—	87	126
4′ 11″	—	—	89	128
5′ 0″	100	153	92	130
5′ 1″	102	155	95	132
5′ 2″	103	158	97	134
5′ 3″	104	160	100	136
5′ 4″	105	164	103	139
5′ 5″	106	169	106	144
5′ 6″	109	174	108	148
5′ 7″	111	179	111	152
5′ 8″	115	184	114	156
5′ 9″	119	189	117	161
5′ 10″	123	194	119	165
5′ 11″	127	199	122	169
6′ 0″	131	205	125	174
6′ 1″	135	211	128	179
6′ 2″	139	218	130	185
6′ 3″	143	224	133	190
6′ 4″	147	230	136	196
6′ 5″	151	236	139	201
6′ 6″	153	242	141	206
6′ 7″	157	248	144	211
6′ 8″	161	254	147	216

6. Practice good genital hygiene. Increasing evidence suggests that childbearing at a very early age increases the chance of developing cervical cancer. All women who started their families early in life should, more than any other group, have gynecological examinations and Pap smears regularly. Do not use talc near body openings.

7. Avoid chemical carcinogens in any form when possible. Some carcinogens and precarcinogens in foods were mentioned earlier. However, many other chemicals in the environment have been identified as cancer-causing agents. Control of carcinogenic contamination of the environment, however, is no longer a matter of individual choice. Reducing the significance of this problem will take continuing federal, state, and community vigilance and action. Financial and political support for the control efforts of agencies monitoring the carcinogenic composition of man's environment is necessary from everyone.

A position paper by Bridbord and associates (1978) regarding the important relationship between occupational factors and cancer constitutes an authoritative critical review of this important issue. The industrial health physicians and nurses and the safety officers in your place of employment should obtain a copy of this study and review it with respect to your specific work environment. Important regulations and standards intended to reduce exposure to cancer-causing agents in the workplace are originating from the Occupational Safety and Health Administration (OSHA) and the Food and Drug Administration (FDA).

Following the preceding suggestions, including adhering to a proper diet, cannot eliminate cancer. However, if the scientists' observations and numerous isolated reports are correct, people could theoretically reduce their chances of getting cancer by the lifelong practice of the dietary and behavioral habits suggested.

One of the most important approaches to the correction of bad habits involves the retraining of one's tastes and interests. One of the first questions many people ask is, "What's left to do and eat?" The answer is that there are more interesting things to do and more good things to eat than you have ever tried before if you will open your eyes and your mind to them.

In addition, you should have a prompt examination if any of the following symptoms develop between your periodic examinations:

1. Unusual bleeding or discharge.
2. A lump or thickening in the breast or elsewhere.
3. A sore that does not heal.
4. Change in bowel or bladder habits.
5. Hoarseness or cough.
6. Indigestion or difficulty of swallowing.
7. Change in wart or mole.

If your symptom lasts longer than two weeks, go to your doctor and have it evaluated. Regular examinations result in some cancers being found while still asymptomatic. This early detection is the best chance for effective treatment. If you have already had a cancer or a precancerous condition, all these suggestions still apply. In addition, you need to review with your physician the follow-up plan specific for your problem. Remember, cancer is the most preventable and in many cases the most curable of all chronic diseases.

Physical Conditioning and Weight Control

Along with making the suggested dietary and behavioral changes you should follow general physical conditioning and weight control programs. The interrelationship of all these factors is stressed in the following plan for general fitness.

Everyone is susceptible to the insidious effects of sedentary jobs, excessive calorie intake, and lack of proper exercise. Excess body fat is a serious detriment to health, longevity, stamina, and appearance. The need to maintain a high state of health and physical fitness is essential to ensure personal effectiveness.

A program can be followed to maintain health and physical fitness. A major emphasis is placed on a vigorous and active health and fitness programs. These programs include weight control/nutrition, smoking cessation, hypertension control, stress management, and substance abuse prevention as well as exercise. Additionally, self-testing can be done against the standards outlined in Table 3 using the procedures described in the outline that follows. All people, except those excused for medical reasons, should attain and maintain a condition of health and physical fitness. Physical readiness cannot be developed by prescription or by medical advice. Progression to each level must be gradual, particularly for the previously unconditioned, through self-motivation.

Special requirements for certain specialized occupations may necessitate more stringent standards than those outlined here. When this situation exists, more stringent requirements can be established as long as they do not violate the health of the individual. All people should utilize the testing criteria and institute programs to assist them in meeting or exceeding the requirements.

If any of the suggestions contained in this article are different from instructions you have from your physician, consult your physician, since other medical problems may require approaches other than those suggested here.

The following is a description of the performance items in Table 3.

Table 3. **PHYSICAL READINESS CLASSIFICATION TABLE AND TEST REQUIREMENTS***

Classification*	Under 30		30–34		35–39		40–44		45–49		50 and Older	
	Men	*Women*	*Men*	*Women*	*Men*	*Women*	*Men*	*Women*	*Men*	*Women*	*Men*	*Women*
Outstanding												
1.5 mi run	9:45	11:30	10:00	12:00	10:30	12:30	11:00	11:30	11:30	13:30	12:00	14:00
Sit ups	100	84	90	75	85	71	80	67	80	67	80	67
Sit reach	+2.0	+4.0	+2.0	+3.5	+1.5	+3.0	+1.5	+3.0	+1.0	+2.0	+1.0	+2.0
Percentage fat	14	18	14	18	14	18	14	18	14	18	14	18
Excellent												
1.5 mi run	10:45	13:00	11:00	13:30	11:30	14:00	12:00	14:30	12:30	15:00	13:00	15:30
Sit ups	75	63	68	56	64	53	60	50	60	50	60	50
Sit reach	+1.0	+3.0	0	+2.0	0	+1.5	0	+1.0	−0.5	+1.0	−0.5	+1.0
Percentage fat	16	22	16	22	16	22	16	22	16	22	16	22
Good												
1.5 mi run	13:00	15:00	14:00	15:30	14:30	16:00	15:00	16:30	15:30	17:00	16:00	17:30
Run in place	350	300	325	280	300	260	300	260	280	200	280	200
Sit ups	50	42	45	38	43	36	40	34	40	34	40	34
Sit reach	0	+2.0	−1.0	0	−1.0	0	−1.0	0	−1.0	0	−1.0	0
Percentage fat	18	24	18	24	18	24	18	24	18	24	18	24
Satisfactory												
1.5 mi run	14:30	16:30	15:30	17:30	16:00	18:00	16:30	18:30	17:00	19:00	17:30	20:00
Run in place	310	260	280	220	260	200	260	200	240	180	240	180
Sit ups	36	30	34	28	32	26	30	25	30	25	30	25
Sit reach	−1.0	0	−1.5	−0.5	−1.5	−1.0	−1.5	−1.0	−2.0	−1.5	−2.0	−1.5
Percentage fat	20	29	20	29	20	29	20	29	20	29	20	29
Minimum Standard												
1.5 mi run	15:00	17:00	16:00	18:00	16:30	18:30	17:00	19:00	17:30	19:30	18:00	20:30
Run in place	280	235	250	200	230	180	230	180	210	160	210	160
Sit ups	33	27	31	25	29	23	27	22	27	22	27	22
Sit reach	−1.5	−0.5	−2.0	−1.0	−2.0	−1.5	−2.0	−1.5	−2.5	−2.0	−2.5	−2.0
Percentage fat	22	30	22	30	22	30	22	30	22	30	22	30

*From OPNAVINST 6110.1B.

†Classification Criteria: Only one classification applies to an individual, and each individual must meet or exceed each and every criteria to achieve the classification.

I. Stamina and cardiorespiratory endurance*
   A. Definition: The ability to persist in physical activity that demands the delivery and utilization of large amounts of oxygen.
   B. Run-walk test (1.5 miles): A course of 1.5 miles should be selected that is relatively free of steep inclines, surface irregularities, and sharp turns. Any combination of running or walking is permitted to achieve the best time. Performances should be recorded with a stopwatch to the nearest second.
   C. Run in place. On an individual basis, running in place may be substituted for the timed distance run or walk whenever desired. Running in place cannot be used to qualify for the excellent or outstanding category. The test consists of running in place with knees up and feet raised approximately 8 in. off the floor on each step. A count is made every time the left foot hits the floor. The score is the number of counts completed in 3 minutes.

II. Strength and muscular endurance*
   A. Definition: The maximum force that can be exerted in a single voluntary contraction and the ability to continue contracting a muscle or muscle group without fatigue.
   B. Sit ups
      1. Lie flat on back with knees bent, heels close to buttocks (approximately 10 in.), and arms folded across chest; feet should be held to floor by a partner or be placed under a structure that will keep them on the floor.
      2. Curl up touching elbows to thighs.
      3. Lie back touching shoulders to floor.
      4. Repeat as many times as possible in 2 minutes.
      5. Caution. It is advisable to perform this excercise on a blanket or other suitable padding to prevent injuries.

III. Flexibility
   A. Definition: The functional capacity of a joint to move through the range of motion.
   B. Sit and reach test
      1. Sit on floor with legs straight, feet spread 6 in. apart, with shoes off.
      2. Keeping legs straight, reach as far forward as possible, touching the floor between legs with fingertips of both hands. Hold the reach at least 3 seconds—do not bounce.
      3. Measure the distance from a line at the heels to the point of touch in inches short (e.g., −2.0 in.) or inches beyond (e.g., +2.0 in.) the line.
      4. Caution. Warm up sufficiently by gradually stretching the back and leg muscle groups before doing the test.

IV. Body composition (percentage of fat)
   A. Definition: The body is composed of fat and lean weight. Body fat is expressed as a percentage of total weight.
   B. Body fat measures should be taken when a person exceeds the height-weight standards outlined in Table 2.
   C. The estimate and measurement of the percentage of body fat are the responsibilities of each individual, with the physician's assistance when

---

*Training effect occurs when an exercise, conducted with sufficient regularity, intensity, and duration, results in improvement in the efficiency of the cardiorespiratory system and/or muscular strength and endurance. The exercise that produces a training effect must be performed a minimum of three times per week, preferably on alternate days, must raise the exerciser's heart rate to 60 to 80 percent of maximum for his or her age, and must maintain the heart rate at that elevated level for 20 to 30 minutes.

necessary. Individuals who exceed the standards should initiate a remedial program. Medical consultation is required only when a concomitant medical condition is suspected.

D. Recommended procedures for estimating body fat require the use of a standard tape measure. The tape should be applied to certain body landmarks (Fig. 1), with sufficient tension to keep it in place without indenting the skin surface. Measures should be recorded to the nearest eighth of an inch.

E. Table 4 is used to estimate the percentage of body fat in men.
   1. Measurement of the neck is taken at a point just below the larynx (Adam's apple).
   2. Measurement of the abdomen is taken at the navel, with the tape level to the floor.
   3. Convert all measurements to percentage points using Table 4. Record the figures on a chart (see Fig. 2).

F. Table 5 is used to estimate the percentage of body fat in women.
   1. Measurement of the neck is taken at a point just below the larynx (Adam's apple).
   2. Measurement of the abdomen is taken at the navel, with the tape level to the floor.
   3. Measurement of the biceps is taken with the arm fully extended, level to the floor, with the palm facing up. Place the tape over the largest circumference of the biceps-triceps muscle group (upper arm).
   4. Measurement of the forearm is taken with the arm fully extended, level to the floor, with the palm facing up. Place the tape over the largest circumference of the forearm.
   5. Measurement of the thigh is taken with the feet slightly apart. Place the tape just below the left buttock and around the thigh, level to the floor.
   6. Convert all measurements to percentage points using Table 5. Record figures on a chart (see Fig. 3). Add the five percentage points. Subtract

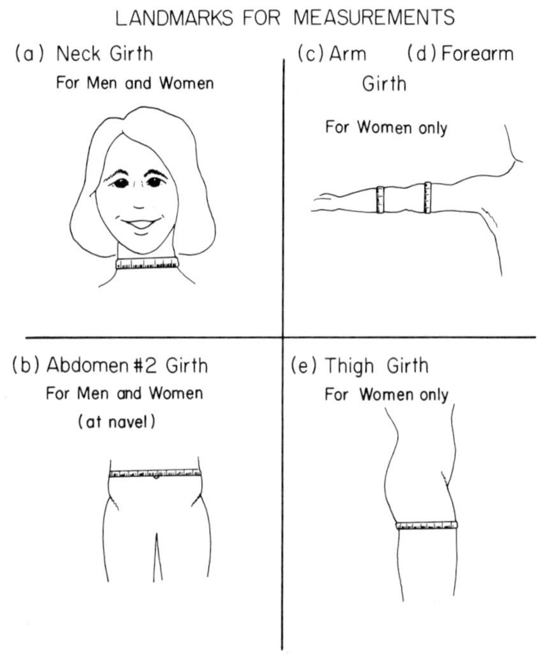

Figure 1. Landmarks for measurements.

Table 4. **ESTIMATION OF THE PERCENTAGE OF FAT IN MEN, USING ABDOMEN AND NECK MEASUREMENTS**

	Neck (in.)								
Abdomen (in.)	*13.00*	*13.25*	*13.50*	*13.75*	*14.00*	*14.25*	*14.50*	*14.75*	*15.00*
25.0	6.3	5.5	4.7	3.9	3.1	2.3	1.5	.7	
25.5	7.2	6.4	5.6	4.8	4.0	3.3	2.5	1.7	.9
26.0	8.2	7.4	6.6	5.8	5.0	4.2	3.4	2.6	1.8
26.5	9.1	8.3	7.5	6.7	5.9	5.1	4.3	3.5	2.8
27.0	10.0	9.2	8.4	7.7	6.9	6.1	5.3	4.5	3.7
27.5	11.0	10.2	9.4	8.6	7.8	7.0	6.2	5.4	4.6
28.0	11.9	11.1	10.3	9.5	8.7	7.9	7.2	6.4	5.6
28.5	12.9	12.1	11.3	10.5	9.7	8.9	8.1	7.3	6.5
29.0	13.8	13.0	12.2	11.4	10.6	9.8	9.0	8.2	7.4
29.5	14.7	13.9	13.1	12.4	11.6	10.8	10.0	9.2	8.4
30.0	15.7	14.9	14.1	13.3	12.5	11.7	10.9	10.1	9.3
30.5	16.6	15.8	15.0	14.2	13.4	12.6	11.9	11.1	10.3
31.0	17.6	16.8	16.0	15.2	14.4	13.6	12.8	12.0	11.2
31.5	18.5	17.7	16.9	16.1	15.3	14.5	13.7	12.9	12.1
32.0	19.4	18.6	17.8	17.1	16.3	15.5	14.7	13.9	13.1
32.5	20.4	19.6	18.8	18.0	17.2	16.4	15.6	14.8	14.0
33.0	21.3	20.5	19.7	18.9	18.1	17.3	16.6	15.8	15.0
33.5	22.3	21.5	20.7	19.9	19.1	18.3	17.5	16.7	15.9
34.0	23.2	22.4	21.6	20.8	20.0	19.2	18.4	17.6	16.8
34.5	24.1	23.3	22.5	21.8	21.0	20.2	19.4	18.6	17.8
35.0	25.1	24.3	23.5	22.7	21.9	21.1	20.3	19.5	18.7
35.5	26.0	25.2	24.4	23.6	22.8	22.0	21.3	20.5	19.7
36.0	27.0	26.2	25.4	24.6	23.8	23.0	22.2	21.4	20.6
36.5	27.9	27.1	26.3	25.5	24.7	23.9	23.1	22.3	21.5
37.0	28.8	28.0	27.2	26.5	25.7	24.9	24.1	23.3	22.5
37.5	29.8	29.0	28.2	27.4	26.6	25.8	25.0	24.2	23.4
38.0	30.7	29.9	29.1	28.3	27.5	26.7	26.0	25.2	24.4
38.5	31.7	30.9	30.1	29.3	28.5	27.7	26.9	26.1	25.3
39.0	32.6	31.8	31.0	30.2	29.4	28.6	27.8	27.0	26.2
39.5	33.5	32.7	31.9	31.2	30.4	29.6	28.8	28.0	27.2
40.0	34.5	33.7	32.9	32.1	31.3	30.5	29.7	28.9	28.1
40.5	35.4	34.6	33.8	33.0	32.2	31.4	30.7	29.9	29.1
41.0	36.3	35.6	34.8	34.0	33.2	32.4	31.6	30.8	30.0
41.5	37.3	36.5	35.7	34.9	34.1	33.3	32.5	31.7	30.9
42.0	38.2	37.4	36.6	35.8	35.1	34.3	33.5	32.7	31.9
42.5	39.2	38.4	37.6	36.8	36.0	35.2	34.4	33.6	32.8
43.0	40.1	39.3	38.5	37.7	36.9	36.1	35.4	34.6	33.8

43.5	41.0	40.3	39.5	38.7	37.9	37.1	36.3	35.5	34.7
44.0	42.0	41.2	40.4	39.6	38.8	38.0	37.2	36.4	35.6
44.5	42.9	42.1	41.3	40.5	39.8	39.0	38.2	37.4	36.6
45.0	43.9	43.1	42.3	41.5	40.7	39.9	39.1	38.3	37.5
45.5	44.8	44.0	43.2	42.4	41.6	40.8	40.0	39.3	38.5
46.0	45.7	45.0	44.2	43.4	42.6	41.8	41.0	40.2	39.4
46.5	46.7	45.9	45.1	44.3	43.5	42.7	41.9	41.1	40.3
47.0	47.6	46.8	46.0	45.2	44.5	43.7	42.9	42.1	41.3
47.5	48.6	47.8	47.0	46.2	45.4	44.6	43.8	43.0	42.2
48.0	49.5	48.7	47.9	47.1	46.3	45.5	44.7	44.0	43.2
48.5	50.4	49.7	48.9	48.1	47.3	46.5	45.7	44.9	44.1
49.0	51.4	50.6	49.8	49.0	48.2	47.4	46.6	45.8	45.0
49.5	52.3	51.5	50.7	49.9	49.2	48.4	47.6	46.8	46.0
50.0	53.3	52.5	51.7	50.9	50.1	49.3	48.5	47.7	46.9

	Neck (in.)								
Abdomen (in.)	*15.25*	*15.50*	*15.75*	*16.00*	*16.25*	*16.50*	*16.75*	*17.00*	*17.25*
25.0									
25.5	0.1								
26.0	1.0	0.2							
26.5	2.0	1.2	0.4						
27.0	2.9	2.1	1.3	0.5					
27.5	3.8	3.0	2.3	1.5	0.7				
28.0	4.8	4.0	3.2	2.4	1.6	0.8	0.0		
28.5	5.7	4.9	4.1	3.3	2.5	1.8	1.0	0.2	
29.0	6.7	5.9	5.1	4.3	3.5	2.7	1.9	1.1	0.3
29.5	7.6	6.8	6.0	5.2	4.4	3.6	2.8	2.0	1.3
30.0	8.5	7.7	6.9	6.2	5.4	4.6	3.8	3.0	2.2
30.5	9.5	8.7	7.9	7.1	6.3	5.5	4.7	3.9	3.1
31.0	10.4	9.6	8.8	8.0	7.2	6.5	5.7	4.9	4.1
31.5	11.4	10.6	9.8	9.0	8.2	7.4	6.6	5.8	5.0
32.0	12.3	11.5	10.7	9.9	9.1	8.3	7.5	6.7	6.0
32.5	13.2	12.4	11.6	10.9	10.1	9.3	8.5	7.7	6.9
33.0	14.2	13.4	12.6	11.8	11.0	10.2	9.4	8.6	7.8
33.5	15.1	14.3	13.5	12.7	11.9	11.1	10.4	9.6	8.8
34.0	16.1	15.3	14.5	13.7	12.9	12.1	11.3	10.5	9.7
34.5	17.0	16.2	15.4	14.6	13.8	13.0	12.2	11.4	10.6
35.0	17.9	17.1	16.3	15.6	14.8	14.0	13.2	12.4	11.6
35.5	18.9	18.1	17.3	16.5	15.7	14.9	14.1	13.3	12.5
36.0	19.8	19.0	18.2	17.4	16.6	15.8	15.1	14.3	13.5
36.5	20.8	20.0	19.2	18.4	17.6	16.8	16.0	15.2	14.4
37.0	21.7	20.9	20.1	19.3	18.5	17.7	16.9	16.1	15.3
37.5	22.6	21.8	21.0	20.3	19.5	18.7	17.9	17.1	16.3
38.0	23.6	22.8	22.0	21.2	20.4	19.6	18.8	18.0	17.2
38.5	24.5	23.7	22.9	22.1	21.3	20.5	19.8	19.0	18.2

Table 4. **ESTIMATION OF THE PERCENTAGE OF FAT IN MEN, USING ABDOMEN AND NECK MEASUREMENTS** *(Continued)*

	Neck (in.)								
Abdomen (in.)	*15.25*	*15.50*	*15.75*	*16.00*	*16.25*	*16.50*	*16.75*	*17.00*	*17.25*
39.0	25.5	24.7	23.9	23.1	22.3	21.5	20.7	19.9	19.1
39.5	26.4	25.6	24.8	24.0	23.2	22.4	21.6	20.8	20.0
40.0	27.3	26.5	25.7	25.0	24.2	23.4	22.6	21.8	21.0
40.5	28.3	27.5	26.7	25.9	25.1	24.3	23.5	22.7	21.9
41.0	29.2	28.4	27.6	26.8	26.0	25.2	24.5	23.7	22.9
41.5	30.2	29.4	28.6	27.8	27.0	26.2	25.4	24.6	23.8
42.0	31.1	30.3	29.5	28.7	27.9	27.1	26.3	25.5	24.7
42.5	32.0	31.2	30.4	29.7	28.9	28.1	27.3	26.5	25.7
43.0	33.0	32.2	31.4	30.6	29.8	29.0	28.2	27.4	26.6
43.5	33.9	33.1	32.3	31.5	30.7	29.9	29.2	28.4	27.6
44.0	34.9	34.1	33.3	32.5	31.7	30.9	30.1	29.3	28.5
44.5	35.8	35.0	34.2	33.4	32.6	31.8	31.0	30.2	29.4
45.0	36.7	35.9	35.1	34.4	33.6	32.8	32.0	31.2	30.4
45.5	37.7	36.9	36.1	35.3	34.5	33.7	32.9	32.1	31.3
46.0	38.6	37.8	37.0	36.2	35.4	34.6	33.9	33.1	32.3
46.5	39.5	38.8	38.0	37.2	36.4	35.6	34.8	34.0	33.2
47.0	40.5	39.7	38.9	38.1	37.3	36.5	35.7	34.9	34.1
47.5	41.4	40.6	39.8	39.0	38.3	37.5	36.7	35.9	35.1
48.0	42.4	41.6	40.8	40.0	39.2	38.4	37.6	36.8	36.0
48.5	43.3	42.5	41.7	40.9	40.1	39.3	38.5	37.8	37.0
49.0	44.2	43.5	42.7	41.9	41.1	40.3	39.5	38.7	37.9
49.5	45.2	44.4	43.6	42.8	42.0	41.2	40.4	39.6	38.8
50.0	46.1	45.3	44.5	43.7	43.0	42.2	41.4	40.6	39.8

	Neck (in.)									
Abdomen (in.)	*17.50*	*17.75*	*18.00*	*18.25*	*18.50*	*18.75*	*19.00*	*19.25*	*19.50*	*19.75*
29.5	0.5									
30.0	1.4	0.6								
30.5	2.3	1.5	0.8							
31.0	3.3	2.5	1.7	0.9	0.1					
31.5	4.2	3.4	2.6	1.8	1.0	0.3				
32.0	5.2	4.4	3.6	2.8	2.0	1.2	0.4			
32.5	6.1	5.3	4.5	3.7	2.9	2.1	1.3	0.5		
33.0	7.0	6.2	5.5	4.7	3.9	3.1	2.3	1.5	0.7	
33.5	8.0	7.2	6.4	5.6	4.8	4.0	3.2	2.4	1.6	0.8
34.0	8.9	8.1	7.3	6.5	5.7	5.0	4.2	3.4	2.6	1.8
34.5	9.9	9.1	8.3	7.5	6.7	5.9	5.1	4.3	3.5	2.7
35.0	10.8	10.0	9.2	8.4	7.6	6.8	6.0	5.2	4.5	3.7
35.5	11.7	10.9	10.1	9.4	8.6	7.8	7.0	6.2	5.4	4.6
36.0	12.7	11.9	11.1	10.3	9.5	8.7	7.9	7.1	6.3	5.5
36.5	13.6	12.8	12.0	11.2	10.4	9.6	8.9	8.1	7.3	6.5
37.0	14.6	13.8	13.0	12.2	11.4	10.6	9.8	9.0	8.2	7.4

37.5	15.5	14.7	13.9	13.1	12.3	11.5	10.7	9.9	9.2	8.4
38.0	16.4	15.6	14.8	14.1	13.3	12.5	11.7	10.9	10.1	9.3
38.5	17.4	16.6	15.8	15.0	14.2	13.4	12.6	11.8	11.0	10.2
39.0	18.3	17.5	16.7	15.9	15.1	14.3	13.6	12.8	12.0	11.2
39.5	19.3	18.5	17.7	16.9	16.1	15.3	14.5	13.7	12.9	12.1
40.0	20.2	19.4	18.6	17.8	17.0	16.2	15.4	14.6	13.8	13.1
40.5	21.1	20.3	19.5	18.8	18.0	17.2	16.4	15.6	14.8	14.0
41.0	22.1	21.3	20.5	19.7	18.9	18.1	17.3	16.5	15.7	14.9
41.5	23.0	22.2	21.4	20.6	19.8	19.0	18.3	17.5	16.7	15.9
42.0	24.0	23.2	22.4	21.6	20.8	20.0	19.2	18.4	17.6	16.8
42.5	24.9	24.1	23.3	22.5	21.7	20.9	20.1	19.3	18.5	17.8
43.0	25.8	25.0	24.2	23.5	22.7	21.9	21.1	20.3	19.5	18.7
43.5	26.8	26.0	25.2	24.4	23.6	22.8	22.0	21.2	20.4	19.6
44.0	27.7	26.9	26.1	25.3	24.5	23.7	23.0	22.2	21.4	20.6
44.5	28.7	27.9	27.1	26.3	25.5	24.7	23.9	23.1	22.3	21.5
45.0	29.6	28.8	28.0	27.2	26.4	25.6	24.8	24.0	23.2	22.5
45.5	30.5	29.7	28.9	28.2	27.4	26.6	25.8	25.0	24.2	23.4
46.0	31.5	30.7	29.9	29.1	28.3	27.5	26.7	25.9	25.1	24.3
46.5	32.4	31.6	30.8	30.0	29.2	28.4	27.7	26.9	26.1	25.3
47.0	33.4	32.6	31.8	31.0	30.2	29.4	28.6	27.8	27.0	26.2
47.5	34.3	33.5	32.7	31.9	31.1	30.3	29.5	28.7	27.9	27.2
48.0	35.2	34.4	33.6	32.9	32.1	31.3	30.5	29.7	28.9	28.1
48.5	36.2	35.4	34.6	33.8	33.0	32.2	31.4	30.6	29.8	29.0
49.0	37.1	36.3	35.5	34.7	33.9	33.1	32.4	31.6	30.8	30.0
49.5	38.1	37.3	36.5	35.7	34.9	34.1	33.3	32.5	31.7	30.9
50.0	39.0	38.2	37.4	36.6	35.8	35.0	34.2	33.4	32.6	31.9

Table 5. **ESTIMATION OF THE PERCENTAGE OF FAT IN WOMEN**

Neck (in.)	%	Neck (in.)	%	Neck (in.)	%	Neck (in.)	%	Neck (in.)	%
15 5/8	0.1	13 7/8	4.1	12 1/8	8.0	10 3/8	11.9	8 5/8	15.4
15 4/8	0.4	13 6/8	4.3	12 0/8	8.2	10 2/8	12.1	8 4/8	16.1
15 3/8	0.7	13 5/8	4.6	11 7/8	8.5	10 1/8	12.4	8 3/8	16.3
15 2/8	1.0	13 4/8	4.9	11 6/8	8.8	10 0/8	12.7	8 2/8	16.7
15 1/8	1.3	13 3/8	5.2	11 5/8	9.1	9 7/8	13.0	8 1/8	16.9
15 0/8	1.5	13 2/8	5.4	11 4/8	9.4	9 6/8	13.3	8 0/8	17.2
14 7/8	1.8	13 1/8	5.7	11 3/8	9.6	9 5/8	13.5	7 7/8	17.4
14 6/8	2.1	13 0/8	6.0	11 2/8	9.9	9 4/8	13.8	7 6/8	17.7
14 5/8	2.4	12 7/8	6.3	11 1/8	10.2	9 3/8	14.1	7 5/8	18.0
14 4/8	2.7	12 6/8	6.6	11 0/8	10.6	9 2/8	14.4	7 4/8	18.3
14 3/8	2.9	12 5/8	6.8	10 7/8	10.8	9 1/8	14.7	7 3/8	18.6
14 2/8	3.2	12 4/8	7.1	10 6/8	11.0	9 0/8	14.9		
14 1/8	3.5	12 3/8	7.4	10 5/8	11.3	8 7/8	15.2		
14 0/8	3.8	12 2/8	7.7	10 4/8	11.6	8 6/8	15.5		

Biceps (in.)	%	Biceps (in.)	%	Biceps (in.)	%	Biceps (in.)	%	Biceps (in.)	%
5 7/8	0.1	7 5/8	4.8	9 3/8	9.4	11 1/8	14.1	12 7/8	18.8
6 0/8	0.4	7 6/8	5.1	9 4/8	9.8	11 2/8	14.5	13 0/8	19.1
6 1/8	0.8	7 7/8	5.4	9 5/8	10.1	11 3/8	14.8	13 1/8	19.5
6 2/8	1.1	8 0/8	5.8	9 6/8	10.4	11 4/8	15.1	13 2/8	19.8
6 3/8	1.4	8 1/8	6.1	9 7/8	10.8	11 5/8	15.5	13 3/8	20.1
6 4/8	1.8	8 2/8	6.4	10 0/8	11.1	11 6/8	15.8	13 4/8	20.5
6 5/8	2.1	8 3/8	6.8	10 1/8	11.4	11 7/8	16.1	13 5/8	20.8
6 6/8	2.4	8 4/8	7.1	10 2/8	11.8	12 0/8	16.5	13 6/8	21.1
6 7/8	2.8	8 5/8	7.4	10 3/8	12.1	12 1/8	16.8		
7 0/8	3.1	8 6/8	7.8	10 4/8	12.4	12 2/8	17.1		
7 1/8	3.4	8 7/8	8.1	10 5/8	12.8	12 3/8	17.5		
7 2/8	3.8	9 0/8	8.4	10 6/8	13.1	12 4/8	17.8		
7 3/8	4.1	9 1/8	8.8	10 7/8	13.5	12 5/8	18.1		
7 4/8	4.4	9 2/8	9.1	11 0/8	13.8	12 6/8	18.5		

Forearm (in.)	%	Forearm (in.)	%	Forearm (in.)	%	Forearm (in.)	%)	Forearm (in.)	%
17 5/8	.2	15 2/8	9.3	12 7/8	18.5	10 4/8	27.7	8 1/8	36.8
17 4/8	.6	15 1/8	9.8	12 6/8	19.0	10 3/8	28.1	8 0/8	37.3
17 3/8	1.1	15 0/8	10.3	12 5/8	19.5	10 2/8	28.5	7 7/8	37.8
17 2/8	1.6	14 7/8	10.8	12 4/8	19.9	10 1/8	29.1	7 6/8	38.3
17 1/8	2.1	14 6/8	11.2	12 3/8	20.4	10 0/8	29.6	7 5/8	38.8
17 0/8	2.5	14 5/8	11.7	12 2/8	20.9	9 7/8	30.1	7 4/8	39.3
16 7/8	3.0	14 4/8	12.2	12 1/8	21.4	9 6/8	30.6	7 3/8	39.7
16 6/8	3.5	14 3/8	12.7	12 0/8	21.9	9 5/8	31.0	7 2/8	40.2
16 5/8	4.0	14 2/8	13.2	11 7/8	22.3	9 4/8	31.5	7 1/8	40.7
16 4/8	4.5	14 1/8	13.7	11 6/8	22.8	9 3/8	32.0	7 0/8	41.2
16 3/8	5.0	14 0/8	14.1	11 5/8	23.3	9 2/8	32.5	6 7/8	41.7
16 2/8	5.4	13 7/8	14.6	11 4/8	23.8	9 1/8	33.0	6 6/8	42.2
16 1/8	5.9	13 6/8	15.1	11 3/8	24.3	9 0/8	33.5	6 5/8	42.5
16 0/8	6.4	13 5/8	15.6	11 2/8	24.9	8 7/8	33.9	0 0/8	.0
15 7/8	6.9	13 4/8	16.1	11 1/8	25.2	8 6/8	34.4		
15 6/8	7.4	13 3/8	16.6	11 0/8	25.7	8 5/8	34.9		
15 5/8	7.9	13 2/8	17.0	10 7/8	26.2	8 4/8	35.4		
15 4/8	8.3	13 1/8	17.5	10 6/8	26.7	8 3/8	36.0		
15 3/8	8.8	13 0/8	18.0	10 5/8	27.2	8 2/8	36.4		

Table 5. **ESTIMATION OF THE PERCENTAGE OF FAT IN WOMEN** *(Continued)*

Abdomen (in.)	%	Abdomen (in.)	%	Abdomen (in.)	%	Abdomen (in.)	%	Abdomen (in.)	%	Abdomen (in.)	%
17 5/8	0.0	23 0/8	4.4	28 3/8	8.9	33 6/8	13.3	39 1/8	17.8	44 4/8	22.2
17 6/8	0.1	23 1/8	4.5	28 4/8	9.0	33 7/8	13.4	39 2/8	17.9	44 5/8	22.3
17 7/8	0.2	23 2/8	4.6	28 5/8	9.1	34 0/8	13.5	39 3/8	18.0	44 6/8	22.4
18 0/8	0.3	23 3/8	4.7	28 6/8	9.2	34 1/8	13.6	39 4/8	18.1	44 7/8	22.5
18 1/8	0.4	23 4/8	4.8	28 7/8	9.3	34 2/8	13.7	39 5/8	18.2	45 0/8	22.6
18 2/8	0.5	23 5/8	4.9	29 0/8	9.4	34 3/8	13.8	39 6/8	18.3	45 1/8	22.7
18 3/8	0.6	23 6/8	5.0	29 1/8	9.5	34 4/8	14.0	39 7/8	18.4	45 2/8	22.9
18 4/8	0.7	23 7/8	5.2	29 2/8	9.6	34 5/8	14.1	40 0/8	18.5	45 3/8	23.0
18 5/8	0.8	24 0/8	5.3	29 3/8	9.7	34 6/8	14.2	40 1/8	18.6	45 4/8	23.1
18 6/8	0.9	24 1/8	5.4	29 4/8	9.8	34 7/8	14.3	40 2/8	18.7	45 5/8	23.2
18 7/8	1.0	24 2/8	5.5	29 5/8	9.9	35 0/8	14.4	40 3/8	18.8	45 6/8	23.3
19 0/8	1.1	24 3/8	5.6	29 6/8	10.0	35 1/8	14.5	40 4/8	18.9	45 7/8	23.4
19 1/8	1.2	24 4/8	5.7	29 7/8	10.1	35 2/8	14.6	40 5/8	19.0	46 0/8	23.5
19 2/8	1.3	24 5/8	5.8	30 0/8	10.2	35 3/8	14.7	40 6/8	19.1	46 1/8	23.6
19 3/8	1.4	24 6/8	5.9	30 1/8	10.3	35 4/8	14.8	40 7/8	19.2	46 2/8	23.7
19 4/8	1.5	24 7/8	6.0	30 2/8	10.4	35 5/8	14.9	41 0/8	19.3	46 3/8	23.8
19 5/8	1.6	25 0/8	6.1	30 3/8	10.5	35 6/8	15.0	41 1/8	19.4	46 4/8	23.9
19 6/8	1.7	25 1/8	6.2	30 4/8	10.6	35 7/8	15.1	41 2/8	19.5	46 5/8	24.0
19 7/8	1.8	25 2/8	6.3	30 5/8	10.7	36 0/8	15.2	41 3/8	19.6	46 6/8	24.1
20 0/8	1.9	25 3/8	6.4	30 6/8	10.8	36 1/8	15.3	41 4/8	19.7	46 7/8	24.2
20 1/8	2.0	25 4/8	6.5	30 7/8	10.9	36 2/8	15.4	41 5/8	19.9	47 0/8	24.3
20 2/8	2.2	25 5/8	6.6	31 0/8	11.1	36 3/8	15.5	41 6/8	20.0	47 1/8	24.4
20 3/8	2.3	25 6/8	6.7	31 1/8	11.2	35 4/8	15.6	41 7/8	20.1	47 2/8	24.5
20 4/8	2.4	25 7/8	6.8	31 2/8	11.3	36 5/8	15.7	42 0/8	20.2	47 3/8	24.6
20 5/8	2.5	26 0/8	6.9	31 3/8	11.4	36 6/8	15.8	42 1/8	20.3	47 4/8	24.7
20 6/8	2.6	26 1/8	7.0	31 4/8	11.5	36 7/8	15.9	42 2/8	20.4	47 5/8	24.8
20 7/8	2.7	26 2/8	7.1	31 5/8	11.6	37 0/8	16.0	42 3/8	20.5	47 6/8	24.9
21 0/8	2.8	26 3/8	7.2	31 6/8	11.7	37 1/8	16.1	42 4/8	20.6	47 7/8	25.0
21 1/8	2.9	26 4/8	7.3	31 7/8	11.8	37 2/8	16.2	42 5/8	20.7	48 0/8	25.1
21 2/8	3.0	26 5/8	7.4	32 0/8	11.9	37 3/8	16.3	42 6/8	20.8	48 1/8	25.2
21 3/8	3.1	26 6/8	7.5	32 1/8	12.0	37 4/8	16.4	42 7/8	20.9	48 2/8	25.3
21 4/8	3.2	26 7/8	7.6	32 2/8	12.1	37 5/8	16.5	43 0/8	21.0	48 3/8	25.4
21 5/8	3.3	27 0/8	7.7	32 3/8	12.2	37 6/8	16.6	43 1/8	21.1	48 4/8	25.5
21 6/8	3.4	27 1/8	7.8	32 4/8	12.3	37 7/8	16.7	43 2/8	21.2	48 5/8	25.6
21 7/8	3.5	27 2/8	7.9	32 5/8	12.4	38 0/8	16.8	43 3/8	21.3	48 6/8	25.8
22 0/8	3.6	27 3/8	8.1	32 6/8	12.5	38 1/8	17.0	43 4/8	21.4	48 7/8	25.9
22 1/8	3.7	27 4/8	8.2	32 7/8	12.6	38 2/8	17.1	43 5/8	21.5	49 0/8	26.0
22 2/8	3.8	27 5/8	8.3	33 0/8	12.7	38 3/8	17.2	43 6/8	21.6	49 1/8	26.
22 3/8	3.9	27 6/8	8.4	33 1/8	12.8	38 4/8	17.3	43 7/8	21.7		
22 4/8	4.0	27 7/8	8.5	33 2/8	12.9	38 5/8	17.4	44 0/8	21.8		
22 5/8	4.1	28 0/8	8.6	33 3/8	13.0	38 6/8	17.5	44 1/8	21.9		
22 6/8	4.2	28 1/8	8.7	33 4/8	13.1	38 7/8	17.6	44 2/8	22.0		
22 7/8	4.3	28 2/8	8.8	33 5/8	13.2	39 0/8	17.7	44 3/8	22.1		

Table 5. **ESTIMATION OF THE PERCENTAGE OF FAT IN WOMEN** *(Continued)*

Thigh (in.)	%	Thigh (in.)	%	Thigh (in.)	%	Thigh (in.)	%	Thigh (in.)	%
11 6/8	0.0	16 2/8	7.0	20 6/8	13.7	25 2/8	20.5	29 6/8	27.3
11 7/8	0.2	16 3/8	7.1	20 7/8	13.9	25 3/8	20.7	29 7/8	27.5
12 0/8	0.4	16 4/8	7.3	21 0/8	14.1	25 4/8	20.9	30 0/8	27.7
12 1/8	0.6	16 5/8	7.4	21 1/8	14.3	25 5/8	21.1	30 1/8	27.9
12 2/8	0.8	16 6/8	7.6	21 2/8	14.5	25 6/8	21.3	30 2/8	28.1
12 3/8	1.0	16 7/8	7.8	21 3/8	14.6	25 7/8	21.5	30 3/8	28.3
12 4/8	1.2	17 0/8	8.0	21 4/8	14.8	26 0/8	21.7	30 4/8	28.5
12 5/8	1.4	17 1/8	8.2	21 5/8	15.0	26 1/8	21.8	30 6/8	28.9
12 6/8	1.6	17 2/8	8.4	21 6/8	15.2	26 2/8	22.0	30 7/8	29.0
12 7/8	1.8	17 3/8	8.6	21 7/8	15.4	26 3/8	22.2	31 0/8	29.2
13 0/8	1.9	17 4/8	8.8	22 0/8	15.6	26 4/8	22.4	31 1/8	29.4
13 1/8	2.1	17 5/8	9.0	22 1/8	15.8	26 5/8	22.6	31 2/8	29.6
13 2/8	2.3	17 6/8	9.1	22 2/8	16.0	26 6/8	22.8	31 3/8	29.8
13 3/8	2.5	17 7/8	9.3	22 3/8	16.2	26 7/8	23.0	31 4/8	30.0
13 4/8	2.7	18 0/8	9.5	22 4/8	16.3	27 0/8	23.2	31 5/8	30.2
13 5/8	2.9	18 1/8	9.7	22 5/8	16.5	27 1/8	23.4	31 6/8	30.4
13 6/8	3.1	18 2/8	9.9	22 6/8	16.7	27 2/8	23.6	31 7/8	30.6
13 7/8	3.3	18 3/8	10.1	22 7/8	16.9	27 3/8	23.7	32 0/8	30.8
14 0/8	3.5	18 4/8	10.3	23 0/8	17.1	27 4/8	23.9	32 1/8	30.9
14 1/8	3.6	18 5/8	10.5	23 1/8	17.3	27 5/8	24.1	32 2/8	31.1
14 2/8	3.8	18 6/8	10.7	23 2/8	17.5	27 6/8	24.3	32 3/8	31.3
14 3/8	4.0	18 7/8	10.9	23 3/8	17.7	27 7/8	24.5	32 4/8	31.5
14 4/8	4.2	19 0/8	11.0	23 4/8	17.9	28 0/8	24.7	32 5/8	31.7
14 5/8	4.4	19 1/8	11.2	23 5/8	18.1	28 1/8	24.9	32 6/8	31.9
14 6/8	4.6	19 2/8	11.4	23 6/8	18.2	28 2/8	25.1	32 7/8	32.1
14 7/8	4.8	19 3/8	11.6	23 7/8	18.4	28 3/8	25.3	33 0/8	32.3
15 0/8	5.0	19 4/8	11.8	24 0/8	18.6	28 4/8	25.4	33 1/8	32.5
15 1/8	5.2	19 5/8	12.0	24 1/8	18.8	28 5/8	25.6	33 2/8	32.7
15 2/8	5.4	19 6/8	12.2	24 2/8	19.0	28 6/8	25.8	33 3/8	32.8
15 3/8	5.5	19 7/8	12.4	24 3/8	19.2	28 7/8	26.0	33 4/8	32.9
15 4/8	5.7	20 0/8	12.6	24 4/8	19.4	28 0/8	26.2		
15 5/8	5.9	20 1/8	12.7	24 5/8	19.6	29 1/8	26.4		
15 6/8	6.1	20 2/8	12.9	24 6/8	19.8	29 2/8	26.6		
15 7/8	6.3	20 3/8	13.1	24 7/8	20.0	29 3/8	26.8		
16 0/8	6.5	20 4/8	13.3	25 0/8	20.1	29 4/8	27.0		
16 1/8	6.7	20 5/8	13.5	25 1/8	20.3	29 5/8	27.2		

Name: ______ Date: ______

Birthdate: ______ Ht: ____ in. ____ cm. Wgt: ____ lb ____ kg

DATE	WEIGHT	NECK	ABDOMEN	% BODY FAT	1.5 MILE RUN MIN.	SEC.	IN 2 MIN.	SIT REACH

Figure 2. Chart for recording data for males.

Name: ______ Date: ______

Birthdate: ______ Ht: ____ in. ____ cm. Wgt: ____ lb ____ kg

DATE	WEIGHT	NECK	ABDOMEN	BICEPS	FOREARM	THIGH	TOTAL POINTS	% BODY FAT

Figure 3. Chart for recording data for females. The percentage of body fat is determined by adding the five percentage points and subtracting 54.598 from the total.

a correction factor of 54.598 from the total. The difference is the percentage of fat.

G. All percent values should be reported to the nearest tenth of 1 percent.

Each individual is responsible for the following: (1) Achieving and maintaining a fitness level equal to, or above, prescribed minimal standards. (2) Putting himself through a readiness test at monthly intervals. (3) Utilizing resource information and the assistance of the physician in the development of personal weight control and physical fitness programs.

A very gradual progression to each performance level is recommended, with maintenance for several weeks at each level before building up gradually to the next level.

References

Ames BN: Dietary carcinogens and anticarcinogens—oxygen radicals and degenerative diseases. Science 221:1256–1264, 1983.

Bridbord K, Decoufle P, Fraumeni JD Jr, et al: Estimates of the fraction of cancer in the United States related to occupational factors. Presented at the Occupational Safety and Health Administration (OSHA) Hearings, Washington, DC, 1978.

Fratkin LB: Influence of diet on breast cancer and the relationship to blood estradiol levels. Presented at Workshop No. 7, Analytical Epidemiology, XII International Cancer Congress, Buenos Aires, October, 1978.

Gaskill SP, McGuire WL, Osborne CK, Stern MP: Breast cancer mortality and diet in the United States. Cancer Res 39:3628–3637, 1979.

Harvey RG: Polycyclic hydrocarbons and cancer. Am Sci 70:386–393, 1982.

Health and Physical Readiness Program. Chief of Naval Operations Instruction 6110.1B, October 19, 1982.

Minton JP: Personal communication, 1983.

Schrauzer GN (ed): Inorganic and Nutritional Aspects of Cancer. Advances in Experimental Medicine and Biology. Vol. 91. New York, Plenum Publishing, 1978.

Spratt JS, Greenberg R: Epidemiology and etiology. *In* Spratt JS (ed): Neoplasms of the Colon, Rectum, and Anus. Philadelphia, WB Saunders Company, 1984.

Spratt JS: The primary and secondary prevention of cancer. J Surg Oncol 18:219–230, 1981.

Stich HF: Carcinogens and Mutagens in the Environment. Food Products. Vol. 1. Boca Raton, FL, CRC Press, 1982.

Weinberg RA: A molecular basis of cancer. Sci Am 249:126–142, 1983.

Yunis JJ: Chromosomal basis of neoplasia. Science 22:227–236, 1983.

Yussman MA, Rao CV: Personal communication, 1983.

INDEX

Note: Page numbers in *italics* refer to illustrations.
Page numbers followed by t refer to tables.